● -- In this book, an expert who is independent of the radiation community provides the human and physical evidence proving that carcinogenesis from ionizing radiation does occur at the lowest conceivable doses and dose-rates. This finding refutes current claims by parts of the radiation community that very low doses or dose-rates may be safe.

● -- The magnitude of hazard per dose-unit is evaluated in this book step-by-step from the newest evidence, and the magnitude is shown to be considerably higher than the 1988 and 1990 estimates from the quasi-official radiation committees.

● -- Because ionizing radiation may turn out to be the MOST important single carcinogen to which huge numbers of humans are actually exposed (environmentally, occupationally, and medically), the practical implications of this book for cancer prevention are very great.

Radiation-Induced Cancer

from

Low-Dose Exposure :

AN INDEPENDENT ANALYSIS

John W. Gofman, M.D., Ph.D.

1990 : First Edition

Committee for Nuclear Responsibility, Inc.

C.N.R. Book Division

Post Office Box 11207

San Francisco, California 94101

U.S.A.

Edited by Egan O'Connor

Publisher's Cataloging-in-Publication Data.
(Library of Congress CIP program currently accepting no new participants.)

Gofman, John William
Radiation-Induced Cancer from Low-Dose Exposure, An Independent Analysis.

Includes bibliographical references and index.

1. Ionizing radiation -- Toxicology.
2. X-rays -- Toxicology.
3. Tumors, Radiation-induced.
4. Radiation injuries.
5. Research methods -- Epidemiology.
6. Nuclear pollution.

[Alternate indexing system.]

1. Radiation injuries, Prevention and control.
2. Tumors, Radiation-induced.
3. Neoplasms, Prevention and control.
4. Dose-response relationship, Radiation.
5. Radiography -- Adverse effects.
6. Radioactive pollutants -- Adverse effects.
7. Nuclear reactors, Chernobyl.

Dewey classification number: 616.9

Library of Congress Catalog Card Number 89-62431.

International Standard Book Number: 0-932682-89-8.

Manufactured in the United States of America.

Printing (on acid-free paper) and binding by Consolidated Printers of Berkeley, California.
Preparation of text, tables, and figures on the Lotus 123 spreadsheet.
Cover and book design by F. Urry.

Previous books (still in print) on this topic by the author:

RADIATION AND HUMAN HEALTH, 1981. ISBN 0-87156-275-8. LC 80-26484.

X-RAYS: HEALTH EFFECTS OF COMMON EXAMS, 1985. ISBN 0-87156-838-1. LC 84-23527.

CONTENTS :   (Longer chapters begin with their own table of contents.)

Pagination starts newly with each chapter.
Tables and figures are assembled at each chapter's end.

More ------->

Contents (Continued)

SOME POSSIBLE CONVENIENCES :

==

● – Many terms are defined right in the Index and Glossary. Additional terms are explained in the text, and the explanation will be found via the flagged entry in the Index and Glossary.

● – The meaning of an acronym or other abbreviation is given next to its own entry in the Index.

● – The equivalence between rads, grays, millisieverts, etc. is shown in a tabulation at the end of the Index.

● – The symbols used for exponents (^ or E+), the rounding-off of numbers, and similar matters are explained on page one of the Index.

About the Author :

John William Gofman is Professor Emeritus of Medical Physics at the University of California at Berkeley, and Lecturer at the Department of Medicine, University of California School of Medicine at San Francisco.

He is the author of several books and more than a hundred scientific papers in peer-review journals, in the fields of nuclear/physical chemistry, coronary heart disease, ultracentrifugal analysis of the serum lipoproteins, the relationship of human chromosomes to cancer, and the biological effects of ionizing radiation with particular reference to cancer-induction.

A Narrative Chronology :

While a graduate student at Berkeley, Gofman co-discovered protactinium-232 and uranium-232, protactinium-233 and uranium-233, and proved the slow and fast neutron fissionability of uranium-233.

Post-doctorally, he continued work related to the atomic bomb. Prior to operation of plutonium-producing reactors at Hanford, plutonium was so rare that not even a quarter-milligram existed, but half a milligram was urgently needed for making measurements in the Manhattan Project. At the request of J. Robert Oppenheimer, Gofman and Robert Connick irradiated a ton of uranyl nitrate by placing it around the Berkeley cyclotron night and day. In 110 Gilman Hall, they scaled up Gofman's previous test-tube-sized sodium uranyl acetate process for the plutonium's chemical extraction. Dissolving 10-pound batches of the "hot" ton in big Pyrex jars, and working around the clock with the help of eight or ten others, in about three weeks they reduced the ton to a half cc of liquid containing 1.2 milligram of plutonium (twice as much as expected).

After the plutonium work, Gofman completed medical school. In 1947, he began his research on coronary heart disease and, by developing special flotation ultracentrifugal techniques, demonstrated the existence of low-density lipoproteins (LDL) and high-density lipoproteins (HDL). His work on their chemistry and health consequences included the first prospective studies demonstrating that high LDL levels represent a risk-factor for coronary heart disease (Co56) and that low HDL levels represent a risk-factor for coronary heart disease (1966, CIRCULATION 34: 679-697). His principal book on the heart disease research is CORONARY HEART DISEASE (1959, Charles C. Thomas, Publisher).

In the early 1960s, the Atomic Energy Commission (AEC) asked him if he would establish the Biomedical Research Division at the Lawrence Livermore National Laboratory, for the purpose of evaluating the health effects of all types of nuclear activities. From 1963-1965, he served as the division's first director, and then stepped down in order to have more time for his own laboratory research in cancer, chromosomes, and radiation, as well as his analytical work on the data from the Japanese atomic-bomb survivors and other irradiated human populations.

In 1965, Dr. Ian MacKenzie had published an elegant report entitled "Breast Cancer Following Multiple Fluoroscopies" (BRITISH J. OF CANCER 19: 1-8), and in 1968, Wanebo and co-workers had reported on "Breast Cancer after Exposure to the Atomic Bombings of Hiroshima and Nagasaki" (NEW ENGLAND J. OF MED. 279: 667-671), but few were willing to concede that breast-cancer could be induced by low-LET radiation.

Gofman and his colleague, Dr. Arthur Tamplin, quantified the breast-cancer risk (1970, LANCET 1: 297), looked at the other available evidence, and concluded overall that human exposure to ionizing radiation was much more serious than previously recognized (Go69; Go71).

Because of this finding, Gofman and Tamplin spoke out publicly in favor of re-examining two programs which they had previously accepted. One was the AEC's "Project Plowshare," a program to use hundreds or thousands of nuclear explosions to liberate natural gas in the Rocky Mountains and to excavate harbors and canals. Experimental shots had already been done in Colorado and Nevada. The second program was the AEC's plan to license about 1,000 nuclear power plants as quickly as possible and to build a "plutonium economy" based on breeder reactors. In 1970, Gofman and Tamplin proposed a five-year moratorium on licensing of commercial nuclear power plants.

In 1973, Gofman returned to full-time teaching at the University of California at Berkeley, until choosing an early and active "retirement."

Next Page -- Curriculum Vitae :

Birth: September 21, 1918 in Cleveland, Ohio.
Education :
===

Grade and high school in Cleveland. A.B. in Chemistry from Oberlin College, 1939.

Ph.D. in Nuclear/Physical Chemistry from the University of California at Berkeley, 1943. Dissertation: Discovery of Pa-232, U-232, Pa-233, and U-233. Proof of the slow and fast neutron fissionability of U-233. Discovery of the 4n + 1 radioactive series.

M.D. from the School of Medicine, University of California at San Francisco, 1946. Internship in internal medicine at the University of California Hospital, San Francisco, 1946-1947.

Positions :
===

Academic appointment in 1947 in the Division of Medical Physics, Department of Physics, University of California at Berkeley. Advancement in 1954 to the full professorship, a position held to the present time, with shift to Emeritus status in December, 1973. Under recent University re-organization, the affiliation is now the Division of Biophysics, Department of Molecular and Cell Biology.

Concurrent appointment since 1947 as either Instructor or Lecturer in Medicine in the Department of Medicine, University of California, San Francisco.

Additional appointments held :
===

Associate Director, Lawrence Livermore National Laboratory, 1963-1969. Resigned this post to gain more time for research and teaching. Remained as Research Associate at Livermore through February, 1973.

Founder and first Director of the Biomedical Research Division of the Lawrence Livermore National Laboratory, 1963-1965. This work was done at the request of the Atomic Energy Commission.

Member, Advisory Board for NERVA (Nuclear Engine Rocket Vehicle Application), approximately 1963-1966.

Member of the Reactor Safeguard Committee, University of California, Berkeley, approximately 1955-1960.

Group Co-Leader of the Plutonium Project (for the Manhattan Project) at the University of California, Berkeley, 1941-1943. This work included meetings at Chicago and Oak Ridge to exchange information and to help DuPont engineers prepare for the reprocessing operations at Hanford, Washington.

Physician in Radioisotope Therapy, Donner Clinic, University of California, Berkeley, 1947-1951.

Medical Director, Lawrence Radiation Laboratory (Livermore), 1954-1957.

Medical consultant to the Aerojet-General Nucleonics Corporation, with special emphasis on the hazards of ionizing radiation, for approximately eight years during the 1960s.

Consultant to the Research Division of the Lederle Laboratories, American Cyanimid, 1952-1955.

Consultant to the Research Division of Riker Laboratories, approximately 1962-1966.

Scientific consultant to Vida Medical Systems, 1970-1974; co-invented the VIDA heart monitor, a pocket-worn computer to detect and announce the occurrence of serious cardiac arrhythmias; invented a skin cardiographic electrode subsequently used widely throughout the USA.

Chairman of the Committee for Nuclear Responsibility, 1971 to the present; pro-bono work; no compensation of any type has ever been accepted.

Patents :
===

3,123,535 (Glenn T. Seaborg, John W. Gofman, Raymond W. Stoughton) : The slow and fast neutron fissionability of uranium-233, with its application to production of nuclear power or nuclear weapons.

2,871,251 (John W. Gofman, Robert E. Connick, Arthur C. Wahl) : The sodium uranyl acetate process for the separation of plutonium in irradiated fuel from uranium and fission products.

2,912,302 (Robert E. Connick, John W. Gofman, George C. Pimentel) : The columbium oxide process for the separation of plutonium in irradiated fuel from uranium and fission products.

Honors and awards :
===

Gold-Headed Cane Award, University of California Medical School, 1946, presented to the graduating senior who most fully personifies the qualities of a "true physician."

Modern Medicine Award, 1954, for outstanding contributions to heart disease research.

The Lyman Duff Lectureship Award of the American Heart Association in 1965, for research in atherosclerosis and coronary heart disease; lecture published in 1966 as "Ischemic Heart Disease, Atherosclerosis, and Longevity," in CIRCULATION 34: 679-697.

The Stouffer Prize (shared) 1972, for outstanding contributions to research in arteriosclerosis.

American College of Cardiology, 1974; selection as one of twenty-five leading researchers in cardiology of the past quarter-century.

University of California, Berkeley, Bancroft Library, 1988; announcement of "the Gofman Papers" established in the History of Science and Technology Special Collection (October 1988, BANCROFTIANA, No.97: 10-11).

Foreword to the First Edition

The nature of this subject is such that new data, and new analyses, and new claims made by other analysts, appear all the time. Therefore, it is our intention to up-date this book whenever it would be appropriate -- either because of new evidence, or because of new claims made by others.

While we were writing this book, the United Nations' radiation committee, UNSCEAR, released its new report in early 1989 (the reference is Un88). And on December 19, 1989, the (U.S.) National Academy of Sciences's radiation committee, BEIR-5, released its new report too (Beir90).

After studying those two updates from the radiation community, I find the need for an independent analysis to be as great as when I began. Perhaps greater. The UNSCEAR and BEIR reports do not examine some of the central issues in this field.

Comparisons Made :

For the convenience of readers, we have set forth the key differences between this book and those two reports in Chapter 25. Although the differences are mentioned in Chapter 1 also, very few readers can expect to understand the origin or consequences of the differences until Chapter 25. After all, if such matters were self-evident, the intervening chapters could have been omitted.

The topic of radiation-induced cancer from low-dose exposure is obviously not closed. In the most valuable low-dose study of all -- the Atomic Bomb Survivors -- more than half the people are still alive. The full radiation-response of the most important group -- those under 20 years of age, at the time of bombing -- is far from established in terms of excess fatal cancers.

This edition of our book carries its analysis through the most recent epidemiologically VALID data from the A-Bomb Study (1950-1982). We have addressed the issue of why the data between 1982-1985, as currently available, cannot be regarded as valid by the common standards of epidemiological science.

Indeed, one purpose of this first edition is to help re-direct the reporting of data from the A-Bomb Study into sound epidemiological lines, for otherwise, this uniquely valuable study can become scientifically meaningless. Our position on this fundamental issue constitutes a profound difference with the 1988

UNSCEAR and the 1990 BEIR reports, both of which accept the practices to which we object. In our judgment, such practices can lead to the DEATH of epidemiology as a science.

"Questionable Practices" Examined :

Partly because radiation research has been so well funded, there are far more data about ionizing radiation as a potentially toxic agent than there are about many other agents to which entire populations are exposed. Thus the field can be regarded as the "canary" which can warn humanity about practices which mean "trouble ahead," if adopted in other fields of toxicology.

The hazard which society needs to recognize is that there are ways in which preconceived notions can enter into scientific health matters, and that, in all research concerned with toxic assaults on health, it is possible to stand medical knowledge on its head. Indeed, medical "unknowledge" can become dominant, if certain practices are handled in scientifically inappropriate ways.

Among the practices questioned by this book are the retroactive alteration of databases, the replacement of actual observations by preferred hypotheses, the artificial constraint of equations to rule out certain dose-responses, the subdivision of data until even the largest database becomes inconclusive, and more (see Index, "Scientifically Questionable Practices").

It is possible to mishandle the evidence concerning radiation injury in such a manner that the next 100 years of human history will be characterized by total medical "unknowledge" in this field, instead of knowledge.

In this first edition, we have endeavored to suggest differences between some sound and unsound practices in epidemiological research.

In subsequent editions of this book, we intend to add an examination of whatever new evidence and new reports warrant consideration, and to state our evaluation of whether the field is moving in the direction of reality-based estimates of hazard, or in the direction of estimates based on unfounded conjecture.

The period ahead may be particularly difficult for keeping the record straight, with regard to radiation risk. Those seriously concerned with realistic estimates will need to be careful in separating speculation from real evidence -- a topic examined in Chapter 35. I predict the pitfalls here are going to grow, rather than diminish.

No Retreat from Human Evidence :

In this book, we have not glossed over uncertainties which presently exist in quantifying the cancer-hazard from exposure to ionizing radiation. Only time -- and the preservation of scientific legitimacy for important studies like the A-Bomb Study -- can resolve them.

However, the fact that there is a range of uncertainty in current risk-estimates cannot justify a retreat to wishful thinking, and cannot justify the replacement of the disturbing human data by more "optimistic" (less disturbing) data from other species. When human evidence of good quality is available -- and it is -- then human evidence is the substrate from which we will derive our estimates of risk. Readers will see those estimates emerge from the current evidence, step-by-step.

By contrast, the 1988 UNSCEAR and 1990 BEIR-5 reports rely heavily on non-human evidence to arrive at their recommended risk-estimates for low dose-rates and (UNSCEAR only) for low total doses.

Semi-Prudence versus Prudence :

The human evidence has developed over time and will continue to do so. At each new stage in its development, the growing body of evidence yields a better and better estimate of risk. The estimate which "falls out of the data" at any stage is the so-called "central value" and it is also called "the best estimate" because it is the value most likely to be right, within the evidence. So this "best estimate" is the appropriate one for use, of course. And it has a range of uncertainty, indicated by upper and lower confidence limits.

Nonetheless, there are people who try to focus the public's attention on only the LOWER limit of the current estimate. Therefore, a reminder is needed: If a central estimate is "off," the health risk may not be LOWER than the central estimate. The health risk may be GREATER than the central value which is being used.

Thus, from the point of view of health, the scientifically best estimate is only SEMI-prudent.

John W. Gofman, January 1990.

CHAPTER 1

The Five Most Important Conclusions of This Book

Before summarizing the five key findings of this book, we need to specify what we mean by a few terms.

The term "radiation" in the title of this book refers to X-rays, gamma rays, and beta particles -- in other words, to IONIZING radiation in the low-LET class (LET, or Linear Energy Transfer). The very special nature of IONIZING radiation and of Linear Energy Transfer, with respect to biological injury, is discussed in Chapter 19.

The term "low-dose exposure" in this field refers to internal organ-doses below about 20 centi-grays (a centi-gray or cGy is the same as a rad). The estimates derived in this book, of cancer-risk per centi-gray, apply to the dose-range between zero and five centi-grays of internal organ-dose. And our risk-estimates apply to such doses received slowly as well as to such doses received instantaneously (acutely).

Our range of zero to five centi-grays is the applicable low-dose range for most environmental, occupational, medical (diagnostic), and dental exposures.

The term "an independent analysis" in the title refers to independence from the radiation community. We use the term "radiation community" in this book to mean all the industries, professions, and governments engaged in activities which CAUSE exposure to ionizing radiation, plus the individuals who regard their jobs, their research grants, or their personal advancement as dependent on such sources.

The leading members of the radiation community are (A) governments -- which sponsor civilian and/or military uses of nuclear energy, and sponsor the overwhelming share of all research on radiation's health-hazards -- plus (B) the nuclear electric industry and (C) the professions of nuclear medicine and radiology.

The Prominent Radiation Committees :

The radiation community's most prominent committees on health effects are four: BEIR, ICRP, NCRP, and UNSCEAR, and they each issue sporadic reports. Their individual members receive recognition in our Chapter 37. BEIR and NCRP are American committees, and ICRP and UNSCEAR are international.

BEIR stands for Biological Effects of Ionizing

Radiations, and the BEIR Committee is organized under the auspices of the National Research Council of the National Academy of Sciences, at the request and expense of the federal government, now via its Office of Science and Technology Policy, Committee on Interagency Radiation Research and Policy Coordination. NCRP stands for National Council on Radiation Protection, and the NCRP is funded by the radiation community too.

ICRP stands for International Commission on Radiological Protection. Founded in 1928 by radiologists, it continues to select its own members from various segments of the radiation community. UNSCEAR stands for United Nations Scientific Committee on Effects of Atomic Radiation, and it reports to the U.N. General Assembly.

The Atomic-Bomb
Survivors of Hiroshima and Nagasaki :

Of the five key findings in this book, the first three are directly related to the on-going Lifespan Study of 91,231 atomic-bomb survivors. Contrary to common assumption, the A-Bomb Study is primarily a low-dose study; very few of the survivors at Hiroshima and Nagasaki received high doses. Over half of the 91,231 survivors in this study are still alive, so the Lifespan Study is far from completed.

The A-Bomb Study is maintained in Hiroshima by the Radiation Effects Research Foundation (RERF), which is sponsored equally by the U.S. Department of Energy (through a contract with the National Academy of Sciences) and the Japanese Ministry of Health and Welfare.

Currently, there are two sets of dose-estimates in the A-Bomb Study. The set established in 1965 is called T65DR. A partial, interim set of new dose-estimates, introduced in 1986, is called DS86. In making our point about how few of the survivors received HIGH doses, we will state the dose-estimates in both dosimetries. Doses shown on the next page refer to average whole-body internal organ-doses, and they are given in centi-sieverts (rems) instead of centi-grays (rads). This change is just the signal that adjustment for the survivors' small exposure to neutrons has been made, and that the doses are equivalent to doses in centi-grays (rads).

===

Initial Persons	T65DR: Mean Organ-Dose (cSv or rems)	DS86: Mean Organ-Dose (cSv or rems)
66,028	0.66	0.88
14,943	10.99	14.56
4,225	35.36	40.62
6,035	71.31 and up	74.24 and up

91,231		

The five most important conclusions of this book follow sequentially, below.

● -- *Finding (1)* :
Method for Handling
the Retroactive Alteration
of Dose-Estimates in the A-Bomb Study :

A clear rule in epidemiological research is that one does not change input to a study after any of the study's output is known. Such rules have been established in research not in order to be bureaucratic, but only to ensure believability for the results. It is virtually self-evident that retroactive revisions of a study's input can create Orwellian opportunities to alter the meaning of the existing results.

Nonetheless, the new DS86 dosimetry for the A-Bomb Study has become the occasion for retroactively altering the entire architecture of this study, and destroying its continuity. The details are thoroughly documented in our Chapters 5 and 10.

There is a "right" way and a "wrong" way to handle new insights about dosimetry in any study.

We emphatically welcome new insights, and Finding Number One of this book is the demonstration of a method for introducing the new DS86 dosimetry into the A-Bomb Study WITHOUT putting the study's scientific credibility into peril. Our way of handling the new DS86 dosimetry is very different from its current handling elsewhere -- handling which we regard as at variance with acceptable practice in prospective epidemiologic research.

In Chapter 25, we show that the "wrong" approach to the new DS86 dosimetry has ALREADY raised a puzzling inconsistency on a key risk-issue, and that the problem can be resolved only by restoring the study's legitimate continuity.

We do not think that the meaningful rules of research can just be disregarded in this field. We consider our Finding Number One as more important than ever, because the 1988 UNSCEAR and 1990 BEIR-5 reports do not question the current handling of the retroactive alterations at all.

==

● -- *Finding (2)* :
Cancer-Risk at Moderate
and High Dose-Levels, Acute Delivery Only :

Substantial agreement exists between this book and the
new UNSCEAR and BEIR reports with respect to cancer-risk
per rad from moderate and high doses acutely delivered, now
that those committees have greatly increased their past
estimates. This finding indicates that our independent
methods and theirs can lead to the same results.

● -- *Finding (3)* :
Cancer-Risk at Low Doses,
Acutely and Slowly Delivered :

Serious disagreement exists between this book and the
radiation committees about the cancer-risk from low-dose
exposure, either acutely or slowly received -- and acute-low
and slow-low doses are the ones which occur in the
overwhelming share of human exposures.

This book, using human evidence exclusively, arrives at
risk-estimates for acute-low and slow-low exposures which
are up to 30-fold higher than the wide range of values
provided by UNSCEAR and BEIR. Chapters 22,23, and 25
show that there is no mystery about the source of
disagreement. The record shows that the radiation
committees reach approximately the same conclusions as we
do with respect to the relevant human evidence, but then the
committees recommend use of what we call more
"optimistic" (less disturbing) findings based on OTHER
species.

We wish our own risk-estimates were lower -- for no one
welcomes potency in a carcinogen -- but we cannot ignore
the direct human evidence.

● -- Finding (4) :
<u>Disproof of Any Safe Dose or Dose-Rate :</u>

Influential segments of the radiation community have been speculating (especially since the Chernobyl accident) about a "threshold" -- namely the notion that low doses and dose-rates may be completely safe. Indeed, some segments are speculating in print that there may be a positive net benefit for human health from low-dose exposure -- a speculation known as "hormesis." The 1988 UNSCEAR Report does not challenge either of the two speculations.

By contrast, we do.

In Chapter 35, we examine studies which are invoked in the name of hormesis, and we find that they provide no scientific basis to support such speculation.

In Chapters 18 through 21, we prove beyond reasonable doubt that no safe dose or dose-rate exists with respect to radiogenic cancer. Our disproof of a threshold is based on human evidence. Both the 1988 UNSCEAR and 1990 BEIR reports fail to address our disproof, although an earlier version of the disproof circulated widely in the radiation community.

In 1987, the U.S. Department of Energy or DOE released its report on the estimated health effects from the Chernobyl accident. The report, which we discuss in detail in our Chapter 24, asserts at every occasion that fallout from the accident may cause no extra cancers at all beyond the immediate vicinity -- which is the same as asserting that there may be a safe dose and dose-rate. The authors (one of whom is on the 1988 UNSCEAR Committee) call this the "zero risk model" (Doe87, p.J.8) and elsewhere, they state that, "There are no direct data that confirm that a few random ionizations in tissue cause fatal cancers" (Doe87, p.7.5).

This book provides those data. And, by reasonable scientific standards, these data rule out the threshold idea with regard to the radiation-induction of human cancer.

==

● -- *Finding (5) :*
The Practical
Implications for Human Health :

The practical implications for human health, of
realistic versus mistaken risk-estimates in this field, can
be illustrated by evaluation of the Chernobyl accident,
but this accident is just "the tip of the iceberg."

Proposals are pending to EXCLUDE very low-dose
exposure of entire populations from consideration in
risk-estimates, and also to handle a large share of
radioactive waste as if it were NOT radioactive -- in
other words, to declare a threshold by using edict to
over-rule evidence.

It is self-evident that if a mistaken notion about safe
doses and dose-rates prevails in this field, human
exposures to ionizing radiation will rise dramatically --
from occupational, environmental, and medical doses.
Quite aside from heritable genetic consequences, which
are not discussed in this book, such a mistake would be
far from trivial. Over time, it could mean cancer inflicted
on a hundred million or more humans.

Indeed, low-dose ionizing radiation may turn out to
be the MOST important single carcinogen to which huge
numbers of humans are actually exposed. No one can
possibly be sure yet, in the absence of comparable data
on all the other human carcinogens and on the
magnitude of exposure to them.

In short, Finding Number Five is that the practical
implications for human health are extremely high in the
so-called "radiation controversy."

Our independent analysis of the human evidence arrives at seriously
different conclusions from those put forth by the radiation community.
Readers who take our step-by-step journey in this book, from the evidence
to the conclusions, will be in a position to judge for themselves whether or
not our conclusions are believable.

The five key findings are reviewed in greater detail in our Closing
Statement (Chapter 25).

1-empty, after 1-5.
===

CHAPTER 2

The Role of Independent Analyses in Research on Toxic Agents

If we let "XYZ" be the generic name for some specific chemical or physical toxic agent -- explicitly excluding ionizing radiation -- we can briefly examine the role of independent analyses in research on the carcinogenicity of XYZ. One opinion is that conflict-of-interest creates no problem in scientific research. A different opinion, however, is that conflict-of-interest in research constitutes a legitimate concern and legitimate topic for open discussion.

Position of Medical Journal Editors :

The International Committee of Medical Journal Editors considers conflict-of-interest so important that the Committee recently moved to bring the topic into full view when the Committee amended its "Uniform Requirements for Manuscripts Submitted to Biomedical Journals." The new passages on conflict-of-interest are quoted by LANCET in its issue of September 14, 1985, page 595 (we are omitting other new passages on true authorship, for instance):

In every article, "one or more statements should specify ... (c) acknowledgements of financial and material support, and (d) financial relationships that may constitute a conflict of interest ... Financial or material support from any source must be specified. If a paper is accepted it may also be appropriate to include mention of other financial relationships that raise a conflict of interest, but initially these should be outlined in the covering letter."

"Manuscripts must be accompanied by a covering letter. This must include: ... (b) a statement of financial or other relationships that might lead to a conflict of interests ..."

After quoting these and other new passages from the "Uniform Requirements," LANCET explicitly states that an author's financial sponsorship may be a potential source of bias when LANCET says:

"On conflict of interest, firm guidelines are even more difficult to formulate; as a first step, perhaps authors should ask themselves whether they would be embarrassed if financial or other potential sources of bias came to light after publication."

Sponsorship of XYZ Research :

Both logic and observation confirm that most people who need to expose other people to XYZ (either directly or environmentally) have a preference for analysts who say such exposures create a negligible amount of cancer -- or better still, none at all.

Therefore, in terms of protecting human health, it would be inherently unsafe if the XYZ community sponsored and thus controlled nearly all research on the carcinogenicity of XYZ. Scientists in the XYZ field would quickly learn the need for prudence about anything which would upset such sponsors -- if the scientists wished to have their grants renewed, their papers published, their nominations to XYZ advisory committees approved, and generally wished to have a comfortable future in their field.

If You Own the Consensus, How Can You Lose ?

In such a situation, one predictable result of the funding would be the extreme scarcity of "boat-rockers" and the extreme abundance of sponsor-friendly and self-censoring XYZ experts.

Similar statements from the latter about the cancer-hazard from XYZ exposure would indeed constitute the overwhelming consensus in the field. Moreover, due to the very wide distribution of grants by the XYZ community, the consensus would appear to arise from a great variety of disinterested sources: Medical centers, schools of public health, schools of veterinary science, departments of environmental sciences, epidemiology, biostatistics, physics, biology, toxicology.

Nonetheless, an "overwhelming consensus of XYZ experts" might be artificial, under the circumstances.

Who Controls the Input ?

The situation would be even more menacing, in terms of undistorted estimates of XYZ carcinogenicity, if the XYZ promoters also tightly controlled the raw data which analysts must use to reach any conclusions at all. To the extent that only sponsor-friendly insiders would be enabled to generate, collect, sort, or revise the actual observations, then anyone using those data -- dependent and independent analysts alike -- would be at the mercy of XYZ partisans.

With all the revelations during recent years -- in field after field -- about falsified research, falsified safety-testing, falsified performance-testing, falsified cost-reports, and falsified pollution-reports, there is nothing far-fetched about the prospect in XYZ research that both dependent and independent analysts could get deceived by falsified databases (see Chapter 24, Part 1). However, chances are high that only the independent analysts would ever raise such a question. The sky almost always falls on anyone who does (Nova88).

The Role in One Sentence :

The role of independent analysts in research on toxic agents is this: They try to find out if evaluation of XYZ toxicity is the same -- when conflict-of-interest is missing -- as the evaluation when conflict-of-interest is present.

It must be emphasized that the PRESENCE of conflict-of-interest does not automatically make every dependent analysis wrong. Of course not. And it must be equally emphasized that the ABSENCE of conflict-of-interest does not automatically make every independent analysis right. Independent analysts can suffer from OTHER biases, and we can make occasional mistakes as readily as ANYONE.

Substance, Not Source :

When I was entering science in the late 1930s, it seemed to be understood that what matters in any analysis is its scientific merit -- its substance, not its source. Readers do not need a "double standard." The first question about independent and dependent analyses alike is: Do the authors show how they proceed, step-by-step, from the raw data to the arrival at their conclusions? If they do not, they are expecting you to care more about the source than the substance.

Complaints about Independence :

Taught by fifty years of observation, we know that many members of the XYZ community use innuendo to cope with independent analysts: "But some of their methods are not the methods WE use," or "Their work is not peer-reviewed."

Such complaints are meant to suggest that the independent methods and results are wrong. But it is not good enough for critics to cast aspersions over a whole analysis unless they are prepared to debate its substance on a SCIENTIFIC level.

When independent analysts take an independent look at a problem, they well may use independent methods. A presumption that independent methods are inferior to the conventional approach would be an

unwarranted bias. After all, independent methods may be more appropriate and SUPERIOR to conventional approaches, especially if conventional approaches were chosen in order to miss or obscure an unwelcome reality.

With regard to peer-review, the peer-review system itself is under serious criticism for inattention to scientific standards (see, for instance, Renn86, Renn88). In any case, XYZ committees can and do self-publish their own work without any control or veto-power from independent peers. Likewise, independent peers may publish their work in channels located beyond the veto-power of the XYZ community.

Whether a report is by an XYZ committee or by an independent analyst, what will count in the end -- with regard to human health -- is the work's scientific content. The rest is noise.

CHAPTER 3

The Intended Readership

Levels of Prior Knowledge :

This book has been written for everyone who has either a professional or a personal interest in the subject, and wants an independent analysis, as defined in Chapter 1.

The book does not require readers to have prior knowledge in this particular field. However, because this is a scientifically rigorous piece of work, it demands some concentration from all its readers, regardless of their background.

Potential readers who lack comfort with numbers may be pleasantly surprised by the book, despite all its digits and tables. They will understand the most important parts of all the chapters, even if they decide in advance to pass over everything which they find intimidating.

Readers whose first language is not English, and readers who are not familiar with this field, can find the meaning of various terms and abbreviations by consulting the entries flagged by (*) in the Index.

Anyone who handles computations easily -- whether in chemistry, physics, engineering, accounting, computer science, marketing, or for any other purpose -- should have no trouble following all aspects of this book. I particularly hope, of course, that it will be useful in the fields of epidemiology, public health, environmental sciences, internal medicine, occupational medicine, nuclear medicine, radiology, dentistry, health physics, nuclear engineering, and radiobiology.

The Most Important Carcinogen?
====================================

The evidence in this book speaks directly to everyone who is interested in specific SUCCESSFUL ways to prevent part of the human misery called cancer. The evidence in this book means that one effective way to prevent a large number of cancers would be to reduce human exposures to low-dose ionizing radiation.

To support this conclusion, we do not depend on expectations based on other species, cell-studies, or high-dose data. The evidence proving that LOW-dose ionizing radiation is a human carcinogen comes from epidemiological records -- from real, whole human beings.

Indeed, ionizing radiation may be the single most important carcinogen to which humans are actually exposed. It may account for a significant share of today's entire cancer problem (see Chapter 24, Part 10).

It is difficult, however, to compare the impact of ionizing radiation with the impact of other carcinogens because there is so little quantitative human evidence on the other carcinogens (see Chapter 25, Part 5). By contrast, we know about ionizing radiation directly from human evidence.

● -- Human evidence shows conclusively that no threshold exists with respect to induction of cancer by the lowest conceivable doses and dose-rates of low-LET ionizing radiation. There is no safe dose or dose-rate.

● -- The new A-bomb evidence shows, when all ages are considered together, that the cancer-hazard per dose-unit is more severe at LOW doses than at intermediate and high doses; the dose-response curve is supra-linear. (See Figure 13-C).

● -- The new A-bomb evidence confirms that the cancer-risk is much higher for younger people than for older people, when they receive the same dose.

Who Receives the Exposures?
=======================================

Medical-Dental Diagnostic Doses :

A surprising number of Americans -- estimated at about 7 out of 10 every year -- receives some exposure to ionizing radiation from diagnostic X-rays in medicine and dentistry (Phs80). Such exams can have real benefits for patients.

But the same diagnostic benefits are often obtainable with much lower doses. Elsewhere, I have estimated that unnecessarily high X-ray doses cause about 1.5 million unnecessary cancers per generation in the United States alone (Go85, Chapter 17). The estimate excludes cancers induced by diagnostic nuclear medicine, and excludes all second cancers induced by therapeutic radiation.

Except for not smoking, probably the single most effective step which people could take, in order to reduce their chance of cancer, is to resist referrals to diagnostic X-ray facilities which cannot provide credible evidence that the doses which they give are well below

===

(not well above) the national average. The carcinogenicity of X-rays is even greater than the carcinogenicity of A-bomb radiation (see Chapter 13).

Occupational Exposures :

According to a governmental estimate, about 1.5 million Americans receive occupational exposure to ionizing radiation. I wonder how many young workers in transport know what doses they receive from radioactive packages and cargo ... how many young nurses know what doses they receive from the patients who contain gamma-emitting radionuclides after having some procedure in nuclear medicine ... and how many young lab technicians who work on radioactive labeling experiments, with beta-emitters, are aware that beta-emitters produce X-rays especially when they interact with materials of high atomic number (the bremsstrahlung mechanism).

Of course, as long as a person's consent to occupational exposure is not based on deception, there is no fraud and therefore, in my view, outsiders have no right to do anything more than provide honest information to workers and employers alike. An independent analysis is an appropriate resource in such circumstances.

Environmental Exposures :

The environment is contaminated by two classes of radioactive isotopes: Those placed there by nature, and those placed there by human activities. The living cells which become irradiated by such contaminants cannot tell the difference, of course (see Chapter 19).

All people on earth receive environmental doses of low-LET ionizing radiation from nature-placed radioisotopes like potassium-40 and carbon-14, and man-placed radioisotopes like strontium-90 and cesium-137 (distributed globally by atomic bomb tests above ground, for instance).

There seems to be less recognition that we all receive some low-LET exposure also from various radionuclides in the decay-chains of uranium and thorium, two substances released into the biosphere by human activity as well as by nature. For instance, in the decay-chain of radon-220 (thoron gas), there is lead-212, which emits both gamma and beta radiations. Moreover, some of the alpha-emitters -- like radium-224 and radon-220 -- emit significant gamma rays of their own, in addition to alpha-particles.

The risk-estimates in this book apply to all low-LET environmental exposures, whether caused by man or by nature.

Effect of Wrong Information :
===

The effort which individuals, families, physicians, health physicists, engineers, and some public officials make -- in order to reduce exposures to ionizing radiation -- is directly related to their perception of the health risk.

The link between perception and probable effort may be illustrated by statements from Robert E. Alexander, who is identified (Alex88a) as a scientist with the U.S. Nuclear Regulatory Commission and the 1988-89 president of the Health Physics Society -- the society whose official journal calls itself "the radiation protection journal."

Alexander's perception seems to be that low doses are probably safe doses with zero health effects. He calls this a "highly significant probability" (Alex88a, p.144). He reports, "Many health physicists are dismayed by the now-common practice of including extremely low doses in health effects estimations" (Alex88a, p.145). "Reasonable people will not knowingly want to support proposals for large expenditures to protect against risks that have an entirely theoretical basis, that may not exist, and that can never be demonstrated" (Alex88b, p.594).

Similar views are illustrated at length in Chapter 24, Parts 8,9, and 10, because perceptions of this type have already culminated in two proposals which are now pending in the U.S.:

● (1) The exclusion of very low-dose exposure when estimates are made of the health-consequences from various radiation-related activities.

● (2) The de-regulation of a large fraction of radioactive waste, so that it can be "disposed of" in landfills and incinerators just like non-radioactive waste (see Chapter 24, Part 10).

Outcome of "the Controversy" :
===

If underestimates prevail concerning the health consequences from low-dose exposure, a realistic prediction is that doses received by the public will rise, and not only in the United States. I would hesitate to predict the limit.

So it seems self-evident that over time, the cancer-risk for everyone in the world (with the emphasis on children) is going to be affected by the outcome of

===

the so-called "radiation controversy" -- by whether or not scientifically reasonable estimates of cancer-risk from low doses replace the widely used underestimates and threshold-claims.

This book results from an independent effort to find out what the scientifically reasonable estimates really are, in view of new data. The key findings were described in Chapter 1.

3-empty, after 3-3.
==

Overview of a Uniquely Valuable Database

Since 1950, more than 90,000 of the survivors of the atomic bombings at Hiroshima and Nagasaki have been enrolled in a lifetime study of their health. (Details are in Chapter 5.) The study, first conducted by the Atomic Bomb Casualty Commission (ABCC), was transferred in 1975 to control by the Radiation Effects Research Foundation (RERF), which has its headquarters at 5-2 Hijiyama Park, Minami-Ku, Hiroshima 732, Japan.

RERF is equally funded by the government of Japan through its Ministry of Health and Welfare and by the government of the United States via the National Academy of Sciences (NAS) under contract with the Department of Energy (DOE).

Cancer-observations among the survivors are reported by RERF in a series of Technical Reports (TR). Generally, these reports also appear in the journal RADIATION RESEARCH, but usually in abbreviated form and after considerable delay. The two versions do not necessarily report identical conclusions (TR-9-87, p.35 versus Pr88, p.458).

The major follow-up reports on cancer-mortality among the survivors have been made, for the past sixteen years, in four-year increments as indicated below:

1950-1966 follow-up.
    (Data published in 1970: TR-11-70; Bee71.)
1950-1970 follow-up.
    (Data published in 1971: TR-10-71; Jab72.)
1950-1974 follow-up.
    (Data published in 1977: TR-1-77; Bee78.)
1950-1978 follow-up.
    (Data published in 1980: TR-12-80; Kato82.)
1950-1982 follow-up.
    (Data published in 1986: TR-1-86; Pr87a.)

Lifespan Follow-Up :

One of the enormous scientific merits of this study is the plan to follow-up these individuals for their complete lifespans. With the A-Bomb Study's follow-up already extended for 37 years after the exposure to radiation, the study is telling us far more about cancer-induction by ionizing radiation than several other studies whose follow-up extends only 15 or 20 years beyond an exposure.

Nonetheless, the A-bomb follow-up is far from complete. Readers can see from Tables 4-A and 4-B that almost two-thirds of the participating A-bomb survivors were still alive in 1982. Those who were young, during the 1945 bombings, account for an ever-growing share of the cancer-observations, of course. In the coming decades of the study, they will contribute very important information on the duration and true magnitude of the radiation risk.

All Dose-Levels :

A unique scientific merit of this study can be seen from the entries in Table 4-A, Column D: The study includes a large unexposed group and a very great range of doses. This permits examination of dose versus cancer-response within a single study. If cancer-rate rises with dose in successively higher Dose-Groups, the argument for causality is stronger than if there were only one exposed group to compare with an unexposed Reference Group.

In the T65DR dosimetry, the average internal organ-dose in Dose-Group 3 is estimated at only 11 centi-sieverts or rems. This is an organ-dose commonly received, medically, in special diagnostic procedures such as fluoroscopy, angiography, and in some isotope procedures such as radio-iodine uptake studies. At the other extreme is an average organ-dose of about 264 cSv (rems), a very high dose indeed when it is received by the entire body.

Because the study also includes exposures between these extremes, it is one of the very few studies capable of revealing whether the cancer-risk per dose-unit is the same at all dose-levels or not. If it is the same, then the dose-response is linear. But if the cancer-risk per dose-unit is more severe at low total doses than at high doses, humanity needs to know it badly, because most human exposures occur at low total doses.

All Ages :

The A-Bomb Survivor Study is uniquely valuable in additional ways. It is the only careful long-term study which includes persons at all ages at the time of exposure (ATE); see Table 4-B, Column A. Thus it has already been capable of revealing what other studies could only suggest: Relative to the spontaneous cancer-rate, the cancer-risk per dose-unit is higher for persons who are young ATE than for persons who are old ATE. As the follow-up period extends beyond its current limit, the A-Bomb Study will enable analysts to quantify age-sensitivity with far more certitude than is possible now.

Both Sexes :

In addition to the inclusion of all doses and all ages, the A-Bomb Study includes both sexes. This is not the case in many studies. Studies which are based on occupational or medical exposures are often limited or nearly limited to one sex.

All Cancer-Sites :

Moreover, the A-Bomb Study is a study following exposure of the entire body to ionizing radiation. Thus, the study can address the problem of radiation-induced cancer in general. By contrast, studies of equal population-size which involve the exposure of only a few organs will necessarily have many fewer cancer-cases to evaluate, and thus findings from such studies will be inherently less reliable due to random fluctuations in small numbers.

Even in the A-Bomb Study, analysts can create a "small-numbers problem" if they practice excessive subdivision of the data by cancer-type, dose, age, sex. It is in the nature of numbers that any database can be rendered inconclusive by excessive subdivision. However, when analysts refrain from such questionable practices, the A-bomb database is a uniquely powerful resource for conclusive human evidence.

Definite Exposure-Date :

Another enormous scientific merit of the A-Bomb Study is the relative absence of confounding variables, which can muddy and even invalidate so many other studies.

For instance, in the A-Bomb Study, all the exposed groups received a single acute dose at the same time. In spite of some doses from residual radioactivity, no one doubts that the dominant exposure was from the explosion and fireball (Chapter 8). The definite exposure-date eliminates the problems which plague studies based on occupational exposures, where there is no clearly defined time-interval between exposure (which takes place over years) and death from cancer. Such studies can provide no reliable indication of the latency period or the duration of radiation's carcinogenic effect. (Even the dosimetry becomes muddier than usual, if cancer occurs during the period of exposure.)

By contrast, the A-Bomb Study is capable of revealing, over its course, some valuable information about the duration of the carcinogenic effect, and about minimum, maximum and average latency periods.

Its Own Internal Control-Group :

The most important confounding variable which is ABSENT from the A-Bomb Study is the need to use an outside control-group (a group not closely related to the exposed group).

Unlike studies which must rely on Vital Statistics for cancer-rates among unexposed population-samples, the A-Bomb Study provides its own control or reference group, internal to the study. Thus, if there is something peculiar and special about the 1945 populations of Hiroshima and Nagasaki -- something which would give them spontaneous cancer-rates unlike the rates elsewhere in Japan -- we can expect such a factor to be randomly distributed at the same rate among those who happened to be exposed by the bombs at one dose-level or any other dose-level, or not to have been exposed at all. (Radial distance, from where the bombs happened to drop, is the prime determinant of dose in the overall study.)

Summary :

The A-bomb database is so valuable that it would be a real blow against human welfare if its scientific worth were undermined by irregular handling -- a danger discussed in detail by Chapters 5 and 6.

Table 4-A

Overview by Dose-Groups of the A-Bomb Study, 1950-1982 (T65DR Dosimetry). Raw Data.

Col.A RERF'S EIGHT DOSE-GROUPS	Col.B KERMA RANGE (RADS)	Col.C TRUE MEAN KERMA (RADS)	Col.D RBE=2 MEAN ORGAN-DOSE (cSv)	Col.E TRUE MEAN AGE ATB (YEARS)	Col.F INITIAL PERSONS IN 1950	Col.G TOTAL DEATHS 1950-1982	Col.H PERSONS STILL ALIVE 1982	Col.I (RAW VALUE) FATAL CANCERS 1950-1982
1	0	0.0	0.0	28.7	37173	12798	24375	2376
2	1-9	3.0	1.5	27.8	28855	9563	19292	1779
3	10-49	21.8	11.0	28.9	14943	5170	9773	1055
4	50-99	70.6	35.4	29.1	4225	1476	2749	314
5	100-199	142.5	71.4	27.9	3128	1029	2099	253
6	200-299	243.6	122.1	26.1	1381	455	926	131
7	300-399	345.2	173.2	26.6	639	215	424	51
8	400+	526.4	264.1	27.1	887	337	550	91
					91231	31043	60188	6050

NOTES ----- ATB means "at time of bombing" in 1945. Cancers exclude leukemia.
Columns B, C, E, and F come from Table 26-E.
Column D comes from Table 9-C, Row 11.
Columns G and I are sums coming from RERF's diskette "R10ALL" (see Tables 26-A,B,C,D).
Column H is Column F minus Column G.
Reminder: Fatal cancers are absolute numbers, not rates per 10,000 initial persons.

Table 4-B

Overview by Age-Bands of the A-Bomb Study, 1950-1982 (T65DR Dosimetry). Raw Data.

Col.A RERF'S FIVE AGE-BANDS IN YEARS, ATB	Col.B KERMA RANGE (RADS)	Col.C TRUE MEAN KERMA (RADS)	Col.D RBE=2 MEAN ORGAN-DOSE (cSv)	Col.E TRUE MEAN AGE ATB (YEARS)	Col.F INITIAL PERSONS IN 1950	Col.G TOTAL DEATHS 1950-1982	Col.H PERSONS STILL ALIVE 1982	Col.I (RAW VALUE) FATAL CANCERS 1950-1982
0-9 YR	0-400+	18.4	9.23	4.1	18402	728	17674	93
10-19 YR	0-400+	29.8	14.95	14.6	19224	1715	17509	349
20-34 YR	0-400+	27.1	13.58	27.0	17691	3075	14616	949
35-49 YR	0-400+	24.1	12.07	42.0	20903	11234	9669	2788
50+ YR	0-400+	19.1	9.58	58.5	15011	14291	720	1871
					91231	31043	60188	6050

Columns A, B, C, and E come from Table 26-E.
Columns D, F, G, and I are calculated from the Master File 26 (A,B,C,D).
Column H is Column F minus Column G.
  Reminder: Entries for mean doses and for fatal cancers include the entire study-population -- the unexposed groups as well as the exposed. Column I excludes leukemia. The radiation-sensitivity of the young, not apparent here, becomes clear in Chapter 15.

4-empty, after tables.

A Growing Problem: Retroactive Alteration of the Study

This chapter is arranged in six parts:

1. Necessity of Basic Rules

Epidemiologists worldwide appreciate the need for certain fundamental rules of research, four of which are described below. The need exists because scientists are neither saints nor robots. Scientists, like the people who are supposed to trust their work, have personal needs, hopes, and wishes which constantly threaten to undermine their scientific objectivity.

The rules of research, needed as barriers to both the unintentional and intentional introduction of bias into research, ordinarily provide the basis on which scientists trust each other's results. Scientists who, and institutions which, are casual about such rules can destroy the credibility of major databases and lengthy research projects.

This chapter documents the current menace to the A-Bomb Study in these respects.

In order to assure readers that I have direct experience with what is and is not required, in order to maintain the credibility of a research project, I will mention a piece of my personal history. When I was proposing that certain blood-lipid measurements are predictors of human atherosclerosis (Go50a, Go50b), I helped to persuade the National Heart Institute to support a multi-center prospective study to test the hypotheses (Co56).

Felix Moore, biostatistician at the National Heart Institute, helped to develop protocols, and I will feel forever grateful to him for his explicit insistence that every possible barrier to bias be built into the procedures, so that no one could dismiss the results -- however they might turn out -- by raising the question

of possible bias. His toughness paid off. No one raised the question, and although the absence of bias cannot guarantee correct results, the results of that study have stood the tests of time very well.

Rule -- Change No Input :

Prospective studies, like the A-Bomb Study, have a supreme virtue which normally gives them greater scientific weight than retrospective studies: Their input is "set in concrete" BEFORE any results from the follow-up are known. Since there is supposed to be no later opportunity whatsoever to ALTER any of the input (for instance, measurements, diagnoses, cohorts), there is supposed to be no chance that unhappiness -- about the study's true outcome -- could affect the results or their meaning via retroactive revisions of the input.

In short, results are supposed to have no influence upon the input. In prospective studies, the lesser opportunity for bias to operate is a major basis for their greater scientific credibility compared with retrospective studies. For convenience in further discussion, we can refer to the rule against fixing up input, after any results are known, as the "change no input" rule.

Rule -- Use Blinding :

In the prospective studies where investigators feel compelled to disregard the "change no input" rule, care must be taken so that the changes are never made by anyone who is familiar with the results of the existing follow-up. We can think of this as the "use blinding" rule.

Rule -- Explain Everything :

Because retroactive alterations of the input weaken

the credibility of any study, investigators are expected to justify the scientific need for each change and to show how it could not have introduced any bias. They often do this with great attention to detail. We can refer to this standard as the "explain everything" rule.

Every UNexplained change in input inevitably raises doubts, including the question: What motivated the investigators to review one particular aspect of the input in the first place? Was something about the outcome -- absent the alteration -- making them unhappy?

Rule -- Keep Cohorts Intact :

We must emphasize the importance of keeping a constant structure and keeping the same people together throughout the full course of a prospective study. In order to illustrate why this is so important for the believability of any study, we shall refer again to Chapter 2's hypothetical compound "XYZ," which explicitly excludes ionizing radiation.

2. Worst-Case Scenarios with Hypothetical Compound "XYZ"

We shall suppose that, in a study of XYZ carcinogenicity, there are five cohorts of 20,000 persons each: An unexposed control-group (Dose-Group 1), plus Dose-Groups 2, 3, 4, and 5 which each received progressively higher doses of XYZ, but which otherwise are just like Dose-Group 1. And we shall suppose that, 35 years after exposure to XYZ, the true results are that cancer-rates rise above the spontaneous rate in direct proportion to the dose of XYZ received.

Now, in order to make the point clear about intact cohorts, we will create worst-case hypothetical scenarios.

Because these are worst-case scenarios, we will say that the XYZ study is controlled by unscrupulous persons who have an interest in making XYZ look less carcinogenic than they know it to be. Having specified that they are unscrupulous, we can say that they would not hesitate to conceal the carcinogenicity by shuffling the persons with cancer, in the study, until cancer-rates were very similar in all five dose-groups. Before moving a cancer-case to the dose-group where it was "needed," the XYZ partisans would assign the appropriate new dose to the person. And in order to create "noise" in the system, the handlers could assign new doses to a lot of cancer-free persons also. If the handlers of the XYZ study were to establish perpetual alteration of the cohorts and dosimetry as an acceptable policy for their study, they could continue shuffling

people, as needed, with each subsequent follow-up.

Of course, a study's meaning can be fixed, retroactively, by adjustments of its input other than the moving of cancer-cases. For instance, without changing the dose of a single CANCER-case, the handlers of the XYZ study could arrange "evidence" even for a safe threshold, just by changing the doses of enough elderly cancer-FREE participants. Since the "expected" cancer mortality-rate (without XYZ exposure) is higher among older people than younger people, the handlers of the study would benefit by moving some cancer-free ELDERLY participants into Dose-Group 2. This would simultaneously raise the mean age of Dose-Group 2, and lower its cancer-rate per 10,000 persons. The excess cancer-deaths really caused by XYZ exposure in Dose-Group 2 would be hidden, because a residual higher cancer-rate in Group 2 than in Group 1 would appear to be simply the natural consequence of Dose-Group 2's older mean age, compared with Dose-Group 1.

With variations on these scenarios, handlers of the XYZ study could obscure the true carcinogenicity of XYZ at low doses for decades.

If the membership of XYZ cohorts is treated as fluid, there are countless ways for the handlers of the XYZ study to obtain whatever results they want, by moving either cancer cases or cancer-free participants -- or both -- from cohort to cohort, after assigning them new doses as needed. By contrast, when cohorts are "set in concrete" early in a study, their constancy becomes a formidable barrier against such behavior.

3. Constant Cohorts and Credibility

The discussion of "Worst-Case Scenarios" with XYZ indicates why the scientific community appropriately has more confidence in the results of studies where investigators provide assurance that cohorts are never disturbed (or only minimally disturbed), than in studies where investigators retroactively and repeatedly change the membership of their cohorts. Continuity is the main barrier against the entry of bias, both conscious and unconscious.

If cohorts are kept intact throughout the course of a prospective study, regardless of retroactive improvement of dosimetry, then everyone knows that (A) the mean age at exposure and the sex-ratio of the cohorts cannot be improperly used as described above in the XYZ study, and (B) a cancer-death occurring in a cohort belongs to that cohort forever, and subsequent follow-ups of that cohort will include every previously recorded case, because cases are permitted to "go" nowhere else.

When cohorts are kept constant, even retroactive improvements in dosimetry can be handled without damaging the integrity and credibility of a prospective study. However, as we shall see in this chapter and in the next one, revision of doses has created a crisis for the A-Bomb Study because cohorts are NOT being kept constant.

4. Criticism of the A-Bomb Study

In contrast to all the virtues described in Chapter 4, the A-Bomb Study appears to grow increasingly deficient in adherence to the basic and meaningful standards of continuity in prospective research, in my opinion.

I arrived reluctantly at this view. It arises from events described in this chapter's "Brief Chronology" -- especially events since the mid-1970s. I have said elsewhere that everyone who follows this field -- myself included -- should have spoken up earlier (Go88b).

Now, with some 40 years of follow-up results on hand for the A-bomb survivors, the dosimetry and the cohorts of the study are being retroactively revised in major ways.

I do not object at all to possible improvements in the study's dosimetry; on the contrary, I welcome every genuine improvement. The problem is not the new dose-estimates. But very serious problems arise from the current and planned HANDLING of such changes -- handling which is described in the years 1987 and 1988 of the "Brief Chronology."

It would be tragic if the credibility of this honestly done study -- a study which has such importance for human health everywhere -- were to be unnecessarily and unfairly undermined by irregular practices which could so easily be unfavorably interpreted.

5. A Brief Chronology

● 1950:

Japan's National Census of 1950 identified 284,000 A-bomb survivors throughout Japan, of which about 195,000 were enumerated in Hiroshima or Nagasaki (Bee71, p.615). Not all 195,000 were enrolled in the follow-up study. One initial criterion for inclusion was that the place of family registration (honseki) be in or adjacent to Hiroshima or Nagasaki; survivors with more distant honseki were put into a "reserve" (Bee71, p.615).

Beebe and co-workers state that all eligible persons who were within 2.5 kilometers of a bomb's hypocenter at the time of bombing (ATB) were included, plus "about 20 % of those more distally exposed, the latter selection being made at random, within restraints as to age, sex, and city, that ensured comparability with those under 2.0 km [kilometers] ATB" (Bee71, p.615).

A "Not in City" (NIC) group of over 26,000 persons was identified and enrolled too; it consists of persons who were away from the cities ATB or were located farther than 10 kilometers from the hypocenters ATB (Bee71, p.616). This group is not called "A-bomb survivors" and is not merged with the nominal "zero dose" cohort of A-bomb survivors in recent RERF reports.

● Mid-1950s:

Excess leukemia -- meaning radiation-induced leukemia -- was showing up undeniably in the A-bomb survivors. "An organized dosimetry study was judged necessary," (Kerr87a, p.3).

● 1957:

Participants in the A-Bomb Study were assigned doses in the T57D dosimetry (Tentative 1957 Doses). T57D doses were based largely on distance from the hypocenter and on measurements made during post-war bomb-testing, at the Nevada Test Site, for instance.

● 1963:

The 1950-1960 follow-up on mortality in the study was published (TR-15-63; Jab65). It covered a total of 99,389 persons: About 73,000 A-bomb survivors and about 26,000 "Not in City" (NIC) persons.

● Mid-1960s:

Excess solid cancers also had started showing up in the A-bomb survivors (Maki68; Go69) -- not just excess leukemia.

A more sophisticated dosimetry was worked out, largely by workers at the Oak Ridge National Lab, and the dosimetry was designated T65D -- Tentative 1965 Doses (Kerr87a, p.3-4).

● 1970 :

The 1950-1966 follow-up on cancer-mortality was released (TR-11-70; Bee71). This follow-up introduced the T65D dosimetry. The survivors were divided into four kerma dose-groups: 0-9 rads, 10-39 rads, 40-179 rads, and 180+ rads.

The report changed the input of persons in a large way. A group of 9,513 A-bomb survivors, who had been ATB within 2.5 kilometers of a hypocenter, was added from the "reserve" of survivors whose honseki was not in or adjacent to either city (see 1950, above). Minor changes in the previous sample of 99,389 persons occurred too: "56 subjects have been excluded because they emigrated from Japan, and 22 have been dropped for such reasons as duplication, error in identification, and failure to possess a family register" (Bee71, p.615). As a result, the sample of the 1950-1966 follow-up report consisted of:

```
A-bomb survivors from the
      previous follow-up...          72758
A-bomb survivors newly added
                   .........          9513

Combined A-bomb survivors in the report... 82271
The number 82271 includes 3791 individuals
with unknown doses.

Not-in-city (NIC) group......          26553

Total sample in 1950-1966 report ...   108824
```

● 1971 :

The 1950-1970 follow-up report on cancer-mortality was published (TR-10-71; Jab72). The number of dose-groups was changed from four to five. About 650 persons were transferred from "dose unknown" into various dose-groups. The "Life Span Study Cohort Extended" was composed as follows:

```
A-bomb survivors with known doses
      (see Table 5-A).......          79113
A-bomb survivors with unknown doses    3131
NIC group (20176 Hiroshima;
      6347 Nagasaki).....             26523

Total sample in 1950-1970 report ...   108767
```

● 1977 & 1978 :

The 1950-1974 follow-up report on cancer-mortality was published (TR-1-77; Bee78). The Not in City or NIC group was omitted. Although the

number of survivors (82242) hardly differed from the previous report, about 625 persons were transferred from "dose unknown" into various dose-groups. The number of dose-groups was changed from five to eight.

```
A-bomb survivors with known doses
      (see Table 5-A)     ...........   79736
A-bomb survivors with unknown doses ..   2506
```

Status of Existing Outcome, 1950-74 :

The supra-linear, concave-downward shape of dose-response for cancer-mortality was already showing up in the 1950-1974 observations (Go81, p.380-85; Go89a), and the record shows that the radiation community also saw indication of this curvature in the evidence (details in Chapter 22, Part 2).

Call to Re-Examine the Dosimetry:

George D. Kerr of the Oak Ridge National Lab (ORNL) reported to the Defense Nuclear Agency (DNA) that at Hiroshima, neutron-exposure might have been overestimated two-fold and distal gamma-exposure might have been underestimated by two-fold. "These differences are too important in the investigations of the effects of radiation on man by the RERF to be treated lightly," Kerr told the DNA (Kerr87a, p.5).

● 1979 :

The Department of Energy funded Kerr to complete an inquiry into the accuracy of the T65D dosimetry. Other analysts were added to the inquiry, partly funded by the Defense Nuclear Agency (Kerr87a, p.5). Work was also underway at the Livermore National Lab on revised estimates of the neutron-exposure.

● 1980 :

The Livermore analysts, Loewe and Mendelsohn, issued their report entitled "Revised Estimates of Dose at Hiroshima and Nagasaki, and Possible Consequences for Radiation Induced Leukemia (Preliminary)" (Lo80). Thereafter, the literature became well furnished with published preliminary estimates from various sources, and they did not agree with each other in some important aspects (Kerr87a, p.7).

The different impact which the competing proposals about dosimetry would have, upon estimates of cancer-hazard, was an obvious part of the debate from the beginning (see 1978 above).

The Blinding Issue :

It would appear impossible to have achieved "blinding" for every physicist who helped to create the new DS86 dosimetry, because a proposed change in a physical parameter (e.g., gamma-ray energies, transport, or transmission-factors; see Chapter 8) would have predictable consequences for raising and lowering doses, or for changing the shape of the dose-response relationship. For instance, a sufficiently large net increase in gamma dose for the distal exposed people would necessarily lessen the estimated cancer-risk per rem and steep supra-linearity of dose-response at low doses.

RERF appears (A) not to see any problem in this aspect of "blinding," and (B) to regard the U.S. and Japanese sponsors of such work as disinterested. See the letter dated June 13, 1988 from RERF to the author, at the end of this chapter.

The T65DR Dosimetry:
The 1950-1978 follow-up on cancer-mortality was released by RERF (TR-12-80; Kato82). The input was altered in two important ways, which changed the term T65D into T65DR dosimetry (R for revised).

First, Kato and Schull tell us (Kato82, p.396): "Recently, as a result of further analysis of the physical evidence, the hypocenter in Nagasaki has been relocated 37 m [meters] to the southwest of the location used in computing the original T65 dose (3) and the dose estimates based on this new hypocenter have been used here."

Second, Kato and Schull tell us that the rounding process used in the calculation of individual doses was changed to the method of half-adjustment (rounding to the nearest rad), instead of rounding down (dropping fractional values of a rad). They say (Kato82, p.396): "... as interest has mounted in the possible consequences of exposure to doses of less than 10 rad, this practice [of rounding down] could obscure an effect through the systematic underestimation, admittedly small but possibly nonnegligible, of the exposure of individuals in the low-dose groups."

[We would like to warn readers against inferring, from the statement above, that small dose-distinctions -- like a fraction of a rad -- can ever be taken seriously in the A-Bomb Study; see Chapter 8, Part 4.]

Discontinuity of Cohorts:
The two changes described above, though small, required RERF to recalculate all the individual doses. Of course, as a result, each of the eight cohorts of survivors necessarily acquired a slightly altered mean dose. However, instead of maintaining continuity by keeping the 1974 cohorts intact -- while using each cohort's NEW mean dose in calculations -- RERF

chose to shift thousands of persons from from one cohort to another before computing the new mean doses. Table 5-A shows the net changes in the cohorts (by comparison with the 1950-1974 cohorts).

Status of Existing Outcome, 1950-78:
The supra-linear dose-response for cancer-mortality, seen in the previous follow-up, was persisting (Go88c, Go89a).

● 1981:

DOE convened a symposium to review what further work was needed on a new dosimetry, and several teams of analysts were established under DOE, NAS, and the Japanese Ministry of Health and Welfare to reassess the dosimetry for A-bomb survivors. Kerr87a lists the membership of each team; some of RERF's leading analysts of the cancer-results were included, which necessarily involves the "blinding" issue again.

● 1983 & 1984 & 1985:

In the book which introduces the new DS86 dosimetry (Roes87), a chapter by Woolson and co-workers describes the very close coordination between those who developed the dosimetry and those who intimately know the results of the follow-up.

Such practices certainly raise the "blinding" issue again. Indeed, in 1984, RERF inspected "the impact of the new dosimetry" on a segment of the survivors, and this "initial look" guided "further developments in dosimetry." To avoid any distortion of these phrases, we provide their exact context below (from Woo87, pp.405-406):

"In May 1983, the authors proposed a dosimetry system for use by the Radiation Effects Research Foundation (RERF) that would incorporate the new findings and calculations of the joint United States-Japan working groups on the reassessment of A-bomb dosimetry. The proposed dosimetry system evolved from extensive discussions with RERF personnel, numerous meetings of the scientists from Japan and the United States involved in the dosimetry reassessment research, and requirements expressed by epidemiologists and radiobiologists on the various review panels ... These discussions and our own experience indicated that, in the light of the expansion of computer and radiation technologies and the desire for more detail in the dosimetry, an entirely new approach to the dosimetry system was appropriate. This resulted in a complete replacement of the T65D system as distinguished from a simpler approach involving a renormalization of T65D parameters to reflect the new dosimetry.

"The proposed dosimetry system for RERF and the plan for implementation was accepted by the Department of Energy (DOE) Working Group on A-bomb Dosimetry chaired by Dr. R.F. Christy. The dosimetry system plan was also presented to the binational A-bomb dosimetry review groups for critical comment and was discussed at joint US-Japan workshop. [sic]

"A prototype dosimetry system incorporating preliminary dosimetry estimates and applicable to only a limited set of A-bomb survivors was installed on the RERF computer system in the fall of 1984. This system was successfully operated at RERF and provided an initial look at the impact of the new dosimetry [1]. [The reference is to Dale L. Preston; see Pr85.] The experience gained by the use of this prototype paved the way for an improved system called Dosimetry System 1986 (DS86), which incorporated further developments in dosimetry and treated a more extensive set of survivors in the RERF data base.

"The fourth joint dosimetry workshop, held in Hiroshima on 16 and 17 March 1986, reviewed the results and findings of the research to assess the A-bomb dose estimates and their incorporation into DS86. As a result, the US-Japan A-bomb radiation dosimetry committees formally approved replacement of T65D with DS86 for use by RERF for computation of doses to A-bomb survivors. The purpose of this chapter is to provide a description of DS86."

● 1986 :

The 1950-1982 follow-up on cancer-mortality, by Preston and co-workers, was released by RERF (TR-1-86; Pr87a). The study has additional names and numbers in the RERF system: "Life Span Study, Report 10, Part 1," and also "Studies of the Mortality of A-Bomb Survivors, Report 8."

The 1950-1982 report used the T65DR dosimetry exclusively.

New Discontinuities in the Cohorts :
This follow-up report retroactively changed the input of persons in a big way: It added 11,393 Nagasaki survivors who were exposed at a distance of 2500 to 9999 meters from the hypocenter "and for whom complete follow-up during 1950-1982 was available" (Pr87a, p.153). Preston and co-workers say:

"These survivors, about half of whom have T65DR

dose estimates of 0 centi-gray (cGy), were added to the cohort to increase the precision of the background (0 cGy) mortality rate estimates and, consequently, the excess risk estimates in Nagasaki. Although a comparable group of survivors is available in Hiroshima, it was felt that, since the Hiroshima 0 cGy group was relatively large already, little improvement in precision would result from the addition of these survivors to the LSS cohort" (Pr87a, p.153). Elsewhere (TR-1-86, draft), they say that the comparable group of Hiroshima survivors consists of 23,000 persons.

A Special "Reserve" of Input :
It seems as if RERF has been conducting one public study, with 80,000 survivors on view (see Table 5-A), plus another study with over 34,000 additional A-bomb survivors in reserve, who are followed-up and selectively added to the public study as needed. These reserves are clearly NOT from the "Not in City" group, which was beyond 10,000 meters ATB from a hypocenter (see 1950).

In addition, some minor changes of the cohorts occurred. According to TR-1-86 (draft): "A total of 21 subjects were lost to follow-up due to emigration. In addition, a small number of subjects were reassigned among city, sex, age ATB, and radiation exposure categories on the basis of information received since the preparation of the last report."

As a result of the changes described above, the expanded Life Span Study cohort (now designated LSS-E85) is composed as follows:

```
A-bomb survivors with known doses
      (see Table 5-A)      ............    91231
A-bomb survivors with unknown doses ..     2384
Not-in-City (NIC) group ..............    26517

Total sample in the 1950-1982 report .   120132
```

Status of Existing Outcome, 1950-82 :
The radiation-induction of fatal cancer from mean internal organ-doses as low as 11 rems was evident, the supra-linear shape of dose-response for cancer-mortality became unmistakable, and the widely suggested concave-upward shape became provably in error (see Chapters 14, 27, 29, and 30 of this book).

● 1987 :

In 1987, RERF and NAS began revealing DS86, "the new dosimetry." [As stated earlier, the National Academy of Sciences (NAS) handles the U.S. Department of Energy's share of RERF sponsorship.]

The main publications were Roes87, Elle87, TR-9-87, and TR-12-87.

Using those publications, we have provided (Chapter 8, Parts 3 and 4) an overview of how DS86 differs from T65DR, and of some important questions which may never be settled, like the explosive yield of the Hiroshima bomb and the magnitude of unmeasured doses from fallout and activation products. In Table 5-B (this chapter), we provide an overview of how many A-bomb survivors do not yet have any place in the DS86 database.

Assignment of New Doses :
From a NAS publication (Elle87, p.22-24), we learn that individual cases can receive very close attention, from someone, before they receive a new DS86 dose:

"The desired end result of the dose reassessment is reliable estimates of the doses delivered to the various organs within a specified survivor. This aspect of the reassessment was performed with particular care ... Three anthropomorphic models were selected ... Several different postures e.g., standing, kneeling, etc., are considered in applying these models. Because dose to some organs, e.g., the breast, varies considerably depending on the orientation of the survivor relative to line of sight to the weapon, a special effort was undertaken by RERF to recover this information from the survivor shielding history ..." (Elle87, p.24).

Woolson confirms that cases receive close, individual attention (Woo87, p.430): "Since complete and detailed drawings exist in RERF files depicting the survivor's location and surrounding neighborhood (see Appendix 7-2) [2], the largest reduction in the uncertainty of the dosimetry from DS86 can be accomplished by a better description of the survivor configuration in a new computer data base."

The "DS86 Subcohort" (Table 5-B) :
Cases which were "difficult," in terms of estimating a new DS86 dose, have been suspended from reports, at least temporarily. Table 5-B shows that suspensions of Nagasaki survivors are high in all dose-groups, but are concentrated in Hiroshima in Dose-Group 2, where an astonishing 31 % is "missing in action" (our term). In all, 15,240 persons out of the total 91,231 persons (about one-sixth of the study-sample) were transferred into suspension -- another reserve of potential input.

RERF calls the remaining 75,991 persons the "DS86 subcohort."

TR-9-87 also reports, "... no efforts have yet been made by RERF to develop ad hoc procedures to assign environmental transmission factors to survivors shielded by terrain or in factories. However, as part of the continuing work of the reassessment committee special consideration is being given to dose estimation procedures for Nagasaki survivors in these important categories" (Pr87b, p12).

We have another indication that suspension of 15,000 persons from the study is temporary. In a letter (August 11, 1988) to myself from the co-author of TR-9-87, Dr. Donald Pierce, we learn: "... it appears that in the near future the DS86 subcohort will be very substantially extended, by computing doses for a large fraction of the remainder of the T65D cohort" (Pier88).

Under the circumstances, it is far from clear what accounted for RERF's rush to introduce the DS86 dosimetry when so much of the study-sample still lacked doses in the new system.

Perpetual Enhancement of the Dosimetry:
In both Elle87 and TR-9-87, we learn that the DS86 dosimetry is not only incomplete, but also provisional:

TR-9-87, p.9: "Work on the new dosimetry system is still in progress. It is certain that various aspects of the basic dosimetry system and the way in which this system is used will be modified over the next few years."

TR-9-87, p.40: "It is certain that over the next few years the DS86 system will be modified and enhanced. In addition, there will be changes in the ways in which this system is used at RERF to provide dose estimates for individual survivors."

TR-9-87, p.46: "It should be kept in mind that the DS86 dosimetry and the way in which it is used at RERF will change with time. These changes will arise because of enhancements and extensions to the original system and RERF's further development of procedures for computation of indirect estimates."

Perpetual revision of DS86 is also suggested by NAS (Elle87, p.27): "The DS86 dosimetry system is well conceived to fulfill the needs of the RERF. It is amenable to future development and should serve as the basis for any future amendments to the A-bomb survivor dosimetry that may be desirable."

The U.S. review panel on the dose-reassessment project apparently expects future changes too: "... the panel recommends that DS86 be reviewed periodically so that it does not become obsolete ... It is not unlikely that additional dose estimates for A-bomb survivors will

===

be put forward from time to time as new information becomes available" (Elle87, p.30).

Oblivion Coming for the T65DR Database:

R.J.M. Fry of the Oak Ridge National Lab (ORNL), and Warren K. Sinclair of the National Council on Radiation Protection (NCRP), presented an "Occasional Survey" in the October 10, 1987 issue of LANCET. Entitled "New Dosimetry of Atomic Bomb Radiations," their survey states that the DS86 dosimetry will REPLACE the T65DR dosimetry: "DS86 completely replaces the T65D system; it is not merely an adjustment, and there have been major changes in dose estimates" (Fry87, p.847). Their statement is consistent with the "replacement" statements by Woolson (Woo87), already quoted in the 1983 segment of this chapter.

Oblivion for the T65DR dosimetry is suggested also by a NAS report. On page 1 of AN ASSESSMENT OF THE NEW DOSIMETRY FOR A-BOMB SURVIVORS, the editor, William H. Ellett writes: "The T65D estimates are now being replaced, but they have had a long and useful life that amply justifies the considerable intellectual and financial effort that went into their development" (Elle87, p.1).

These statements all refer to REPLACING the T65DR doses, instead of keeping them and simply providing each cohort with an ADDITIONAL entry, called mean dose in the DS86 system.

The statements do not hint that the ENTIRE T65DR database (doses, cohorts, structure, and all) has been directed toward oblivion, but the direction seems confirmed in 1988.

● 1988 :

In 1988, RERF released Technical Report TR-5-88 (Shi88). It is "based on the recently revised dose system, called DS86, that has replaced previous estimates of individual exposures ... Here, the focus is on cancer mortality among the 76,000 A-bomb survivors within the LSS sample for whom DS86 doses have been estimated ..." (Shi88, p.1). Some 15,000 LSS members were omitted because, although they had T65DR doses, they had no DS86 doses while TR-5-88 (Shi88) was in preparation.

A Completely New Architecture :

In TR-5-88, which covers 1950-1985, the doses are not the only things which are new.

Many of the remaining 75,991 persons have been moved into new cohorts (see Tables 10-A and 10-B).

This means new groupings of the cancers which had been previously enumerated (1950-1982) among those 75,991 persons, and of course, it means new mean ages ATB and new sex-ratios in each cohort, too. TR-5-88 also introduces the subdivision of Dose-Groups 2 and 3, and changes the age-bands from five to six. Even the follow-up periods from 1950 onward are treated in units of 5-years instead of 4-years.

In summary, the architecture of the A-Bomb Study is now completely altered -- not just the doses -- and the T65DR database has been removed from the public's sight.

6. Summary on the Growing Problem

The circumstances, events, and plans associated with "the new dosimetry" and described above would be an extraordinary threat to the credibility of any prospective study, no matter how disinterested its sponsors might be in the study's outcome.

We have no evidence that bias has been introduced into the A-Bomb Study up to this point, and one of our main objectives is to help see that the future handling of the study is such that no one will ever be able to introduce a criticism of bias against it. It is self-evident that as the crucial second half of this study is unfolding over the next 10, 20, and 30 years, new personnel will take over its handling, and -- unless current practices are changed -- they will inherit a study in which continuity will be lacking and in which the changing of dosimetry-inputs may be more the rule than the exception.

At the beginning of this chapter, I objected NOT to genuine improvements in A-bomb dosimetry, but to the way in which retroactive changes of many types are unnecessarily disrupting the continuity of this study.

The chapter's title called it "a growing problem." It is growing not only because of all the recent disconnections between the study's past and its future, but also because of the explicitly expressed intention (see 1987) to CONTINUE altering the study's input, even as more and more of the cancer-outcome is at hand in the future. Such practices would unavoidably create a real threat to the scientific credibility of the whole study.

In research, enthusiasm for improved accuracy -- in dosimetry, for instance -- is natural, and I share it too. However, we must not allow this type of enthusiasm ever to blind us to unintended, but nonetheless devastating, consequences of using the new insights in ways which would be certain to undermine the credibility of the entire effort.

A Reasonable Solution :

A major thrust of this book is to propose and demonstrate a very different approach to handling the A-bomb database and to using the new DS86 dosimetry. We will show how an improved dosimetry can be ADDED to the A-Bomb Study while preserving the study's continuity and valid prospective structure.

RERF's Point of View :

We have, of course, expressed our concerns to RERF, and we present the gracious response from RERF's chairman at the end of this chapter's text. His letter makes three major points:

(1) The subject we raise is of great importance, and our concerns are scientifically legitimate, because retroactive alterations of a study's input can create opportunities for existing results to influence such alterations.

(2) But RERF feels the procedures associated with design and application of the new dosimetry are adequate to protect the study against bias and to maintain its credibility.

(3) Nonetheless, RERF will think over the need to maintain the T65DR database.

Telephone: 082-261-3131
Facsimile: 082-263-7279
Cable: RERF HIROSHIMA

財団法人　放射線影響研究所
RADIATION EFFECTS RESEARCH FOUNDATION

広島市南区比治山公園５番２号
**5-2 Hijiyama Park, Minami-Ku
Hiroshima, 732 Japan**

A Cooperative Japan - United States Research Organization
日 米 共 同 研 究 機 関

13 June 1988

John W. Gofman, M.D., Ph.D.
102 Donner Laboratory
Department of Biophysics
  and Medical Physics
University of California, Berkeley
Berkeley, CA 94720 U.S.A.

Dear Dr. Gofman:

Your letter of March 31, 1988 was recently forwarded to me, as it raises an important policy issue to which Mr. Usagawa is unable to respond. The issue that you discuss relates to the recently concluded dose reassessment effort, resulting in the DS86 dosimetry system. It appears to be your feeling that this system should not be used exclusively, as a replacement of the T65D dosimetry system, but that any future evaluations of dose-response relationships on the Hiroshima and Nagasaki databases should be performed using both systems so as to avoid bias to enter the study.

We fully endorse the view, of course, that it is essential for the dosimetry system to be designed and operated in such a way that there is no chance that the cancer data can affect the exposure estimates. This is true whether one applies T65D or DS86. The concerns expressed in your letter, however, suggest that you may not be fully aware of the way the dosimetry systems operate. First, the design of the new system was done entirely outside this Foundation, by U.S. and Japanese scientists, both groups with their own scientific oversight committees, and with no knowledge of, or access to individual survival information. Second, as far as calculation of individual exposures at RERF is concerned, this is done by well-defined computerized calculations, involving only the original shielding histories from which the T65D estimates were computed. There are no individual judgements made in which cancer results, or other biological endpoints, might come into play. This includes decisions regarding survivors for whom DS86 estimates cannot yet be computed, as these are made on classes of survivors, not individuals, defined by shielding histories alone.

The history of the entire effort is contained in the final report, entitled "US - Japan Joint Reassessment of Atomic Bomb Radiation Dosimetry in Hiroshima and Nagasaki", a report that was published by this Foundation as a matter of convenience, not because it had any rights of authorship. I enclose a copy of the relevant section of this report for your information.

I believe that, given the careful way in which the dose reassessment was carried out, with publication in the open scientific literature and continuous oversight as its significant features, your concern about bias does not appear to be justified. We shall, however, be sure to consider the necessity, and if so, the feasibility of dual analyses of our data. Please

John W. Gofman, M.D., Ph.D.   -2-   13 June 1988

note that many of our recent Technical Reports have contained analyses
involving both T65D and DS86.

     Thank you very much for your interest in our studies, and for your
thoughtful remarks on a subject that is of great importance to both of us.

                              Sincerely,

                              J. W. Thiessen, Vice Chairman

                         For Itsuzo Shigematsu, M.D.
                              Chairman

Encl.

IS:hs

Table 5-A

Number and Distribution of A–Bomb Survivors : Changes of Input in Four Consecutive RERF Reports.

	Col.A Dose-Group 1	Col.B Dose-Group 2	Col.C Dose-Group 3	Col.D Dose-Group 4	Col.E Dose-Group 5	Col.F Dose-Group 6	Col.G Dose-Group 7	Col.H Dose-Group 8	Col.I Unknown Doses
1950-1970 Follow-up	Grps 1 + 2					Grps 6 + 7 + 8			
HIROSHIMA Persons	43730		10707	2665	1677		1460		1670
NAGASAKI Persons	11404		3700	1231	1229		1310		1461
BOTH CITIES Persons	55134		14407	3896	2906		2770		3131
Persons with Doses: 79113									Source: Jab72.
1950-1974 Follow-up									
HIROSHIMA Persons	29943	13796	10761	2718	1721	656	370	505	1441
NAGASAKI Persons	4700	6706	3759	1314	1391	748	270	378	1065
BOTH CITIES Persons	34643	20502	14520	4032	3112	1404	640	883	2506
Persons with Doses: 79736									Source: Bee78.
1950-1978 Follow-up									
HIROSHIMA Persons	27577	15933	10911	2783	1740	659	369	510	1429
NAGASAKI Persons	4004	7140	4031	1442	1388	722	270	377	957
BOTH CITIES Persons	31581	23073	14942	4225	3128	1381	639	887	2386
Persons with Doses: 79856									Source: Kato82.
1950-1982 Follow-up									
HIROSHIMA Persons	27569	15931	10909	2783	1740	659	369	510	
NAGASAKI Persons	9604	12924	4034	1442	1388	722	270	377	
BOTH CITIES Persons	37173	28855	14943	4225	3128	1381	639	887	2384
Persons with Doses: 91231									Source: Tables 26-H, 26-I, Pr87a.

NOTES -----

1. There is substantial continuity of cohorts in these four follow-ups, although the continuity is certainly not perfect. Altered cohorts in each follow-up mean that analysts are dealing with new mean doses, new mean ages ATB, new male-female ratios, and new distributions of previously reported cancers. Such changes are a serious matter, for the reasons discussed in the text.

----

2. Table 5-B discusses the 1950-1985 cohorts for the T65DR database.

Table 5-B
Persons Missing from the DS86 Dosimetry, As Introduced in 1987, Plus New Alteration of T65DR Cohorts

Col.A	Col.B	Col.C	Col.D	Col.E	Col.F	Col.G	Col.H	Col.I	Col.J	Col.K
T65D Dose-Group	LSS Persons 1950-82 T65DR	LSS Persons 1950-85 T65DR	LSS Persons Omitted by DS86	1950-85 Persons with DS86 Doses	Percent 1950-85 LSS Omitted by DS86	LSS Persons 1950-82 T65DR	LSS Persons 1950-85 T65DR	LSS Persons Omitted by DS86	1950-85 Persons with DS86 Doses	Percent 1950-85 LSS Omitted by DS86
	---------------- HIROSHIMA ----------------					---------------- NAGASAKI ----------------				
1	27569	27568	2324	25244	8.4	9604	9603	172	9431	1.8
2	15931	16573	5155	11418	31.1	12924	13194	3218	9976	24.4
3	10909	10363	1209	9154	11.7	4034	3805	1068	2737	28.1
4	2783	2707	113	2594	4.2	1442	1417	485	932	34.2
5	1740	1725	99	1626	5.7	1388	1375	718	657	52.2
6	659	657	63	594	9.6	722	723	295	428	40.8
7	369	369	41	328	11.1	270	267	95	172	35.6
8	510	506	74	432	14.6	377	376	108	268	28.7
SUMS	60470	60468	9078	51390		30761	30760	6159	24601	

LSS = Life Span Study.
All the entries in this table were generated by RERF:
Col.B entries come from Table 26-H in this book; Col.G entries come from Table 26-I.
All the other columns (except A) come directly from TR-9-87, Tables 3 and 4, p.11, for 1950-1985.
 At page 7, TR-9-87 says that it means T65DR whenever it writes T65D.

 It is evident from Columns F and K that the DS86 dosimetry was far from complete at the time of its first use by RERF. Indeed, one-quarter to one-half of the Nagasaki cohorts was in suspension, and an astonishing 31 % of Dose-Group 2 in Hiroshima was likewise "missing in action."

 Thus the initial "DS86 Subcohort" consists of only 75,991 persons who have both a T65DR and a DS86 dose-assignment (51,390 persons from Col.E + 24,601 persons from Col.J).

 The FULL cohort of 91,231 persons, in the 1950-1982 follow-up (T65DR database), is described by Columns B and G. Columns C and H describe the full cohort for 1950-1985 (T65DR database), according to TR-9-87. However, TR-9-87 does not explain the puzzling differences, which are rather substantial in Hiroshima's low-dose groups.

 For instance, Dose-Group 2 increases by (16,573 - 15,931) or 642 persons. Dose-Group 3 decreases by (10,909 - 10,363) or 546 persons. Dose-Group 4 decreases by (2,783 - 2,707) or 76 persons. Since all that anyone can observe here is the final NET change in the size of various T65DR cohorts, it is conceivable that the number of affected persons was many THOUSANDS. Net changes occur in Nagasaki too. The consequence is that, in Dose-Groups 2, 3 and 4, the T65DR full cohorts in 1985 no longer have the same membership, mean age ATB, mean dose, or sex-ratio in Dose-Groups 2, 3 and 4 as the T65DR full cohorts had in 1982. Changes like this are a serious matter, for the reasons discussed in the text.

 However, we think that the disruption in continuity of the T65DR cohorts may be accidental and therefore temporary. A similar discontinuity within the DS86 dosimetry became evident in comparing TR-9-87 (p.11) with TR-12-87 (p.8). Those disparities were explained in a footnote in TR-12-87 (p.8) as the result of different RERF analysts using different rounding procedures for doses. The footnote states that "a consensus" among analysts there has now been reached.

5-empty, after tables.

==

What Will Happen to the A–Bomb Database? A Pending Proposal

Right now, the A–Bomb Study has reached a crossroad where decisions must be made by RERF and RERF's sponsors on how to preserve the study's legitimacy as a prospective epidemiological inquiry -- with all the normal continuity and safeguards expected of such a study -- and how not to sacrifice it (needlessly) in the quest for a better dosimetry.

We say "needlessly" because this book will show how improved dosimetries can be ADDED to the A–Bomb Study without destroying its continuity and its legitimacy as a first-class prospective inquiry.

Key Role of the 1950–1982 Follow–Up :

The first step in our proposal is to identify the study's valid prospective structure. Chapter 5 demonstrates that there has been substantial continuity of doses, cohorts, and structure of the study during the 1950–1970, 1950–1974, 1950–1978, and 1950–1982 follow-ups (Table 5–A).

Although the "change no input" rule and others were bent in the handling of this database during those follow-ups, the rules were not broken badly enough to nullify the study's credibility as a uniquely valuable prospective inquiry into the effect of ionizing radiation upon human cancer-rates. We reach this conclusion largely because the rule-bending occurred while relatively little of the cancer-outcome was known. Even by late 1982, about two-thirds of the study's population was still alive, and more of the cancer-story lay in the study's future than in its past.

It is clear from Chapter 5 that the 1950–1982 follow-up is currently the LAST complete follow-up where there is substantial continuity of doses, cohorts, and structure. Therefore, the 1950–1982 follow-up represents the proper base for subsequent follow-ups, if the A–Bomb Study is going to maintain the continuity which is required of all prospective studies.

A Simple Proposal :

Our proposal is that the eight 1950–1982 dose-cohorts of A-bomb survivors (Table 5–A) now be "frozen" and kept intact as the base for all the remaining follow-ups of the Life Span Study. Membership in a cohort would be virtually immutable from 1982 onward, in the normal manner of a prospective study. Thus, there would be no change in any cohort's mean age at the time of bombing, no

change in any cohort's initial male-female ratio, and no movement of any cancer-deaths from one cohort to another. Of course, there would also be no further alteration of any cohort's mean T65DR dose.

These eight stable dose-cohorts would be "set in concrete" and observed for health effects for their full remaining lifespans as "constant cohorts." The five existing age-bands would also remain undisturbed. If the study is continued in this manner, no one would be entitled to "raise an eyebrow" skeptically about the objectivity of the T65DR database, or to question its scientific worth due to irregular, unacceptable, or sub-standard handling.

Then, as SUPPLEMENTAL information appended to the study, the new DS86 dose-estimates for these same cohorts of persons could be (and should be) provided.

This "dual dosimetry" would permit everyone to benefit from the insights about dosimetry which occurred AFTER the eight cohorts were established. Indeed, the proposal could easily handle the continual "enhancing" of the current DS86 dosimetry which is planned for the future. With this approach, even a possible 24th iteration of DS86 would in no way disrupt the permanent architecture of the T65DR database.

In short, we propose to append the DS86 dosimetry to the EXISTING structure of the A–Bomb Study, without sacrificing the study's T65DR anchor into the world of legitimate prospective research.

Demonstration of the Proposal :

The simplicity of the proposal is demonstrated in Chapters 13, 14, 15, and 16 of this book, where we do analyses in BOTH dosimetries for the SAME sets of persons. While only the T65DR results have the standing of a prospective study, the supplemental and parallel DS86 results provide a basis on which analysts can properly propose any hypothesis which they regard as justified by the results in DS86.

We repeat a reminder published elsewhere: Under the basic rules of research, the DS86 database can never have legitimacy as an integral part -- much less the only part -- of a prospective inquiry (Go89b).

Everything to Gain, Nothing to Lose :

The "constant-cohort, dual-dosimetry" proposal

offers everything to gain, and nothing to lose. By keeping the T65DR dosimetry and database intact, one gains both the scientific credibility which belongs to a well-conducted prospective study, and yet one is able to find out what the results would be with a different dosimetry.

By contrast, one loses everything if the T65DR database is sent to oblivion and if it is replaced by a new dosimetry and a new structure. In effect, the on-going study would be terminated and a new one would begin -- not with a clean slate, but with all the cumulative results through 1982 at hand.

In addition, RERF and NAS have stated the intention to continue altering the study's input indefinitely, even after introducing the DS86 database. Their enthusiasm for an ever-improving dosimetry may have caused them to give insufficient weight to the unwanted consequences of such practices upon the future scientific credibility of the whole effort.

A Pending Decision :

After all the suffering in Hiroshima and Nagasaki, and after all the decades of hard work to extract important biomedical information for humanity from that experience, the A-Bomb Study has now reached the crossroad which we have described in this chapter and the previous one.

No one wants to throw away the chance to continue this uniquely valuable A-Bomb Study as a first-class prospective inquiry. Surely everyone must want to help protect it from being subjected, needlessly and forever, to the criticism that its handling was epidemiologically unacceptable. And skepticism about standards in health research is becoming very common (see Chapter 24, Part 1, "A Distasteful Subject").

Following our correspondence with RERF on this issue in 1988 (see Chapter 5), we opted to leave the matter at rest until we were able to DEMONSTRATE our proposal to RERF, NAS, and interested epidemiologists. This book provides the demonstration. Neither we nor anyone else can ever use this "constant-cohort, dual-dosimetry" approach beyond the 1982 follow-up, unless RERF and RERF's sponsors make a favorable decision about our proposal.

The decision may affect more than the A-Bomb Study. Practices affecting a world-famous database are likely also to have international repercussions for the standards of biomedical research in general -- far beyond the single field of ionizing radiation.

For both reasons, we regard the issue as one of the most important topics of this book.

CHAPTER 7

Collecting All the Required Data from RERF

In order to evaluate cancer-risk and dose-response from the A-Bomb Study (1950-1982), we needed to assemble the raw data from RERF. Since RERF had not published all of them, this task was not routine. It involved four sets of source-material:

● (1)
The Written Technical Report (TR) :

The RERF Technical Report for the 1950-1982 cancer follow-up is TR-1-86 by Preston and Pierce (Pr86). TR-1-86 is also called Life Span Study (LSS) Report 10. An abbreviated version of TR-1-86 was published in the journal RADIATION RESEARCH in 1987 (Pr87a).

Analysts using these publications, however, need to avoid three erroneous entries in their Table I:

ERROR No.1: Hiroshima subjects in the 1-9 kerma-rad dose-category are given as 15,391. This is an error. The correct number is 15,931.

ERROR No. 2: The mean dose for Hiroshima in the 300-399 kerma-rad dose-category is given as 364.4. This is an error. The correct value is 346.4.

ERROR No. 3: The mean dose for Hiroshima in the 400+ kerma-rad dose-category is given as 524.2. This is a small error. The correct number is 524.4.

This book uses the correct numbers, of course; they will be seen as entries in our special Table 26-H, which also comes from RERF.

Welcoming Input from Readers :
In mentioning these slips in the the RERF report, we intend no criticism. We certainly hope that anyone who notices such slips in THIS book will inform us, so that we may correct them before another printing and can thus prevent trouble for others who may use our numbers "downstream." Other types of comment also are welcome.

● (2)
The Corresponding Floppy Diskette :

Most commendably, RERF has started to make available floppy diskettes which contain far more data than do the written reports. For the 1950-1982 follow-up, we used the RERF diskette entitled "Cancer and Non-Cancer Mortality, R10ALL.DAT" (R-Ten-All). The diskette reports the observations for the 91,231 A-bomb survivors in the Life Span Study, but omits the "Not in City" or NIC group (see Chapter 5).

On the diskette, the 1950-1982 data are arranged in 1,280 rows of entries. The number 1,280 is the product of 2 cities, times 2 sexes, times 5 age-bands, times 8 dose-classes, times 8 four-year follow-ups.

Except for Chapter 17 in this book, we always deal with the aggregate or cumulative observations from 1950-1982. Therefore, we have summed the entries for the eight separate follow-ups, and this reduces the file from 1,280 to 160 rows, or subsets.

We have reproduced these 160 rows of raw data in this book's Chapter 26 as Master Table 26-A,B,C,D as follows:

Table 26-A : Hiroshima Males (40 lines).
Table 26-B : Nagasaki Males (40 lines).
Table 26-C : Hiroshima Females (40 lines).
Table 26-D : Nagasaki Females (40 lines).

● (3) Previously Missing Data --
Persons, True Doses, True Ages ATB

We (and other analysts) also need the actual numbers of persons initially in each of the 160 subsets, their true mean doses, and their true mean ages ATB. These three crucial types of data are not provided on the RERF diskette.

We requested the missing data from RERF, and we received it as nine printout sheets, which are reproduced in Chapter 26 as Tables 26-E through 26-M. This information is not available (as we go to press) anywhere else in the literature. Except for reduction in size and addition of some identifying titles, the sheets are exactly what RERF provided (final version, August 29, 1988).

We would like to express our appreciation for the excellent cooperation of Dr. Donald A. Pierce, who was Chief of RERF's Department of Statistics at that time.

Initial Persons :
The RERF diskette provides person-years (PYR), but not the number of persons initially in each subset in 1950. Therefore the persons in our Master Table

===

26-A,B,C,D come from the special Tables 26-E through 26-M (where they are called "cases").

True Mean Doses :

The diskette provides fictitious or nominal doses. It uses the mean dose of an entire dose-group whether or not it really describes a particular subset of that dose-group. Therefore, the true mean kerma-doses in Master Table 26-A,B,C,D (Column G) were added by us from the special Tables 26-E through 26-M.

True Mean Ages At-Time-Of-Bombing :

The diskette provides fictitious or nominal ages ATB. It uses the midpoint of an age-band whether or not the midpoint really describes a particular subset of that age-band. Therefore the true mean ages ATB in our Master Table 26-A,B,C,D (Column D) were put there by us from the special Tables 26-E through 26-M.

The data which we received from RERF, on the true mean ages ATB, apply to RERF's customary eight dose-groups. It is easy to see in Table 26-E (and even easier in Table 4-A) that true mean age ATB is not the same in all eight dose-groups. In view of RERF's new practice of subdividing Dose-Groups 2 and 3, the following point deserves emphasis.

A Warning about Subdivision :

If a dose-group is divided into halves (its lower dose-range and its upper dose-range), its two cohorts will probably have different mean ages. When Dose-Group 2 is divided, it is impossible to predict whether the people falling into its lower dose-range are younger, or older, than the people falling into its upper dose-range. The same uncertainty exists about any division of Dose-Group 3.

For the reasons explained in Chapter 11, and demonstrated in Chapter 13, no analysis of risk or dose-response could be properly done with subdivided groups in the absence of the necessary adjustments for age-differences.

The problem does not arise in this book, because we use the customary undivided dose-groups for which true age-data now have been provided by RERF. In our judgment, the number of cancer cases and the dosimetry in this database do not permit subdivision (see Chapter 8, Part 4).

● (4) Missing Data for DS86 Subsets -- Neutron and Gamma Components of Dose

Our approach to application of the new dosimetry was described in Chapter 6. In order to use our approach, we needed to obtain data which have not been published by RERF: The DS86 neutron and gamma components for each subset of persons shown in RERF Technical Report TR-12-87, Appendix Table 2 (Shi87).

We requested this information from J.W. Thiessen, M.D., the Vice-Chairman of RERF and representative of the (U.S.) Department of Energy, Office of Health and Environmental Research (Doe87, p.xvii). He graciously provided it in December 1988.

The printouts from RERF are reproduced in Chapter 26 as our Tables 26-N and 26-"O". Chapter 10 shows the steps which lead from the special Tables 26-N and 26-"O" to the entries in Columns I (Eye) and J of the Master Table 26-A,B,C,D.

A Word of Appreciation :
===========================

RERF holds in trust, for humans everywhere, a unique database of great importance for human health. With regard to the courtesy and attention which RERF gives to meeting requests from outside analysts, RERF sets a fine standard indeed for other research institutions.

========================

CHAPTER 8

Dosimetry : From Bomb, to Kerma, to Internal Organ–Dose

This chapter is divided into five parts:

Introduction :

No quantification of cancer-risk from low-dose ionizing radiation can begin, of course, without an estimate of the mean dose received by the internal organs from which the fatal cancers arise. What is needed is an estimate which can be reasonably used for all internal organs.

We show exactly how such estimates are obtained in Chapter 9 for the T65DR cohorts (1950-1982). Then in Chapter 10, we show exactly how they are obtained in the DS86 dosimetry for the SAME cohorts -- for the SAME people.

The foundation for those two chapters is laid by this chapter.

1. Sources of Ionizing Radiation from an Atomic Bomb

Kerr and colleagues provide a handy summary of the sources of neutrons and gamma rays from an atomic explosion (Kerr87b). From their Table 1, we have made the listing below.

● PROMPT NEUTRONS from fission (weapon still intact and still able to sustain the fission process).
TIME EMITTED after detonation: < one microsecond.

● DELAYED NEUTRONS emitted by the fission-products (after explosion and burn-up of the weapon).
TIME EMITTED after detonation: < one minute.

● PROMPT GAMMA RAYS from the fission process itself.
TIME EMITTED after detonation: < one microsecond.

● SECONDARY-ORIGIN GAMMA RAYS resulting from the interaction of neutrons with the weapon itself, with air, or with ground.

TIME EMITTED after detonation: From < one microsecond (for gammas resulting from neutron interaction with the weapon) to 0.2 seconds (from neutron interaction with air or ground).

● ACTIVATION GAMMA RAYS, produced by neutron-activation of ground or other materials.
TIME EMITTED after detonation: Initial, 0.2 seconds to 1 minute. Residual, 1 minute to years.

● DELAYED GAMMA RAYS from fission-products.
TIME EMITTED after detonation: Initial, 0.2 seconds to 1 minute. Residual, 1 minute to years.

Kerr points out, "Because the fission products are contained in the fireball formed after the weapon explodes and because the rapidly-rising fireball reaches an altitude of about two miles (3000 m) by the end of one minute, irradiation by delayed neutrons and gamma rays soon ceases at ground level" (Kerr87b).

At Hiroshima and Nagasaki, the extremely early gamma rays and neutrons, transported from the explosion-region outward, dominate the doses received by survivors who were located at various distances from the hypocenter of the bomb. Thus, the exposure of survivors is properly regarded as acute exposure.

2. The Relationship of Kerma and Internal Organ–Dose

RERF Technical Reports use terms whose meaning is fairly constant: Kerma, free-in-air kerma, environmental transmission-factor, shielded kerma, body-transmission/ organ-absorption factor, and internal organ-dose.

Kerma :

Kerma is the acronym for "kinetic energy released in material" (Elle87, p.6). For a discussion of "kerma," we can rely on William C. Roesch, editor of RERF's Volume 1 about the DS86 dosimetry (Roes87). He states the following, in the Editor's Note on an unnumbered page before its table of contents (his italics are capitalized by us):

"The object of the reassessment program is to determine the ABSORBED DOSE (or simply the DOSE) in certain organs of the people exposed to the bombs. For practicality, determination of a quantity often approximately equal to the dose, the KERMA, is usually made instead. The concept of absorbed dose deals with the energy imparted by ionizing radiation to a medium per unit of mass. 'Energy imparted' means the difference in energy of the particles and quanta entering and leaving a small test volume. For the particles and quanta encountered in A-bomb dosimetry, the energy difference for photons and neutrons equals the energy they give to the charged particles they produce by interactions in the volume. This difference, per unit mass, is the quantity called the kerma."

There is more to it than that -- much more -- and for an advanced discussion of the exact relationship of kerma to dose, Roesch refers to an earlier work (Roes68).

However, his Editor's Note provides explicit assurance that, in most of the organs of interest in A-bomb dosimetry, "the kerma gives a sufficiently accurate approximation to the dose" (Roes87).

Free-in-Air Kerma :

In physics, it is common to estimate quantities (such as dose) for some imaginary, "ideal" circumstances. The term "free-in-air kerma" is one such term. Roesch, still in the Editor's Note, defines the term as follows:

"For example, in this report, it is common to determine the kerma that would be produced in tissue by the radiations at a point in air. One such condition is used so often that its kerma is given a special name: the kerma-in-tissue at a point in air over bare ground (i.e. no person present and not in or near a building) is called the FREE-IN-AIR (FIA) KERMA or the FREE-FIELD KERMA."

The ability to compute the dose to a gram of flesh suspended in air without a body present, at a given distance from a given explosion, is important, but still it is just an early step on the way to computing something which counts -- say, the average dose to the intestines of a whole, irradiated person who was shielded by a wooden house, or by a concrete factory, or by a hill.

Organ-Dose in Relation to Kerma and Transmission-Factors :

In TR-9-87 (p.6), Preston and Pierce devote a paragraph to terms which we shall quote verbatim (their underlining is capitalized by us):

"The tissue kerma in air at specific locations unadjusted for the effect of shielding by structures or terrain will be called the FREE-IN-AIR (FIA) KERMA. The tissue kerma in air at the survivor location after adjustment for the effects of shielding by structures or terrain will be called KERMA. ORGAN DOSE will be used to refer to the mean absorbed dose for specific organs. The terms TOTAL KERMA and TOTAL ORGAN DOSE will be used to mean the sum of gamma-ray and neutron kerma or organ dose, respectively. In analyses which make use of assumed or estimated RBE values the level of radiation is expressed in terms of DOSE EQUIVALENT. FIA kerma, kerma, and organ dose is [sic] given in SI units, gray (Gy) or milligray (mGy), while dose equivalent is expressed in sieverts (Sv) or millisieverts (mSv). The ratio of kerma to FIA kerma will be called the ENVIRONMENTAL TRANSMISSION FACTOR while the ratio of organ dose to kerma will be referred to as the BODY TRANSMISSION/ORGAN ABSORPTION FACTOR."

In this book, we shall abbreviate the last term as "body transmission-factor."

Shielded Kerma :

Elsewhere in RERF reports, what is defined above as "kerma" is sometimes explicitly called "shielded kerma."

Absorbed Dose :

In some other RERF reports -- for instance, in discussion of doses from fallout in the DS86 book, Volume 1 -- the term "absorbed dose" is often used. The meaning there is explicitly an average internal organ-dose (Roes87, p.224).

• Summary -- Two Modifiers for Kerma, to Obtain Organ-Dose :

When RERF reports provide values for "shielded kerma" or just "kerma" (which is the same), the kerma values need two kinds of modification in order to obtain the corresponding internal organ-doses.

One adjustment is for attenuation of both neutron and gamma dose by the body (the appropriate body transmission-factors). The other adjustment is only for the neutron component of the dose; it is the application of the factor which converts doses from high-LET neutrons to their dose-equivalents in low-LET units, according to the higher presumed Relative Biological Effectiveness (RBE) of neutrons.

3. Comparison of T65DR and DS86 Dosimetries

● *Neutron FIA Kerma at Hiroshima :*
"Hiroshima DS86 FIA neutron kerma estimates are about 10 % of the T65D estimates at all ground ranges" (TR-9-87, p.9; at page 7, TR-9-87 says that it means T65DR whenever it says T65D).

● *Neutron FIA Kerma at Nagasaki :*
In Nagasaki, neutrons were unimportant even in the T65DR dosimetry. In the DS86 dosimetry, there is "a reduction of about 30 % in the neutron kerma" (TR-9-87, p.9).

● *Gamma FIA Kerma at Hiroshima :*
"The DS86 FIA gamma kerma estimates in Hiroshima are larger than the corresponding T65D estimates. This difference increases with distance. Thus at a distance of 700 m from the hypocenter the ratio of the DS86 FIA gamma kerma estimate to the T65D value is 1.3 while at 2,000 m the ratio is 3.7" (TR-9-87, p.9).

● *Gamma FIA Kerma at Nagasaki :*
The DS86 system introduces "little change" in the FIA gamma kerma for this city (TR-9-87, p.9).

● *Environmental Transmission-Factors :*
According to TR-9-87 (p.9-10), the factors for neutrons changed very little in DS86 from their T65DR values, but "the average DS86 environmental transmission factor for gamma radiation is about 50 % of that for T65D in Hiroshima and about 60 % in Nagasaki" and this change "has a dramatic impact on gamma kerma estimates."

It should be noted that "the current DS86 system" appears to cope with shielding by wooden houses, but not with shielding by concrete factories or by all types of terrain (TR-9-87, p.9,10,12). Factories and terrain account for the omission of about one thousand of the Nagasaki survivors, in Dose-Groups 4 and 5, from the current DS86 dosimetry (TR-9-87, p.12). Such omissions were shown in detail in our Table 5-B.

● *Gamma Shielded Kerma at Hiroshima :*
"In Hiroshima the average DS86 gamma kerma estimate is less than the T65D estimate for ground

ranges of less than about 1,300 m and greater than the T65D estimate at larger ground ranges" (TR-9-87, p.10).

● *Gamma Shielded Kerma at Nagasaki :*
In Nagasaki, at all distances, the DS86 gamma kerma is lower than it was in the T65D dosimetry (TR-9-87, p.10).

● *Neutron Shielded Kerma in DS86 :*
"The ratio of neutron to total kerma increases smoothly with kerma from less than 1 % to about 6.5 % in Hiroshima and from less than 1 % to about 1.5 % in Nagasaki" (TR-9-87, p.10).

● *Body Transmission-Factors, Gamma Dose :*
Preston and Pierce choose the dose to the large intestine (colon) as "a representative dose" for internal organs in general (TR-9-87, p.3). They report that "For intestinal doses, the DS86 body transmission/organ absorption factor is 80 % larger than the T65D factor" (TR-9-87, p.13). We agree with Preston and Pierce that this change in body transmission-factors for gamma dose is "a large effect"; it almost doubles the organ-dose from any particular shielded gamma kerma.

A comparison of old and new body transmission-factors for neutrons as well as gammas is provided in the next chapter by our Table 9-A.

The Net Effect on Organ-Doses :

It has been noted by others (TR-9-87, p.3; Fry87, p.845) that several aspects of the dosimetry-revision tend to cancel each other out -- to offset each other. For instance, in Hiroshima, organ-doses from neutrons decrease in DS86, but organ-doses from gamma rays increase -- especially in the low-dose classes.

The net effect of the new dosimetry (current version), on organ-doses in each RERF Dose-Group, can be seen from the next two chapters by comparing Table 9-C with Table 10-E.

4. Uncertainties about Doses from Weapon-Yield, Fallout, and Activation Products

Anyone who reads Volume 1 of RERF's DS86 book (Roes87) will realize that the dosimetry of the A-bomb survivors will always be approximate -- which is typical of just about every human study in the field of ionizing radiation.

The DS86 dosimetry leaves many, many questions

unsettled, including the yield of the Hiroshima bomb -- which remains uncertain with a range of 12-18 kilotons (Elle87, p.8-9). Also unresolved is the question of doses from "residual radioactivity" (neutron-activation products and fallout).

Activation Products :

RERF's DS86 book points out that the creation of activation products, resulting from neutron-capture by substances in or above the ground, decreases as distance from the hypocenter increases. Near the hypocenter at Hiroshima, activation products produced an upper limit for absorbed dose of about 50 rads (50 centi-gray, or 0.5 Gray), and near the hypocenter at Nagasaki, about 18 to 24 rads (Chris87, p.21). "The cumulative exposure would be about one-third as large after a day and only a few percent after a week" (Oka87, p.223).

According to Sztanyik (Sz78), "Shortly after the detonation, thousands of people entered the affected areas in both cities for rescue work, in search of their relatives and to assist in removal of ruins." This means that an LSS survivor who was up to 10,000 meters from groundzero ATB (a presumably unexposed survivor, for instance), and who then tried to help within 1000 meters of the hypocenter, could have received an unquantifiable or poorly quantified dose of radiation.

Fission-Product Fallout :

In both Hiroshima and Nagasaki, there were regions of fallout at quite a distance from the hypocenter. In Nagasaki, the Nishiyama area received fallout about one hour after the bombing. "The upper limits on absorbed dose from gamma rays for persons continuously in the fallout area at Nagasaki ranged from about 12 to 24 rad" (Chris87, p.21). An exposure of at least one-fifth the maximum extended over some 1,000 hectares (Chris87, p.21). For Hiroshima, the estimated absorbed doses from fallout may have ranged from about 0.6 to 2 rads for those with continuous residence in the Koi-Takasu region (Chris87, p.21).

External doses in the fallout areas were first measured "some weeks or months" after the bombing. Approximate initial levels could be back-calculated "providing storms had not washed away a large portion of the activity" (Chris87, p.20).

The Missing Information :

According to the chapter on residual radioactivity in RERF's DS86 Volume 1, "Many factors affecting the accuracy of the measurements are not well known 40 years after the bombs, therefore exposure estimates must be rough approximations. In general, the exposure rates were not measured soon enough to avoid some weathering and they were not repeated often enough to account for subsequent weathering or to provide a time distribution of radioactivity. The number of sites monitored was too small to develop a good estimate of detailed geographical distribution of the radioactivity. Also, in such surveys, it is difficult to avoid unrepresentative sampling and it is not known whether such a sampling bias exists. Finally, the details of calibration and measurement are not always available" (Oka87, p.206).

Handling of This Confounding Variable :
===

The likelihood that the "unexposed" group (Dose-Group 1) is NOT a group with zero dose has needed facing for a long time (Go81). The radiation community is starting to acknowledge it:

"At the present time doses due to residual activity are not calculated by the DS86 system. It is recommended that the few individuals from areas of high residual radioactivity not be included in the nonexposed cohort for epidemiological studies" (Chris87, p.21).

"The individual exposures from residual radiation may not be significant compared with the direct radiation at the time of the bomb. On the other hand, individuals with potential exposure from these sources are dubious candidates for inclusion in a cohort that was presumably not exposed" (Oka87, p.224).

"Care has to be taken to exclude those exposed in this way from the control population" (Fry87, p.847).

The words sound fine, but one must wonder why the exclusions were not made 30 years ago. It would be a very questionable practice indeed to make additional exclusions now, when 40 years of outcome are at hand.

Steps in the Wrong Direction :

The nominally "unexposed" Dose-Group 1 is not the only group affected by permanent uncertainties about activation products, fallout, and even the size of the bomb at Hiroshima -- the city which provides 60,470 of the 91,231 survivors (from Table 9-D).

The lower is the Dose-Group, however, the greater is the accuracy of dosimetry required, before a

Dose-Group could conceivably be subdivided -- even prospectively. Nonetheless, RERF has recently started to subdivide Dose-Groups 2 and 3 into lower-dose and upper-dose halves (see Tables 26-N and 26-O, and Kato87). We regard this as a move in the wrong direction, scientifically.

The undivided Dose-Group 2 has a shielded kerma range of 1-9 rads, with a mean internal organ-dose of only l.5 to 1.9 rems (see Row 11 in Tables 9-C and 10-E). In other words, in both dosimetries, there is a very small difference in mean dose between Dose-Group 1 (nominally "zero" dose) and the undivided Dose-Group 2. The doses from fallout and/or from activation products encountered during rescue-work could easily be bigger than this dose-difference for thousands of people in Dose-Groups 1 and 2.

The idea that reliable dose-differences can be created within this small dose-range in the future -- by perpetual adjustment of the input -- strains belief. Under the circumstances, we see no way for scientists ever to have confidence in alleged dose-differences between Dose-Group 1 and Dose-Group 2.

Reasonable Handling of Dose-Groups 1 + 2 :

Hidden doses from residual radioactivity are a confounding variable of relatively small importance in the cohorts where a few rads more, or a few rads less, in a group's mean dose cannot have much of an impact on results. But for Dose-Groups 1 and 2, permanent and well-founded uncertainty about true doses can result in uncertainty about which cohort really received the higher dose.

The realistic solution is both scientifically solid and simple: It consists of treating Dose-Groups 1 and 2 as not provably different, and just combining them into a single, very low-dose Reference Group. In the T65DR dosimetry, this dose would be only 654 millirems (see Table 9-C, Row 11, far right); in the DS86 dosimetry, this dose would be only 861 millrems (see Table 10-E, Row 11, far right.)

Dose-Groups 1 and 2 very often need to be combined ANYWAY for a different purpose: To reduce the small-numbers problem. The combination has frequently been used by analysts of the A-Bomb Study (Bee78; Kato82; Land84; Toku84; Waka83; also Beir80 at p.155).

The combination of Dose-Groups 1 and 2 is scientifically strong, and seems far more likely to produce believable results, under the circumstances,

than subdivision. It is not clear why anyone is suddenly moving in the less credible direction, of sub-division.

5. Choice of RBE Values for the Neutron-Component

It is now recognized that exposure of the A-bomb survivors by neutrons is a very small part of their total exposure. Part 3 of this chapter reported that, in Hiroshima, neutrons account for less than 1 % up to about 6.5 % of the total shielded kerma doses; in Nagasaki, the range is less than 1 % up to about 1.5 % of the total shielded kerma doses. The percentage of total organ-dose which comes from neutrons is even lower, after shielded kermas are adjusted by the body transmission-factors, because those factors are much lower for neutrons than for gammas (Table 9-A). The overwhelming part of the exposure in both cities was caused by gamma rays.

On the other hand, per rad of dose delivered to an organ, a large body of radiobiological evidence indicates that radiations of high-LET (Linear Energy Transfer), like neutrons and alpha particles, are more potent in causing biological effects than low-LET radiations like gamma-rays and X-rays. Therefore, every analyst of the A-Bomb Study confronts the question: For human carcinogenesis, what is the relative biological effectiveness (RBE) of a rad from fission neutrons versus a rad from A-bomb gamma-rays?

A Formal Definition of RBE :

George Kerr provides one common definition of RBE, as follows:

"The RBE is defined as the absorbed dose from orthovoltage x rays, divided by the absorbed dose from another radiation needed to produce the same level of biological effect" (Kerr88, p.242).

(Orthovoltage X-rays, also called medium voltage X-rays, fall in the range of about 180-400 kilovolts (Des89, p.656).)

The definition of RBE means that, if one rad of neutron exposure produces the same level of biological effect as 10 rads of orthovoltage X-rays, then the RBE value for neutrons would be 10, relative to the X-rays. However, if two rads of gamma radiation are required to produce the same level of biological effect as one rad of orthovoltage X-rays, then the RBE of the gamma rays would be 0.5, and the RBE of neutrons relative to the GAMMA RAYS would be 20, not 10.

===

The biological effect which this book considers among A-bomb survivors is the increase in the cancer mortality-rate, per unit dose of acute low-LET exposure. There is no theory or body of evidence which permits any generalization that RBE for cancer-induction will be the same as RBE for some other biological endpoint, or that RBEs for humans will be comparable to RBEs for other species.

Below, we shall briefly review the types of evidence which might provide guidance on the RBE of fission-neutrons versus gamma exposure, for cancer-induction in the human.

Past Evidence -- A-Bomb Study :

==============================

By 1965, the T65D system of dosimetry was in place, with its estimates of neutron and gamma doses to the survivors of the A-bombing. Readers who examine Table 9-B will see that the shielded kerma doses (T65DR) estimated for neutrons -- relative to the corresponding gamma doses -- are very low at Nagasaki, and quite important at Hiroshima.

Among analysts of the study, it became conventional practice to multiply the shielded kerma doses from neutrons by an RBE factor of 5 or 10 for greater carcinogenic potency, compared with gamma rays. As we shall see, however, the evidence soon cast doubt on 5 to 10 as the proper RBE range for neutrons, within the T65DR dosimetry.

In 1977, McGregor and co-workers published findings on breast-cancer in Hiroshima and Nagasaki survivors. A major finding of their study was stated twice, as follows:

"The Hiroshima and Nagasaki dose-response curves were similar, which suggested approximate equivalence of neutron and gamma radiations in their carcinogenic effect on breast tissue, and were consistent with a linear model" (McGr77, p.799).

"The dose-response function was reasonably linear and was similar in the two cities. There was no evidence suggesting that gamma and neutron radiations entail different risks per rad" (McGr77, p.808).

In 1978, Mole published a review on the subject of breast-cancer induction by ionizing radiation, in which he stated the following: "The incidence of breast cancer per rad was closely similar at Hiroshima and Nagasaki, for deaths (Mole, 1975) and for diagnoses (McGregor et al., 1977), showing that the RBE of fission neutrons cannot much exceed one for induction of breast cancer in women" (Mole78, p.402).

In 1979, Land and McGregor further amplified their conclusion concerning the RBE of neutrons in breast-cancer induction by radiation: "... For breast cancer there was no epidemiological evidence that the effects of neutron and gamma radiation were markedly different. Therefore, no account was taken of radiation quality in the present report" (Land79, p.17). And, indeed they did not take any account of RBE; all their calculations used breast-dose in rads (total gamma plus neutron dose).

Plentiful Flags of Warning :

It is amazing that these findings did not produce great flags of warning that something was radically wrong. The findings indicated that (A) either the estimate of neutron RBE values like 10 must be seriously wrong for carcinogenesis in humans, or (B) the estimate of neutron fluences at Hiroshima must be seriously exaggerated.

In 1980, while writing RADIATION AND HUMAN HEALTH (Go81), I examined all the evidence and concluded there was something radically wrong with the neutron story -- a conclusion based not only on the breast-cancer findings but also on the leukemia findings and on frequency of small head-size for those irradiated in utero. These concerns were discussed in Go81 under the listing "Neutron Issue at Hiroshima-Nagasaki" (brain-damage data at pp.730-3 and pp.736-7; breast-cancer data at p.246; leukemia data at p.380 and pp.668-9). At page 246, I stated the following explicitly:

"The paper by McGregor and co-workers showed that there is no significant difference between the findings from Hiroshima and those from Nagasaki, and that there is no evidence to suggest that an RBE value for neutrons other than 1.0 (indicating no difference in effectiveness) is needed. A higher RBE had been suggested earlier because there was a higher neutron component in the radiation at Hiroshima than at Nagasaki. Like McGregor and co-workers, we shall use an RBE of 1.0 for neutrons and we can therefore combine the Hiroshima and Nagasaki findings. In other words, we shall treat rads absorbed from neutrons just like rads absorbed from gamma rays, in terms of their cancer-producing effects. However, in correcting kerma doses in air to absorbed tissue doses, we shall use appropriate factors for gamma rays and neutrons (see chapter 6)."

I made the choice of assigning RBE = 1.0 to neutrons for all cancers and leukemia in the A-bomb experience, since that was the only rational choice at the time.

Of course I recognized that the true RBE could be much higher than 1.0, but if that were the case, then the neutron-component must have been grossly exaggerated in the T65DR dosimetry for Hiroshima. Since there was no way for me to prove that the neutron-component at Hiroshima was much too high, assigning RBE = 1.0 for neutrons was a reasonable way not to participate in an obvious error. If I had blindly accepted both RBE = 10 and what turned out to be a 10-fold overestimation of neutrons at Hiroshima, I would have used the equivalent of RBE = 100 for Hiroshima neutrons. Within a year, I learned that neutrons had indeed been overestimated at Hiroshima by about 10-fold (Lo81, Fig. 1, p.663).

Current Evidence -- A-Bomb Study :

When the DS86 dosimetry corrected the neutron errors in the A-Bomb Study, one consequence was to lessen the difference between Hiroshima and Nagasaki in their neutron-to-gamma ratios. In addition, the organ-doses from neutrons are extremely low compared with the organ-doses from gamma-rays, as noted at the beginning of this section.

Under the circumstances, it is hardly surprising that analysts are unable to learn anything from the study about the true neutron RBE for cancer-induction. The inquiry requires a level of accuracy and precision which the data cannot possibly meet.

In TR-9-87, Preston and Pierce comment: "It is well-understood that RBE cannot be usefully estimated from the cancer mortality data, because the gamma-ray and neutron exposures to individuals are very highly correlated. What little information on this [which] was available within the T65D dosimetry was largely due to the ratio of neutron to gamma-ray exposures differing substantially between cities. Since this is no longer the case in the DS86 dosimetry, even less information is now available about RBE in these data" (Pr87b, p.27).

Preston and Pierce relate that they tested constant RBE values from 1 to 50 in the DS86 system, and could not find evidence that one value was better than another (Pr87b, p.27).

Their colleagues at RERF, Shimizu and co-workers, also attempted to evaluate neutron RBE, in TR-5-88. They comment: "Since the neutron dose is very small under the DS86 system, an analysis of the dose response using the gamma and neutron doses separately or to estimate the neutron RBE is difficult" (Shi88, p.36). After making extensive efforts and producing sets of estimates, they conclude: "However, the uncertainties in these estimates are too large to permit serious consideration of these RBEs" (Shi88, p.36-37).

In order to make their own estimates of lifetime fatal cancer-risks in the DS86 dosimetry, Shimizu and co-workers ended up by using a constant neutron RBE value of 10, and going ahead with their calculations.

Elsewhere, Fry and Sinclair also acknowledge that neutrons in the A-Bomb Study are so sparse that "... direct estimates of neutron relative biological effectiveness may be precluded or be much more difficult" (Fry87, p.845).

Other Types of Evidence :

With respect to the correct RBE value for neutrons, there simply exists no relevant human epidemiological evidence -- a conclusion reached also by Warren Sinclair, who says "there are no human data" (Sin88, p.151).

Analysts might hope to put some upper limits on RBE values for neutron exposure, by examining RBE values for ALPHA exposure versus low-LET exposure. Unfortunately, the human epidemiological evidence on the proper RBE for alpha exposure is still cloudy, at best.

One contribution to the uncertainty comes from human evidence which suggests that radiation-induced cancer from alpha exposure may show up EARLIER than from low-LET exposure (Go83; Go85). If RBE is going to reflect LIFETIME excess cancer-risk per rad, but if the existing follow-ups are all incomplete, RBEs based on incomplete follow-ups will overestimate the carcinogenic potency per rad of the radiations which induce cancers earlier. (This situation may be analogous to the tendency to overstate the relative radiation-inducibility of leukemia per rad, just because leukemia shows up EARLIER than most of the solid tumors.)

Since the correct RBE values for alpha exposure are still so uncertain, they cannot provide much guidance for inferring correct RBE values for neutrons.

Then what kind of evidence can be used, for estimating the RBE of neutrons?

Although the relevance of experiments with

cell-studies and with other species is always uncertain, there is no other guidance on neutrons. Radiobiological experiments have been indicating that biological dose-responses from neutrons are usually linear at low doses, and then begin to flatten.

Fry (Fry81, p.232) has stated that, for experimental animal data, "... results consistently show that the dose-response curve for tumor incidence after exposure to neutron radiation bends over at relatively low doses." Kerr (Kerr88, Fig.3, p.245) cites one mouse-study of female mammary adenocarcinomas where the linear dose-response from neutron irradiation appears to be shifting to supra-linearity (concavity-downward) in the region of 10-20 rads of neutron dose.

Is RBE Constant or Variable, in the A-Bomb Study?
==========================

In the absence of any human evidence contradicting the experiments referred to above, we are going to assume that dose-response for neutrons in the A-Bomb Study is linear. The neutron doses received by the A-bomb survivors are so low that they would certainly lie in the linear segment of the neutron dose-response curve.

We can ascertain their values in DS86, if we look ahead to Chapter 10. We take the shielded kerma values from Table 10-D, Rows 2 and 6, and multiply them by the body transmission-factor of 0.19 from Table 9-A, in order to obtain mean organ-doses. The results, below, show that the highest mean neutron organ-dose is about 4.369 rads. Indeed, very few people in the study received an organ-dose over one rad from neutrons.

Dose-Group	Hiroshima Neutron Organ-Dose	Nagasaki Neutron Organ-Dose
1	0 rad	0 rad
2	0.009 rad	0 rad
3	0.058 rad	0.002 rad
4	0.270 rad	0.050 rad
5	0.620 rad	0.126 rad
6	1.330 rad	0.243 rad
7	2.165 rads	0.410 rad
8	4.369 rads	0.994 rad

With respect to the GAMMA dose in the A-Bomb Study, the shape of dose-response for cancer-induction is supra-linear (concave-downward), as will be shown in Chapter 14. Nonetheless, for the short dose-segment below 5 rads, we can make the simplification that dose-response is linear.

If the dose-response below 5 rads is linear for both the neutrons and the gamma-rays, and if neither has a threshold, it follows that the RBE-value of neutrons will be constant at all neutron doses which occur in the A-Bomb Study. With respect to human carcinogenesis, we have shown elsewhere in this book that no threshold exists for low-LET radiations.

Therefore, in our analyses of the A-Bomb Study, we use a constant RBE value for neutrons. The remaining question is simply: What value should we use?

The Fallacy of RBE = 100 :
==========================

As noted above, Shimizu and co-workers use the constant RBE value of 10 for neutrons with the DS86 dosimetry. We do not fault that choice. Almost any choice is arbitrary, in the absence of relevant human evidence.

But some choices can and should be ruled out, because real-world human evidence invalidates a key premise on which they rest. We refer to suggestions (for instance, in Beir80) that the RBE for neutrons versus low-LET radiations is destined to rise progressively as total dose goes down toward zero dose.

The suggestion would be valid, of course, if dose-response were linear for neutrons, and concave-UPWARD for low-LET radiation. Under such circumstances, the neutron RBE would necessarily vary with dose-level, and would increase at lower doses. If the dose-response curve of the low-LET radiation were presumed to have a very flat region near zero dose, then the ratio of slopes (or biological effect) at equal doses of the two radiations could easily rise to 100 or more, in the zero-dose region. Indeed, if the low-LET dose-response were assigned a threshold, the neutron RBE would rise to infinitely high values at doses below the alleged threshold-dose for the low-LET radiation.

The reasoning above, however, is simply inapplicable and irrelevant here. For human carcinogenesis, there is no threshold dose, and the evidence from the A-Bomb Study has clearly shown for a long time that dose-response from gamma rays is NOT concave-upward (see Chapters 14 and 22).

The human epidemiological evidence on gamma dose-response overrules any suggestion that the neutron RBE might need to be raised to very high values in the A-Bomb Study. Moreover, such evidence from

===

real, whole humans must prevail over data from the lab, where radiobiologists have generated every dose-response one could imagine or desire, in their experiments.

Describing experimental work, Fry says "Because of the marked variation in the shape of dose-response curves for low-LET radiation, RBE values vary almost infinitely" (Fry81, p.224). Indeed, in his discussion of possibilities, Fry includes the non-linear threshold model for carcinogenesis by low-LET radiation (Fry81, Fig.4, p.228) -- the model which leads to the infinite RBE value for neutrons.

But it is now 1990, and we must dismiss that model (and many others) for human carcinogenesis, because we have human data which provide a reality-based answer about low-LET dose-response and about the absence of any threshold. There is simply no basis for accepting the suggestion that neutron RBE always rises to very high values at low doses.

Current ICRP-NCRP Position on Neutron RBE :

=======================================

Kerr reports that "Both the ICRP and the NCRP are now recommending essentially the same guidance with respect to the quality factor for fast neutrons: an increase by a factor of two" (Kerr88, p.242).

(Quality factor, Q, is the term used for RBE in radiation protection, while the term RBE is often reserved for radiobiological experiments. ICRP stands for International Commission on Radiological Protection, and NCRP stands for (USA) National Council on Radiation Protection and Measurements.)

The recommended two-fold increase is necessarily made in the absence of any direct human evidence on neutron-potency. Kerr acknowledges that "The Q for neutrons is based on a large, unfocused body of experimental data on RBE. Orthovoltage x rays are the usual reference radiation, but gamma rays from 137-Cesium and 60-Cobalt have also been widely used as reference radiations. The mixed use of reference radiations, acute versus fractionated exposures, and high versus low dose rates, can easily result in a factor of 2, or more, discrepancy in the measured values of RBE for the same biological end point" (Kerr88, p.243).

In circumstances like this, it is fair to say that the scientific basis for increasing RBE by a factor of two is thin, and that the basis for the customary value of 10 is also thin.

Nonetheless, there is a persuasive basis for

assigning SOME value to RBE when one is dealing with credible dose-estimates for radiations having LET values which differ greatly. After all, Linear Energy Transfer is a measure of spatial concentration of energy-transfers, and there is no doubt that the biological impact of ionizing radiation is strongly tied to the spatial concentration of its energy-depositions.

The RBE Values Chosen for This Book :

=======================================

In our analyses of the A-Bomb Study, we are using a constant RBE value of 20 for neutron organ-doses in the DS86 dosimetry. Therefore, we are using a constant RBE value of 2 in the T65DR dosimetry. The RBE of 2, combined with the mistaken T65DR estimates of neutrons, is about equivalent to RBE = 20 with the correct estimate of neutrons. By contrast, if we were to use RBE = 20 in the T65DR dosimetry, it would be equivalent to using a constant RBE value approaching 200, because the neutrons at Hiroshima were overestimated by about 10-fold, and were nearly negligible at Nagasaki.

All our analyses will use a neutron RBE of 2 for the T65DR dosimetry, with its overestimate of neutron doses unaltered, and a neutron RBE of 20 for the DS86 dosimetry, where neutron doses are supposed to be correct.

In the T65DR dosimetry, even though some of the neutron organ-doses (in rads, or centi-grays) appear to lie beyond the linear segment of the presumed neutron dose-response curve, in reality they did not lie beyond it. Therefore we again avoid participating in the dosimetry error when we presume -- in both dosimetries alike -- that neutron dose-response is linear in the study's neutron dose-range.

Because the RBE of 2, combined with the mistaken T65DR estimates of neutrons, is about equivalent to the RBE of 20 with the correct estimate of neutrons, the differences (if any) between our findings in the T65DR and in the DS86 systems cannot be blamed on a use of different values for neutron RBE. We have, in effect, used the constant RBE of 20 in both dosimetries.

If the RBE of 20 is too high for neutrons -- and it may well be too high -- it will lead to an underestimate of radiation-induced cancer-risk in this book, since a higher RBE value raises the total dose in rems (centi-sieverts) without increasing the observed cancers at all.

=====================

8-empty, after 8-9.
===

Converting T65DR Mean Kerma Values to Mean Internal Organ-Doses

In this chapter, we shall obtain average internal organ-doses in the T65DR dosimetry. Chapter 8, Part 2, has already indicated that this step simply consists of multiplying the shielded kerma values by two types of factor: The body transmission-factor and (for neutrons only) an RBE factor.

The Body Transmission-Factors :

The body transmission-factors are provided in our Table 9-A, for obtaining whole-body internal organ-doses from mean kerma values.

In reality, no individual can receive a uniform whole-body organ-dose from an external source of radiation, since a beam of radiation diminishes as it travels through the body. However, this problem of dosimetry is reduced in the A-Bomb Study because people were randomly oriented with respect to the bomb; some received higher doses in the front, others in the back, and others in the side. Thus the approximation of a mean whole-body internal organ-dose may be better in this study than for some other types of studies involving whole-body irradiation by external sources.

The Shielded Neutron Kermas :

In reporting the 1950-1982 follow-up, RERF did not show the gamma and neutron shielded kerma values separately -- only the total (TR-1-86, Pr86, Pr87a). This omission creates no problem, however, because the necessary shielded neutron values are provided in an earlier RERF follow-up, 1950-1974 (Bee78), and subsequent changes in the cohorts would cause only trivial changes. Of course the shielded GAMMA kermas can be obtained too, by subtraction of the neutrons from the total.

Both the neutron and gamma shielded kerma values are provided in Table 9-B.

Internal Organ-Dose for RERF's Eight Dose-Groups :

============================

Table 9-C performs the conversion, from shielded kerma in rads, to mean internal organ-dose in rems (or cSv), for RERF's eight dose-groups. Table 9-C is based on the constant RBE value of 2 for neutrons, which is a reasonable value with the T65DR dosimetry

(see Chapter 8, Part 5).

Reference Group -- 1 + 2 :

Two important reasons exist for the common practice of combining Dose-Groups 1 and 2, and they were given already in Chapter 8, Part 4: Realism about hidden doses from residual radioactivity, and achievement of a statistically more reliable control-group.

In Table 9-C, the combination of Dose-Groups 1 and 2 (in the righthand column) produces a mean internal organ-dose of only 0.654 cSv or 654 millirems. In other words, we obtain a control-group or Reference Group with much greater stability than Dose-Group 1 alone, yet its members received only a very low internal organ-dose.

Whenever analysts must subdivide the control-group by age-bands or sex, having the extra people and cancer-cases from both dose-groups is particularly important. Analysts who seek scientifically strong results would combine the two dose-groups, even if the uncertainty about doses (including the yield of the Hiroshima bomb) were absent. And the uncertainty will never be absent (Chapter 8, Part 4).

Internal Organ-Dose for RERF's 160 Subsets :

==========================

As readers will see in Chapter 15, full analysis of cancer-risk requires separate mean organ-doses for each of RERF's 160 subsets of the database (see Master Table 26-A,B,C,D). Our method for obtaining these organ-doses is illustrated below for RBE = 2.

The first step is tabulating the correlation between the mean total kerma-doses (neutron plus gamma) and the corresponding mean total organ-doses (neutron plus gamma). This is done for RBE = 2 in Table 9-D.

Now, if we go to the Master Table 26-A, for Hiroshima males, we find that the average of 3.3 kerma rads (from Table 9-D, Col.C) shows up in Column F five times -- once for each of RERF's five age-bands. But in Table 26-A, Column G, we see how the average varies with each age-band. Let us consider the 42-year-old age-band ATB. It includes ages 35 through 49 years at the time of bombing (Table 4-B).

===

For the 42-year-old age-band, we see the true kerma-dose is 3.5 rads instead of 3.3. In other words, it is (3.5 / 3.3) or 1.0606 times the overall average for Dose-Group 2. We obtain the corresponding organ-dose for Table 26-A, Column H, by saying:

Since 3.3 kerma rads at Hiroshima correspond with 1.658 organ cSv (from Table 9-D), then (3.5 / 3.3) x (1.658 cSv), or 1.76 cSv, is the appropriate organ-dose for that subset of Hiroshima males (age 42 ATB).

And so 1.76 cSv (rem) becomes the entry, for males age 42 ATB, in Column H of Table 26-A.

This is the method by which all 160 organ-doses for the T65DR dosimetry were obtained for Column H of the Master Table 26-A,B,C,D. Care was taken to use the Hiroshima pairs from Table 9-D for calculating the 80 HIROSHIMA subsets, and Nagasaki pairs for the 80 NAGASAKI subsets. Later, when we analyse RERF's five age-bands separately, we make special organ-dose adjustments for the small body-size of those who were age 0-9 years ATB (Chapter 31).

Table 9-A
Body Transmission-Factors, to Obtain Internal Organ-Doses from Mean Shielded Kerma Values.

Row	Col.A Dosimetry and Source	Col.B Internal Organ	Col.C Gamma Absorption	Col.D Direct Neutron Absorption	Col.E Neutron-Capture Gamma
1	T65DR (Kerr79) (Beir80, p.197)	Combined Cancer-Sites Excl. Leuk.	0.50	0.22	0.07
2	T65DR (Shi87, p.43)	Colon Large Intestine	0.40	0.14	0.08
3	DS86 (Shi87, p.43; see also p.14)	Colon Large Intestine	0.74	0.19	0.41

These factors, for Hiroshima and Nagasaki persons combined, are used to obtain "whole-body" internal organ-doses (see text).

----

1. For our T65DR analysis (Table 9-C), we use the factors in Row 1.
    For our DS86 analysis (Table 10-E), we use the factors in Row 3.

In Row 3, the choice of large intestine (colon) is not arbitrary. RERF analysts report that the dose absorbed by this organ is the best approximation of internal dose absorbed by all the cancer-sites, excluding leukemia (TR-9-87, p.3, and TR-5-88, p.50). Preston and Pierce, and Shimizu and co-workers, all use colon-dose in their own DS86 estimates of Lifetime Fatal Cancer-Yields arising from whole-body exposure (combined cancer-sites).

----

2. In Table 9-C, we use the transmission-factors from Row 1 instead of Row 2 for the T65DR dosimetry. Using Row 1 increases mean organ-dose (relative to using Row 2), without increasing the corresponding cancer-mortalities, so lower Cancer-Yields are the net effect of the choice.

----

3. Column E provides the body transmission-factor for the n,gamma reaction, in which neutrons are captured in tissue, and gamma rays are emitted.

Table 9-B
Mean Shielded Kerma-Doses (T65DR) in Rads, with Neutron and Gamma Components, by Separate Cities and by Cities Combined.

Row		Col.A Dose-Group 1	Col.B Dose-Group 2	Col.C Dose-Group 3	Col.D Dose-Group 4	Col.E Dose-Group 5	Col.F Dose-Group 6	Col.G Dose-Group 7	Col.H Dose-Group 8
1	HIROSHIMA Persons	27569	15931	10909	2783	1740	659	369	510
2	Mean Dose (n)	0.0	0.8	4.3	13.4	30.3	56.8	92.1	144.1
3	Mean Dose (g)	0.0	2.5	17.8	56.9	108.7	186.7	254.3	380.3
4	Mean Dose (n+g)	0.0	3.3	22.1	70.3	139.0	243.5	346.4	524.4
5	NAGASAKI Persons	9604	12924	4034	1442	1388	722	270	377
6	Mean Dose (n)	0.0	0.0	0.0	0.2	1.3	3.4	5.4	10.5
7	Mean Dose (g)	0.0	2.6	21.2	71.0	145.6	240.3	338.3	518.7
8	Mean Dose (n+g)	0.0	2.6	21.2	71.2	146.9	243.7	343.7	529.2
	BOTH CITIES Persons	37173	28855	14943	4225	3128	1381	639	887
9	Kerma-Dose, calc.	0	3.0	21.9	70.6	142.5	243.6	345.3	526.4
10	Kerma-Dose from 26-E	0	3.0	21.8	70.6	142.5	243.6	345.2	526.4

NOTES -----   (n) = NEUTRONS   (g) = GAMMA

1. The entries in Rows 1 and 5 for Persons are "cases" from Tables 26-H and 26-I (26-Eye).

----

2. The entries in Rows 4 and 8 for total Mean Dose, neutron and gamma components combined, come from "Meandose" in Tables 26-H and 26-I (26-Eye). Also they match the entries in Master Table 26-A,B,C,D, Column F, for "Disk Kerma-Dose" as provided by RERF diskette R10ALL.

----

3. The entries in Rows 2 and 6 for the mean neutron shielded kerma-dose come from Bee78. The gamma values in Rows 3 and 7 are obtained by subtraction of the neutron values from the totals (n+g).

----

4. The entries in Row 9 are calculated from the entries in Rows 1, 4, 5, and 8 directly above them. The entries in Row 10, taken from Table 26-E, are provided as a check; Rows 9 and 10 are the same, except for very small rounding-artifacts.

Table 9–C
Mean Organ–Doses (T65DR) in Centi–Sieverts, for Neutron RBE = 2, by Separate Cities and by Cities Combined.

Row	T65DR, RBE = 2	Col.A Dose-Group 1	Col.B Dose-Group 2	Col.C Dose-Group 3	Col.D Dose-Group 4	Col.E Dose-Group 5	Col.F Dose-Group 6	Col.G Dose-Group 7	Col.H Dose-Group 8	Col.I Ref. Group (1 + 2)
1	HIROSHIMA Persons	27569	15931	10909	2783	1740	659	369	510	43500
2	Organ-Dose (n) RBE=2	0	0.352	1.892	5.896	13.332	24.992	40.524	63.404	
3	Organ-Dose (n,gamma)	0	0.056	0.301	0.938	2.121	3.976	6.447	10.087	
4	Organ-Dose (g)	0	1.250	8.900	28.450	54.350	93.350	127.150	190.150	
5	Total Organ-Dose, cSv	0	1.658	11.093	35.284	69.803	122.318	174.121	263.641	0.607
6	NAGASAKI Persons	9604	12924	4034	1442	1388	722	270	377	22528
7	Organ-Dose (n) RBE=2	0	0.000	0.000	0.088	0.572	1.496	2.376	4.620	
8	Organ-Dose (n,gamma)	0	0.000	0.000	0.014	0.091	0.238	0.378	0.735	
9	Organ-Dose (g)	0	1.300	10.600	35.500	72.800	120.150	169.150	259.350	
10	Total Organ-Dose, cSv	0	1.300	10.600	35.602	73.463	121.884	171.904	264.705	0.746
	BOTH CITIES Persons	37173	28855	14943	4225	3128	1381	639	887	66028
11	Total Organ-Dose, cSv	0	1.498	10.960	35.393	71.427	122.091	173.184	264.093	0.654
12	Organ-Dose from Neut.	0	0.194	1.381	3.914	7.670	12.708	24.405	38.419	0.085
13	Organ-Dose from Gamma	0	1.303	9.579	31.479	63.757	109.383	148.779	225.674	0.570
14	Neutron cSv / Total cSv	0	0.130	0.126	0.111	0.107	0.104	0.141	0.145	0.130

NOTES FOR T65DR, neutron RBE = 2 -----   (n) = NEUTRONS   (g) = GAMMA

1. Table 9-C corresponds with Table 9-B, except that all entries in Table 9-C are now whole-body internal organ-doses, not shielded kerma-doses.

----

2. The entries in Rows 2 and 7 for the neutron-component are the corresponding neutron entries in Table 9-B times 0.44 (which is two times the conversion factor of 0.22 from Table 9-A, Col.D). The extra factor of two is necessary because calculations are for neutron RBE = 2.

----

3. The entries in Rows 3 and 8 are the entries for neutrons in Table 9-B times the conversion factor of 0.07 (from Table 9-A, Col.E). No RBE factor of 2 is used because, after the n,gamma reaction has occurred (see Table 9-A), the dose is delivered by GAMMA radiation.

----

4. The entries in Rows 4 and 9 for the direct gamma component are the corresponding gamma entries in Table 9-B times the conversion factor of 0.50 (from Table 9-A, Col.C).

----

5. The entries in Row 11, for mean organ-dose in the combined cities, are calculated for each column by the formula [(Row 1 times Row 5) + (Row 6 times Row 10)] / (Row 1 + Row 6).
    The entries in Row 12 are [(Row 1 times Row 2) + (Row 6 times Row 7)] / (Row 1 + Row 6).
    The entries in Row 13 are obtained by subtracting Row 12 from Row 11.
    The entries in Row 14 are, of course, Row 12 / Row 11.
Ostensible errors in the third decimal place of Row 13 come from rounding after making a calculation with longer strings of digits.

----

6. Doses in Row 11 will undergo slight adjustment in the course of the age-and-sex normalization process of Chapter 11.

Table 9-D
(T65DR Dosimetry) Correlation of Kerma–Doses with Organ–Doses, RBE = 2.

Col.A	Col.B	Col.C	Col.D		Col.E	Col.F	Col.G		Col.H
		HIRO	HIRO			NAGA	NAGA		BOTH
	HIRO	KERMA	ORGAN		NAGA	KERMA	ORGAN		CITIES
	PERSONS	(RADS)	(cSv)		PERSONS	(RADS)	(cSv)		PERSONS
Dose-Grp 1	27569	0	0		9604	0	0		37173
Dose-Grp 2	15931	3.3	1.658		12924	2.6	1.300		28855
Dose-Grp 3	10909	22.1	11.093		4034	21.2	10.600		14943
Dose-Grp 4	2783	70.3	35.284		1442	71.2	35.602		4225
Dose-Grp 5	1740	139.0	69.803		1388	146.9	73.463		3128
Dose-Grp 6	659	243.5	122.318		722	243.7	121.884		1381
Dose-Grp 7	369	346.4	174.121		270	343.7	171.904		639
Dose-Grp 8	510	524.4	263.641		377	529.2	264.705		887
SUM,Pers.	60470				30761				91231

Columns C and F come from Table 9-B.   Columns D and G come from Table 9-C.
Persons are included in this table just for reference.

CHAPTER 10

Obtaining Mean DS86 Doses for the T65DR Cohorts

For the reasons fully discussed in Chapters 5 and 6, we propose to use the new DS86 dosimetry by leaving the T65DR dose-cohorts intact, and simply providing each cohort with the appropriate DS86 mean dose in ADDITION to its T65DR mean dose. By contrast, the approach taken so far by RERF to using the new dosimetry, as shown below, would leave no continuity between the DS86 cohorts and the study's previous cohorts.

RERF's Way of Using the DS86 Dosimetry :

Table 10-A shows how RERF plans to redistribute Hiroshima survivors into new cohorts, and Table 10-B shows how RERF plans to redistribute Nagasaki survivors into new cohorts. Tables 10-A and 10-B refer to RERF's "DS86 Subcohort" of 75,991 survivors (see our Table 5-B), not to the full 91,231 study-sample (see our Table 5-A, 1950-1982).

The distribution of individuals in the T65DR system is shown on the lefthand side, in ten ROWS (because RERF is subdividing two of the eight Dose-Groups). The distribution of persons in the new cohorts is shown in ten COLUMNS. We are not responsible for the slight disparities between Table 5-B and these tables. The disparities originate with RERF.

To illustrate what Tables 10-A and 10-B are showing about the discontinuity of proposed cohorts, we will examine Hiroshima Dose-Group 4 in Table 10-A. In the new subcohort of 75,991 persons, 2,670 individuals remain in the T65DR Hiroshima Group 4 (lefthand side).

But these 2,670 individuals will not stay together as a cohort, after RERF's proposed handling. Instead, with RERF's approach, the New Group 4 will have 2,911 members (see center of the bottom row) -- and only 1,806 of the 2,911 members will come from the previous Group 4. The vertical column entitled "New Group 4" shows that 291 members will come from the previous Group 3-B, and 1,806 members will come from the previous Group 4, and 814 members will come from previous Group 5.

All the vertical columns in Tables 10-A and 10-B show similar alteration of the T65DR cohorts.

Tables 10-A and 10-B make it clear that RERF is using the shielded kerma-ranges (for instance, 1-5 rads, 6-9 rads, 10-19 rads, 20-49 rads, 50-99 rads,

etc.) as the basis for composing its totally new cohorts for the DS86 database. But no need exists to treat these particular dose-ranges as inviolable. Treating them this way means sacrificing the continuity of the study's cohorts, the continuity of their prior cancer-counts, the continuity of their true mean ages ATB, and the continuity of their male-female ratios, while saving only the continuity of something which has no importance at all -- the arbitrary dividing-lines in the shielded kerma dose-range.

Our Way of Using the DS86 Dosimetry :

The "constant-cohort, dual-dosimetry" approach, proposed in Chapter 6, begins here, by answering the question: "After the individuals who compose a T65DR cohort have each been assigned a new DS86 dose by RERF, what is the NEW average dose -- in the DS86 system -- for the original group of people?"

The key to obtaining DS86 doses for the full, unaltered T65DR cohorts lies in Tables 10-A and 10-B, where the crucial parts are Columns A and B. These columns show both the mean T65DR and the mean DS86 shielded kerma-doses for the SAME people. That dose-correspondence is the key.

The entries for Column A come directly from TR-12-87, Appendix Table 2, p.42. Neutrons and gammas are shown separately. The entries for Column B are calculated from the entries to their right, which are supplementary information provided by RERF at our request (see Chapter 7 and Tables 26-N and 26-"O" in this book).

Partial versus Full Cohorts :

Table 10-C, which assembles the needed entries from Tables 9-B, 10-A, and 10-B, performs the next step in obtaining DS86 kerma-doses for the FULL, unaltered T65DR cohorts.

Because Tables 10-A and 10-B come from the PARTIAL cohorts, their Columns B (mean shielded kerma-values in the DS86 dosimetry) should not be directly matched with Table 9-B's T65DR kerma values, which come from the FULL cohorts.

Table 10-C uses straight-forward proportion to adjust the DS86 kerma-doses from Tables 10-A and 10-B so that they CAN be properly paired with the

T65DR kerma-doses from Table 9-B for the full cohorts. Note 1 of Table 10-C provides the details.

The operation in Table 10-C incorporates the approximation that the T65DR-DS86 dose-correspondence, shown for 75,991 study-participants in Tables 10-A and 10-B, will be similar for the 15,240 persons who do not yet have any DS86 dose.

This approximation cannot affect our findings in the T65DR dosimetry at all, of course. Moreover, it will be quite surprising if the future DS86 doses, for the 15,240 persons presently without them, are so "out of line" that they can appreciably alter any of the findings in this book with respect to the DS86 dosimetry. Whenever we receive the missing information from Dr. Thiessen at RERF, we can check this assumption. During preparation of this analysis, RERF provided no DS86 data beyond its "subcohort."

DS86 Version
of T65DR Tables 9-B and 9-C :

Table 10-D uses the entries from Table 10-C, Columns F and J, to present the DS86 shielded kerma-doses for the full T65DR cohorts, in the format which is directly comparable to T65DR Table 9-B.

Table 10-E takes the DS86 mean shielded kerma-values from Table 10-D, and converts them into mean internal organ-doses. This is done by using the appropriate DS86 body transmission-factors and the neutron RBE factor of 20. Details are in the Notes of Table 10-E. Table 10-E is the DS86 counterpart of T65DR Table 9-C.

Constant Cohorts with Dual Dosimetry :

With Table 10-E plus Table 9-C (from the previous chapter), we end up with mean internal whole-body doses for the SAME cohorts of people, in both the T65DR and DS86 dosimetries.

Table 10-F demonstrates how we use simple proportions to obtain DS86 doses for all 160 rows of the Master Table 26-A,B,C,D.

====================

Table 10-A

Hiroshima: Correlation of Mean T65DR Doses (Shielded Kerma) with Mean DS86 Doses (Shielded Kerma).

All doses and dose-ranges are in centi-grays; n = neutrons; g = gammas.

OLD AND NEW DOSES IN THE OLD T65DR COHORTS (51,390 PERSONS). | RERF'S PROPOSED REDISTRIBUTION OF THE SAME 51,390 PERSONS INTO NEW COHORTS. (All doses in cGy)

	Persons	Col.A T65DR (cGy)	Col.B DS86 (cGy)	NEW GRP 1 · 0	NEW GRP 2-A · 1-5	NEW GRP 2-B · 6-9	NEW GRP 3-A · 10-19	NEW GRP 3-B · 20-49	NEW GRP 4 · 50-99	NEW GRP 5 · 100-199	NEW GRP 6 · 200-299	NEW GRP 7 · 300-399	NEW GRP 8 · 400+
GROUP 1	25244			20346	4898								
n =		0.0	0.00	0 n	0.0 n								
g =		0.0	0.16	0 g	0.8 g								
GROUP 2-A	8903				7716	1074	113						
n =		0.0	0.00		0.0 n	0.0 n	0.1 n						
g =		2.0	3.23		2.7 g	6.2 g	10.9 g						
GROUP 2-B	1984				130	1631	221	2					
n =		2.0	0.09		0.0 n	0.1 n	0.1 n	0.2 n					
g =		6.0	7.78		4.8 g	7.4 g	12.2 g	19.5 g					
GROUP 3-A	4904				1	671	3668	564					
n =		3.0	0.12		0.1 n	0.1 n	0.1 n	0.3 n					
g =		11.0	13.90		5.0 g	8.2 g	13.5 g	23.3 g					
GROUP 3-B	4684						358	4035	291				
n =		6.0	0.52				0.3 n	0.5 n	1.1 n				
g =		26.0	31.12				17.2 g	30.5 g	56.8 g				
GROUP 4	2670							806	1806	58			
n =		13.0	1.38					1.0 n	1.5 n	2.7 n			
g =		57.0	57.39					41.4 g	63.0 g	104.8 g			
GROUP 5	1642								814	819	9		
n =		30.0	3.23						2.4 n	4.0 n	7.7 n		
g =		109.0	101.75						79.2 g	123.1 g	199.1 g		
GROUP 6	595									475	118	2	
n =		55.0	6.78							6.1 n	9.4 n	14.2 n	
g =		188.0	165.47							151.0 g	221.6 g	290.7 g	
GROUP 7	328									63	214	51	
n =		89.0	11.01							8.1 n	10.8 n	15.5 n	
g =		257.0	230.05							168.7 g	228.6 g	311.9 g	
GROUP 8	436									7	142	114	173
n =		140.0	22.34							8.7 n	13.0 n	18.2 n	33.3 n
g =		383.0	362.86							182.6 g	245.9 g	323.5 g	492.1 g
BOTH TOTALS = 51,390 PERSONS.	51,390			20346	12745	3376	4360	5407	2911	1422	483	167	173

NOTES: The entries in Column A come directly from TR-12-87, Appendix Table 2, p.42. The entries for "n" and "g" in the ten righthand columns were provided to this author by RERF (see Table 26-N of this book). The entries in Column B are calculated from the entries to their right, weighted by the persons directly above those entries.

Table 10-B

Nagasaki: Correlation of Mean T65DR Doses (Shielded Kerma) with Mean DS86 Doses (Shielded Kerma).

All doses and dose-ranges are in centi-grays; n = neutrons; g = gammas.

```
OLD AND NEW DOSES IN THE OLD     | RERF'S PROPOSED REDISTRIBUTION OF THE SAME 24,601 PERSONS INTO NEW COHORTS.
T65DR COHORTS (24,601 PERSONS).  |  NEW    NEW    NEW    NEW    NEW    NEW    NEW    NEW    NEW    NEW
                                 |  GRP    GRP    GRP    GRP    GRP    GRP    GRP    GRP    GRP    GRP
RERF      Col.A  |     Col.B   |   1     2-A    2-B    3-A    3-B     4      5      6      7      8
DOSE-     T65DR  |     DS86    |
GROUPS    (cGy)  |     (cGy)   |   0     1-5    6-9    10-    20-    50-    100-   200-   300-   400+
                                  All doses in cGy        19     49     99     199    299    399

==============================================================================================================

GROUP 1    9431  PERSONS          9431
   n =  0.0 | n =  0.00 |    0 n    |      |      |      |      |      |      |      |      |
   g =  0.0 | g =  0.00 |    0 g    |      |      |      |      |      |      |      |      |

==============================================================================================================

GROUP 2-A  8744  PERSONS          4495   4249
   n =  0.0 | n =  0.00 |    0 n   0.0 n  |      |      |      |      |      |      |      |
   g =  2.0 | g =  0.44 |    0 g   0.9 g  |      |      |      |      |      |      |      |

==============================================================================================================

GROUP 2-B  1069  PERSONS                 1069
   n =  0.0 | n =  0.00 |         0.0 n    |      |      |      |      |      |      |      |
   g =  7.0 | g =  2.50 |         2.5 g    |      |      |      |      |      |      |      |

==============================================================================================================

GROUP 3-A  1702  PERSONS                 1124   506    72
   n =  0.0 | n =  0.00 |         0.0 n  0.0 n  0.0 n  |      |      |      |      |      |
   g = 14.0 | g =  5.33 |         4.3 g  6.8 g 11.1 g  |      |      |      |      |      |

==============================================================================================================

GROUP 3-B  1165  PERSONS                  5      247    676    237
   n =  0.0 | n =  0.02 |         0.0 n  0.0 n  0.0 n  0.1 n  |      |      |      |      |
   g = 31.0 | g = 14.95 |         5.2 g  8.1 g 14.1 g 24.7 g  |      |      |      |      |

==============================================================================================================

GROUP 4     953  PERSONS                               64     805    84
   n =  0.0 | n =  0.20 |                       0.1 n  0.2 n  0.3 n  |      |      |      |
   g = 70.0 | g = 33.35 |                      17.4 g 32.0 g 58.4 g  |      |      |      |

==============================================================================================================

GROUP 5     667  PERSONS                                     109    479    79
   n =  1.0 | n =  0.51 |                              0.3 n  0.5 n  0.9 n  |      |      |
   g =147.0 | g = 70.62 |                             41.9 g 69.5 g117.0 g  |      |      |

==============================================================================================================

GROUP 6     426  PERSONS                                            140    273    13
   n =  3.0 | n =  1.13 |                                     0.9 n  1.2 n  2.2 n  |      |
   g =241.0 | g =115.61 |                                    86.7 g125.7 g215.2 g  |      |

==============================================================================================================

GROUP 7     175  PERSONS                                                   2      134    38     1
   n =  5.0 | n =  2.00 |                                            1.0 n  1.8 n  2.7 n  3.8 n  |
   g =343.0 | g =176.35 |                                           95.5 g157.2 g244.5 g314.0 g  |

==============================================================================================================

GROUP 8     269  PERSONS                                                          38    103    43    85
   n = 10.0 | n =  4.98 |                                                   2.4 n  3.1 n  4.8 n  8.5 n
   g =514.0 | g =337.25 |                                                 168.9 g239.6 g337.9 g530.5 g

==============================================================================================================

BOTH TOTALS = 24,601 PERSONS.    13926  6447   753    812   1151   705    524    154    44     85

==============================================================================================================
```

NOTES: The entries in Column A come directly from TR-12-87, Appendix Table 2, p.42. The entries for "n" and "g" in the ten righthand columns were provided to this author by RERF (see Table 26-"O" of this book). The entries in Column B are calculated from the entries to their right, weighted by the persons directly above those entries.

Table 10–C
T65DR and DS86, Mean Shielded Kerma–Doses: Comparison of Partial and Full Cohorts.
Doses are in cGy (rads); n = neutrons; g = gammas.

Col.A	Col.B	Col.C T65DR KERMA, PARTIAL COHORT	Col.D DS86 KERMA, PARTIAL COHORT	Col.E T65DR KERMA, FULL COHORT	Col.F DS86 KERMA, FULL COHORT	Col.G T65DR KERMA, PARTIAL COHORT	Col.H DS86 KERMA, PARTIAL COHORT	Col.I T65DR KERMA, FULL COHORT	Col.J DS86 KERMA, FULL COHORT
	neutron and gamma								
		========================= HIROSHIMA ==============				============ NAGASAKI ============			
DOSE- GROUP 1	n=	0	0	0	0	0	0	0	0
	g=	0	0.16	0	0.16	0	0	0	0
DOSE- GROUP 2	n=	0.36447	0.01640	0.8	0.048	0	0	0	0
	g=	2.72894	4.05917	2.5	3.719	2.54469	0.66441	2.6	0.679
DOSE- GROUP 3	n=	4.46558	0.31541	4.3	0.304	0	0.00813	0	0.00813
	g=	18.32791	22.31244	17.8	21.670	20.9079	9.23906	21.2	9.368
DOSE- GROUP 4	n=	13	1.38	13.4	1.422	0	0.20	0.2	0.262
	g=	57	57.39	56.9	57.289	70.0	33.35	71.0	33.826
DOSE- GROUP 5	n=	30	3.23	30.3	3.262	1.0	0.51	1.3	0.663
	g=	109	101.75	108.7	101.470	147.0	70.62	145.6	69.947
DOSE- GROUP 6	n=	55	6.78	56.8	7.002	3.0	1.13	3.4	1.281
	g=	188	165.47	186.7	164.326	241.0	115.61	240.3	115.274
DOSE- GROUP 7	n=	89	11.01	92.1	11.393	5.0	2.00	5.4	2.16
	g=	257	230.05	254.3	227.633	343.0	176.35	338.3	173.934
DOSE- GROUP 8	n=	140	22.34	144.1	22.994	10.0	4.98	10.5	5.229
	g=	383	362.86	380.3	360.302	514.0	337.25	518.7	340.334

1. The entries in Cols. C and D come from Table 10-A (Cols. A and B). See Note 2 below.
   The entries in Cols. G and H come from Table 10-B (Cols. A and B). See Note 2 below.
   The entries in Cols. E and I come from Table 9-B.
   The entries in Col. F are calculated: (Col.D) x the ratio (Col.E / Col.C).
      Exception: Group 2 neutrons were related to Dose-Group 3 and calculated as follows:
      (0.01640) + [(0.8 - 0.36447) / (4.46558 - 0.36447)] x (0.31541 - 0.01640).
   The entries in Col. J are calculated: (Col.H) x the ratio (Col.I / Col.G).
      Exception: Group 4 neutrons were related to Dose-Group 5 (because of the zero-entry in
      Col.G) and calculated as follows: (0.2) + (0.2 / 1.0)(0.51 - 0.2).

----

2. The extra digits in Dose-Groups 2 and 3 come from calculating the weighted average values
when combining Dose-Group 2-A with 2-B, and Dose-Group 3-A with 3-B. The digits are maintained
for calculating the DS86 values in Cols. F and J.

----

3. Comparison of Cols.E and F, for Hiroshima gamma kerma, shows that at low doses (far from the
hypocenter), DS86 exceeds T65DR. At higher doses (closer to the hypocenter), the opposite is
true. This cross-over is confirmed in Shi87, Fig.2, p.12.

----

4. Comparison of Cols.I and J, for Nagasaki neutron kerma, shows that at low doses (far from the
hypocenter), DS86 exceeds T65DR. At higher doses (closer to the hypocenter), the opposite is
true. This cross-over is confirmed in Shi87, Fig.2, p.12.

----

5. Irregularities and cross-overs, like the ones described in Notes 3 and 4, account for some
otherwise unexpected T65DR-DS86 dose-correlations in subsequent tables.

Table 10-D
Mean Shielded Kerma–Doses (DS86) in Rads, for the Original Full T65DR Cohorts, With Neutron and Gamma Components.

Row		Col.A Dose- Group 1	Col.B Dose- Group 2	Col.C Dose- Group 3	Col.D Dose- Group 4	Col.E Dose- Group 5	Col.F Dose- Group 6	Col.G Dose- Group 7	Col.H Dose- Group 8
1	HIROSHIMA Persons	27569	15931	10909	2783	1740	659	369	510
2	Mean Dose (n)	0.0	0.048	0.304	1.422	3.262	7.002	11.393	22.994
3	Mean Dose (g)	0.16	3.719	21.67	57.289	101.47	164.326	227.633	360.302
4	Mean Dose (n+g)	0.16	3.77	21.97	58.71	104.73	171.33	239.03	383.30
5	NAGASAKI Persons	9604	12924	4034	1442	1388	722	270	377
6	Mean Dose (n)	0.0	0.0	0.008	0.262	0.663	1.281	2.160	5.229
7	Mean Dose (g)	0.0	0.679	9.368	33.826	69.947	115.274	173.934	340.334
8	Mean Dose (n+g)	0.0	0.679	9.38	34.09	70.61	116.56	176.09	345.56
	BOTH CITIES Persons	37173	28855	14943	4225	3128	1381	639	887
9	Kerma-Dose, calc.	0.12	2.38	18.57	50.31	89.59	142.69	212.44	367.26

NOTES -----   (n) = NEUTRONS   (g) = GAMMA

This table is the DS86 counterpart of Table 9-B.
It provides mean shielded kerma-doses for the SAME cohorts of persons.

----

1. The entries in Rows 1 and 5 for Persons are "cases" from Tables 26-H and 26-I.

----

2. The entries in Rows 2, 3, 6, and 7 for the mean neutron and gamma components are all taken from the DS86 values calculated in Table 10-C, Columns F and J, for the full T65DR cohorts.

----

3. The entries in Row 9 are calculated from the entries in Rows 1, 4, 5, and 8 directly above them.

Table 10-E

Table 10-E
Mean Organ-Doses (DS86) for the Full T65DR Cohorts, with Neutron RBE = 20, in Centi-Sieverts.

Row	DS86, RBE = 20	Col.A Dose-Group 1	Col.B Dose-Group 2	Col.C Dose-Group 3	Col.D Dose-Group 4	Col.E Dose-Group 5	Col.F Dose-Group 6	Col.G Dose-Group 7	Col.H Dose-Group 8	Col.I Ref. Group (1 + 2)
1	HIROSHIMA Persons	27569	15931	10909	2783	1740	659	369	510	43500
2	Organ-Dose (n) RBE=20	0	0.182	1.155	5.404	12.396	26.608	43.293	87.377	
3	Organ-Dose (n,gamma)	0	0.020	0.125	0.583	1.337	2.871	4.671	9.428	
4	Organ-Dose (g)	0.12	2.752	16.036	42.394	75.088	121.601	168.448	266.623	
5	Total Organ-Dose, cSv	0.12	2.95	17.32	48.38	88.82	151.08	216.41	363.43	1.157
6	NAGASAKI Persons	9604	12924	4034	1442	1388	722	270	377	22528
7	Organ-Dose (n) RBE=20	0	0.0	0.030	0.996	2.519	4.868	8.208	19.870	
8	Organ-Dose (n,gamma)	0	0.0	0.003	0.107	0.272	0.525	0.886	2.144	
9	Organ-Dose (g)	0	0.502	6.932	25.031	51.761	85.303	128.711	251.847	
10	Total Organ-Dose, cSv	0.00	0.50	6.97	26.13	54.55	90.70	137.80	273.86	0.288
	BOTH CITIES Persons	37173	28855	14943	4225	3128	1381	639	887	66028
11	Total Organ-Dose, cSv	0.088	1.856	14.522	40.788	73.615	119.510	183.198	325.360	0.861
12	Organ-Dose from Neut.	0.000	0.101	0.852	3.899	8.013	15.242	28.469	58.685	0.044
13	Organ-Dose from Gamma	0.088	1.755	13.670	36.889	65.602	104.269	154.730	266.675	0.817
14	Neutron cSv / Total cSv	0.000	0.054	0.059	0.096	0.109	0.128	0.155	0.180	0.051

NOTES FOR DS86, neutron RBE = 20 -----   (n) = NEUTRONS   (g) = GAMMA

This table is the DS86 counterpart of Table 9-C.
It provides mean internal organ-doses for the SAME cohorts of persons as Table 9-C.

----

1. The entries in Rows 2 and 7 for the neutron-component are the corresponding neutron entries in Table 10-D times 3.8 (which is 20 times the conversion factor of 0.19 from Table 9-A, Row 3). The extra factor of twenty is necessary because calculations are for neutron RBE = 20. Note that the body transmission-factors are not the same for the T65DR and DS86 dosimetries.

----

2. The entries in Rows 3 and 8 are the entries for neutrons from Table 10-D times the conversion factor of 0.41 (from Table 9-A, Col.E). Note that the factor for DS86 is nearly 6-fold higher than for T65DR. No RBE factor of 20 is used because, after the n,gamma reaction has occurred, the dose is delivered by GAMMA radiation.

----

3. The entries in Rows 4 and 9 for the direct gamma component are the corresponding gamma entries in Table 10-D times the conversion factor of 0.74 (from Table 9-A, Row 3). Note that the transmission-factor is appreciably higher for DS86 than for T65DR.

----

4. The entries in Row 11, for mean organ-dose in the combined cities, are calculated for each column by the formula [(Row 1 times Row 5) + (Row 6 times Row 10)] / (Row 1 + Row 6).
   The entries in Row 12 are [(Row 1 times Row 2) + (Row 6 times Row 7)] / (Row 1 + Row 6).
   The entries in Row 13 are obtained by subtracting Row 12 from Row 11.
   The entries in Row 14 are, of course, Row 12 / Row 11.

----

5. Doses in Row 11 will undergo slight adjustment in the course of the age-and-sex normalization process of Chapter 11.

Table 10-F
Correlations Needed To Calculate Kerma–Doses and Organ–Doses in DS–86 Dosimetry, for the 160 Rows of the Master Table 26–A,B,C,D.

Row	FULL COHORTS Kerma doses in rads (cGy) Organ-doses in rems (cSv)	Col.A Dose-Group 1	Col.B Dose-Group 2	Col.C Dose-Group 3	Col.D Dose-Group 4	Col.E Dose-Group 5	Col.F Dose-Group 6	Col.G Dose-Group 7	Col.H Dose-Group 8
1	HIROSHIMA Persons	27569	15931	10909	2783	1740	659	369	510
2	T65DR Shielded Kerma Mean Dose	0.00	3.30	22.10	70.30	139.00	243.50	346.40	524.40
3	DS86 Shielded Kerma Mean Dose	0.16	3.77	21.97	58.71	104.73	171.33	239.03	383.30
4	DS86 Mean Internal Organ-Dose (Neutron RBE = 20.)	0.12	2.95	17.32	48.38	88.82	151.08	216.41	363.43
5	NAGASAKI Persons	9604	12924	4034	1442	1388	722	270	377
6	T65DR Shielded Kerma Mean Dose	0.00	2.60	21.20	71.20	146.90	243.70	343.70	529.20
7	DS86 Shielded Kerma Mean Dose	0.00	0.68	9.38	34.09	70.61	116.56	176.09	345.56
8	DS86 Mean Internal Organ-Dose (Neutron RBE = 20.)	0.00	0.50	6.97	26.13	54.55	90.70	137.80	273.86
9	BOTH CITIES Persons	37173	28855	14943	4225	3128	1381	639	887

Persons are provided here as a possible convenience; they are not involved in the calculations below.

    Entries for Rows 2 and 6 come from Table 9-B, Rows 4 and 8.
    Entries for Rows 3 and 7 come from Table 10-D, Rows 4 and 8.
    Entries for Rows 4 and 8 come from Table 10-E, Rows 5 and 10.

HOW ENTRIES FOR TABLE 26-A,B,C,D, Columns I (Eye) and J, WERE OBTAINED FOR ADDITIONAL DS86 KERMA DOSES:

In the illustration below, we shall consider only Dose-Group 4 in Hiroshima. In Row 2, above, we see that the T65DR mean kerma-dose is 70.30 rads, and that it corresponds with a DS86 mean kerma-dose of 58.71 rads (Row 3). These are the average values derived from all 2,783 Hiroshima survivors in this Dose-Group -- all ages and both sexes.

Now, if we go to Master Table 26-A, for Hiroshima Males, we will calculate the DS86 doses for the males who were age 27 years ATB (Column C) and who are in Dose-Group 4 (Column E).

We find that their true T65DR mean kerma-dose is 68.0 rads, which is lower than the 70.30 rads above in Row 2. Therefore, we know that the corresponding DS86 mean kerma-dose will also be lower than the 58.71 rads above in Row 3. So we multiply 58.71 rads by the factor (68.0 rads / 70.30 rads), and we enter 56.79 rads in Column I (Eye) as the true DS86 kerma-dose.

To obtain the corresponding internal organ-dose, we start again with the anchor in Table 10-F above. We see in Row 3 that, in Dose-Group 4, the DS86 mean kerma-dose is 58.71 rads, and that it corresponds with a DS86 mean internal organ-dose in Row 4 of 48.38 rems.

However, for the males who were age 27 years ATB, we determined above that the DS86 mean kerma-dose is 56.79 rads, which is lower than 58.71 rads. Therefore, we multiply 48.38 rems by the factor (56.79 rads / 58.71 rads), and we enter 46.80 rems in Column J as the DS86 internal organ-dose.

In the same steps, values were determined for all the rows of Columns I and J in Master Table 26-A,B,C,D.

Achievement of Age– and Sex–Matching across RERF's Eight Dose-Groups

The Importance of Matching :

When analysts approach the A-Bomb Survivor database for the purpose of learning how cancer-risk varies with radiation-dose, they need reasonable assurance that persons in each of RERF'S Dose-Groups are alike in their cancer-risk -- except for radiation dose. In other words, analysts need a sound basis for thinking that the SPONTANEOUS cancer-rates would be the same in all eight RERF Dose-Groups in the ABSENCE of any radiation exposure from the bomb.

Age and sex are features having a profound influence on spontaneous cancer-rates. Age and sex can also affect spontaneous cancer-rates indirectly, by affecting rates at which the NON-cancer causes of death compete with cancer.

Therefore, we must ask, "Are the Dose-Groups in the A-Bomb Study alike in the age and sex of their members?"

A Possible Misinterpretation :

Analysts must avoid misinterpreting RERF allusions to "comparability" of age and sex between heavily and lightly irradiated survivors (Bee71, p.615), and to "sex- and age-matched" samples in the A-Bomb Study (Pr87a, p.153). Given the history of the study (Chapter 5), it is understandable that there are important differences across the eight RERF Dose-Groups in both age-distribution at the time of bombing (ATB) and in male-female ratios.

These differences mean that it would be FALSE to assume that the observed cancer-rates in the eight Dose-Groups incorporate comparable spontaneous rates, and therefore it would be FALSE to assume that the differences in observed cancer-rates are exclusively due to radiation.

Unfortunately, the dissimilar distributions of age and sex in RERF's eight Dose-Groups may not be evident, to outside analysts, from RERF reports. As noted in Chapter 7, RERF was very cooperative about supplying the necessary data, and those data are incorporated into our Master Table 26-A,B,C,D and all the tables derived therefrom.

Illustration of the Need for Matching :

============================

We will use some entries in Table 11-B to illustrate that problems would arise from using the RAW data, unmatched for age and sex. (Table 11-B comes from Master Table 26-A,B for males; column-headings are more fully described there.)

In Table 11-B, Column C identifies the RERF Dose-Group. Columns A and B show that every Dose-Group is composed of persons in five age-bands, according to age at the time of bombing (ATB); the age-bands are described in Table 11-A. For brevity, the RERF diskette named each age-band by the midpoint of its age-range (Column A).

In Table 11-B, Column F tells the number of persons initially in each age-band when the follow-up began in 1950, and the total initial persons in each Dose-Group. The number of persons in an age-band over the total persons in its Dose-Group is the fraction entered in Column G. For instance, the entry G17 is entry F17 divided by entry F23.

Now, if we compare the fractions in G17-G21 with the fractions in G41-G45, we see that the age-distribution in the male Reference Group (Dose-Groups 1+2) is quite different from the age-distribution in Dose-Group 5. This means that at the end of the 1982 follow-up, these two groups of persons are bound to have different cancer-rates per 10,000 initial persons, even if BOTH groups were unexposed by the bombing, simply because their age-distributions differ. In other words, the cancer-risk of these two groups is NOT alike, except for radiation dose.

When we turn to Table 11-D and make the same comparison for the females (entries G17-G21 versus G41-G45), we find that their distribution of ages is also NOT alike across Dose-Groups. Nor is it like the male distribution.

The problem is compounded when we discover that the male-female ratio is not the same across Dose-Groups either. For instance, in the Reference Group, the ratio is (27585 males / 38443 females), or 0.7176, whereas in Dose-Group 5, the ratio is (1386 males / 1742 females), or 0.7956.

Conclusion about the Need :

Dissimilarities like this pervade the database. Therefore we can be certain that the eight RERF Dose-Groups do NOT share the same spontaneous cancer death-rate, and that the eight groups would show different cancer death-rates during the follow-up even if no group had been exposed to bomb radiation at all. Therefore, it is imperative for every analyst to develop some method to overcome these confounding variables. Otherwise, it would be impossible to distinguish the age and sex effect on cancer death-rate from the radiation effect.

Our Method
of Matching for Age and Sex :
============================

Combination of Dose-Groups :

Like many other analysts, we combine Dose-Groups 1+2 to make the Reference Group. The reasons were discussed earlier: Realism about hidden doses from residual radioactivity, and achievement of a statistically more reliable control group (see Chapters 8 and 9).

We make another combination of Dose-Groups at the outset: Dose-Groups 6+7+8. If readers look again at Table 4-A, Column F, they will see that very few persons are in the three highest Dose-Groups. Death from acute radiation sickness probably accounts for the sparsity. It should be remembered that the Lifespan Study, of potential delayed radiation effects, did not begin until 1950 -- after the acute effects from radiation had already occurred.

By combining Dose-Groups 6+7+8, we achieve a Dose-Group almost comparable to Dose-Group 5 in size and statistical reliability, and we reduce the hazard of attributing biological meaning to the random fluctuations of small numbers.

Guiding Principles :

Our method of matching the Dose-Groups for age and sex distribution follows two principles.

(1) We want to achieve a database in which all Dose-Groups enter the lifespan follow-up in 1950 as directly comparable cohorts, alike in both age-distribution and sex-distribution. In other words, all Dose-Groups must be alike in the fraction of their total initial persons who are males age-5-ATB, alike in the fraction of their total initial persons who are females age-5-ATB, alike in the fraction of their total initial persons who are males age-15-ATB, females age-15-ATB, and so forth.

(2) We want to stay as close to the original raw

numbers as possible.

The result is achieved by taking care of the age-normalization first, and then the sex-normalization. The notes of Tables 11-A through 11-H explain the logic and process step by step.

Net Result
of Proper Matching :
==========================

Table 11-H presents the data after both age and sex matching have been achieved, and male and female observations have been combined.

Spontaneous cancer-rates, in-so-far as they are affected by age-distribution and sex-ratio, have been rendered identical from Dose-Group to Dose-Group by the normalization process. Moreover, age- or sex-related sensitivity to induction of cancer by radiation itself will not differ across Dose-Groups, because age-distribution and sex-ratio across Dose-Groups have been rendered the same.

The cancer death-rates labeled "observed" in this book are the values from Table 11-H.

Comparison of
Raw and Normalized Observations :

Comparison of the raw and normalized observations is readily made by a comparison of data from Table 4-A with those of Table 11-H. The number of initial persons in each dose-group is the same in both tables. The doses remain very nearly the same. The comparison is made in the tabulation which follows.

Dose-Group	Initial Persons	Observed Cancer Deaths (Raw)	Observed Cancer Deaths Normalized	Change in Ca-Deaths	Percent Change
Ref 1+2	66,028	4,155	4,297.1	+142.1	+ 3.42%
Exposed	25,203	1,895	1,918.7	+ 23.7	+ 1.25%
SUM	91,231	6,050	6,215.8		
1+2	66,028	4,155	4,297.1	+142.1	+ 3.42%
3	14,943	1,055	1,064.0	+ 9.0	+ 0.85%
4	4,225	314	305.8	- 8.2	- 2.55%
5	3,128	253	261.6	+ 8.6	+ 3.40%
6-8	2,907	273	287.3	+14.3	+ 5.25%
SUM	91,231	6,050	6,215.8		

===

Preventing Overestimation
of Radiation-Risk at Low Doses :

The two top rows in the tabulation show that the normalized data have resulted in a larger percentage increase in cancer-deaths in the Reference Group (1+2) than in the exposed groups. Since mean doses are virtually unaffected by normalization, this means that there will be a smaller increment in cancer-deaths per centi-sievert (rem) among exposed persons in the normalized database than in the raw database.

We have also made the comparison of raw and normalized data for the exposed groups separately, in the tabulation.

For Dose-Group 3 (the lowest exposure), normalization has resulted in a far smaller percentage increase in cancer-deaths than in the Reference Group. The net effect will be to lessen the radiation-induction of cancer per rem for that comparison. Chapter 13, Part 3, will show this in detail.

Similarly, for Dose-Groups 4 and 5, the effect of normalization will be to lessen the radiation-induction of cancer or to leave it unchanged. For the very high-dose group of exposed (6+7+8), normalization will produce an increase in radiation-induction of cancer per rem.

Overall, the effects of matching for age and sex are (A) a decrease in risk-estimates for low-dose exposure, and (B) a decrease in the supra-linear curvature of the dose-response relationship.

The Missing Data from RERF :

It should be noted that the ability to do age-sex matching in this manner depended on the cooperation of RERF in supplying the data on initial persons -- data now provided to additional analysts by the tables in this book.

While I was still without the extra data from RERF, I used the "raw" database to make some interim estimates of risk (Go88c; Go89a). Where space permitted (Go88c), I warned readers that the missing data might either raise or lower the interim values. Those interim values are now superseded and replaced by the values in this book, which are based upon the data which I sought.

After receiving the data from RERF, I developed more than one method for using them to make age and sex adjustments, and the methods produce closely similar results.

Results from a method which is not shown in this book assured me that it would be unnecessary to do additional matching for the age-variation across the various Dose-Groups WITHIN each separate age-band. It turns out that such adjustments -- which would alter cancer-observations by small fractions of one case -- are too small to matter and can be neglected. However, a responsible analyst does not leave the issue in doubt. The doubt necessarily persisted in my own mind, until RERF supplied the data I requested, which included the TRUE mean ages ATB instead of the midpoints of the age-ranges. In Table 11-B, for instance, a comparison of entries B17, B25, B33, B41, and B49, shows that the true mean age of males age 5 ATB varies across Dose-Groups from 3.92 years old to 4.64 years old. Readers can see the variation within other age-bands too.

Correction-Factor of 1.23
for Underascertainment of Cancer

===

Recent RERF reports (Pr87b, p.35; and Shi88, p.41, pp.49-50) as well as the BEIR-3 Report (Beir80) indicate that, in the Japanese experience, cancer-deaths are underestimated. They use the estimate that measured cancer-deaths in any dose-group -- including Dose-Group 1, of course -- should be multiplied by 1.23. BEIR-3, referring to its own risk-estimates for cancer, says:

"Finally, the mortality coefficients were expanded by a factor of 1.23 (derived from comparison of autopsy and death-certificate diagnoses) to adjust for incomplete death-certificate ascertainment of cancer" (Beir80, p.196 at the bottom). BEIR-3 cites the RERF study of this issue, by Steer and co-workers (Steer73).

We, too, have applied the underascertainment factor of 1.23 in this book. Readers will see where we have handled it, in each of our analyses.

Site-Specific Errors :

Earlier in its report, BEIR-3 states: "Death-certificate diagnoses differ greatly in their accuracy, even within the set of neoplastic diseases; but for the A-bomb survivors, an active autopsy program in the period 1961-1969 has provided unusually good information on errors in death-certificate diagnoses" (Beir80, p.154).

● -- Lung-Cancer : "Autopsy studies have also confirmed that in the study population [the A-bomb survivors] lung cancer is misdiagnosed on death certificates in over half the cases, with over 1/3 of cases

===

not even coded as cancer" (Beir80, p.239; see also pp. 313-314).

● -- Esophageal-Cancer : "... esophageal cancer has a 70 % detection rate by death certificate and 70 % of such death certificate diagnoses are confirmed by autopsy in the experience of the ABCC..." (Beir80, p.360).

● -- Pancreatic-Cancer : "... cancer of the pancreas is often poorly diagnosed on death certificates in Japan, and death certificates are commonly completed before autopsy findings become known" (Beir80, p.386).

● -- Urinary Organs : "... the death certificate has a very low detection rate for cancers of urinary organs in the Japanese experience" (Beir80, p.402-403).

Site-Specific Risk-Analysis :

It should be noted that underascertainment of cancer as the cause of death is not the same issue as misdiagnosis of the original site of a fatal cancer. Error about original site matters only if an analysis is attempting to determine cancer-risk or dose-response for a single site of cancer (say, lung-cancer) or a group of cancers (say, respiratory cancers).

Whenever overall risk of fatal cancer is the information sought by an analysis, subdivision of the cancers by site can be and should be avoided (see Chapter 12). This book contains no site-specific analysis.

Table 11-A

Notes for Tables 11-B,C,D,E : Age-Normalization of Observations across Dose-Groups.

1. SOURCE OF THE DATA: In Table 11-B for males, all the data in Columns A through N (other than Col.G) come from Master Tables 26-A for Hiroshima and 26-B for Nagasaki. The Master Tables have been re-arranged by Dose-Group. Within a Dose-Group, the dose received by a particular age-band was not the same in the two cities. In combining the cities to make Table 11-B, we weighted each dose by the number of persons who received it. We have combined the observations for Dose-Groups 6+7+8 to lessen the instability of small numbers (see text). We have combined Dose-Groups 1+2 for use as our Reference Group (see text), and also preserved them separately for other purposes. In Table 11-D, female entries come in similar fashion from Master Tables 26-C and 26-D. (In all tables, "per 10K init" means "per 10,000 initial persons" in the row.)

==

2. OVERVIEW: We are going to convert Table 11-B into Table 11-C (and Table 11-D into Table 11-E). The purpose of this conversion or normalization is to insure that we will examine groups of people who are truly comparable with respect to their cancer-risk, except for their different radiation doses. To be comparable, RERF's eight Dose-Groups must start the lifespan follow-up with the same distribution of ages in each Dose-Group.

We will use the fractions in the raw female Reference Group as the standard to which all other Dose-Groups, both male and female, will conform with respect to age-distribution within a Dose-Group. Those fractions have been calculated in Table 11-D, Col.G, Rows 17-21. The denominator for each calculation was 38,443 persons -- the total number in the Dose-Group. For instance, the fraction entered in Col.G, Row 21, is (6007 / 38443), or 0.156.

==

THE TWO-STEP CONVERSION-PROCESS : For brevity, these notes will describe only the conversion of Table 11-B into 11-C (males). Exactly the same simple process converts Table 11-D into Table 11-E (females).

==

STEP 1 :
======== In each Dose-Group, we are going to keep the total number of initial persons the same as in the raw data. Above, we specified that in each age-normalized Dose-Group, fractions of total persons from each age-band will be like the Female Reference Group:

0.180 from the age-band 5 years ATB (0 through 9 years old ATB);   from Table 11-D, entry G17.
0.193 from the age-band 15 years ATB (10 through 19 years old ATB); from Table 11-D, entry G18.
0.241 from the age-band 27 years ATB (20 through 34 years old ATB); from Table 11-D, entry G19.
0.230 from the age-band 42 years ATB (35 through 49 years old ATB); from Table 11-D, entry G20.
0.156 from the age-band 60 years ATB (50 years and older ATB);   from Table 11-D, entry G21.

In Table 11-C, we fill Col.G with these fractions, and then calculate appropriate new entries for Col.F.

EXAMPLE USING MALE DOSE-GROUP 1 : To obtain entry F60 for Table 11-C, we calculate the number which is 0.156 times the total 15,406 male persons initially in Dose-Group 1, and enter 2407.30 initial persons. (Note: our calculations were done with fractions having many more than three decimal places; calculations done without the extra digits will not match the entries exactly. The entry 2407.30 comes from multiplying 15,406 initial persons by the fraction 0.156257316.) Step 1 completes such calculations for Table 11-C, Column F.

==

STEP 2 :
======== The observations in Table 11-B, Cols. H through N, must be adjusted up or down accordingly. The conversion is simply the ratio of (new number of persons / old number of persons) times (old observation).

EXAMPLE USING MALE DOSE-GROUP 1, OBSERVED CANCER-DEATHS :
  The new number of initial persons = 2407.30 persons (from Table 11-C, entry F60).
  The old number of initial persons = 2946 persons (from Table 11-B, entry F5).
  The old number of cancer-deaths = 447 cancer deaths (from Table 11-B, entry N5).
  The new number of cancer-deaths = (2407.30 persons / 2946 persons) x (447 cancer-deaths) = 365.26 cancer-deaths.
Thus, 365.26 cancer-deaths is the age-normalized entry N60 for Table 11-C.

In that fashion, all the age-normalized entries for Columns H through N were calculated for Table 11-C. Thereafter, all the rates in Columns P through T were newly calculated. For each age-band within a Dose-Group, the observed rates still match the corresponding entries in Table 11-B, and are undistorted by the normalization. The appropriate effect of age-normalization is seen only in a Dose-Group's summary row. In Table 11-C (Rows 62,70,78,86,94,102,110), doses have also been adjusted accordingly. In Table 11-E (females), Row 78 shows no dose change because this group is the standard.

Table 11-B
Raw Data for Males, by Dose-Groups : Hiroshima + Nagasaki Combined, 1950–1982.

	A	B	C	D	E	F	G	H	I	J	K	L	M	N		P	Q	R		T
				RBE=2	RBE=20		INIT.									CANC	CANC	ALL	ALL DEATH	
		MALE		T65DR	DS86		PERS				ALL			ALL CANC		DEATHS	DEATHS	DEATH	MINUS	PYR
	DISK	TRUE	RERF	ORGAN	ORGAN	MALES	OVER	PERS.			NEO-	ALL		EXCEPT		/10K	PER	/10K	ALL	PER
Row	AGE	AGE	DOSE-	DOSE	DOSE	INITIAL	TOTAL	YEARS	ALL	ALL	PLASM	MALIG	LEUK	LEUK		INIT.	10K	INIT.	MALIG	INIT.
No.	ATB	ATB	GRP	(rems)	(rems)	PERS.	PERS.	(PYR)	CAUSE	DISEASE						PERSONS	PYR	PERS.	/ 10K INIT.	PERS.
1	5	4.13	1	0.000	0.082	3787	0.246	119484	178	107	15	14	4	10		26.41	0.84	470	433	31.55
2	15	13.99	1	0.000	0.084	3290	0.214	100188	392	263	57	53	4	49		148.94	4.89	1191	1030	30.45
3	27	28.20	1	0.000	0.092	1860	0.121	53743	512	470	148	140	7	133		715.05	24.75	2753	2000	28.89
4	42	42.57	1	0.000	0.092	3523	0.229	82845	2295	2169	606	581	15	566		1606.59	68.32	6514	4865	23.52
5	60	58.18	1	0.000	0.091	2946	0.191	38168	2869	2774	471	450	3	447		1517.31	117.11	9739	8211	12.96
6																				
7	MALE, RAW		1	0.000	0.088	15406	1.000	394429	6246	5783	1297	1238	33	1205		782.16	30.55	4054	3251	25.60
9	5	4.21	2	1.449	1.595	3031	0.249	95555	152	89	19	17	2	15		49.49	1.57	501	445	31.53
10	15	13.91	2	1.707	2.195	3088	0.254	94585	356	272	73	68	4	64		207.25	6.77	1153	933	30.63
11	27	27.83	2	1.533	2.149	1433	0.118	41127	372	338	97	94	3	91		635.03	22.13	2596	1940	28.70
12	42	42.67	2	1.572	2.160	2476	0.203	57506	1672	1582	424	402	5	397		1603.39	69.04	6753	5129	23.23
13	60	58.10	2	1.502	2.006	2151	0.177	27959	2088	2021	320	304	4	300		1394.70	107.30	9707	8294	13.00
14																				
15	MALE, RAW		2	1.559	2.000	12179	1.000	316732	4640	4302	933	885	18	867		711.88	27.37	3810	3083	26.01
17	5	4.16	1+2	0.644	0.755	6818	0.247	215039	330	196	34	31	6	25		36.67	1.16	484	439	31.54
18	15	13.95	1+2	0.827	1.106	6378	0.231	194773	748	535	130	121	8	113		177.17	5.80	1173	983	30.54
19	27	28.04	1+2	0.667	0.987	3293	0.119	94870	884	808	245	234	10	224		680.23	23.61	2684	1974	28.81
20	42	42.61	1+2	0.649	0.945	5999	0.217	140351	3967	3751	1030	983	20	963		1605.27	68.61	6613	4974	23.40
21	60	58.14	1+2	0.634	0.899	5097	0.185	66127	4957	4795	791	754	7	747		1465.57	112.96	9725	8246	12.97
22																				
23	MALE, RAW		1+2	0.688	0.932	27585	1.000	711161	10886	10085	2230	2123	51	2072		751.13	29.14	3946	3177	25.78
25	5	4.10	3	10.491	13.323	1547	0.263	48977	64	36	5	3	2	1		6.46	0.20	414	394	31.66
26	15	14.09	3	11.111	13.918	1112	0.189	34398	106	86	27	25	6	19		170.86	5.52	953	728	30.93
27	27	28.21	3	11.568	15.341	703	0.119	20191	199	178	57	56	2	54		768.14	26.74	2831	2034	28.72
28	42	42.73	3	11.470	15.466	1381	0.235	32453	898	849	255	247	7	240		1737.87	73.95	6503	4714	23.50
29	60	58.16	3	11.055	14.809	1145	0.194	15625	1106	1085	166	160	5	155		1353.71	99.20	9659	8262	13.65
30																				
31	MALE, RAW		3	11.076	14.468	5888	1.000	151644	2373	2234	510	491	22	469		796.54	30.93	4030	3196	25.75
33	5	3.92	4	34.784	39.792	359	0.213	11247	16	8	0	0	0	0		0.00	0.00	446	446	31.33
34	15	14.55	4	35.238	36.527	342	0.203	10540	38	29	10	10	1	9		263.16	8.54	1111	819	30.82
35	27	27.30	4	35.539	38.013	237	0.141	6869	63	59	13	12	1	11		464.14	16.01	2658	2152	28.98
36	42	42.49	4	35.665	40.562	438	0.260	10251	288	278	85	84	2	82		1872.15	79.99	6575	4658	23.40
37	60	57.14	4	35.662	42.639	308	0.183	4633	293	287	53	51	0	51		1655.84	110.09	9513	7857	15.04
38																				
39	MALE, RAW		4	35.372	39.600	1684	1.000	43540	698	661	161	157	4	153		908.55	35.14	4145	3213	25.86
41	5	4.64	5	71.647	72.789	189	0.136	5966	8	6	5	4	2	2		105.82	3.35	423	212	31.56
42	15	15.20	5	71.796	67.754	371	0.268	11368	40	33	7	6	1	5		134.77	4.40	1078	916	30.64
43	27	27.79	5	71.154	70.735	224	0.162	6307	72	66	28	25	3	22		982.14	34.88	3214	2098	28.15
44	42	42.26	5	69.453	74.855	368	0.266	8805	233	224	73	73	1	72		1956.52	81.77	6332	4348	23.93
45	60	56.48	5	72.237	81.509	234	0.169	3061	228	219	43	41	1	40		1709.40	130.67	9744	7991	13.08
46																				
47	MALE, RAW		5	71.124	73.130	1386	1.000	35507	581	548	156	149	8	141		1017.32	39.71	4192	3117	25.62
49	5	3.98	6-8	171.56	185.85	212	0.164	6393	27	21	16	15	9	6		283.02	9.38	1274	566	30.16
50	15	15.29	6-8	182.90	201.84	363	0.281	10947	54	47	21	20	3	17		468.32	15.53	1488	937	30.16
51	27	27.96	6-8	171.10	184.68	232	0.179	6752	64	60	27	27	5	22		948.28	32.58	2759	1595	29.10
52	42	42.31	6-8	183.50	205.62	314	0.243	6822	231	226	76	74	10	64		2038.22	93.81	7357	5000	21.73
53	60	56.17	6-8	188.68	221.49	173	0.134	2446	167	164	31	30	4	26		1502.89	106.29	9653	7919	14.14
54																				
55	MALE, RAW		6-8	179.84	199.69	1294	1.000	33360	543	518	171	166	31	135		1043.28	40.47	4196	2913	25.78

[--Various Causes of Death--]

Abbreviations: PERS. = PERSON(S) ; PYR = PERSON-YEARS ; MALIG = MALIGNANCIES ; LEUK = LEUKEMIA ; CANC = CANCER;
INIT. = INITIAL ; /10K = per 10,000 .

Table 11–C
Age–Normalized Data for Males, by Dose–Groups : Hiroshima + Nagasaki Combined, 1950–1982.

ROW NO.	A DIS AG AT	B MALE TRUE AGE ATB	C RERF DOSE-GRP	D RBE=2 T65DR ORGAN DOSE (rems)	E RBE=20 DS86 ORGAN DOSE (rems)	F MALES INIT. PERS.	G INIT. PERS OVER TOTAL PERS	H PERS. YEARS (PYR)	I ALL CAUSE	J ALL DIS-EASE	K ALL NEO-PLASM	L ALL MALIG	M LEUK	N ALL CANC EXCEPT LEUK	P CANC DEATHS /10K INIT. PERSONS	Q CANC DEATHS PER 10K PYR	R ALL DEATH /10K INIT. PERS.	All Death - ALL MALIG /10K INIT.	T PYR PER INIT. PERS
56	5	4.13	1	0.000	0.082	2779.20	0.180	87687	131	79	11	10	3	7.34	26.41	0.84	470	433	31.55
57	15	13.99	1	0.000	0.084	2966.75	0.193	90344	353	237	51	48	4	44.19	148.94	4.89	1191	1030	30.45
58	27	28.20	1	0.000	0.092	3710.94	0.241	107225	1022	938	295	279	14	265.35	715.05	24.75	2753	2000	28.89
59	42	42.57	1	0.000	0.092	3541.82	0.230	83287	2307	2181	609	584	15	569.02	1606.59	68.32	6514	4865	23.52
60	60	58.18	1	0.000	0.091	2407.30	0.156	31189	2344	2267	385	368	2	365.26	1517.31	117.11	9739	8211	12.96
61																			
62	MALE, NORM		1	0.000	0.089	15406.00	1.000	399732	6157	5701	1352	1289	38	1251.16	812.13	31.30	3997	3160	25.95
64	5	4.21	2	1.449	1.595	2197.05	0.180	69264	110	65	14	12	1	10.87	49.49	1.57	501	445	31.53
65	15	13.91	2	1.707	2.195	2345.32	0.193	71837	270	207	55	52	3	48.61	207.25	6.77	1153	933	30.63
66	27	27.83	2	1.533	2.149	2933.63	0.241	84195	762	692	199	192	6	186.29	635.03	22.13	2596	1940	28.70
67	42	42.67	2	1.572	2.160	2799.94	0.230	65029	1891	1789	479	455	6	448.94	1603.39	69.04	6753	5129	23.23
68	60	58.10	2	1.502	2.006	1903.06	0.156	24736	1847	1788	283	269	4	265.42	1394.70	107.30	9707	8294	13.00
69																			
70	MALE, NORM		2	1.556	2.038	12179.00	1.000	315062	4880	4540	1030	980	20	960.13	788.35	30.47	4007	3202	25.87
72	5	4.16	1+2	0.644	0.755	4976.25	0.180	156951	241	143	25	23	4	18.25	36.67	1.16	484	439	31.54
73	15	13.95	1+2	0.827	1.106	5312.07	0.193	162221	623	446	108	101	7	94.11	177.17	5.80	1173	983	30.54
74	27	28.04	1+2	0.667	0.987	6644.57	0.241	191428	1784	1630	494	472	20	451.98	680.23	23.61	2684	1974	28.81
75	42	42.61	1+2	0.649	0.945	6341.76	0.230	148370	4194	3965	1089	1039	21	1018.02	1605.27	68.61	6613	4974	23.40
76	60	58.14	1+2	0.634	0.899	4310.36	0.156	55922	4192	4055	669	638	6	631.71	1465.57	112.96	9725	8246	12.97
77																			
78	MALE, NORM		1+2	0.684	0.945	27585.00	1.000	714891	11033	10239	2385	2272	58	2214.08	802.64	30.97	4000	3176	25.92
80	5	4.10	3	10.491	13.323	1062.18	0.180	33628	44	25	3	2	1	0.69	6.46	0.20	414	394	31.66
81	15	14.09	3	11.111	13.918	1133.86	0.193	35075	108	88	28	25	6	19.37	170.86	5.52	953	728	30.93
82	27	28.21	3	11.568	15.341	1418.28	0.241	40734	401	359	115	113	4	108.94	768.14	26.74	2831	2034	28.72
83	42	42.73	3	11.470	15.466	1353.64	0.230	31810	880	832	250	242	7	235.25	1737.87	73.95	6503	4714	23.50
84	60	58.16	3	11.055	14.809	920.04	0.156	12555	889	872	133	129	4	124.55	1353.71	99.20	9659	8262	13.65
85																			
86	MALE, NORM		3	11.183	14.648	5888.00	1.000	153802	2322	2176	529	511	22	488.80	830.16	31.78	3944	3076	26.12
88	5	3.92	4	34.784	39.792	303.79	0.180	9517	14	7	0	0	0	0.00	0.00	0.00	446	446	31.33
89	15	14.55	4	35.238	36.527	324.29	0.193	9995	36	27	9	9	1	8.53	263.16	8.54	1111	819	30.82
90	27	27.30	4	35.539	38.013	405.64	0.241	11756	108	101	22	21	2	18.83	464.14	16.01	2658	2152	28.98
91	42	42.49	4	35.665	40.562	387.15	0.230	9061	255	246	75	74	2	72.48	1872.15	79.99	6575	4658	23.40
92	60	57.14	4	35.662	42.639	263.14	0.156	3958	250	245	45	44	0	43.57	1655.84	110.09	9513	7857	15.04
93																			
94	MALE, NORM		4	35.393	39.357	1684.00	1.000	44287	662	626	152	148	4	143.41	851.62	32.38	3933	3055	26.30
96	5	4.64	5	71.647	72.789	250.03	0.180	7892	11	8	7	5	3	2.65	105.82	3.35	423	212	31.56
97	15	15.20	5	71.796	67.754	266.90	0.193	8178	29	24	5	4	1	3.60	134.77	4.40	1078	916	30.64
98	27	27.79	5	71.154	70.735	333.85	0.241	9400	107	98	42	37	4	32.79	982.14	34.88	3214	2098	28.15
99	42	42.26	5	69.453	74.855	318.64	0.230	7624	202	194	63	63	1	62.34	1956.52	81.77	6332	4348	23.93
100	60	56.48	5	72.237	81.509	216.57	0.156	2833	211	203	40	38	1	37.02	1709.40	130.67	9744	7991	13.08
101																			
102	MALE, NORM		5	71.145	73.162	1386.00	1.000	35927	559	527	156	148	10	138.40	998.53	38.52	4036	2968	25.92
104	5	3.98	6-8	171.56	185.85	233.43	0.180	7040	30	23	18	17	10	6.61	283.02	9.38	1274	566	30.16
105	15	15.29	6-8	182.90	201.84	249.19	0.193	7515	37	32	14	14	2	11.67	468.32	15.53	1488	937	30.16
106	27	27.96	6-8	171.10	184.68	311.69	0.241	9071	86	81	36	36	7	29.56	948.28	32.58	2759	1595	29.10
107	42	42.31	6-8	183.50	205.62	297.49	0.230	6463	219	214	72	70	9	60.63	2038.22	93.81	7357	5000	21.73
108	60	56.17	6-8	188.68	221.49	202.20	0.156	2859	195	192	36	35	5	30.39	1502.89	106.29	9653	7919	14.14
109																			
110	MALE, NORM		6-8	179.05	198.76	1294.00	1.000	32947	567	542	177	172	33	138.86	1073.08	42.14	4380	3054	25.46

Abbreviations: PERS. = PERSON(S) ; PYR = PERSON-YEARS ; MALIG = MALIGNANCIES ; LEUK = LEUKEMIA ; CANC = CANCER ; INIT. = INITIAL ; /10K = per 10,000 .

Table 11-D
Raw Data for Females, by Dose-Groups : Hiroshima and Nagasaki Combined, 1950–1982.

Row No.	A DISK AGE ATB	B Fem. TRUE AGE ATB	C RERF DOSE-GRP	D RBE=2 T65DR ORGAN DOSE (rems)	E RBE=20 DS86 ORGAN DOSE (rems)	F FE-MALES INIT. PERS.	G INIT. PERS. OVER TOTAL PERS.	H PERS. YEARS (PYR)	I ALL CAUSE	J ALL DIS-EASE	K ALL NEO-PLASM	L ALL MALIG	M LEUK	N ALL CANC EXCEPT LEUK	P CANC DEATHS /10K INIT. PERS.	Q CANC DEATHS per 10K PYR	R ALL DEATH /10K INIT. PERS.	ALL DEATH MINUS ALL MALIG /10K Init.	T PYR PER INIT. PERS.
1	5	4.09	1	0.000	0.082	3842	0.177	122363	102	79	23	20	2	18	46.85	1.47	265	213	31.85
2	15	14.95	1	0.000	0.087	4185	0.192	130296	280	233	73	70	4	66	157.71	5.07	669	502	31.13
3	27	26.71	1	0.000	0.093	5193	0.239	158651	670	646	227	219	6	213	410.17	13.43	1290	868	30.55
4	42	41.70	1	0.000	0.095	5084	0.234	136916	2241	2165	543	515	14	501	985.44	36.59	4408	3395	26.93
5	60	59.00	1	0.000	0.091	3463	0.159	53998	3259	3168	393	376	3	373	1077.10	69.08	9411	8325	15.59
6																			
7	FEMALE, RAW		1	0.000	0.090	21767	1.000	602224	6552	6291	1259	1200	29	1171	537.97	19.44	3010	2459	27.67
9	5	4.06	2	1.427	1.584	3093	0.185	98447	91	64	23	22	2	20	64.66	2.03	294	223	31.83
10	15	14.80	2	1.502	1.721	3218	0.193	100803	196	168	58	51	1	50	155.38	4.96	609	451	31.32
11	27	26.67	2	1.505	1.903	4067	0.244	123272	563	533	200	188	5	183	449.96	14.85	1384	922	30.31
12	42	41.71	2	1.475	1.848	3754	0.225	100120	1709	1640	448	431	7	424	1129.46	42.35	4552	3404	26.67
13	60	59.13	2	1.471	1.815	2544	0.153	39086	2364	2312	258	238	3	235	923.74	60.12	9292	8357	15.36
14																			
15	FEMALE, RAW		2	1.478	1.783	16676	1.000	461729	4923	4717	987	930	18	912	546.89	19.75	2952	2394	27.69
17	5	4.08	1+2	0.637	0.752	6935	0.180	220810	193	143	46	42	4	38	54.79	1.72	278	218	31.84
18	15	14.88	1+2	0.653	0.797	7403	0.193	231099	476	401	131	121	5	116	156.69	5.02	643	480	31.22
19	27	26.69	1+2	0.661	0.888	9260	0.241	281923	1233	1179	427	407	11	396	427.65	14.05	1332	892	30.45
20	42	41.71	1+2	0.627	0.840	8838	0.230	237037	3950	3805	991	946	21	925	1046.62	39.02	4469	3399	26.82
21	60	59.05	1+2	0.623	0.821	6007	0.156	93084	5623	5480	651	614	6	608	1012.15	65.32	9361	8339	15.50
22																			
23	FEMALE, RAW		1+2	0.641	0.824	38443	1.000	1063953	11475	11008	2246	2130	47	2083	541.84	19.58	2985	2431	27.68
25	5	3.98	3	10.702	13.548	1547	0.171	49157	52	42	13	13	4	9	58.18	1.83	336	252	31.78
26	15	14.86	3	10.714	13.790	1663	0.184	51876	115	97	27	26	3	23	138.30	4.43	692	535	31.19
27	27	26.82	3	10.987	14.848	2189	0.242	66414	301	278	131	126	5	121	552.76	18.22	1375	799	30.34
28	42	41.60	3	10.989	15.224	2291	0.253	61023	1050	1014	287	278	4	274	1195.98	44.90	4583	3370	26.64
29	60	58.71	3	10.826	14.896	1365	0.151	21653	1279	1247	175	161	2	159	1164.84	73.43	9370	8190	15.86
30																			
31	FEMALE, RAW		3	10.864	14.534	9055	1.000	250123	2797	2678	633	604	18	586	647.16	23.43	3089	2422	27.62
33	5	4.17	4	34.652	39.233	372	0.146	11771	12	11	4	4	1	3	80.65	2.55	323	215	31.64
34	15	15.16	4	36.457	39.149	543	0.214	17078	30	23	7	7	0	7	128.91	4.10	552	424	31.45
35	27	26.60	4	35.604	42.377	670	0.264	20277	109	104	42	38	2	36	537.31	17.75	1627	1060	30.26
36	42	41.64	4	34.654	43.001	582	0.229	15535	276	258	81	79	3	76	1305.84	48.92	4742	3385	26.69
37	60	58.50	4	35.351	43.680	374	0.147	5770	351	338	44	41	2	39	1042.78	67.60	9385	8289	15.43
38																			
39	FEMALE, RAW		4	35.392	41.562	2541	1.000	70431	778	734	178	169	8	161	633.61	22.86	3062	2397	27.72
41	5	4.34	5	70.310	74.071	213	0.122	6663	11	9	5	5	2	3	140.85	4.50	516	282	31.28
42	15	15.14	5	72.440	68.103	556	0.319	17255	51	42	22	21	3	18	323.74	10.43	917	540	31.03
43	27	25.67	5	72.590	75.907	436	0.250	13275	55	52	27	24	2	22	504.59	16.57	1261	711	30.45
44	42	41.87	5	70.016	78.935	366	0.210	9741	174	169	47	43	1	42	1147.54	43.12	4754	3579	26.62
45	60	58.15	5	71.744	77.444	171	0.098	2549	157	153	28	28	1	27	1578.95	105.91	9181	7544	14.91
46																			
47	FEMALE, RAW		5	71.639	73.979	1742	1.000	49483	448	425	129	121	9	112	642.94	22.63	2572	1877	28.41
49	5		6-8	180.94	197.66	210	0.130	6503	15	12	9	9	3	6	285.71	9.23	714	286	30.97
50	15		6-8	166.18	176.34	493	0.306	15168	57	53	27	26	4	22	446.25	14.50	1156	629	30.77
51	27		6-8	179.41	203.47	447	0.277	13171	95	90	50	48	7	41	917.23	31.13	2125	1051	29.46
52	42		6-8	175.59	202.90	326	0.202	8532	167	163	58	56	6	50	1533.74	58.60	5123	3405	26.17
53	60		6-8	171.02	195.56	137	0.085	2035	130	126	24	21	2	19	1386.86	93.35	9489	7956	14.86
54																			
55	FEMALE, RAW		6-8	174.08	193.63	1613	1.000	45408	464	444	168	160	22	138	855.55	30.39	2877	1885	28.15

Abbreviations: PERS. = PERSON(S) ; PYR = PERSON-YEARS ; MALIG = MALIGNANCIES ; LEUK = LEUKEMIA ; CANC = CANCER ;
INIT. = INITIAL ; /10K = per 10,000 ; Fem = FEMALES .

Table 11-E

Age-Normalized Data for Females, by Dose-Groups : Hiroshima and Nagasaki Combined, 1950-1982.

Row No.	A DISK AGE ATB	B Fem. TRUE AGE ATB	C RERF DOSE-GRP	D RBE=2 T65DR ORGAN DOSE (rems)	E DS86 ORGAN DOSE (rems)	F FE-MALES INIT. PERS.	G INIT. PERS. OVER TOTAL PERS	H PERS. YEARS (PYR)	[--VARIOUS CAUSES OF DEATH--] I ALL CAUSE	J ALL DIS-EASE	K ALL NEO-PLASM	L ALL MALIG	M LEUK	N ALL CANC EXCEPT LEUK	P CANC DEATHS /10K INIT. PERS.	Q CANC DEATHS PER 10K PYR	R ALL DEATH /10K INIT. PERS	ALL DEATH MINUS All MALIG /10K INIT	T PYR PER Init. PERS
56	5	4.09	1	0.000	0.082	3926.70	0.180	125060	104	81	24	20	2	18.40	46.85	1.47	265	213	31.85
57	15	14.95	1	0.000	0.087	4191.69	0.193	130505	280	233	73	70	4	66.11	157.71	5.07	669	502	31.13
58	27	26.71	1	0.000	0.093	5243.15	0.241	160183	676	652	229	221	6	215.06	410.17	13.43	1290	868	30.55
59	42	41.70	1	0.000	0.095	5004.21	0.230	134767	2206	2131	534	507	14	493.14	985.44	36.59	4408	3395	26.93
60	60	59.00	1	0.000	0.091	3401.25	0.156	53035	3201	3112	386	369	3	366.35	1077.10	69.08	9411	8325	15.59
61																			
62	FEMALE, NORM		1	0.000	0.090	21767.00	1.000	603550	6468	6209	1246	1188	29	1159.05	532.48	19.20	2971	2426	27.73
64	5	4.06	2	1.427	1.584	3008.30	0.180	95751	89	62	22	21	2	19.45	64.66	2.03	294	223	31.83
65	15	14.80	2	1.502	1.721	3211.31	0.193	100593	196	168	58	51	1	49.90	155.38	4.96	609	451	31.32
66	27	26.67	2	1.505	1.903	4016.85	0.241	121752	556	526	198	186	5	180.74	449.96	14.85	1384	922	30.31
67	42	41.71	2	1.475	1.848	3833.79	0.230	102249	1745	1675	458	440	7	433.01	1129.46	42.35	4552	3404	26.67
68	60	59.13	2	1.471	1.815	2605.75	0.156	40035	2421	2368	264	244	3	240.70	923.74	60.12	9292	8357	15.36
69																			
70	FEMALE, NORM		2	1.478	1.784	16676.00	1.000	460380	5007	4799	1000	942	18	923.81	553.97	20.07	3002	2438	27.61
72	5	4.08	1+2	0.637	0.752	6935.00	0.180	220810	193	143	46	42	4	38.00	54.79	1.72	278	218	31.84
73	15	14.88	1+2	0.653	0.797	7403.00	0.193	231099	476	401	131	121	5	116.00	156.69	5.02	643	480	31.22
74	27	26.69	1+2	0.661	0.888	9260.00	0.241	281923	1233	1179	427	407	11	396.00	427.65	14.05	1332	892	30.45
75	42	41.71	1+2	0.627	0.840	8838.00	0.230	237037	3950	3805	991	946	21	925.00	1046.62	39.02	4469	3399	26.82
76	60	59.05	1+2	0.623	0.821	6007.00	0.156	93084	5623	5480	651	614	6	608.00	1012.15	65.32	9361	8339	15.50
77																			
78	FEMALE, NORM		1+2	0.641	0.824	38443.00	1.000	1063953	11475	11008	2246	2130	47	2083.00	541.84	19.58	2985	2431	27.68
80	5	3.98	3	10.702	13.548	1633.49	0.180	51905	55	44	14	14	4	9.50	58.18	1.83	336	252	31.78
81	15	14.86	3	10.714	13.790	1743.73	0.193	54394	121	102	28	27	3	24.12	138.30	4.43	692	535	31.19
82	27	26.82	3	10.987	14.848	2181.13	0.241	66176	300	277	131	126	5	120.57	552.76	18.22	1375	799	30.34
83	42	41.60	3	10.989	15.224	2081.73	0.230	55449	954	921	261	253	4	248.97	1195.98	44.90	4583	3370	26.64
84	60	58.71	3	10.826	14.896	1414.91	0.156	22445	1326	1293	181	167	2	164.81	1164.84	73.43	9370	8190	15.86
85																			
86	FEMALE, NORM		3	10.858	14.504	9055.00	1.000	250369	2755	2637	615	586	18	567.97	627.25	22.69	3043	2396	27.65
88	5	4.17	4	34.652	39.233	458.39	0.180	14504	15	14	5	5	1	3.70	80.65	2.55	323	215	31.64
89	15	15.16	4	36.457	39.149	489.32	0.193	15390	27	21	6	6	0	6.31	128.91	4.10	552	424	31.45
90	27	26.60	4	35.604	42.377	612.07	0.241	18523	100	95	38	35	2	32.89	537.31	17.75	1627	1060	30.26
91	42	41.64	4	34.654	43.001	584.17	0.230	15593	277	259	81	79	3	76.28	1305.84	48.92	4742	3385	26.69
92	60	58.50	4	35.351	43.680	397.05	0.156	6125	373	359	47	44	2	41.40	1042.78	67.60	9385	8289	15.43
93																			
94	FEMALE, NORM		4	35.339	41.535	2541.00	1.000	70136	791	747	178	169	8	160.58	631.95	22.90	3113	2449	27.60
96	5	4.34	5	70.310	74.071	314.25	0.180	9831	16	13	7	7	3	4.43	140.85	4.50	516	282	31.28
97	15	15.14	5	72.440	68.103	335.46	0.193	10411	31	25	13	13	2	10.86	323.74	10.43	917	540	31.03
98	27	25.67	5	72.590	75.907	419.61	0.241	12776	53	50	26	23	2	21.17	504.59	16.57	1261	711	30.45
99	42	41.87	5	70.016	78.935	400.48	0.230	10659	190	185	51	47	1	45.96	1147.54	43.12	4754	3579	26.62
100	60	58.15	5	71.744	77.444	272.20	0.156	4058	250	244	45	45	2	42.98	1578.95	105.91	9181	7544	14.91
101			5																
102	FEMALE, NORM		5	71.426	75.009	1742.00	1.000	47734	540	517	143	135	9	125.40	719.83	26.27	3101	2328	27.40
104	5		6-8	180.94	197.66	290.98	0.180	9011	21	17	12	12	4	8.31	285.71	9.23	714	286	30.97
105	15		6-8	166.18	176.34	310.62	0.193	9556	36	33	17	16	3	13.86	446.25	14.50	1156	629	30.77
106	27		6-8	179.41	203.47	388.53	0.241	11448	83	78	43	42	6	35.64	917.23	31.13	2125	1051	29.46
107	42		6-8	175.59	202.90	370.83	0.230	9705	190	185	66	64	7	56.88	1533.74	58.60	5123	3405	26.17
108	60		6-8	171.02	195.56	252.04	0.156	3744	239	232	44	39	4	34.95	1386.86	93.35	9489	7956	14.86
109																			
110	FEMALE, NORM		6-8	174.95	195.83	1613.00	1.000	43464	568	545	183	173	23	149.64	927.73	34.43	3524	2452	26.95

Abbreviations: PERS. = PERSON(S) ; PYR = PERSON-YEARS ; MALIG = MALIGNANCIES ; LEUK = LEUKEMIA ; CANC = CANCER :
INIT. = INITIAL ; /10K = per 10,000 .

Table 11-F
Male and Female Summary Data, Age-Normalized Values. 1950-1982, Cities Combined.

ROW NO.	SEX	C RERF DOSE GRP	D RBE=2 T65DR ORGAN DOSE (rems)	E RBE=20 DS86 ORGAN DOSE (rems)	F INITIAL PERSONS	H PERSON YEARS (PYR)	I ALL CAUSE	J ALL DIS- EASE	K ALL NEO- PLASM	L ALL MALIG	M LEUK	N ALL CANC EXCEPT LEUK	P CANC DEATHS /10K INIT. PERSONS	Q CANC DEATHS PER 10K PYR	R ALL DEATH /10K INIT. PERS.	ALL DEATH MINUS ALL MALIG /10K INIT.	T PYR PER INIT. PERS.
111	M	1	0.000	0.089	15406	399732	6157	5701	1352	1289	38	1251.16	812.13	31.30	3997	3160	25.95
112	M	2	1.556	2.038	12179	315062	4880	4540	1030	980	20	960.13	788.35	30.47	4007	3202	25.87
113	M	1+2	0.684	0.945	27585	714891	11033	10239	2385	2272	58	2214.08	802.64	30.97	4000	3176	25.92
114	M	3	11.183	14.648	5888	153802	2322	2176	529	511	22	488.80	830.16	31.78	3944	3076	26.12
115	M	4	35.393	39.357	1684	44287	662	626	152	148	4	143.41	851.62	32.38	3933	3055	26.30
116	M	5	71.145	73.162	1386	35927	559	527	156	148	10	138.40	998.53	38.52	4036	2968	25.92
117	M	6-8	179.05	198.76	1294	32947	567	542	177	172	33	138.86	1073.08	42.14	4380	3054	25.46
118																	
119	M	1-8			37837	981855	15144	14109	3400	3251	128	3123.54					
121	F	1	0.000	0.090	21767	603550	6468	6209	1246	1188	29	1159.05	532.48	19.20	2971	2426	27.73
122	F	2	1.478	1.784	16676	460380	5007	4799	1000	942	18	923.81	553.97	20.07	3002	2438	27.61
123	F	1+2	0.641	0.824	38443	1063953	11475	11008	2246	2130	47	2083.00	541.84	19.58	2985	2431	27.68
124	F	3	10.858	14.504	9055	250369	2755	2637	615	586	18	567.97	627.25	22.69	3043	2396	27.65
125	F	4	35.339	41.535	2541	70136	791	747	178	169	8	160.58	631.95	22.90	3113	2449	27.60
126	F	5	71.426	75.009	1742	47734	540	517	143	135	9	125.40	719.83	26.27	3101	2328	27.40
127	F	6-8	174.95	195.83	1613	43464	568	545	183	173	23	149.64	927.73	34.43	3524	2452	26.95
128																	
129	F	1-8			53394	1475656	16130	15455	3364	3192	106	3086.59					
131	M+F	1-8			91231	2457511	31274	29564	6764	6444	233	6210.13					

NOTES FOR CONVERSION OF TABLE 11-F INTO TABLE 11-G :

1. Rows 111 through 117 (Males) are simply transfers of Rows 62,70,78,86,94,102,110 from Table 11-C.
    Rows 121 through 127 (Females) are simply transfers of Rows 62,70,78,86,94,102,110 from Table 11-E.
Col.B (Age) is omitted because age-bands are now combined.
Col.G (Ratio) is omitted because all the values transferred would be 1.0 .

2. Next, we want to combine the male and female observations. Our objective remains a series of Dose-Groups which are alike in cancer-risk, except for their radiation-doses. Therefore, the proportions of males and females must be normalized to the same ratio in every Dose-Group. These ratios are not the same, in the absence of normalization. For instance, the ratio in the Reference Group is (27585 males / 38,443 females), or 0.717556. The ratio in Dose-Group 3, however, is (5888 / 9055), or 0.650248. In Dose-Group 5, the ratio is (1386 males / 1742 females), or 0.795637. The sex-ratio normalization is a two-step process again.

STEP 1: ESTABLISHING THE SEX-NORMALIZED NUMBERS OF PERSONS.
===

We shall normalize to the standard of the Reference Group; therefore, the male-female ratio in every Dose-Group will be 0.717556. We shall continue preserving the original total number of persons in every Dose-Group. These totals (males + females) are calculated from Column F directly above (see also Table 4-A).

EXAMPLE, USING DOSE-GROUP 1. TOTAL PERSONS = 37,173. (15,406 MALES + 21,767 FEMALES.)
  Let F = age- and sex-normalized number of females in Dose-Group 1.
  Then 0.717556 times F is the age- and sex-normalized number of males in Dose-Group 1.
  F + (0.717556)(F) = 37,173. And (1.717556)(F) = 37,173. And F = (37,173 / 1.717556).
  And finally, F = 21,642.98 age- and sex-normalized females, for Table 11-G, Col.F, Row 142.
  Male persons = (37,173) - (female persons).
  Males = 15,530.02 persons, the entry for Table 11-G, Col.F, Row 132. (Notes continue on next page.)

Table 11-G
Sex-Ratio Normalization, Yielding Age- and Sex-Normalized Data. 1950–1982, Cities Combined.

Notes: See Table 11-F.

ROW NO.	SEX	RERF DOSE-GRP	RBE=2 T65DR ORGAN DOSE (rems)	RBE=20 DS86 ORGAN DOSE (rems)	INITIAL PERSONS	PERSON YEARS (PYR)	ALL CAUSE	ALL DIS-EASE	ALL NEO-PLASM	ALL MALIG	LEUK	ALL CANC EXCEPT LEUK	CANC DEATHS /10K INIT. PERS.	CANC DEATHS PER 10K PYR	ALL DEATH /10K INIT. PERS.	ALL DEATH MINUS ALL MALIG /10k Init	PYR PER INIT PERS.
		A	C	D	E	F	H	I	J	K	L	M	N	P	Q	R	T
132	M	1	0.000	0.089	15530.02	402950	6207	5747	1363	1300	38	1261.23	812.13	31.30	3997	3160	25.95
133	M	2	1.556	2.038	12054.96	311853	4830	4494	1020	970	20	950.36	788.35	30.47	4007	3202	25.87
134	M	1+2	0.684	0.945	27584.98	714891	11033	10239	2385	2272	58	2214.08	802.64	30.97	4000	3176	25.92
135	M	3	11.183	14.648	6242.84	163071	2462	2307	561	542	24	518.25	830.16	31.78	3944	3076	26.12
136	M	4	35.393	39.357	1765.11	46420	694	656	159	155	5	150.32	851.62	32.38	3933	3055	26.30
137	M	5	71.145	73.162	1306.81	33874	527	497	147	140	9	130.49	998.53	38.52	4036	2968	25.92
138	M	6-8	179.05	198.76	1214.48	30923	532	508	166	161	31	130.32	1073.08	42.14	4380	3054	25.46
139																	
140	M				38114.22	989179	15249	14207	3419	3270	127	3143.46					
142	F	1	0.000	0.090	21642.98	600112	6431	6174	1239	1181	29	1152.44	532.48	19.20	2971	2426	27.73
143	F	2	1.478	1.784	16800.04	463804	5044	4835	1007	949	18	930.68	553.97	20.07	3002	2438	27.61
144	F	1+2	0.641	0.824	38443.02	1063953	11475	11008	2246	2130	47	2083.00	541.84	19.58	2985	2431	27.68
145	F	3	10.858	14.504	8700.16	240558	2647	2534	591	563	17	545.71	627.25	22.69	3043	2396	27.65
146	F	4	35.339	41.535	2459.89	67897	766	723	172	163	8	155.45	631.95	22.90	3113	2449	27.60
147	F	5	71.426	75.009	1821.19	49904	565	541	149	141	10	131.10	719.83	26.27	3101	2328	27.40
148	F	6-8	174.95	195.83	1692.52	45607	596	572	192	181	24	157.02	927.73	34.43	3524	2452	26.95
149																	
150	F				53116.78	1467919	16049	15378	3350	3179	106	3072.28					
	M+F	1-8			91231	2457098	31299	29585	6769	6449	233	6215.75					

NOTES FOR CONVERSION OF TABLE 11-F INTO TABLE 11-G, continued.

In this fashion, all the entries for Table 11-G, Col.F, were established.
Checking will show that all male-female ratios in Table 11-G are 0.7176 .
Dose-Group 4 is an example : (F136 / F146) = (1765.11 / 2459.89) = 0.7176 .

STEP 2: SEX-NORMALIZATION OF THE CORRESPONDING OBSERVATIONS.
==

The old observations in Cols. H through N of Table 11-F are normalized by multiplying each one by the ratio of (new persons / old persons).

EXAMPLE, USING MALE DOSE-GROUP 1, OBSERVED PERSON-YEARS :
  The new number of initial persons = 15,530.02 (from Table 11-G, Col.F, Row 132).
  The old number of initial persons = 15,406 (from Table 11-F, Col.F, Row 111).
  The old number of Person-Years = 399,732 (from Table 11-F, Col.H, Row 111).
  The new number of Person-Years = (15530.02 persons / 15406 persons) x (399732 PYR) = 402950 PYR.
That is the new entry for Table 11-G, Col.H, Row 132.

  In that fashion, all the age- and sex-normalized entries for Columns H through N were calculated for Table 11-G. Thereafter, all the rates in Columns P through T were newly calculated, to check that the observed rates still match the corresponding entries in Table 11-F. Mean doses per person (Cols.D,E) remain unchanged.

  Now the data are ready to combine. The combination is shown in Table 11-H.
===

Column S, "All Deaths Minus All Malignancies, per 10,000 Initial Persons," is (for each row) :
[(Col.I - Col.L) / Col.F] times 10,000. All malignancies include leukemia, of course.

Table 11-H
Directly Comparable Dose-Groups, after Combination of Male and Female Data.

Columns A, B, and G are omitted.

Row No.	C RERF DOSE-GRP	D RBE=2 T65DR ORGAN DOSE (rems)	E RBE=20 DS86 ORGAN DOSE (rems)	F M + F INITIAL PERSONS	H PERSON YEARS (PYR)	I ALL CAUSE	J ALL DIS-EASE	K ALL NEO-PLASM	L ALL MALIG	M LEUK	N ALL CANC EXCEPT LEUK	O	P CANC DEATHS /10K INITIAL PERSONS	Q CANC DEATHS PER 10K PYR	R ALL DEATH /10K INIT PERS	ALL DEATH MINUS ALL MALIG /10k INIT	T PYR PER INIT PERS
151	1.00	0.00	0.089	37173	1003062	12638	11920	2602	2481	67	2413.68		649.31	24.06	3400	2732	26.98
152	2	1.511	1.890	28855	775657	9875	9329	2027	1919	38	1881.04		651.89	24.25	3422	2757	26.88
153	1+2	0.659	0.875	66028	1778844	22508	21247	4631	4402	105	4297.08		650.80	24.16	3409	2742	26.94
154	3	10.994	14.564	14943	403628	5110	4840	1152	1105	41	1063.97		712.02	26.36	3419	2680	27.01
155	4	35.361	40.625	4225	114318	1460	1380	331	318	13	305.77		723.72	26.75	3456	2702	27.06
156	5	71.308	74.238	3128	83778	1092	1037	297	280	19	261.58		836.27	31.22	3492	2595	26.78
157	6-8	176.66	197.054	2907	76530	1128	1081	358	343	55	287.34		988.45	37.55	3882	2703	26.33
158	1-8		M + F =	91231	2457098	31299	29585	6769	6449	233	6215.75						

Additional Combinations of Dose-Groups.

Row No.	C	D	E	F	H	I	J	K	L	M	N	O	P	Q	R	S	T
159	3+4	16.365	20.309	19168	517946	6570	6220	1483	1423	54	1369.74		714.60	26.45	3427	2685	27.02
160	3-8	41.673	47.388	25203	678254	8790	8338	2138	2046	128	1918.67		761.29	28.29	3488	2676	26.91
161	4+5	50.653	54.924	7353	198096	2552	2417	628	599	31	567.36		771.60	28.64	3471	2657	26.94
162	5-8	122.06	133.397	6035	160308	2221	2118	654	623	74	548.93		909.57	34.24	3680	2647	26.56

1.   The male and female rows of age-sex normalized data, from Table 11-G, have been combined above in three steps.

STEP 1, USING TABLE 11-G : The observations in Columns F through N were added according to Dose-Group. For example, in Dose-Group 1, to combine male and female observations in those columns, we added Rows 132 and 142. The sums appear in Row 151 of Table 11-H above.

STEP 2, USING TABLE 11-H : We calculated new rates for Columns P through T. ("Per 10,000 initial persons" is abbreviated as "per10K Init Pers" where space is short.)

STEP 3, USING TABLE 11-G : We recalculated the mean doses. For instance, entry D154 above is the weighted mean T65DR dose in Dose-Group 3 for males and females. It is calculated as follows from Table 11-G : [(11.183 rems per male x 6242.84 males) + (10.858 rems per female x 8700.16 females)] / 14,943 total persons in Dose-Group 3.

----

2.   It makes a negligible difference whether Dose-Groups are normalized before they are combined, or normalized after they have been combined. For instance, the difference between the entry N153 above (4297.08 cancer-deaths) and the sum of entries N151 and N152 (sum = 4294.72 cancer-deaths) is 2.36 cases -- a difference of about 0.06 of one percent. When Dose-Groups 6,7,8 are normalized separately, before combination, their combined cancer-deaths are 288.12 compared with 287.34 (entry N157 above) -- a difference of 0.78 cancer-death or about 0.27 of one percent.

----

3.   RESULT OF NORMALIZATION : We can be mathematically assured that all Dose-Groups in Table 11-H (including the additional combinations shown in Rows 159-162) are alike in the fraction of their total initial persons who are males age-5-ATB, alike in the fraction of their total initial persons who are females age-5-ATB, and so forth. In other words, all the Dose-Groups above enter the lifespan follow-up in 1950 as directly comparable cohorts, alike in both age-distribution and sex-distribution.

CHAPTER 12

The Focus on Two Central Questions

This chapter is arranged in five parts:

1. The Focus of Our Analyses

Chapters in the previous section have prepared the A-bomb database for answering some questions about the quantitative aspects of cancer-production in humans by ionizing radiation. The analysis begins in the next chapter. Therefore, it is important to be explicit now about which questions will be examined, because different methods are appropriate for different questions.

Two of the
Central Questions in This Field :

Over the past twenty years, one question has been so commonly asked by analysts in this field that -- for convenience in discussion -- we have given a name to its answer: Lifetime Fatal Cancer-Yield. Although the question is phrased in many ways, it is always a variant of the following:

"How many extra fatal cancers will be produced among a population of 10,000 exposed persons per rem (or centi-sievert) of whole-body exposure, during the remaining lifespan of the entire group?"

Definition of Fatal Cancer-Yield :
Fatal Cancer-Yield is the number of fatal, radiation-induced cancers which occur among a specified number of irradiated people, per unit of dose, during a specified amount of time after the exposure.

Most reports and papers present Lifetime Fatal Cancer-Yield as a Number, N, per 10,000 irradiated persons (or N x 10^-4 persons), but some express it as N per hundred thousand persons (N x 10^-5 persons) or per million persons (N x 10^-6 persons). The radiation unit varies too. We use "per rem" or centi-sievert (rem^-1, or cSv^-1); others sometimes use rads

(rad^-1) or grays (Gy^-1) or milli-grays (mGy^-1). A table of dose-equivalents is located at the end of our Index.

Initial Persons and Cancer in General :
Regardless of the units chosen, the analysts share a common thrust in their question: How many extra cancer-deaths, of all types combined, will occur in a specified number of initial persons per unit of radiation exposure to the entire body, during the post-exposure lifespan of the group?

Analysts addressing this question include, among many, the UNSCEAR and BEIR-3 radiation committees, myself, Hoffman and Radford (Hoff85), and RERF analysts Preston and Pierce (Pr87b; Pr88) and Shimizu and co-workers (Shi88). A directly related and very important second question is:

"Is the Fatal Cancer-Yield the same at all dose-levels and dose-rates, or is the risk per rem at low doses and dose-rates different from the risk per rem at high doses and high dose-rates?"

The focus of our analyses is on those two questions: The cumulative number of radiation-induced cancer-deaths per 10,000 initial exposed persons, and possible variation in the number of radiation-induced cancers with variation in dose-level or dose-rate.

Additional Questions :

Of course, there are many additional questions which COULD be asked. How many years of lifespan are lost by an individual who dies early of radiation-induced cancer? (This issue was treated in Go81.) Another example: When thirty years have passed since the bombing and some of the initial persons have died from a variety of causes, at what rate per 10,000 residual persons are people dying of radiation-induced cancer per year?

==

These and many other questions are perfectly valid, of course, and are not to be disparaged, but they are wholly separate and simply different from the two main questions which we are asking here.

2. Examination of All Cancer-Deaths Combined

Our analyses quantify radiation-risk to populations from all cancers COMBINED, excluding leukemia, as do many of the analyses by others (recently, the RERF reports TR-1-86, TR-9-87, TR-5-88).

There are three main reasons for handling all cancers combined.

(1) Primary Site Misdiagnosis :
First, by keeping all the cancers combined, analysts avoid the errors originating with misdiagnosis of the cancer's primary site -- errors described near the end of Chapter 11. For instance, if lung-cancers have spread beyond the lung and are mislabeled as brain-cancers or liver-cancers, and if misdiagnosis of the primary site is common (see Chapter 11), then some serious errors are going to be made about site-specific rates, site-specific latency periods, site-specific sex-and-age differences, and so forth. Analysts invite error if they ask a database to answer questions which it is not capable of answering, or if they ask a question too early in a follow-up.

(2) Small-Numbers Problem :
Second, by keeping all the cancers combined, analysts avoid creating a small-numbers problem of real severity. As noted in Chapter 4, even the biggest database can be rendered inconclusive by excessive subdivision. The most reliable results come from the least possible subdivision.

When we look at the entries for cancer-deaths in Column N of Tables 11-B (males) and 11-D (females), we are impressed with the very small numbers of cases in many of the rows -- and these entries are for all types of cancer COMBINED. This may surprise some people, who may have assumed that a study with 91,231 participants and a follow-up already lasting 37 years post-irradiation would NOT present analysts with the small-numbers problem.

What we all need to recognize is that 66,028 out of the 91,231 initial persons are in Dose-Groups 1 and 2, and they received almost NO DOSE. When analysts attempt to subdivide the EXPOSED groups by specific cancer-sites (or by age and sex), it is not surprising at all that we are still fighting the small-numbers problem,

and the statistical instability inherent in such data. Column N in Tables 11-B and 11-D stands as a reminder that we cannot ask more from the A-Bomb Study than its database is presently able to answer.

(3) Scientific Believability :
Third, by keeping all the cancers combined, analysts may provide what many people desire: A believable estimate of how many people die from radiation-induced cancer of ANY type, per rem of whole-body exposure. Until THIS question can be answered in a scientifically credible way, it would be a mistake to attempt something inherently less credible: A site-specific analysis.

Moreover, there is no pressing social need to subdivide cancers into sites or classes, because when the issue is DYING from radiation-induced cancer, few people care very much whether the fatal disease arises in one organ or in a different one (unless the time from exposure to death is very different -- an issue which remains clouded by the problems of misdiagnosis and small-numbers).

Exclusion of Leukemia :

It is customary to exclude radiation-induced leukemia from a combined analysis, however, because its distribution in time is CLEARLY much earlier than the other radiation-induced cancers.

Leukemia's exclusion from the combination does not seriously diminish the total number of malignancies in the database, as Row 158 in Table 11-H can show. For the entire 1950-1982 follow-up, Table 11-H, Row 158, shows 233 cumulative deaths from leukemia (normalized data) compared with over 6,000 cumulative deaths from the other cancers combined.

The comparison in no way denigrates the importance of leukemia as a cancer, of course. However, the comparison does illustrate the fact that, when single cancers are considered in isolation, there can be a drastic drop in numbers and an associated drop in reliability for site-specific analyses. Readers might remember the numbers 233 and 6000. Nonetheless, some segments of the radiation community have been giving greater or equal weight to leukemia data than to all cancers combined (Chapters 22,25; recently Mu89).

Exclusion of Non-Fatal Cancers :

Evaluation of Fatal Cancer-Yield, by definition, excludes non-fatal radiation-induced cancer. We would like to make it clear that exclusion of non-fatal radiation-induced cancers from this book is not meant to trivialize the misery and expense caused by non-fatal cancer-cases -- including a high proportion of thyroid-cancers and skin-cancers. The exclusion here is due to the greater reliability, currently, of the available MORTALITY data in the A-Bomb Study.

3. Lifetime versus Minimum Fatal Cancer-Yields

Cancer-induction by ionizing radiation occurs in an exposed population over years and decades. Although, by late 1982, the population of A-bomb survivors has already been observed to a time which is 37 years beyond the bombings, cancer-production by the exposure is definitely not yet finished -- it is persisting (Chapter 17).

At the present time, no analyst can know whether or not a limit exists on the post-irradiation time-period during which radiation-induced cancer-deaths (excess cancer-deaths) will continue to occur. If radiation-induced cancers continue to occur for the full lifespan of those who were only age 5 at the time of the bombings, then about another 37 years will be needed to ascertain with certainty the LIFETIME Fatal Cancer-Yield in this population.

The Minimum Fatal Cancer-Yield :

Meanwhile, along the way to the final count, there is great value in ascertaining how many radiation-induced cancer-deaths per 10,000 initial persons have ALREADY occurred at various times.

We call an interim count the MINIMUM Fatal Cancer-Yield, because every radiation-induced cancer which occurs AFTER an interim count can only increase the interim value. Radiation-induced cancers which have already occurred cannot be undone, so in common parlance, they are "in-the-box."

The cases which are "in-the-box" as of 1982 are not subject to dispute. They are not hypothetical, predicted, or dependent on any choice among competing models of radiation carcinogenesis (for instance, the "absolute" and "relative risk" models). The radiation-induced cases are known to have occurred by a straight-forward method. One can compare real-world events (cumulative cancer death-rates per 10,000 initial persons) in groups whose cancer-risk should be the same except for radiation exposure, and then the difference is the radiation-induced rate. We shall return, below, to the issue of the groups' comparability (see "A Potential Cause").

It is highly unlikely that cases already "in-the-box" are going to climb OUT of "the box." The only way for the final LIFETIME Fatal Cancer-Yield to turn out lower than the interim 1950-1982 Fatal Cancer-Yield would be for the irradiated survivors to start having FEWER cancers per 10,000 initial persons than the Reference Group in subsequent follow-ups. But the evidence in Chapter 17, on the duration of the radiation-effect in the A-Bomb Study, is a powerful indication that EXCESS cancers will continue to occur beyond 1982 in the irradiated groups.

But Just Suppose That ...

Although the odds are heavily against the following scenario, we wish to describe it and to comment on its public health implications.

Let us suppose that at the end of the lifespan follow-up of the A-bomb survivors, when all 91,231 initial persons have died of one cause or another, the cancer death-rates per 10,000 initial persons are the SAME in the Reference Group and in the exposed groups. By definition, the LIFETIME Fatal Cancer-Yield would be zero. On the other hand, we already know (not a speculation) that interim counts along the way show that EXCESS cancer-deaths have been occurring in the exposed groups. Such a combination of findings would probably mean that radiation ACCELERATED fatal cancer in the people who were going to die of cancer anyway, but at some later time.

And we must comment on the meaning of advancing such cancer-deaths by 5, 10, 20, 30, or 40 years through radiation. Dying of cancer at age 20 years, or at age 30, 40, 50 or 60 years, is sharply different for an individual than dying from cancer "anyway" at age 70 years. Acceleration of cancer by radiation would almost make irrelevant whether there were any "extra" fatal cancers or not.

Periodic Examination of Minimum Fatal Cancer-Yields :

By examining the Minimum Fatal Cancer-Yield periodically, we are necessarily moving closer and closer to the ultimate Lifetime Fatal Cancer-Yield. If we reach a time when successive interim counts show no further increase in the Minimum value, this would suggest that we should not expect the final Lifetime value to exceed the most recently found Minimum value.

On the other hand, if successive interim evaluations of Cancer-Yield were to show a steeper rise than expected, or even a fall, predictions of the Lifetime Fatal

===

Cancer-Yield could be appropriately revised up or down, prior to the final counts.

Therefore we think it would be useful, in this field, for analysts to report not only their current predictions about the LIFETIME Fatal Cancer-Yield, but also to state explicitly their findings about the current MINIMUM Fatal Cancer-Yield.

4. Potential Cause of False Answers

We have emphasized, in Chapter 11 and above, the importance of comparing Dose-Groups whose cancer-risk, at any interim time during the lifetime follow-up, would be alike (except for sampling variation) in the ABSENCE of exposure to the bombings. Otherwise, Cancer-Yields could be falsely high or falsely low.

Our normalization process in Chapter 11 ensured that all the Dose-Groups were perfectly matched for age and sex at the outset of the study in 1950. The nature of the study itself makes the presence of additional confounding variables less likely in this study than in some others. In the A-Bomb Study, for instance, dose is related to the survivor's distance from the bomb's hypocenter. Since the radius from the hypocenters extends in all directions (except into the sea), and since two separate cities are involved, Dose-Groups are going to be composed of persons from many neighborhoods and occupations.

It is a reasonable approximation -- but an approximation nonetheless -- that the radiation-exposed and the unexposed groups will have the same exposure to all kinds of hazards which can affect death-rates along the way to the final count.

An Extreme Scenario
Involving a Single Dose-Group :

The importance of this approximation can be readily appreciated by considering an extreme and extremely unlikely scenario. Suppose that one of the exposed groups moves into a single neighborhood sometime after the bombings, and suppose that a disastrous epidemic occurs in this one locale early in the follow-up. Suppose that the epidemic removes half of this particular cohort.

This scenario means that this one Dose-Group is no longer like the others in cancer-risk. Sorely depleted by the epidemic, it simply has many fewer residual persons, per 10,000 initial persons, available to develop cancer. So if we just count cancers, we could find that

this one exposed group has FEWER cancers per 10,000 initial persons at the end of the study than the Reference Group.

The scenario illustrates how fallacious answers could arise if initially comparable groups do not REMAIN comparable during a follow-up.

Guidance from Non-Cancer
Death-Rates and Person-Years :

Readers will have noticed, in Tables 11-B through 11-H, that Column P speaks directly to the central question of cancer death-rate per 10,000 initial persons, whereas Columns Q, R, S and T do not. The function of Columns Q-T, however, can be clarified by reference to the epidemic scenario above.

For instance, if the epidemic scenario had really occurred, the problem would show up almost immediately in Columns R and S, "All Deaths per 10,000 Initial Persons" and "All Deaths Minus All Malignancies per 10,000 initial persons." Both these rates would suddenly soar compared with the rates in the other Dose-Groups. (As noted in Table 11-G, "All Malignancies" include leukemia.)

Somewhat later, the problem would become evident in Column T, the ratio "Person-Years per Initial Person." Every person in a study contributes one person-year for each full year he(she) is alive during the follow-up period. If the epidemic scenario were really to affect one Dose-Group and not the others, the increment in person-years per initial person, in the affected group, would be far lower than in the other groups during each subsequent follow-up. On a cumulative basis (like Column T), the ratio in the group which was depleted by the epidemic would necessarily fall behind the rising ratios in the undepleted groups. (Under some other circumstances, however, a detectable reduction of person-years per initial person can be the result of enough EXTRA cancers, which also cause people to be removed early from a follow-up.)

Eventually Column Q, "Cancer-Deaths per 10,000 Person-Years," may also show anomalies. But as a detector of an "epidemic" catastrophe, it is trickier because the group affected by the epidemic would have both fewer cancers AND fewer person-years.

We have studied Columns Q-T, in Tables 11-G and 11-H for entire Dose-Groups, and in Tables 11-C and 11-E for separate age-bands. In examining the age-bands, one gives particular attention to the two oldest, because they account for the overwhelming share -- 77 % -- of the cancers observed so far in the

==

1950-1982 follow-up period (see Table 4-B).

Of course we see some anomalies, but this is to be expected on the basis of random differences in sampling (sampling variation). Column F provides a reminder of the modest magnitude of the numbers from which such rates arise. We see no indication, in the 1950-1982 follow-up data, that any calamity has occurred which would make it unsuitable to compare cancer-deaths per 10,000 initial persons in the Reference Group with such rates in the various exposed groups.

"Competition" from
Other Radiation-Induced Deaths :

Above, we have discussed defenses against obtaining false Cancer-Yields due to an undetected and competing cause of death which affected one Dose-Group much more than the other Dose-Groups. So we should mention that there is one situation in which false Cancer-Yields would NOT result from a difference across Dose-Groups in non-cancer death rates per 10,000 initial persons.

Suppose that fatal cancer were not the ONLY delayed (beyond 1950) cause of death resulting from exposure to ionizing radiation. For the sake only of illustrating this point, suppose that ionizing radiation also increased or accelerated heart disease. If it truly did so, we would expect to see Column S entries in Table 11-H already rising with dose, somewhat the way the cancer entries in Column P rise with dose. The extra deaths from heart disease would be competing with cancer for potential victims, and therefore we would expect a LOWER Fatal Cancer-Yield than we would see without this radiation-induced competition.

But it would not be a FALSELY low Cancer-Yield. Radiation would be "entitled" to do whatever it does, and if it caused sufficient extra deaths from non-malignant disease to lower the number of extra cancer-deaths per 10,000 initial persons, so be it. It would not cause a FALSE evaluation of the cancer effect.

5. Reasons for Confidence in the A-Bomb Study

In epidemiology, there can never be a guarantee that analysts have detected every confounding variable which is important enough to invalidate the results.

For instance, suppose that all of the Reference Group in the A-Bomb Study has taken up residence next to a "cancer-factory," but no one realizes it. If this highly unlikely situation were real, it would be causing an underestimate of the Minimum Fatal Cancer-Yield from radiation, because the situation would be reducing the observed DIFFERENCE in cancer-deaths, per 10,000 initial persons, between the radiation-exposed groups and the Reference Group. On the other hand, if all of RERF's Dose-Group 3 had taken up residence next to the "cancer-factory" while the other Dose-Groups had not, the result would be an overestimated Minimum Fatal Cancer-Yield at low doses.

As noted earlier, one of the great virtues of the A-Bomb Study is that its very nature protects it quite well (though never perfectly) from such hazards.

There is additional reason for confidence in the Cancer-Yields which will be obtained from the A-Bomb Study. Our normalization process in Chapter 11 ensured that the Dose-Groups were completely comparable in age and sex distributions at the outset of the study, in 1950. Moreover, we have an objective basis for believing that they have remained comparable, between 1950 and 1982. Table 11-H, Column S, certainly affirms that no catastrophe has yet affected one Dose-Group and not the others. So far, "All Deaths Minus All Malignancies, per 10,000 Initial Persons" remains approximately constant, within sampling variation, from one Dose-Group to another.

However, it should be noted that only about a third of the study's initial population has died so far (31,299, normalized, out of 91,231 initial persons). By the time that EVERYONE has died, every excess cancer-death occurring in an exposed Dose-Group will necessarily mean a reduction in that group's NON-cancer death-rate per 10,000 initial persons. There can, of course, be only 10,000 total deaths per 10,000 initial persons.

In the end, everything must add up.

12-empty, after 12-5.

==

Analysis and Results by the Cancer Difference Method

This chapter is arranged in seven parts:

Then tables.
Then figures.

1. Logic of the Cancer Difference Method

In Table 13-A, readers will find all the input-data which are required for using the Cancer Difference Method to extract the Minimum Fatal Cancer-Yield from the evidence provided by the A-Bomb Study, 1950-1982. The data are comprehensive, and include both cities, both sexes, all ages, and all cancer-sites (leukemia excluded). Readers will notice that there are entries (Columns B and C) for both dosimetries. This is the next step in demonstrating our "constant-cohort, dual-dosimetry" proposal for handling the A-bomb database.

The data from Rows 1 through 6 are the input for Figures 13-A and 13-B, which plot cumulative cancer death-rate per 10,000 initial persons versus dose.

The Cancer Difference Method says: If we compare two groups of people who are alike in their cancer-risk, except for their radiation doses, and if their cumulative cancer death-rates per 10,000 initial persons are truly different, then the difference in cancer-rate is due to the difference in radiation dose.

If the higher cancer-rate is associated with the higher dose, then the difference in cancer-rate (the excess cancer-rate) is the RADIATION-induced cancer-rate. When we divide the difference in rate per 10,000 initial persons by the difference in dose, we are obtaining the radiation-induced cancer-rate among 10,000 persons of mixed ages, PER CENTI-SIEVERT OF AVERAGE DOSE (whole-body internal organ-dose). This quantity is, by definition, the Minimum Fatal Cancer-Yield.

It is not necessary for the Reference Group to have no dose at all, since the difference in cumulative cancer death-rate between any two compared groups will be divided by the DIFFERENCE in dose (not by the entire dose of the group with higher exposure).

The Cancer Difference Method can also provide an initial look at the dose-response relationship. An issue of central importance in evaluating the cancer hazard from ionizing radiation is whether the hazard per centi-sievert is LOWER at low total doses, is the SAME at all total doses, or is HIGHER at low total doses.

If we pick one class of people as the Reference Group, and then compare it serially with groups which received progressively higher doses, we can discover whether Cancer-Yield stays the same as total dose increases, or whether Cancer-Yield changes in a single direction as total dose increases. Therefore, we are going to compare six exposed groups (Table 13-A, Rows 8-13) with the Reference Group.

Except for Dose-Group 3, which is big enough to stand alone in terms of statistical strength, the exposed groups in Rows 8-13 consist of combinations. Adjacent Dose-Groups have been combined, as indicated by Column A, Rows 9-13, to reduce the relative instability of the observations in E4, E5, and E6. In Row 10, ALL of the exposed groups have been combined into a single class, and it, too, will be contrasted with the Reference Group.

An Easy Task :
It is hard to imagine an easier task than making these comparisons -- now that the input has been properly prepared. In Chapters 9 and 10, readers have seen the work required to obtain the average

==

organ-doses for all eight of RERF's Dose-Groups, and in both dosimetries. In Chapter 11, readers have seen the work required to overcome the fact that the people in RERF's eight Dose-Groups were NOT "alike except for radiation doses"; in the raw data, the distribution of ages and sexes differed from Dose-Group to Dose-Group.

Now there is only one more requirement to meet: The cancer death-rates in compared groups must be TRULY different, and not explicable as

random differences in sampling (sampling variation). Statistical testing in Chapter 27 has demonstrated that each of the six exposed groups in Rows 8-13 shows a significantly higher cumulative cancer-rate than does the Reference Class. We wish to stress that such tests are reliable because they were made on the normalized numbers of cancers, not on the raw numbers. So, with the assurance that cancer death-rates are truly different in the groups to be compared, the final requirement for analysis by the Cancer Difference Method has been met.

2. Calculation of the Minimum Fatal Cancer-Yield

We are going to illustrate the calculation of Minimum Fatal Cancer-Yields by making three of the six comparisons, in the T65DR dosimetry. For the T65DR dosimetry, calculations take the data from Columns B and F of Table 13-A, whereas for the DS86 dosimetry, calculations take the data from Columns C and F. In "constant-cohorts," there is only ONE set of cohorts and thus only ONE set of cancer-rates (Column F).

● STEP 1: We are asking this question, "How big is the difference in cancer death-rate between the Reference Group and the Low, Mid, and High Dose-Groups?" So, we take the rates from Rows 7, 8, 11, and 12 of Table 13-A:

	Column 1		Column 2		Column 3
Low-Dose Exposed minus Reference Class, in cancers / 10,000	= 712.02	minus	650.80	=	61.22
Mid-Dose Exposed minus Reference Class, in cancers / 10,000	= 771.60	minus	650.80	=	120.80
High-Dose Exposed minus Reference Class, in cancers / 10,000	= 909.57	minus	650.80	=	258.78

Chapter 11 established that it is appropriate to regard the residual differences in cancer-rates per 10,000 initial persons (Column 3) as having been caused by the radiation dose-difference between classes.

==

● STEP 2: So the next question is, "How big (how many rems or cSv) are the dose-differences?" We take the doses from Column B, Rows 7, 8, 11, and 12 of Table 13-A:

Low-Dose Exposed minus Reference Class, in rems (cSv)	= 10.994	minus	0.659	=	10.335
Mid-Dose Exposed minus Reference Class, in rems (cSv)	= 50.653	minus	0.659	=	49.994
High-Dose Exposed minus Reference Class, in rems (cSv)	= 122.056	minus	0.659	=	121.397

==

● STEP 3: We calculate the radiation-induced cancer-rates per rem (cSv):

Comparing Low-Dose with Ref.	Radiation-induced cancer-rate	61.22
	Difference in dose	$\frac{61.22}{10.335} = 5.92$

Comparing Low-Dose with Ref.
$$\frac{\text{Radiation-induced cancer-rate}}{\text{Difference in dose}} = \frac{61.22}{10.335} = 5.92$$

Comparing Mid-Dose with Ref.
$$\frac{\text{Radiation-induced cancer-rate}}{\text{Difference in dose}} = \frac{120.80}{49.99} = 2.42$$

Comparing High-Dose with Ref.
$$\frac{\text{Radiation-induced cancer-rate}}{\text{Difference in dose}} = \frac{258.78}{121.40} = 2.13$$

The analysis is complete for those three comparisons. For three different dose-levels, we have the Minimum Fatal Cancer-Yield, namely the cumulative number of radiation-induced cancer-fatalities which have already occurred (1950-1982) among 10,000 persons of mixed ages, per cSv of whole-body internal organ-dose. Precisely the same steps are used to make the additional comparisons, of course, and the results are entered in Table 13-B, Row 1, Columns B through G.

These are the so-called central values or best estimates. Confidence-limits are provided in Chapter 27, Part 2.

In Row 2 of Table 13-B, the values of Row 1 are increased by the factor of 1.23 used by RERF for underdiagnosis of cancer-death (see the end of Chapter 11).

Columns H through M of Table 13-B present the findings for exactly the SAME cohorts of persons, when their mean doses have been re-estimated under the current version of the DS86 dosimetry.

The parallel analyses demonstrate the "constant-cohort, dual-dosimetry" approach to maintaining the scientific status of the A-Bomb Study as an objective prospective study, while also examining the implications of a new dosimetry.

3. Discussion of the Minimum Values

Reliability of Input and Method :
Because the data in this chapter remain undivided by cancer-site, age, sex, city, or short periods, they suffer the least possible amount from random differences in sampling. Indeed, combination of various adjacent Dose-Groups has produced datapoints with greater stability than Dose-Groups examined singly. Moreover, all the datapoints used in this analysis remain free from the hazard of unintended distortion by elaborate statistical manipulation and "tortured mathematics" -- a phrase appropriately used in the BEIR-3 Report by its chairman (Edward P. Radford, in Beir80, p.239).

In addition, the Minimum Fatal Cancer-Yields in Table 13-B are independent from any model or hypothesis for radiation carcinogenesis. The values are based exclusively on the count of actual cancer-cases which have already occurred, and which cannot be undone or disputed as "hypothetical."

Comparison of Normalized and Raw Data at Low Doses :
In Chapter 11, after matching RERF's Dose-Groups for age and sex distribution, we stated that the effect of the normalization would be to REDUCE the estimates of cancer-hazard from low-dose exposure, by comparison with findings based on the raw data. Now we can show in detail how this happens.

Cancer-Yield is a difference in cancer-rate divided by the corresponding difference in dose. The dose-difference is virtually the SAME in our raw and normalized data. But let us look at cancer-rates.

For low-dose exposure, the relevant rates are in the Reference Group and Dose-Group 3, of course. In the normalized data from Table 13-A, we find that the difference in cumulative cancer death-rates is (712.02 per 10,000 in Dose-Group 3) minus (650.80 per 10,000 in the Reference Group), or a difference of 61.22 cancer-deaths per 10,000 initial persons. What would the difference have been in the raw data?

We can find out most easily by consulting Table 4-A. The rate in Dose-Group 3 is (1055 cancers / 14943 initial persons) x (10000), or 706.02 cancer-deaths per 10,000 initial persons. In the Reference Group (1+2), there are (2376 + 1779), or 4155 cancer-deaths. There are (37173 + 28855), or 66028 initial persons. The rate is (4155 / 66028) x (10000), or 629.28 cancer-deaths per 10,000 initial persons. Therefore, in the raw data, the difference in cancer death-rates would have been (706.02 - 629.28), or 76.74 cancer-deaths per 10,000 initial persons -- which is a greater difference in rate than 61.22, the value from the normalized data.

When the smaller, normalized difference in cancer-rate is divided by a fixed difference in dose, the result is necessarily a smaller increment in cancer-rate per unit dose from the normalized data, than from the raw data -- in other words, a lower Cancer-Yield or risk-estimate.

Comparison of Findings in the T65DR and DS86 Dosimetries :
If one examines Row 1 of Table 13-B, the biggest difference one can find, between results in T65DR and DS86, occurs at the lowest dose-level (entries B1 and H1). There is nothing puzzling about it, in the "constant-cohort, dual-dosimetry" approach.

The individuals in Dose-Group 3, and their observed cancer death-rate, are the same in the two parallel analyses. Likewise, the individuals in the Reference Group, and their observed cancer death-rate, are the same in the two analyses. It follows that the DIFFERENCE in their cancer death-rates is the same in both dosimetries. Indeed, everything is identical in the two analyses except for average dose.

The new dosimetry increases the dose-estimate of the low-dose exposed group from 10.994 rems up to 14.564 rems -- by about 32 percent, which is the largest of any exposed group on a percentage basis (Table 13-A, Rows 1-6). When a fixed difference in cancer-rate is divided by a larger difference in dose, the inevitable consequence is a smaller difference in cancer-rate per unit dose -- in other words, a lower Cancer-Yield or risk-estimate.

Shape of the Dose-Response Relationship :

Along Row 1 of Table 13-B, Cancer-Yield is steadily falling as the dose examined is steadily rising, and this is true in both dosimetries. In other words, everywhere in the dose-range, the average carcinogenic potency per rem of exposure is falling as dose rises.

An approximately constant Cancer-Yield at all dose-levels would suggest the linear dose-response, of course. The observed deviations from constancy in Row 1 are not random at all, however. They occur in a single direction, and strongly suggest a supra-linear dose-response. Figure 13-C contrasts supra-linear vs. concave-upward responses.

In Chapter 14, we shall examine this very important question of shape in quantitative detail. For readers who are curious about shape when cancer-risk is evaluated per 10,000 person-years instead of per 10,000 initial persons, we provide additional analysis and curves in Chapter 30.

Low-Dose Exposures Slowly Delivered :

In Chapters 22 and 23, we show that there is no basis in logic or in human evidence for thinking that the Minimum Fatal Cancer-Yields for LOW-dose exposure in Table 13-B would be lower, if the exposures had been slowly delivered instead of acutely delivered.

4. A Warning about X-Ray versus Gamma Exposure

For medical personnel and patients alike, it is important to note that Cancer-Yields based exclusively on the A-Bomb Study may underestimate -- by about two-fold -- the cancer-hazard per rem from X-ray exposures. In other words, the values in Table 13-B may need doubling.

Although both gamma rays and X-rays are classed as radiations of low-LET (Linear Energy Transfer), readers will see later that medical X-rays transfer a given amount of energy in a much shorter range of tissue than do A-bomb gamma radiations (Table 20-Eye, in our Threshold section). Therefore, the RBE of X-rays is probably higher than the RBE of A-bomb gamma rays. (RBE is defined and discussed in Chapter 8, Part 5.)

In some experimental work, others have tried to quantify the extra potency of orthovoltage X-rays compared with gamma rays of higher energy. For instance, Bond and co-workers state that "... the RBE of 250-kVp X rays compared to Co-60 gamma rays for low doses and dose rates, appears to be of the order of 2" (Bon78, p.433). Sinclair makes a statement which amounts to suggesting the potency of orthovoltage X-rays is twice as high as the potency of gamma rays, when he suggests that the RBE values for neutrons, which are tied to the classic X-ray base, should be multiplied by a factor of TWO to adjust for a gamma-ray base (Sin85). Kerr, referring to Sinclair's 1985 review-paper, concurs about the factor of two (Kerr88, p.243-245).

5. Radiation-Induced Cancer Demonstrated at 11 and 15 Rems

Before we calculated the Minimum Fatal Cancer-Yields in Part 2 of this chapter, we demonstrated that there exists a statistically significant difference between the observations in Dose-Group 3 versus the Reference Group. This fact deserves some emphasis, because it is very commonly and very mistakenly asserted in many circles that there is no evidence of radiation-induced cancer occurring in humans below high doses like 50 cSv (rems) or even 100 cSv. (See Index, "Low-dose human data lacking.")

Contrary to such claims, the evidence is conclusive that low-LET doses far lower than 50 cSv -- indeed, far lower than 10 cSv -- have induced cancer in humans (see Threshold section of this book).

Even if we limit discussion in this chapter to the A-Bomb Study, the evidence in Chapter 27, Part 1, is that cancer death-rates are truly different and HIGHER in Dose-Group 3 compared with the Reference Group (Dose-Groups 1 + 2). This finding is consistent with the work by Preston and co-workers (Pr86), who report finding the difference between Dose-Group 3 and Dose-Group 1 (by itself) to be significant. Since the average organ-dose in Dose-Group 3 is 10.994 cSv in the T65DR dosimetry, and 14.564 cSv in the DS86

===

system, excess cancer has been observed in the A-bomb survivors at these doses -- way below 50 or 100 cSv.

Our testing in Chapter 27, Part 1, yields p-values which are quite low for both the one-tailed and the two-tailed testing. Moreover, our testing is based on the age- and sex-normalized values for cancer cases. It has already been pointed out, in Part 3 of this chapter, that the net effect of normalization was to REDUCE the gap in cancer-rate between Dose-Group 3 and the Reference Group. So it cannot be said that the normalization process caused the difference in cancer-rates to be significant; the adjustments REDUCED the likelihood of finding a significant difference.

6. Lifetime Fatal Cancer-Yield -- Calculation and Discussion

Part 2 of this chapter produced Minimum Fatal Cancer-Yields for low-dose exposure which are very solidly grounded in the available evidence for 1950-1982, in both dosimetries. The data which are required to extend the "constant-cohort, dual-dosimetry" analysis to 1985 are not yet at hand (Chapter 6, page 2).

The next question was already described in Chapter 12: How will the ultimate LIFETIME Fatal Cancer-Yields compare with the MINIMUM Fatal Cancer-Yields now "in-the-box"?

Every analyst who tries to answer this question is necessarily making a prediction. The basis should be careful examination of trends in whatever evidence has already accumulated. Such work is presented in Chapter 17.

How Long Does the Carcinogenic Effect Persist ?

In Chapter 17, readers will see for themselves that the carcinogenic effect of the bombings appears to be INCREASING with time since the exposures, when all age-bands are considered as a unit. On the other hand, when the study's five age-bands are examined separately, the risk-ratio (of cancer death-rates in the exposed groups over cancer death-rates in the Reference Group) appears to be approximately constant through time. The approximate constancy of this ratio is remarkable, because it occurs even in age-bands where the spontaneous cancer death-rate has been tripling, six-folding, or ten-folding during the first 32 years of follow-up.

If the risk-ratio is approximately constant during the first 32 years of follow-up, it suggests that the carcinogenic effect from exposure is probably lifelong. This interim finding from the A-Bomb Study is compared with interim findings from other studies, in Chapter 17.

Only future follow-ups can resolve the issue with certainty. Meanwhile, analysts must use the best available evidence. Therefore, our Lifetime Fatal Cancer-Yields incorporate the presumption that the carcinogenic effect will persist for the full lifespan after exposure -- because no OTHER presumption can be justified by the evidence so far. Incidentally, RERF analysts are now using the same presumption (TR-9-87, p.34; TR-5-88, p.50).

Basis for the Factor of 2.223 :

Table 13-B, Note 4, states that all the Lifetime Cancer-Yields in the table are obtained by multiplying the Minimum Cancer-Yields by 2.223. Where does this factor come from?

It comes from Table 28-D, Row 14. It is the ratio of the ultimate number of spontaneous cancer-deaths expected beyond 1950 in the Reference Group when all participants have died, over the cumulative number of spontaneous cancer-deaths already observed in this group between 1950-1982. Chapter 28 shows, step by step, how we estimated the ultimate number, which we derived from the observations internal to the A-Bomb Study itself.

And why do we use this ratio to convert Minimum Fatal Cancer-Yields into Lifetime values? The answer will emerge from the assumption and relationships described below.

The key assumption here is that the current risk-ratio (exposed cancer-rate over Reference cancer-rate) will persist unchanged. By current risk-ratio, we mean the ratio which describes the entire 1950-1982 follow-up. For brevity, we can call this current ratio "C." For instance, in the low-dose comparison, Column F of Table 13-A shows that "C" is (712.02 / 650.80), or 1.094. In this chapter, we are using the assumption that this ratio will still be about 1.094 when the full lifespan follow-up is complete. Now we will state the fundamental relationships.

Let Ref stand for cancer-rate per 10,000 in the Reference Group.
Let Exp stand for cancer-rate per 10,000 in the radiation-exposed group. (Exp = Exposed.)
Let C = the current risk-ratio of (Exp / Ref).

===

Therefore:
Exp = C times Ref, or CRef.

Thus, in Equation (1) below, we can substitute CRef for Exp. Since Minimum Fatal Cancer-Yield is the difference in cancer-rates over the difference in dose, we can write:

● -- Equation (1) for MINIMUM Fatal Cancer-Yield:

Minimum Fatal Cancer-Yield
    = (Exp - Ref) / Dose-Difference.
    = (CRef - Ref) / Dose-Difference.

If the ultimate spontaneous cancer-rate per 10,000 initial persons is going to become 2.223-fold higher than the cumulative rate through 1982, and if the ultimate risk-ratio of (Exposed Ca-Rate / Reference Ca-Rate) is going to remain "C," then we can write:

Ultimate Ref = 2.223 Ref.
C = (Ultimate Exp / Ultimate Ref).
C = (Ultimate Exp / 2.223 Ref).
Ultimate Exp = C times 2.223 Ref, or 2.223 CRef.
Then we can make substitutions, in Equation (2).

● -- Equation (2) for LIFETIME Fatal Cancer-Yield:

Lifetime Fatal Cancer-Yield
    = (Ult.Exp - Ult.Ref) / Dose-Difference.
    = (2.223 CRef - 2.223 Ref) / Dose-Diff.
    = (2.223)(CRef - Ref) / Dose-Diff.

Comparison of Equations (1) and (2) shows that the Lifetime value would be exactly 2.223 times higher than the Minimum "in-the-box" value, since the dose-difference does not change. And thus one can use the ratio of (ultimate spontaneous cancer-rate / interim spontaneous cancer-rate), which is 2.223, to convert Minimum Fatal Cancer-Yields into Lifetime Fatal Cancer-Yields.

POSSIBLE Underestimation of Lifetime Fatal Cancer-Yields :

From the relationships above, it is obvious that an underestimate of the ultimate spontaneous cancer-rate would result in an underestimate of Lifetime Fatal Cancer-Yield, and an overestimate of ultimate spontaneous cancer-rate would result in an overestimate of Lifetime Fatal Cancer-Yield.

It seems more likely that our method in Chapter 28 UNDERestimates the ultimate spontaneous cancer-rate than OVERestimates it. The basis for this statement is

the fact that our method results in the estimate that only 14.5 percent of the initial persons in the Reference Group will ever die of cancer (Table 28-D, entry G13).

This fraction is substantially lower than the fraction suggested elsewhere. In TR-9-87 (p.34) and TR-5-88 (p.53), RERF has suggested "about 20%" as the appropriate "background lifetime risk for all cancer except leukemia in the LSS sample" (LSS means Life Span Study). Japanese vital statistics show that between 1975 and 1983, cancer was accounting for 19 - 23 % of all deaths (So81; Undemo86).

Only time can reveal whether our estimate of ultimate spontaneous cancer-deaths in the Reference Group has, or has not, introduced a serious underestimate into our Lifetime Fatal Cancer-Yields. Obviously if we had a basis right now for BELIEVING that a higher value for ultimate spontaneous rate would be scientifically superior, we would have presented a higher value.

PROBABLE Underestimation of Lifetime Fatal Cancer-Yields :

There is a wholly separate reason for treating the Lifetime Fatal Cancer-Yields in Table 13-B as probable underestimates: They come from a method which IGNORES what is already known about the greater carcinogenic effect of ionizing radiation upon the young than upon the old. From prior analyses (including Go69, Go81, Beir80, Nih85, etc.), we know that the cancer-risk per centi-sievert of dose is higher, the younger the recipient; this conclusion is confirmed again by the 1950-1982 follow-up of the A-bomb survivors (see Chapter 15).

When we look at the raw data in Table 4-B, we see that almost two-thirds of the 91,231 initial participants are still alive at the end of 1982. Also we see that, out of the 6,050 cancers observed so far, 4,659 or 77 % have come from the two age-bands which were oldest at the time of bombing (ATB).

In the normalized data of Table 28-D, we find the same thing in the Reference Group, which was hardly exposed at all. Out of 4,297.08 spontaneous cancer-deaths observed so far (entry H13), the number which comes from the two oldest age-bands is (1018.02 + 631.71 + 925 + 608), or 3,182.73 cases. This is 74 percent of the total. By contrast, the number of spontaneous cancers coming so far from the two youngest age-bands ATB is still extremely low.

As the older age-bands ATB continue passing from the scene, it is self-evident that both the spontaneous and the radiation-induced cancers coming in the A-bomb survivors, beyond 1982, have to come primarily from the younger age-bands -- in great contrast to the source of the cancers observed between 1950-1982.

Thus it is NOT realistic to assume that the risk-ratio (exposed / Reference Group), as defined earlier in this section, will stay the same beyond 1982 as it was from 1950-1982. The observations prior to the end of 1982 are based on groups with a much lower radiation-risk per centi-sievert than the radiation-risk in the groups which will produce the cancers beyond 1982. In other words, if the carcinogenic effect from exposure is lifelong, the Lifetime Yields in Table 13-B -- and also in Table 14-C -- are unrealistically low.

In Chapter 15, we will examine the age-bands separately (which means confronting the small-numbers problem), and we will make estimates of the Lifetime Fatal Cancer-Yields which DO take age-sensitivity into account.

7. The Bottom Line
from the Cancer Difference Method

1. This chapter is our first demonstration of the "constant-cohort, dual-dosimetry" approach to adding another dosimetry (DS86) to the A-Bomb Study. Our approach leaves the study's existing doses, structure and cohorts intact. Our approach also means that the findings in Table 13-B are directly comparable in the existing dosimetry (T65DR) and in the current version of the revised dosimetry (DS86).

2. The Minimum and Lifetime Fatal Cancer-Yields are presented in Table 13-B, for exposure of a mixed-age population. The findings are based on the 1950-1982 follow-up. Although RERF possesses additional observations through 1985, the data required to do a "constant-cohort, dual-dosimetry" analysis are not yet available to us.

3. In order to evaluate hazard to a population of mixed ages, from low doses of ionizing radiation, there is no need to extrapolate any results from high to low doses. The evidence in this chapter and Chapter 27 (Part 1) shows that excess cancer (radiation-induced cancer) is provably real at average organ-doses at least as low as 11 to 15 rems (centi-sieverts). The A-Bomb Study -- and several others (see Chapter 21) -- simply invalidate the common claim that there exists no human evidence of radiation-induced cancer below high doses like 50 rems (centi-sieverts) or even 100 rems.

4. The low-dose Cancer-Yields in Table 13-B (Columns B and H), already apply to low-dose exposure, and were not extrapolated from high-dose data. Moreover, as we shall show in Chapter 23, the low-dose Cancer-Yields apply to low doses which are SLOWLY delivered, as well as to low doses which are acutely delivered.

5. The evidence in Table 13-B is that cancer-risk per rem of exposure is MORE severe at low doses than at high doses. This very important finding will be explored and validated in quantitative detail in Chapter 14 (and also in Chapter 30, for readers who are interested in person-years).

6. Findings in this chapter are extremely solid for Minimum Fatal Cancer-Yields and for the shape of the dose-response relationship, because the data have not been excessively subdivided, and because all the datapoints remain free from the hazard of unintended distortion by elaborate statistical manipulation. In addition, the Minimum Fatal Cancer-Yields in Table 13-B are independent from any hypotheses. The values are based exclusively on the count of actual cancer-cases which have already occurred, and which cannot be undone or disputed as "hypothetical."

7. The estimated LIFETIME Fatal Cancer-Yields in Table 13-B are unrealistically low, because the method is not the appropriate one for making predictions beyond 1982 (a very different method is used in Chapter 16 to determine the probable Lifetime Fatal Cancer-Yields). Even so, the estimates for low-dose exposure in Table 13-B, entries H4 and B4, are much higher than the lifetime values of 1.0 and 2.0 which have been routinely used by the radiation community for making statements about low-dose exposure.

Table 13-A

Basic Input-Data for Determining Minimum Fatal Cancer-Yield by the Cancer Difference Method.

Source: The A-Bomb Study (1950-1982), Both T65DR and DS86 Dosimetries.

Row	Col.A Dose- Group	Col.B Organ- Dose (cSv). RBE = 2 in T65DR	Col.C Organ- Dose (cSv). RBE = 20 in DS86	Col.D Initial Persons Male+Female in Dose-Group	Col.E Cancer- Deaths (except Leukemia) 1950-82	Col.F Cancer Death-Rate per 10,000 Initial Persons
1	Group 1	0.000	0.089	37173	2413.68	649.31
2	Group 2	1.511	1.890	28855	1881.04	651.89
3	Group 3	10.994	14.564	14943	1063.97	712.02
4	Group 4	35.361	40.625	4225	305.77	723.72
5	Group 5	71.308	74.238	3128	261.58	836.27
6	Group 6+7+8	176.662	197.054	2907	287.34	988.45
	SUM	T65DR	DS86	91231	6213.38	

REFERENCE-CLASS (Dose-Groups 1 + 2) :

Row		Col.B	Col.C	Col.D	Col.E	Col.F
7	Group (1+2)	0.659	0.875	66028	4297.08	650.80

THE SIX EXPOSED DOSE-CLASSES TO BE ANALYZED BY THE CANCER DIFFERENCE METHOD :

Row		Col.B	Col.C	Col.D	Col.E	Col.F
8	Low-Dose: Group 3	10.994	14.564	14943	1063.97	712.02
9	Groups (3+4)	16.365	20.309	19168	1369.74	714.60
10	All: (3+4+5+6+7+8)	41.673	47.388	25203	1918.67	761.29
11	Mid-Dose: (4+5)	50.653	54.924	7353	567.36	771.60
12	High-Dose:(5+6+7+8)	122.056	133.397	6035	548.93	909.57
13	Groups (6+7+8)	176.662	197.054	2907	287.34	988.45

NOTES -----

1. The data above include both cities, both sexes, all ages, and all cancer-sites (leukemia excluded). The cancer death-rate in Column F of each row is (Col.E / Col.D) x (10,000).

----

2. All entries in Rows 1 through 13 come from Table 11-H, and are reproduced here for convenience. (See Table 11-H, Note 2, about the slight disparity between entry E7 above and the sum of entries E1+E2.)

Table 13-B
Cancer–Yields at Different Levels of Exposure, by the Cancer Difference Method.

Basis: A-Bomb survivors, 1950-82. (Cities, sexes, ages, and all cancer-sites combined. Leukemia excluded.)
Cancer-hazard from X-rays may be underestimated by the A-Bomb Study. See this chapter, Part 4.

Cancer-Yields are radiation-induced cancer-deaths among 10,000 persons of mixed ages, per cSv of whole-body internal organ-dose.

Row	A Basis for Cancer-Yield	[----- Fatal Cancer-Yield -----] T65DR Dosimetry, Neutron RBE = 2.0						[------ Fatal Cancer-Yield ------] DS86 Dosimetry, Neutron RBE = 20					
		B Ref. vs. 11 cSv	C Ref. vs. 16 cSv	D Ref. vs. 42 cSv	E Ref. vs. 51 cSv	F Ref. vs. 122 cSv	G Ref. vs. 177 cSv	H Ref. vs. 15 cSv	I Ref. vs. 20 cSv	J Ref. vs. 47 cSv	K Ref. vs. 55 cSv	L Ref. vs. 133 cSv	M Ref. vs. 197 cSv
1	MINIMUM FATAL CANCER-YIELD "IN THE BOX"	5.92	4.06	2.69	2.42	2.13	1.92	4.47	3.28	2.38	2.24	1.95	1.72
2	MINIMUM FATAL CANCER-YIELD "IN THE BOX" Corrected for Underascert.	7.29	5.00	3.31	2.97	2.62	2.36	5.50	4.04	2.92	2.75	2.40	2.12
3	LIFETIME FATAL CANCER-YIELD	13.17	9.03	5.99	5.37	4.74	4.26	9.94	7.30	5.28	4.97	4.34	3.83
4	LIFETIME FATAL CANCER-YIELD Corrected for Underascert.	16.20	11.11	7.37	6.61	5.83	5.25	12.23	8.98	6.50	6.11	5.34	4.71

1. The Cancer-Yields above in Row 1 are each calculated from Table 13-A as demonstrated in the text. For instance, entry B1 above is -- with reference to Table 13-A -- (F8 minus F7) / (B8 minus B7). Each Cancer-Yield is a difference in cancer-rate divided by the corresponding difference in dose. Each value in Row 1 reflects the linear approximation between the Reference Dose (Table 13-A, entries B7, C7) and one specific dose at a time (Table 13-A, entries B8-B13, C8-C13, taken serially).

----

2. However, the findings in Row 1 suggest that dose-response is not linear, but rather is supra-linear everywhere in the dose-range. Along Row 1, the average potency per cSv (rem) is falling as dose rises, instead of showing constancy at all dose-levels.

----

3. Minimum Fatal Cancer-Yields are called "In-the-Box" because they represent no forward projection; they quantify only the radiation-induced deaths already observed 1950-82. The adjustment for under-ascertainment of cancer-deaths is a factor of 1.23, as suggested by RERF and BEIR-3 (see Chapter 11).

----

4. Entries for Lifetime Fatal Cancer-Yields, which are the Minimum values times 2.223 (see text), are probably underestimates (see Table 16-B).

----

5. The central values above represent the best estimates from the Cancer Difference Method, prior to regression analysis. There is, of course, sampling variation in every database. The 90 % confidence-limits on the values above are calculated in Chapter 27, Part 2. It is neither scientifically nor socially responsible to select the lowest value in a confidence-range for use, or the highest value either. The appropriate value to use is the one most likely to be right: The obtained value.

Figure 13–A

T65DR Dosimetry: Cumulative Cancer–Deaths versus Dose.

For the atomic-bomb survivors, this plot shows cumulative cancer-deaths (1950-1982) per 10,000 initial persons, versus mean whole-body internal organ-dose in the T65DR dosimetry (neutron RBE = 2).

Data for the six observations (indicated by the boxes) are from Table 13-A, Rows 1 through 6, Columns B and F.

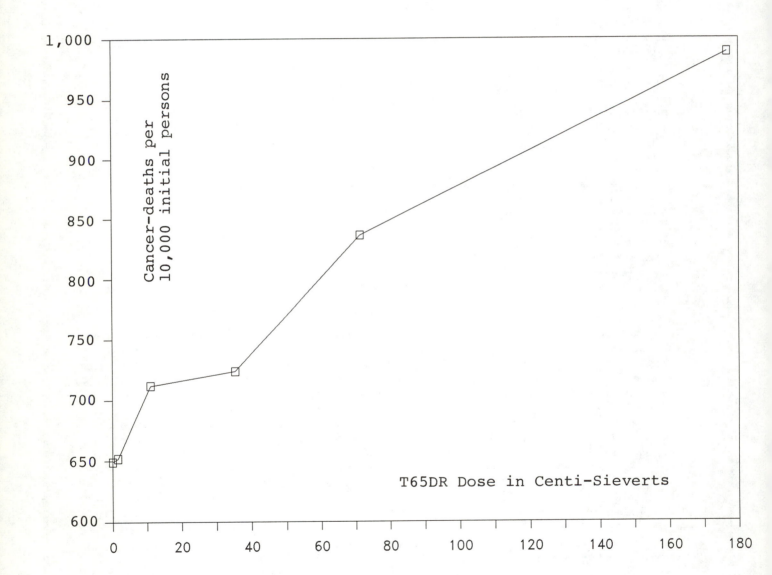

Figure 13-B

DS86 Dosimetry: Cumulative Cancer–Deaths versus Dose.

For the atomic-bomb survivors, this plot shows cumulative cancer-deaths (1950-1982) per 10,000 initial persons, versus mean whole-body internal organ-dose in the DS86 dosimetry (neutron RBE = 20).

Data for the six observations (indicated by the boxes) are from Table 13-A, Rows 1 through 6, Columns C and F.

This plot shows cancer-response versus dose for exactly the SAME cohorts of survivors as Figure 13-A. This is the "constant-cohort, dual-dosimetry" approach to the DS86 dosimetry. The only difference between Figures 13-A and 13-B is the mean internal organ-dose assigned to the cohorts. (The dose-scale in this figure extends up to 200 cSv.)

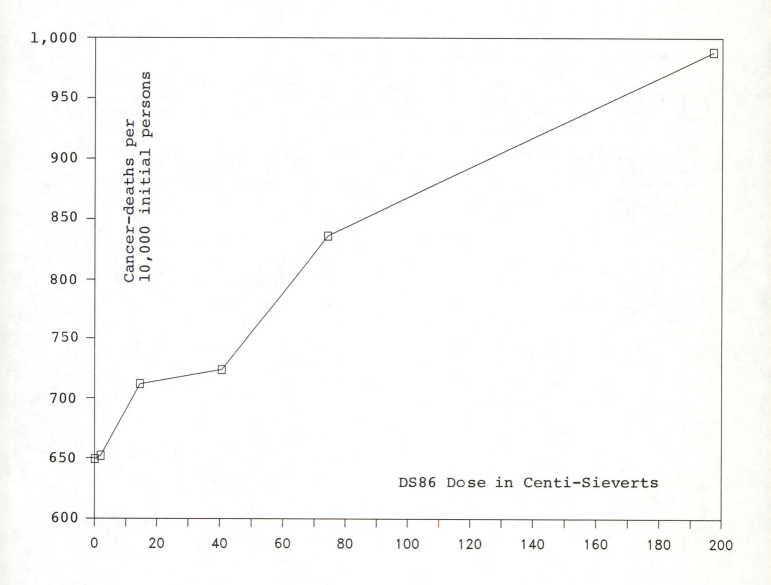

Figure 13–C

Contrast between Concave-Downward (Supra-Linear) and Concave-Upward Dose-Response Relationships.

Both curves A and B, below, depict the behavior of a response (for instance, cancer death-rate) as a dose of something increases. The response need not be cancer death-rate, and the "something" need not be ionizing radiation. Curves A and B are just generic dose-response curves.

Curve A = Supra-Linear Curvature :
===

The shape of Curve A is often called "concave-downward" or supra-linear. It is supra-linear because, if a straight line is drawn between any two points along the curve, the curve will lie ABOVE the line.

In a supra-linear dose-response, the risk per unit of dose is highest in the low dose-range. The magnitude of response, per unit of increase in dose, DECLINES with rising dose.

Curve B = Concave-Upward Curvature :
===

The shape of Curve B is often called "concave-upward." In Curve B, if a straight line is drawn between any two points along the curve, the curve will lie BELOW the line. In a concave-upward dose-response, the risk per unit of dose is lowest in the low dose-range. The magnitude of response, per unit of increase in dose, RISES with rising dose.

The dose-response relationship depicted by Curve B is often called "linear-quadratic" -- which is an ambiguous term unless the sign of the quadratic term is specified. When the quadratic term is positive, the shape is concave-upward, but when the quadratic term is negative, the shape is concave-downward. (This is explained in Chapter 23, Part 2.)

Concave-Downward,
or Supra-Linear
Dose-Response Relationship

Concave-Upward, or
Linear-Quadratic (Q-positive)
Dose-Response Relationship

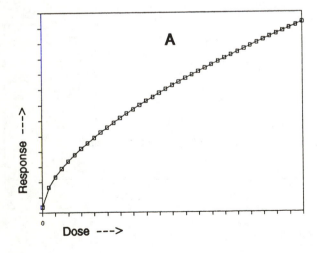

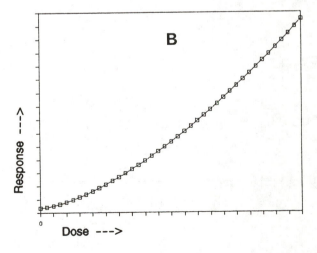

CHAPTER 14

Shape of the Dose-Response Relationship, and Low-Dose Cancer-Yields Based on the Best-Fit Curve

This chapter is arranged in six parts:

In the previous chapter, the Cancer Difference Method gives us Minimum Fatal Cancer-Yields in both the T65DR and DS86 dosimetries, and the results indicate that the cancer-risk is more severe per centi-sievert (rem) at low doses than at high doses. In other words, the findings in the previous chapter strongly suggest that shape of dose versus cancer-response is presently supra-linear. (Other terms for supra-linear, including "concave-downward," "upward convex," and even "sub-linear," are discussed in Chapter 23, Part 4.)

In this chapter, we will use the technique of curvilinear regression analysis for three purposes: (A) to depict the shape of dose-response in the A-bomb survivors, (B) to determine whether or not the supra-linear shape meets the test of statistical significance, and (C) to calculate Cancer-Yields based on the best-fit equation.

1. Supra-Linear Shape of the Dose-Response

In Chapter 29, we have used the data from Table 13-A, Rows 1 through 6, to demonstrate the technique of curvilinear regression. The steps of input, output, writing the best-fit equation, plotting graphs, and statistical testing are all presented in detail in that chapter. Readers who consult Chapter 29 will see for themselves exactly how we obtain the findings which are discussed in this chapter and elsewhere.

Findings from Chapter 29 are brought forward into this chapter. For instance, the equation which best fits the observations, in the T65DR dosimetry, is brought forward from Table 29-B and is presented in the Upper Notes of Table 14-A of this chapter.

Using the equation, we have calculated the predicted cancer-rates in Table 14-A, Column C, for dose-intervals of 10 cSv -- and for even smaller intervals at very low doses. In addition, Column C includes best-fit cancer-rates calculated for the specific organ-doses where we have the observed cancer-rates, so that the observed rate (in Column D) and the rate predicted by the curve (in Column C) can be compared. (Readers can ignore Columns E, F, and G until Part 5 of this chapter.)

Since the best-fit equation can provide predicted cancer-rates at any dose-level, of course Table 14-A includes estimates for 2, 5, and 10 cSv -- doses which lie between the mean doses received by Dose-Group 2 and Dose-Group 3. These estimated rates are interpolations between two actual observations; they are not extrapolations in a direction beyond any observed datapoint.

<u>*Figures 14-E and 14-F :*</u>

The information in Columns A, C, and D is plotted in Figure 14-E, which shows the cumulative cancer death-rate per 10,000 initial persons versus T65DR dose. The boxes are the actual observations, while the smooth curve says: This is what one would most probably see if one had more observations and less sampling variation.

Table 14-B and Figure 14-F provide the comparable information for the DS86 dosimetry.

Figures 14-E and 14-F look very much alike. Indeed, in both dosimetries, the equations which best fit the observations turn out to have the same dose-exponent: Dose^0.75. From Figures 14-E and F, it is self-evident that the dose-response curves are presently concave-downward (supra-linear) in both dosimetries.

(Our analysis has been made in terms of cancer-deaths per 10,000 initial persons. Some readers may be curious about the shape of dose-response if response is measured in cancers per 10,000 person-YEARS. The analysis is provided for them in Chapter 30.)

RERF's Treatment of Dose-Group 8 :

The actual dose-response must be somewhat more supra-linear than we can know. The basis for our statement is a fact found in RERF's report TR-9-87 (p.7). In Dose-Group 8 (the highest Dose-Group), "... the T65D total kerma is set equal to 6 Gy for all survivors whose T65D total kerma estimate is greater than 6 Gy." With this sentence, RERF refers to both TR-1-86 and TR-12-80, so apparently RERF has been throwing out some part of the dose not only in the 1950-1982 follow-up, but also in the previous 1950-1978 follow-up.

It follows that, in our own analysis, the combined Dose-Group 6+7+8 must really have a somewhat higher mean organ-dose than we can know. But, of course, the observed cancer death-rate would not change. Therefore, in Figure 14-E, the uppermost datapoint really needs some sliding to the right (toward higher dose), a move which would operate in the direction of greater supra-linear curvature. We are confident that the effect would be small. However, we do not see how RERF's handling of Dose-Group 8 can IMPROVE anyone's analysis of dose-response.

In Part 3 of this chapter, we identify another factor which also will operate in the direction of underestimating the supra-linearity of low-LET dose-response.

Males and Females Tested Separately :

By definition, the general public includes both sexes. It is impossible to have "population exposure" without irradiating both men and women. Therefore, if analysts are evaluating the dose-response from exposure of a general population, what matters is the NET dose-response. When they treat males and females as a unit in their analyses, the shape they obtain for dose versus cancer-response necessarily incorporates and reflects whatever difference may exist in male versus female response.

For other purposes, however, we may want to know if males and females are alike in the shape of dose-response. Of course, the moment analysts start subdividing the database, they increase the small-numbers problem, and findings are necessarily less reliable.

Using exactly the steps demonstrated in Chapter 29, we did regression analyses for males and females separately. The input data for cancer-rates and mean organ-doses were obtained from Table 11-G. The results are summarized below, in the equations of best fit. All the equations have supra-linear dose-exponents (below 1.0).

● -- MALES :

T65DR: Ca-deaths per 10,000 initial persons
   = $(5.986)(Dose^{0.75}) + 796.389$
DS86: Ca-deaths per 10,000 initial persons
   = $(7.248)(Dose^{0.70}) + 792.248$

● -- FEMALES :

T65DR: Ca-deaths per 10,000 initial persons
   = $(10.086)(Dose^{0.70}) + 540.838$
DS86: Ca-deaths per 10,000 initial persons
   = $(9.463)(Dose^{0.70}) + 538.102$

In other words, examined separately, males and females each show a supra-linear dose-response. The values of R-Squared for males are lower than for females, which means the finding is statistically weaker for males.

2. Basis for Ruling-Out a Concave-Upward Dose-Response

Chapter 29 demonstrates the technique of achieving curvilinear regression by raising a single dose-term, serially, to a variety of dose-exponents. We vary the exponent from Dose^2 (the quadratic dose-response), to Dose^1.4 and Dose^1.16 (linear-quadratic shapes), to Dose^1.0 (the linear dose-response), to Dose^0.85 and lower (supra-linear curves). Let us be explicit about the cancer-risks associated with these terms.

Supra-Linear Dose-Response :
This model of dose-response predicts that, with increase in total dose, the increase in cancer death-rate per cSv of dose will decrease. Each additional cSv of exposure will be less hazardous than the previous cSv. The plot of cancer-rate versus dose is concave-DOWNWARD (illustrated by Figure 14-A), and

==

the dose-exponent is less than 1.0.

Linear Dose-Response :

Here a plot of cancer death-rate versus dose yields a straight line -- hence the name "linear." The increase in cancer-rate per additional unit of dose is the same over the entire dose-range (illustrated by Figure 14-B), and the dose-exponent is 1.0.

Linear-Quadratic Dose-Response :

When the quadratic dose-term (Q) has a positive coefficient, this model predicts that the increase in cancer-rate, per unit increase in dose, will increase as total dose increases. Each additional cSv of exposure will be more hazardous than the previous cSv. The plot of cancer-rate versus dose is concave-UPWARD (illustrated by Figure 14-C). When a single dose-exponent is used, the exponent must be greater than 1.0, but less than 2.0.

However, as emphasized elsewhere (Go89b; also Chapters 23 and 29 of this book), when the quadratic term has a negative coefficient, the net result is a concave-DOWNWARD, supra-linear dose-response (see Figure 23-H).

Pure Quadratic Dose-Response :

This model, whose plot is also concave-UPWARD, bends away even more than the linear-quadratic dose-response from a straight line (illustrated by Figure 14-D), and the dose-exponent is 2.0.

Figures 14-A, B, C, D, for males and females combined, come from the input provided in Table 14-D. The four figures depict how the ACTUAL observations in the T65DR dosimetry relate to the values calculated by best-fit equations having the four shapes described above. Comparable figures are not included for the DS86 dosimetry simply because Figure 14-F already reveals that they would look like the T65DR figures.

Curve Fitting --
Supra-Linear Fit Is Significantly Better

In a good fit, not only should the weightiest observations lie close to the calculated curve, but their scatter (if any) should fall to both sides of it. In addition, it is a sign of poor fit if the observations on both ends lie on the same side of the curve while the observations in the middle all lie on the opposite side.

Inspection of Figures 14-A, B, C, and D shows the greatly inferior fit of both the linear-quadratic (Dose^1.4) and the pure quadratic (Dose^2) models. Indeed, such inspection predicts the results of the

formal statistical testing in Tables 29-D and E.

The results in Tables 29-D and 29-E show that the supra-linear dose-response in the A-Bomb Study (1950-1982), in both the T65DR and the DS86 dosimetries, is significantly better than the linear relationship (p = 0.01).

As for a concave-upward dose-response, statistical testing in Tables 29-D and 29-E simply rules out such a relationship as the plausible choice. Even in the absence of any formal statistical testing, this conclusion is evident from inspection of Figures 14-C and 14-D, compared with Figures 14-A and 14-B.

As an independent check on the statistical significance of the supra-linear fit, we also used the power polynomial method of curve-fitting. It shows that there is both a statistically significant linear dose-term (Dose^1.0) and a statistically significant quadratic dose-term (Dose ^2.0), and that the coefficient of the quadratic term is NEGATIVE. The equation of best fit from the power polynomial method produces a plot of cumulative cancer-rate versus dose which is virtually identical with the plot produced by the best-fit equation containing the Dose^0.75 term (Figures 14-E and 14-F).

Comparison with Statements from RERF :

Readers are in a position to evaluate our analysis of the shape of dose-response, step-by-step, from start to finish. They will not be able to compare it directly with RERF reports, however. RERF analysts are determining dose-response from input which is different from ours. For instance, in TR-5-88, Shimizu and co-workers discard the evidence between 1950-1955, and use only the observations from 1956 onwards. They are using only 75,991 of the initial 91,231 persons. For their 75,991 persons, they have additional observations out to 1985. They are using newly constructed cohorts, not a constant-cohort analysis. In effect, they are using a different database.

Nonetheless, there is a key similarity between our analysis and the analysis by Shimizu and co-workers: The RERF analysts do not find a concave-upward dose-response either. They find the following:

1. When they examine all cancers combined except leukemia as we do, and when they include all the Dose-Groups as we do, they find that their data fit linearity and supra-linearity equally well (Shi87, pp.28-30, and Shi88, pp.50-51).

2. When they examine males and females

separately and include all the evidence, as we do, again they indicate that they find a linear or supra-linear dose-response (Shi88, p.53, Table 19).

However, Shimizu and co-workers never use the term, supra-linear. Their important points about the supra-linear shape might even be missed by any readers who assume that LQ (linear-quadratic) and LQ-L models are always concave-UPWARD. The assumption would be mistaken. If the Q-coefficient for dose is NEGATIVE in an LQ model, the net LQ curvature is concave-DOWNWARD (Figure 23-H, again). Therefore readers of RERF reports need to pay close attention to RERF statements and footnotes such as:

"For those sites other than leukemia and colon, the fitted curve associated with the LQ model is invariably concave downwards, not upwards ..." (Shi87, top p.29).

"... since the curvature is invariably downwards when a curvilinear model gives an acceptable fit, this would imply a higher risk at low doses than that which obtains under a linear model" (Shi87, p.30).

"Coefficient for the Q-term is negative" for the LQ model; this is the footnote which applies to analysis of the full dose-range in Table 19 of TR-5-88 (Shi88, p.53).

A Possible Route to Error :

Having found the dose-response to be linear or supra-linear (concave-downward), Shimizu and co-workers propose an alternative way to determine the dose-response. We quote:

"For all cancers except leukemia, although the L model fits well for both the total dose range and the dose range excluding high doses, the LQ model can not be shown to be inappropriate statistically. It should be noted that Q term in the LQ model is negative when the entire dose range is used, reflecting the level off of the dose-response curve at the higher dose range. In order to obtain useful risk estimates in the low-dose range with the LQ model, we have estimated the risk limiting doses to under 2 Gy, so as to obtain a positive Q term" (Shi88, p.50-51).

Although the paper (Shi88) is unclear on whether 2 Gy is kerma dose or internal organ-dose unadjusted for RBE, the statement quoted above means that they threw away the high Dose-Groups (probably 6,7,8) because, in someone's opinion, supra-linearity (the negative Q-coefficient) is not "useful." Not useful to whom? And for what?

Where does such an approach to evidence end?

It may easily end in error. For instance, it is self-evident from Figures 13-A and 13-B in the previous chapter, that if one discarded Dose-Group 5 as well as Dose-Group 6-8, one would end up with the opposite result: The dose-response would be based on the four residual datapoints, and it would be MORE supra-linear, not less. (This statement is supported by regression analysis which excludes Dose-Groups 5-8).

Moreover, if we look objectively at the entries in Table 13-A, Column E, we see that the absolute number of cancer-deaths observed in Dose-Group 4 is about the same as in Dose-Group 5, and also in the combined Dose-Group 6+7+8. This means that the statistical reliability of each of these three observations is about the same. If analysts are willing to discard one, then on an objective basis, why should they not discard all three?

Suppose the first discarding of data (Dose-Groups 6-8) would result in DECREASING the study's supra-linear curvature, but suppose the next, equally justifiable discarding of data (Dose-Group 5) would result in EXAGGERATING its supra-linear curvature. What is the appropriate choice?

In my opinion, the curvature which is most likely to be right is the curvature which comes from using ALL the available evidence. It would certainly not be science at all, if I were to keep the evidence which leads to answers I may LIKE, while throwing out the evidence which produces answers I may NOT like.

In my judgment, analysts will be most likely to obtain the RIGHT answer about dose-response when they use all of the observations. The reason is this. The jaggedness observed in Figures 13-A and 13-B has virtually no chance of being biologically meaningful. Such jaggedness is almost certainly the result of sampling variation, which means that it would not be there (the dose-response would be smooth) if the study had included a BILLION persons instead of only 91,231. One of the great scientific virtues of the A-Bomb Study is its inclusion of such a vast range of doses. If we USE all the data in regression analysis, the additional observations are likely to help "correct" the jaggedness of sampling variation. But if we start throwing away any of the valuable evidence without a very good reason indeed, we will almost certainly increase the chance of mistaken results.

Conclusion
about Shape in the A-Bomb Study :

Our analysis of dose-response is based on ALL the

evidence. No Dose-Groups (and no follow-up years) have been thrown out. Our findings fit concavity-DOWNWARD (supra-linearity) provably better than linearity, and fit concavity-downward enormously better than concavity-UPWARD.

We are forced to conclude, not by preference but by the evidence currently available to us, that concavity-upward is NOT credible as the shape of dose-response in the A-Bomb Study. The credible choice is presently supra-linearity.

Will supra-linearity persist to the end of the study, decades from now? No one can know. (As we said in Chapter 12, no one can rule out even remote possibilities -- like there being no EXCESS cancer anymore at the end of the study, which would mean a flat dose-response. Of course, in that unlikely case, the INTERIM excess of cancer-deaths would represent a major misery for those who died from the disease 10, 20, 30, 40 years earlier than otherwise.)

Meanwhile, analysts must report whatever is ruled in and out by the CURRENTLY available evidence. This chapter and Chapter 29 rule out the concave-upward shape as a good fit for the 1950-1982 observations. The data say that the dose-response curvature is concave-DOWNWARD.

It should be emphasized that the findings about dose-response -- like the findings for MINIMUM Fatal Cancer-Yields -- involve no forward projections and no hypotheses about radiation carcinogenesis. Our findings simply amount to an objective description of what the present evidence IS on the shape of the dose-response.

3. Purely Low-Let Radiation versus Mixed (Gamma + Neutron)

The dose-response curve which fits the observations best is presently concave-downward or supra-linear (Figure 14-E for the T65DR dosimetry; Figure 14-F for the DS86 dosimetry). In each dosimetry, the equation which generates the best-fit has a dose-exponent of 0.75.

The dose-input for the regression-analysis (Chapter 29) was composed of two types of radiation: Gamma and neutron. (Tables 9-C and 10-E, Row 14, show the small fraction of the internal organ-dose, in rems, which was contributed by neutrons.) Therefore, the curves depict dose-response for a mixture of the two radiations.

Nonetheless, one must conclude that the concave-downward curvature is caused by the low-LET (gamma) component of the exposure, not by the high-LET (neutron) component.

The basis for this conclusion is clear if we start by imagining that the A-bomb survivors received ONLY neutron-exposure, but no gamma exposure. For neutron-exposure, the experimental observation is that dose-response is linear, at least up to 10 rads of total neutron dose (Chapter 8, Part 5). And if we adjust for the greater carcinogenic potency of neutrons, by multiplying neutron doses (below 10 rads) by a constant RBE of 20 to obtain rems, a plot of cancer-rate versus pure neutron doses in rems would still be linear. We have shown (page 8-8) that the highest mean neutron organ-dose was about 4.369 rads in the DS86 dosimetry, where such doses are supposed to be correct; 4.369 is a dose well below 10. Therefore, if the A-bomb survivors had received ONLY neutron-exposure, our plots of cancer-rates versus dose in rems would be LINEAR.

Now, we return to the real situation. The A-bomb survivors ALSO received a gamma dose. And when cancer-rate is plotted versus dose in rems, for the COMBINED neutron and gamma doses, the best fit for the observations becomes supra-linear, even though it would have been linear if only the neutrons had been present. It follows that the curvature is caused by the gamma exposure, not by the neutrons.

Underestimation of the Low-Let Curvature :

Our analyses must somewhat UNDERestimate the true degree of supra-linearity for low-LET (gamma) dose-response. Table 10-E, Row 14, shows that the fraction of total dose, in cSv, contributed by neutrons rises with rising total dose. The rising share from neutrons (from 5.4 % in Dose-Group 2, up to 18 % in Dose-Group 8) prevents the supra-linear curvature for gamma-exposure from being fully seen.

The gamma's supra-linear dose-response means that the percent increase in spontaneous cancer-rate, per average rem of gamma dose, FALLS as gamma-dose rises. By contrast, the neutron's linear dose-response means that the carcinogenicity of neutrons is CONSTANT in all eight dose-groups. As the combined dose from gammas and neutrons is rising, the average carcinogenicity of the gamma rems is falling whereas the carcinogenicity of the neutron rems is NOT falling.

Therefore, when neutrons contribute an "extra" share of the combined dose as the combined dose is rising (Table 10-E, Rows 11 and 14), it means that the observed cancer-rates at the higher doses are somewhat elevated above the rates which would have occurred if the fraction contributed by neutrons had not risen. The result is that the "extra" share from neutrons progressively "lifts" the right-hand half of the curve of Cancer-Rate versus Combined Dose, in the direction of linearity. In other words, the supra-linear curvature would be MORE pronounced if the fraction of combined dose coming from neutrons had not risen. Thus the supra-linearity of low-LET dose-response is somewhat underestimated in our DS86 analyses.

4. Basis for Generalizing from the A-Bomb Study

This chapter and Chapter 29 have confirmed what Table 13-B so strongly suggested: The dose-response is presently supra-linear throughout the dose-range. The result does not depend on high-dose data. If analysts threw out Dose-Groups 5-8, the supra-linearity would be even more pronounced. We would emphatically NOT approve of throwing out data, however.

The finding, that dose-response for low-LET exposure is concave-downward (supra-linear), is based on observation of all fatal cancers COMBINED, with only leukemia excluded. In other words, the finding does not rest on a small study involving just leukemia or a few cancer-sites, or on a study resting on incidence instead of mortality. And the finding is based on two dosimetries. And the finding is not based on a single sex- or age-group. It is broadly based on both sexes and all ages.

In other words, the finding of supra-linearity at low doses is based on excellent human epidemiological evidence -- in our judgment, the best which is available at this time anywhere.

Therefore, it is scientifically reasonable to generalize from the A-Bomb Study, 1950-1982: In humans, the dose-response for induction of fatal cancer by low-LET ionizing radiation is most probably supra-linear in shape, even at low doses. The risk per rem RISES as total dose falls.

This finding is directly at variance with the widely applied presumption -- not based on human epidemiology -- that the human cancer-hazard per centi-sievert of low-LET exposure would go DOWN with decreasing total doses. Readers are referred to Un77, p.414, para.318; Un86, p.191, para.153; Beir80, p.190; Ncrp80, pp.5-9; Nih85, p.iv; Nrc85, p.II-101-103;

Doe87, p.7.3, 7.4; and others. Some of these sources use the presumption, while also acknowledging that the available human epidemiological data do not SUPPORT it (see Chapter 22).

The Past and Future of Supra-Linearity :

The supra-linear shape of dose-response has been showing up in the A-Bomb Study for at least three consecutive follow-ups: 1950-1974, 1950-1978, and 1950-1982 (Go81; Go89a; Ncrp80 -- details in our Chapter 22, Part 2). In other words, supra-linearity is not a characteristic which appeared only with the addition of the 1978-1982 observations. And, according to RERF analysts (Shi87; Shi88), it is still showing up in the revised database when they add some observations through 1985 (see this chapter, Part 2).

Although no one can be sure that supra-linearity will continue its persistence through all future follow-ups, the only reasonable forward projection is the one which rests on the best available evidence. And the best available evidence, from at least three consecutive follow-ups, suggests that supra-linearity will persist.

On the other hand, if the A-Bomb Study itself does not persist with a continuous "constant-cohort, dual-dosimetry" database, it will be hard for anyone to sort out which future findings on dose-response result from extension of the time-interval since the exposure, and which future findings result from perpetual revision of the DS86 doses and cohorts.

5. Low-Dose Cancer-Yields Based on the Best-Fit Curve

When analysts seek to estimate the cancer-hazard from exposing populations of mixed ages to ionizing radiation, the doses received by Dose-Group 3 in the A-Bomb Study are considerably higher than the relevant levels suggested by nuclear accidents like Chernobyl, for example. We should be asking, what are the likely Cancer-Yields if people receive total doses like 5 cSv (or less)?

Tables 14-A and 14-B provide the probable values for the MINIMUM Fatal Cancer-Yields, in Column G. We have starred the entries calculated from 5 cSv of total exposure, because we think those are the appropriate ones to use for low-dose exposures up to 5 cSv and for slow exposures. (We closely examine the issue of slow dose-rates in Chapter 23, Parts 6 and 7.)

The notes of Tables 14-A and 14-B explain exactly how the values were obtained. Readers will see that this is still the Cancer Difference Method: A difference in cancer-rate is divided by the corresponding difference in dose. However, in this version, the cancer-rates are not the direct observations; instead, they are the rates predicted after the actual observations have produced an equation of best fit. In Tables 14-A and 14-B, the division-step for the starred entries at 5 cSv amounts to the approximation that every rem (cSv) between 0 and 5 rems is EQUALLY potent.

Table 14-C assembles the low-dose Cancer-Yields from Table 13-B as well as from Tables 14-A and 14-B, so that they can be easily compared with each other. The net effect of regression-analysis is to reduce the T65DR risk-estimate below its value in Table 13-B, and to render it almost identical with the DS86 estimate.

The Basing of Values
on a Total Dose of 5 Centi-Sieverts :

Readers may wonder why we suggest using Cancer-Yields calculated from a total dose of 5 cSv, even for use with population-exposure which might be lower (say, one centi-sievert or less). At first glance, it may look as if we are deliberately underestimating the likely Minimum Fatal Cancer-Yields from very low-dose exposure, since we are using linearity instead of supra-linearity between 0 dose and 5 rems.

Our reasoning is as follows. The technique of curvilinear regression provides the values of low-dose Cancer-Yield which are most likely to be true, given the evidence at hand. And the equation which has the highest R-Squared value in regression analysis is the equation which is most likely to make the best predictions. Therefore the equation which we should use, and which we DO use, is the one in which the dose-exponent is 0.75. Objectivity requires use of results from available evidence, rather than use of preconceptions about how the curvature "ought" to behave at low doses (see Chapter 23). Unlike the BEIR-3 Committee (see Chapter 22), we do not constrain any regression in order to make it support a pre-judgment.

On the other hand, as we pointed out in Chapter 29, while we know that 0.75 is significantly better than the dose-exponent 1.0, we do not know that 0.75 is significantly better than 0.80, 0.85, 0.70, or 0.65. Yet the shape of the curve is such that small changes in the dose-exponent have a big effect, at one or two cSv, on the values for Cancer-Yield in Columns F and G of Tables 14-A and 14-B. In view of this sensitivity, we want to avoid using any values for Cancer-Yield derived directly from the curve at one or two cSv.

We regard our decision as a scientifically reasonable judgment which simultaneously (A) avoids the irresponsibility of throwing away the low-dose results of regression analysis down to 5 cSv, and (B) avoids the introduction of any unstable element into an analysis which has been securely based in reality.

A Comment by RERF about BEIR Choices :

The shape of dose-response is central to obtaining risk-estimates at low (and slow) doses. If analysts choose unrealistic versions of the dose-response relationship, they will provide unrealistic estimates of cancer-hazard. RERF analysts, in trying to figure out why their own current risk-estimates are so much higher than those of the BEIR-3 Committee, comment (TR-5-88, p.51):

[Some of the disparity] "... may be ascribed to the fact that in BEIR III, the curvature in dose response for leukemia was used for all cancers except leukemia instead of the actual curvature which probably is much closer to linearity, and this may cause much smaller estimates to be produced than if the actual dose-response curve were to be applied."

Venturing below 10 Rems :

Now that we have examined the logic and results of regression analysis, as a tool for obtaining a smooth and probable dose-response at all doses, we can discuss a matter which puzzles us and may puzzle readers too.

In its 1980 report, the BEIR-3 Committee declined to make risk-estimates for acute exposures lower than 10 rems (Beir80, p.144). RERF analysts appear to be split on this issue. In TR-9-87 (Pr87b, p.35), Preston and Pierce present their estimates of Lifetime Fatal Cancer-Yield as cancer deaths per 10 milli-sieverts (per rem). By contrast, in TR-5-88 (Shi88, Table 19, p.53), Shimizu and co-workers explicitly constrain their estimates of Lifetime Fatal Cancer-Yields to acute exposures of 0.1 Sievert (10 rems).

It is puzzling to us that Shimizu and co-workers make a big effort to determine what the dose-response relationship is, starting at zero dose, and then they seem unwilling to USE it in the low dose-range. As we pointed out in Part 1 of this chapter, estimates below 10 rems are not extrapolations in a direction beyond any actual observations. Such estimates are interpolations BETWEEN actual observations in Dose-Group 3 and Dose-Group 2. Indeed, Dose-Groups 1-3 provide the most reliable observations in the whole study, in terms of cancer-cases (not necessarily in dosimetry). If analysts will not use the section of the dose-response

BELOW Dose-Group 3, it would seem they should have no reason to use it ABOVE Dose-Group 3 either, where the datapoints are based on far fewer cancer-deaths.

By contrast, to us it seems highly reasonable -- almost obligatory -- for analysts to presume that the dose-response which derives from the dose-range as a whole ALSO characterizes the little segment between zero dose and 10 rems.

On the other hand, refusal to make estimates below 10 rems could be a way of suggesting that maybe the risk of radiation-induced cancer just disappears somewhere between 10 rems and zero dose.

The human evidence against any harmless dose of ionizing radiation, with respect to carcinogenesis, is examined in detail in the Threshold section of this book (Section 5). Here we shall limit our comments to the A-Bomb Study (see also Chapter 35, Part 9).

The A-Bomb Study, properly handled, certainly offers no basis for belief in a threshold, or a lesser hazard per rem either, anywhere below 10 rems. On the contrary. Its present supra-linear curvature indicates the risk per rem is growing steadily higher as dose approaches zero. Even if its present dose-response were linear (instead of supra-linear), this would be no basis for belief either in a safe threshold somewhere below 10 rems, or a lesser effect per rem.

In short, even if there were no additional evidence in Section 5 against a threshold, and even if the dose-response in the A-Bomb Study were linear instead of supra-linear, we would consider the basis for making risk-estimates below 10 rems to be scientifically compelling.

6. The Bottom Line from Best-Fit Curves

1. This chapter and Chapter 29 show that the relationship between dose and cancer-response per 10,000 initial persons is presently supra-linear (concave-downward). Statistical testing demonstrates that the evidence fits a concave-DOWNWARD curvature significantly better than the evidence fits a linear dose-response, and very much better than it fits a concave-UPWARD shape. See Figures 14-A, B, C, and D. In short, the present evidence from the A-bomb survivors is that cancer-risk is greater per rem (centi-sievert) at low doses than at high doses, in both dosimetries. (Chapter 30 shows the same finding in cancer-response per 10,000 person-YEARS.)

2. The finding of supra-linearity is solidly based in the existing evidence, and does not rely on any forward projections, hypotheses, or models. We have simply presented an objective description of what the available evidence is showing in a database which covers all cancers (leukemia excluded), all doses, all ages, and both sexes. This direct and comprehensive human epidemiological evidence carries great scientific weight compared with observations from other species, of course, or from laboratory experiments.

3. The evidence is at variance with the assumption, almost universally used by the radiation community, that the cancer-risk should be less severe per rem at low acute doses than at high acute doses. With regard to low doses delivered SLOWLY, we show in Chapter 23, Part 7, that there is no reason to reduce the low-dose Cancer-Yields in Table 14-C when exposure is slow instead of acute.

4. Although no one can be certain that the supra-linear curvature will persist through all future follow-ups, the only reasonable forward projection is the one which rests on the best available evidence. And the best available evidence, from at least three consecutive follow-ups, is that supra-linearity is persistent. However, if the A-Bomb Study ITSELF does not persist with a continuous "constant-cohort, dual-dosimetry" database, it will be hard for anyone to sort out which future findings on dose-response result from extension of the time-interval since the bombings, and which future findings result from perpetual revision of the DS86 doses and cohorts.

5. Regression analysis provides the best-fit equation for dose-response, and the equation can predict cancer-rates at any dose-level, including doses like 2, 5, and 10 rems which lie between the mean dose received by Dose-Group 2 and Dose-Group 3. The estimated cancer-rates at these doses are interpolations between two actual observations -- they are not extrapolations in a direction beyond any observed data-point.

6. Unlike some current analysis at RERF, our analysis of dose-response uses ALL of the observations, high-dose and low-dose, and ALL of the follow-up years, in order to obtain the most reliable results. We do not approve of throwing away evidence without a very good reason indeed. It should be noted that the supra-linear curvature of dose versus cancer-response occurs throughout the dose-range. In fact, if the high-dose evidence from Dose-Groups 5-8 were discarded, the low-dose evidence from Dose-Groups 1-4 would produce greater supra-linearity -- not less.

7. The best-fit equation from our regression analysis is used to obtain another set of Minimum and Lifetime Fatal Cancer-Yields by the Cancer Difference Method, for low-dose exposure. Table 14-C compares the new set with the first set, in both T65DR and DS86 dosimetries. The net effect of regression analysis is to REDUCE the estimate in the T65DR dosimetry. In the new set of estimates, the Lifetime Cancer-Yields remain probable underestimates, as they were in Table 13-B.

The Lifetime Fatal Cancer-Yield from the best-fit curve is 12.90 in the T65DR dosimetry, and 12.03 in the current version of the DS86 dosimetry. By contrast, the lifetime values commonly used by the radiation community for statements about low-dose exposure are between 1.0 and 2.0 (see Chapter 24, Part 7, and Chapter 34, Wolfe).

Table 14-A
T65DR Dosimetry: Comparison of Calculated Cancer-Rates with Observed Cancer-Rates.
T65DR Dosimetry: Minimum Fatal Cancer-Yields per Centi-Sievert among 10,000 Persons.

Col.A Dose cSv T65DR	Col.B Dose^0.75	Col.C Cancer-Rate per 10,000 Calculated	Col.D Cancer-Rate per 10,000 Observed	Col.E Calculated Ca-Rate MINUS the Calculated Spontaneous Ca-Rate	Col.F Avg.Incr. in Ca-Rate per cSv	Col.G MINIMUM FATAL CA-YIELD
0	0.00000	649.5440	649.31			
1	1.00000	656.5968		7.053	7.053	8.675
1.511	1.36260	659.1542	651.89	9.610	6.362	7.825
2	1.68179	661.4053		11.861	5.931	7.295
5	3.34370	673.1265		23.582	4.716	5.801 *
10	5.62341	689.2048		39.661	3.966	4.878
10.994	6.03762	692.1261	712.02	42.582	3.873	4.764
20	9.45742	716.2453		66.701	3.335	4.102
30	12.81861	739.9511		90.407	3.014	3.707
35.361	14.50098	751.8165	723.72	102.273	2.892	3.557
40	15.90541	761.7217		112.178	2.804	3.449
50	18.80302	782.1579		132.614	2.652	3.262
60	21.55825	801.5900		152.046	2.534	3.117
70	24.20045	820.2250		170.681	2.438	2.999
71.308	24.53891	822.6120	836.27	173.068	2.427	2.985
80	26.74961	838.2037		188.660	2.358	2.901
90	29.22011	855.6276		206.084	2.290	2.816
100	31.62278	872.5731		223.029	2.230	2.743
110	33.96601	889.0995		239.555	2.178	2.679
120	36.25650	905.2539		255.710	2.131	2.621
130	38.49971	921.0748		271.531	2.089	2.569
140	40.70015	936.5940		287.050	2.050	2.522
150	42.86161	951.8383		302.294	2.015	2.479
160	44.98731	966.8305		317.286	1.983	2.439
170	47.08003	981.5900		332.046	1.953	2.402
176.662	48.45714	991.3025	988.45	341.759	1.935	2.379
180	49.14218	996.1339		346.590	1.925	2.368
190	51.17587	1010.477		360.933	1.900	2.337
200	53.18296	1024.633		375.089	1.875	2.307

UPPER NOTES: -----
   Entries in Col.A come from Table 13-A, with many doses added between observations.
   Entries in Col.C for the predicted rates are calculated, both for observed doses and
interpolated doses, with the equation derived from Table 29-B:
                    Cancer-Rate = (7.0528)(Dose^0.75) + 649.544.
   Values for the term (Dose^0.75) are obtained from Col.B above.
   Entries in Col.D come from Table 13-A, and lie near the calculated values.
   Columns A, C, and D are plotted in Figure 14-E.

-------------------------------- Right-Hand Side of Table ---------------------------------

FATAL CANCER-YIELD = NUMBER OF RADIATION-INDUCED CANCER-DEATHS AMONG 10,000
   INITIAL PERSONS OF MIXED AGES, PER CENTI-SIEVERT OF WHOLE-BODY INTERNAL ORGAN-DOSE.

   Entries in Col.E are Col.C minus 649.544 (which is the calculated spontaneous rate / 10,000).
   Entries in Col.F are Col.E / Col.A.   The entries correspond to the Min. Fatal Cancer-Yield
calculated by the Cancer Difference Method, before the 1.23-fold correction used by RERF for
underascertainment of cancer-deaths (see Chapter 11).   The progressive decline of Col.F entries
with rising dose reflects the supra-linearity of dose-response.
   Entries in Col.G are Col.F entries times 1.23, the underascertainment correction.   The
starred value is the one which we use for low-dose exposure.   In subsequent chapters also, we
use values per cSv based on best-fit at 5 cSv.

Table 14-B
DS86 Dosimetry: Comparison of Calculated Cancer-Rates with Observed Cancer-Rates.
DS86 Dosimetry: Minimum Fatal Cancer-Yields per Centi-Sievert among 10,000 Persons.

Col.A Dose cSv DS86	Col.B Dose^0.75	Col.C Cancer-Rate per 10,000 Calculated	Col.D Cancer-Rate per 10,000 Observed	Col.E Calculated Ca-Rate MINUS the Calculated Spontaneous Ca-Rate	Col.F Avg.Incr. in Ca-Rate per cSv	Col.G MINIMUM FATAL CA-YIELD
0	0.0000	647.693				
0.089	0.1634	648.768	649.31			
1	1.0000	654.272		6.579	6.579	8.093
1.890	1.6121	658.299	651.89	10.606	5.611	6.902
2	1.6818	658.758		11.065	5.533	6.805
5	3.3437	669.692		21.999	4.400	5.412 *
10	5.6234	684.691		36.998	3.700	4.551
14.564	7.4553	696.744	712.02	49.051	3.368	4.143
20	9.4574	709.916		62.223	3.111	3.827
30	12.8186	732.030		84.337	2.811	3.458
40	15.9054	752.339		104.646	2.616	3.218
40.625	16.0915	753.564	723.72	105.871	2.606	3.205
50	18.8030	771.404		123.711	2.474	3.043
60	21.5582	789.531		141.838	2.364	2.908
70	24.2005	806.915		159.222	2.275	2.798
74.238	25.2911	814.091	836.27	166.398	2.241	2.757
80	26.7496	823.687		175.994	2.200	2.706
90	29.2201	839.941		192.248	2.136	2.627
100	31.6228	855.749		208.056	2.081	2.559
110	33.9660	871.166		223.473	2.032	2.499
120	36.2565	886.235		238.542	1.988	2.445
130	38.4997	900.994		253.301	1.948	2.397
140	40.7002	915.472		267.779	1.913	2.353
150	42.8616	929.692		281.999	1.880	2.312
160	44.9873	943.678		295.985	1.850	2.275
170	47.0800	957.447		309.754	1.822	2.241
180	49.1422	971.014		323.321	1.796	2.209
197.054	52.5943	993.727	988.45	346.034	1.756	2.160
200	53.1830	997.600		349.907	1.750	2.152

UPPER NOTES: -----
    Entries in Col.A come from Table 13-A, with many doses added between observations.
    Entries in Col.C for the predicted rates are calculated, both for observed doses and
interpolated doses, with the equation derived from Table 29-C:
$$\text{Cancer-Rate} = (6.5793)(\text{Dose}^{0.75}) + 647.693.$$
    Values for the term (Dose^0.75) are obtained from Col.B above.
    Entries in Col.D come from Table 13-A, and lie near the calculated values.
    Columns A, C, and D are plotted in Figure 14-F.

--------------------------------------- Right-Hand Side of Table ---------------------------------------

FATAL CANCER YIELD = NUMBER OF RADIATION-INDUCED CANCER-DEATHS AMONG
    10,000 PERSONS OF MIXED AGES, PER CENTI-SIEVERT OF WHOLE-BODY INTERNAL ORGAN-DOSE.

    Entries in Col.E are Col.C minus 647.693 (which is the calculated spontaneous rate / 10,000).
    Entries in Col.F are Col.E / Col.A. The entries correspond to the Min. Fatal Cancer-Yield
calculated by the Cancer Difference Method, before the 1.23-fold correction used by RERF for
underascertainment of cancer-deaths (see Chapter 11). The progressive decline of Col.F entries
with rising dose reflects the supra-linearity of dose-response.
    Entries in Col.G are Col.F entries times 1.23, the underascertainment correction. The
starred value is the one which we use for low-dose exposure. In subsequent chapters also, we
use values per cSv based on best-fit at 5 cSv.

Table 14-C

Cancer-Yields at the Low Doses, by the Cancer Difference Method, with and without Curvilinear Regression.

Basis: A-bomb survivors, all ages combined, 1950-1982. Both T65DR and DS86 dosimetries.
Cancer-hazard from X-rays may be underestimated by the A-Bomb Study. See Chapter 13, Part 4.

Cancer-Yields are radiation-induced cancer-deaths among 10,000 persons of mixed ages, per cSv of
whole-body internal organ-dose.
All Cancer-Yields below are corrected for underascertainment of cancer-deaths.

		---Fatal Cancer-Yield--- T65DR Dosimetry Neutron RBE = 2.0			---Fatal Cancer-Yield--- DS86 Dosimetry Neutron RBE = 20	
Col.A		Col.B	Col.C		Col.D	Col.E
Source of Estimate for Minimum Fatal Cancer-Yields		MINIMUM FATAL CANCER- YIELD	LIFETIME FATAL CANCER- YIELD		MINIMUM FATAL CANCER- YIELD	LIFETIME FATAL CANCER- YIELD
Row						
1 Dose-Group 3 versus Ref. Group Table 13-B.		7.29	16.20		5.50	12.23
2 Best-Fit Curve Tables 14-A and 14-B.		5.80	12.90		5.41	12.03

NOTES -----

1. The MINIMUM values above in Row 1 come from Table 13-B, Columns B and H. If there had been no dose-groups higher than Dose-Group 3 in the A-bomb experience, these are the only values which would exist in Table 13-B. The entries in Row 1 above are the values before regression analysis provides a smooth best-fit curve.

----

2. The MINIMUM values in Row 2 above come from the best-fit curves provided by regression analysis, using all dose-groups.
    The MINIMUM value in Row 2, Column B, comes from Table 14-A, Column G (the starred value).
    The MINIMUM value in Row 2, Column D, comes from Table 14-B, Column G (the starred value).

----

3. LIFETIME values (Columns C and E) are always the MINIMUM value times 2.223, in the Cancer Difference Method. The factor 2.223 comes from Table 28-D, Row 14. These LIFETIME entries are probably underestimates (see Chapter 13, Part 6, and Chapter 16, Table 16-B).

Table 14-D

Input Values for Figures 14-A, 14-B, 14-C, and 14-D. T65DR Dosimetry with Neutron RBE = 2.

Input for Figure 14-A

Equation for Dose^0.75 from Table 29-B:

Ca-Rate = (7.0528)(Dose^0.75) + 649.544

Dose cSv	Dose cSv^0.75	Ca-Rate Calc.	Ca-Rate Observed
0.000	0.0000	649.544	649.31
1.511	1.3626	659.154	651.89
10.994	6.0376	692.126	712.02
35.361	14.5010	751.817	723.72
71.308	24.5388	822.611	836.27
130.000	38.4997	921.075	
176.662	48.4571	991.303	988.45

Input for Figure 14-B

Equation for Dose^1 from Table 29-B:

Ca-Rate = (1.947)(Dose^1) + 661.153

Dose cSv	Dose cSv^1	Ca-Rate Calc.	Ca-Rate Observed
0.000	0.000	661.153	649.31
1.511	1.511	664.094	651.89
10.994	10.994	682.558	712.02
35.361	35.361	730.002	723.72
71.308	71.308	799.990	836.27
130.000	130.000	914.263	
176.662	176.662	1005.114	988.45

Input for Figure 14-C

Equation for Dose^1.4 from Table 29-B:

Ca-Rate = (0.242)(Dose^1.4) + 671.922

Dose cSv	Dose cSv^1.4	Ca-Rate Calc.	Ca-Rate Observed
0.000	0.000	671.922	649.31
1.511	1.782	672.353	651.89
10.994	28.682	678.863	712.02
35.361	147.212	707.547	723.72
71.308	393.001	767.028	836.27
130.000	911.005	892.385	
176.662	1399.591	1010.623	988.45

Input for Figure 14-D

Equation for Dose^2 from Table 29-B:

Ca-Rate = (0.01047)(Dose^2) + 680.048

Dose cSv	Dose cSv^2	Ca-Rate Calc.	Ca-Rate Observed
0.000	0.00	680.048	649.31
1.511	2.28	680.072	651.89
10.994	120.87	681.313	712.02
35.361	1250.43	693.140	723.72
71.308	5084.83	733.286	836.27
130.000	16900.00	856.991	
176.662	31209.54	1006.812	988.45

The construction of Table 14-D is described, step-by-step, in Chapter 29.

When the above values are plotted for dose (cSv), calculated cancer-rate, and observed cancer-rate, they demonstrate graphically how closely or how distantly the observed points lie to the corresponding curve calculated by regression analysis.

In a good fit, not only should the weightiest observations lie close to the calculated curve, but their scatter (if any) should fall to both sides of it. In addition, it is a sign of poor fit if the observations on both ends lie on the same side of the curve while the observations in the middle all lie on the opposite side.

Because the dose-response is so similar in T65DR and DS86 (compare Figure 14-E with Figure 14-F), we have not shown graphs comparable to 14-B, 14-C, and 14-D for the DS86 analysis.

Distribution of Datapoints Relative to Four Dose–Response Curves.

Input for the four figures below is provided by Table 14-D. Each figure depicts the SAME observations (indicated by the boxy symbol): Cancer-mortality versus dose in the A-Bomb Study, 1950-1982. What differs is the dose-response curve in each figure.

● -- In Figure 14-A, the "fit" between the observations and the supra-linear curve is good, with datapoints either lying on the curve or falling to both sides of it.

● -- In Figure 14-B, the fit between the observations and the linear "curve" is inferior to the fit in Figure 14-A.

● -- In Figure 14-C, the fit between the observations and the linear-quadratic (Q-positive) curve is very poor, with the observations at both ends lying on the same side of the curve, and the observations in the middle all lying on the opposite side.

● -- In Figure 14-D, the fit between observations and the quadratic dose-response curve is even worse than in Figure 14-C.

● -- Statistical testing (Chapter 29) establishes that the supra-linear dose-response fits the evidence significantly better than the linear dose-response.

Figure 14-A, below: Fit Relative to Supra-Linear (Dose^0.75)

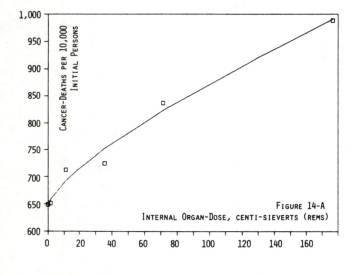

Figure 14-B, below: Fit Relative to Linear (Dose^1.0)

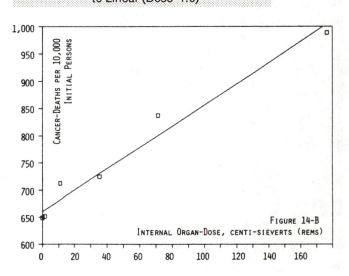

Figure 14-C, below: Fit Relative to Linear-Quadratic (Dose^1.4)

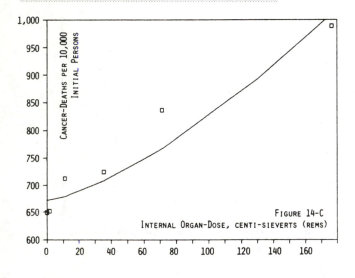

Figure 14-D, below: Fit Relative to Quadratic (Dose^2.0).

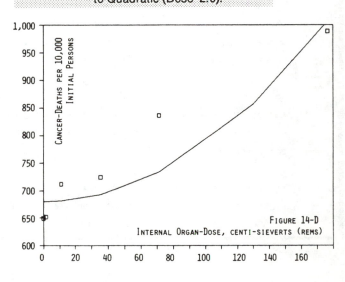

Figure 14-E

T65DR Dosimetry: Best-Fit Curve for Cumulative Cancer-Deaths versus Dose.

For the atomic-bomb survivors, this plot shows cumulative cancer-deaths (1950-1982) per 10,000 initial persons, versus mean whole-body internal organ-dose in the T65DR dosimetry (RBE = 2). Input for this figure comes from Table 14-A, Columns A, C, and D.

● -- The boxy symbols, which show the observed cancer death-rate per 10,000 initial persons versus dose, come from Columns A and D of Table 14-A.

● -- Points along the best-fit curve come from Column C of Table 14-A, and show calculated cancer death-rates per 10,000 initial persons versus dose, based on the equation of best fit, shown below. This curve is the same as the curve in Figure 14-A, of course.

Figure 14-F (next page) will show the best-fit curve for the SAME cohorts of survivors in the supplemental DS86 dosimetry.

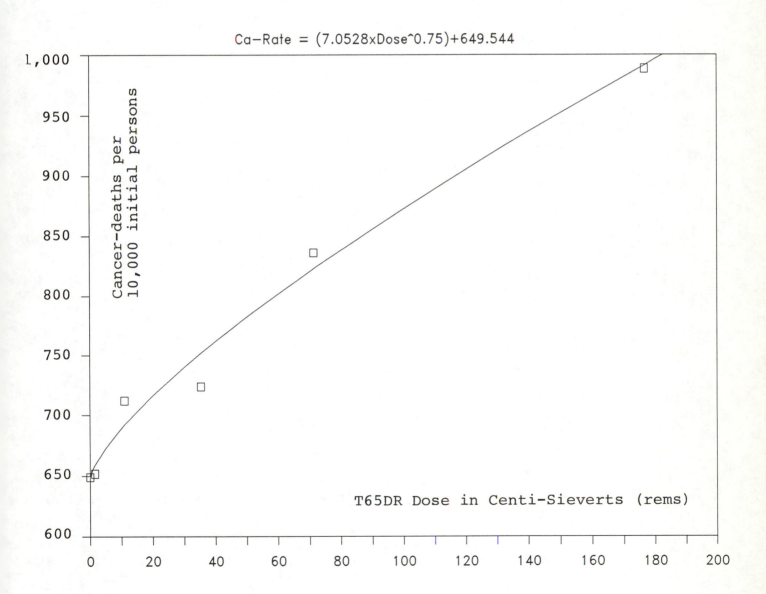

$$Ca-Rate = (7.0528 \times Dose^{0.75}) + 649.544$$

Figure 14-F

DS86 Dosimetry: Best–Fit Curve for Cumulative Cancer–Deaths versus Dose.

For the atomic-bomb survivors, this plot shows cumulative cancer-deaths (1950-1982) per 10,000 initial persons, versus mean whole-body internal organ-dose in the DS86 dosimetry (RBE = 20). Input for this figure comes from Table 14-B, Columns A, C, and D.

● -- The boxy symbols, which show the observed cancer death-rate per 10,000 initial persons versus dose, come from Columns A and D of Table 14-B.

● -- Points along the best-fit curve come from Column C of Table 14-B, and show calculated cancer death-rates per 10,000 initial persons versus dose, based on the equation of best fit.

With our "constant-cohort, dual dosimetry" approach to the DS86 dosimetry, the T65DR cohorts of survivors remain undisturbed, and merely receive a second dose-estimate. Super-imposition of Figures 14-F and 14-E would show that the DS86 dosimetry shifts the boxy symbols somewhat to the right (higher dose) -- as predictable from comparing Column A in Tables 14-A and 14-B. Consequently, the equations of best fit for the T65DR and DS86 dosimetries are somewhat different.

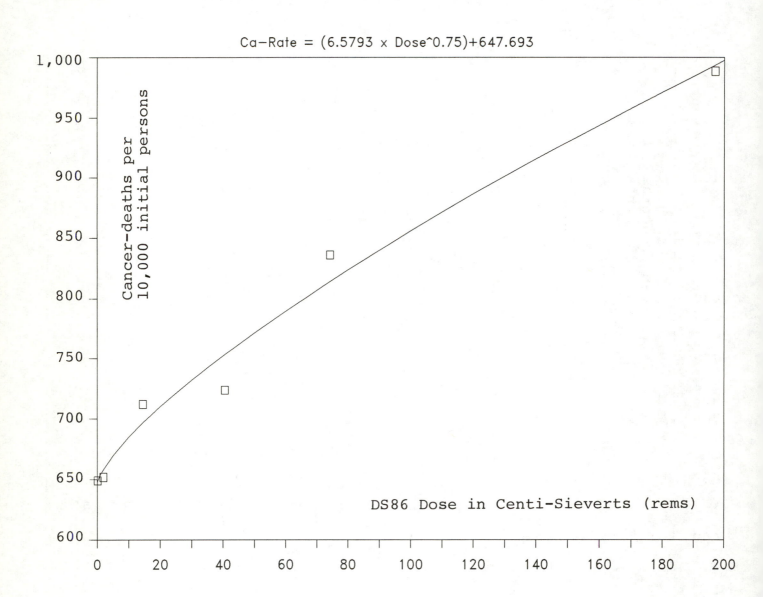

$$Ca-Rate = (6.5793 \times Dose^{0.75}) + 647.693$$

Radiation Risk by Age and Sex, from the Cancer-Rate Ratio Method

This chapter is arranged in eight parts:

Then tables.

1. Overview and Definitions

Unlike the Cancer Difference Method, the Cancer-Rate Ratio Method will obtain Minimum and Lifetime Fatal Cancer-Yields, for a population of mixed ages, by summing the SEPARATE contributions made by distinct age-sex subsets of the population.

This chapter evaluates the risk of radiation-induced cancer observed so far in each of the five age-bands of the A-bomb survivors, males and females separately. The risks are expressed in terms of ten different "K-values" (defined below). The next chapter will use the K-values from this chapter to obtain the Minimum and Lifetime Fatal Cancer-Yields.

The Definition of K-Value :

K is defined here as the fractional increase in the spontaneous cancer death-rate per centi-sievert of whole-body internal organ-dose. (Multiplied by 100, K would be the PERCENT increase in the spontaneous cancer death-rate per cSv.) The definition of K needs comparison with the definition of Fatal Cancer-Yield.

Fatal Cancer-Yield is defined as the number of radiation-induced fatal cancers among 10,000 initial persons per cSv average whole-body internal organ-dose.

Therefore, if the observed K-values are applied to the spontaneous cancer-deaths observed so far in the Reference Group per 10,000 initial persons, the result is the MINIMUM Fatal Cancer-Yield. If these observed K-values are applied to the estimated ULTIMATE spontaneous cancer-deaths per 10,000 initial persons

in the Reference Group, the result is the LIFETIME Fatal Cancer-Yield. Readers who look ahead to Tables 16-A and 16-B, in the next chapter, can see immediately how K-values and spontaneous cancer-rates are used to estimate Cancer-Yields (the "per 10,000" step occurs at the end).

That is the easy part. The work comes beforehand, in obtaining the proper K-values to use in the range of common low-dose exposures, up to 5 cSv.

Raw versus Low-Dose K-Values :

The evidence in Chapters 14 and 29 shows that the dose-response relationship is presently concave-downward (supra-linear), and that the dose-exponent which produces the best-fit is Dose^0.75. Therefore it would be inexcusable -- indeed, a sign of bias -- if we ignored this information in deriving the best estimates we can of K-values.

Our method for taking supra-linearity into account, however, uses a series of linear equations. The analysis begins in Part 2 by developing the simple linear equations which yield Equation (7), which is the key one.

We shall use Equation (7) first to obtain a set of "raw K-values" which do NOT take supra-linearity into account, and then a set of "low-dose K-values" which DO take supra-linearity into account. It is not necessary to obtain the raw K-values in order to obtain the low-dose K-values, but we do it so that everyone (ourselves included) can know how raw and low-dose K-values compare in magnitude.

The input data which are assembled and

consolidated in Tables 15-B through 15-K are needed equally for obtaining raw and low-dose K-values.

2. Origin of the Key Equation

We will use the following symbols; when a digit follows a letter, the digit is serving as a subscript.

```
D2 = some dose of ionizing radiation greater
     than zero-dose.
R2 = cancer death-rate (1950-1982) at D2,
     per 10,000 exposed persons.
D1 = some dose less than D2.
R1 = cancer death-rate (1950-1982) at D1,
     per 10,000 exposed persons.
Ro = spontaneous cancer death-rate (1950-1982)
     when dose is zero.
K  = fractional increase in Ro per cSv of dose.
```

When the dose-response relationship in a set of observations is linear, then the fractional increase in the spontaneous cancer death-rate per cSv of dose is the the same everywhere in the dose-range, high-dose and low-dose alike. Of course, this is definitely not true when dose-response is either concave-downward or concave-upward. But in a linear dose-response, K is a constant.

Equations (1) and (4) below are nothing other than the equation for a straight line, where Ro is the intercept on the y-axis, where the quantity (KRo) is the slope of the straight line, and where the intercept and points (D2,R2) and (D1,R1) all lie along the SAME straight line. Since Equation (7) below is derived from Equations (1) and (4), Equation (7) produces K-values which are valid if the dose-response relationship is LINEAR.

● -- Equation (1) :

   R2 = Ro + (K)(Ro)(D2)

Factoring-out Ro, and then re-arranging, we have

● -- Equation (2) :

   R2 = Ro (1 + KD2) , then

   R2/Ro = 1 + KD2 , then

● -- Equation (3) :

$$K = \frac{(R2/Ro) - 1}{D2}$$

And also for the lower dose, D1, we can write

● -- Equation (4) :

   R1 = Ro + (K)(Ro)(D1)

● -- Then Equation (5) :

   R1 = Ro (1 + KD1)

If we need to solve for K without using Ro at all, it can be done without using Equation (3), if we simply divide Equation (2) by Equation (5) -- which causes Ro to cancel out in Equation (6).

● -- Equation (6) :

$$(R2/R1) = \frac{(1 + KD2)}{(1 + KD1)}$$

And, as we begin to isolate K, we have:

   (R2/R1)(1 + KD1) = (1 + KD2) , then

   (R2/R1) + (R2/R1)(KD1) = 1 + KD2

Transposing terms and factoring-out K, we have:

   (KD2) - (R2/R1)(KD1) = (R2/R1) - 1 , then

   K [D2 - (R2/R1)(D1)] = (R2/R1) - 1 , then

● -- Equation (7) :

$$K = \frac{(R2/R1) - 1}{(D2) - (R2/R1)(D1)}$$

So K can be evaluated with Equation (7) from ANY two observations, since R2, D2, R1, and D1 are all known from two observations. Equation (7) is the one which we will use repeatedly in this chapter. Indeed, its term (R2/R1) is the basis for calling this the Cancer-Rate Ratio Method.

3. Obtaining Raw K-Values for Each Age and Sex

In Part 1 of this chapter, we drew a distinction between two sets of K-values: "Low-dose K-values" which take account of supra-linearity, and "raw K-values" which do NOT take account of supra-linearity. Before this new use of the word "raw" causes any confusion, we must point out that BOTH the low-dose and the raw K-values are derived from the raw (pre-normalized) A-bomb data.

The work in this chapter uses only the raw data. It is completely unnecessary to use age-normalized data when we are keeping each age-band separate, and completely unnecessary to use sex-normalized data when we are keeping males and females separate. Therefore, we are using the raw data from Tables 11-B (males) and 11-D (females). In addition, we use Master Tables 26-A,B,C,D in order to show the data for Dose-Groups 6, 7, and 8 separately.

Elsewhere, we established that WITHIN a single age-band, the slight age-differences ATB across Dose-Groups are appropriately disregarded (see Chapter 11).

Dose-Increment for Small Body-Size :

As indicated by Table 4-B, the average age of the 0-9 year-olds ATB was only 4.1 years. The organ-doses in Master Tables 26-A,B,C,D, and in Tables 11-B and 11-D, do not include any correction for the small body-size of this age-band. Chapter 31 presents the method used for making the adjustment, and the findings are presented in Table 15-A.

In the Cancer-Rate Ratio Method, which examines each age-band separately, the 4-year-olds ATB take on importance in the estimates of LIFETIME Fatal Cancer-Yield for a population of mixed-ages. Therefore, the work in Chapter 31 is worthwhile, in order to avoid preventable error.

The effect of the adjustment is to increase dose by about 13-20 percent for this age-band, without changing the cancer-observations of course. The result is to REDUCE the K-values for the very young children ATB, and thus to REDUCE the Lifetime Fatal Cancer-Yield for the overall population, compared with estimates calculated without this dose-adjustment, in the Cancer-Rate Ratio Method.

The Small-Numbers Problem :

All analysts who begin to subdivide the Dose-Groups of the A-Bomb Study are immediately confronted with the small-numbers problem, especially for RERF's two age-bands who were youngest ATB (0-9 years and 10-19 years).

For example, inspection of Tables 11-B and 11-D, Column N, shows that it would be scientifically meaningless, at this stage of the follow-up, to base K-values on comparing observations in Dose-Group 3 with the Reference Group (1+2) AFTER the database has been subdivided into ten age-sex groups. After

subdivision, analysts are confronted in Dose-Group 3 with statistically unstable numbers of cancer-deaths like 1 cancer for males 0-9 years ATB, 19 cancers for males 10-19 years ATB, 9 cancers for females 0-9 years ATB, and 23 cancers for females 10-19 years ATB.

Therefore the comparison of Dose-Group 3 with the Reference Group, which was statistically strong in the Cancer Difference Method when observations were not subdivided, is ruled out by the small-numbers problem after subdivision. To reduce the instability of small numbers, all good analysts must decide on some combination of age-bands, sexes, or dose-groups (see for instance RERF TR-9-87, Table 7, p.21; and TR-5-88, Table 2-4, p.64).

The Consolidation of Dose-Groups :

This chapter lessens the small-numbers problem by consolidating the observations within each age-sex group into two classes: Low-dose and high-dose. The low-dose class is composed of RERF Dose-Groups 1 + 2 + 3, and represents an average organ-dose in the neighborhood of 3 cSv (specifics are in Tables 15-B through 15-K). The high-dose class is composed of Dose-Groups 4 + 5 + 6 + 7 + 8, and represents an average organ-dose in the neighborhood of 70-100 cSv (specifics are in Tables 15-B through 15-K).

This consolidation provides real-world observations to use for D2, R2, D1, and R1 in Equation (7), and provides them for each of the ten age-sex groups separately.

Calculation of Raw K-Values :

Tables 15-B through 15-K show the derivation of twenty raw K-values (ten in each dosimetry), step-by-step, from the input data to the result. Each calculation amounts to having a two-point dose-response at about 3 cSv and at about 85 cSv. One can imagine a straight line connecting these two points. By using Equation (7), the K-value which applies to this straight line is determined.

4. Discussion of the Raw K-Values

The raw K-values derived in Tables 15-B through 15-K are assembled for convenience at the bottom of Table 15-L (Note 2).

Higher Hazard for
Those Who Are Young at Exposure :

The raw K-values reflect a greater sensitivity to radiation carcinogenesis in those who are young at exposure (the two youngest age-bands ATB) than in those who are older. This is seen in both sexes

independently. It is even seen for each sex in the
age-band 0-9 years ATB, in spite of the severe
small-numbers problem in those groups.

In the females, sensitivity falls with advancing age in
a remarkably regular way. In the males, there is an
irregularity in the age-band 20-34 years ATB. We
regard this as more likely to be an artifact from sampling
than to be biologically meaningful, but only time will tell
with certainty. Meanwhile, we shall not use any
smoothing operation for either the raw K-values or
(later) the low-dose K-values.

Male versus Female K-Values :
When we compare K-values for males and females,
we find that the males seem generally less
radio-sensitive than the females. In the one age-band
(50+) where these are the final results -- because
almost everyone has died -- this is what we see. On
the other hand, the age-band 35-49 years ATB is the
age-band which accounts for the most cancer-deaths in
the study by far (Table 4-B), which makes it the most
reliable to date. In this age-band, radio-sensitivity is
about the SAME in males and females.

Independence from Hypotheses and Models :
It is self-evident that there necessarily exists some
ratio between two cancer-rates (R2 and R1) observed
at two different doses (D2 and D1). The ratio may be
greater than 1.0, equal to 1.0, or less than 1.0, but
whatever its value, it exists. Equation (7) simply uses
the observed ratio and the doses to calculate the value
of K: The fractional increase in the spontaneous
cancer-rate per cSv of dose.

Thus the raw K-values in Table 15-L are
independent from any forward projection, hypothesis, or
model of radiation carcinogenesis. They are
"in-the-box" observations with respect to the follow-up
through 1982. Whether or not they will keep the same
value during the remaining follow-up periods is a
separate question, which no one can answer with
certainty, of course.

Raw K-Values Not Applicable for Low-Doses :
Because dose-response is concave-downward
instead of linear, and because raw K-values are derived
from a D2 in the range of 70-100 cSv of average
organ-dose, the raw K-values would (if used)
necessarily underestimate the Cancer-Yield -- the
radiation hazard -- from low-dose exposure. In Part 6,
we will determine the size of the underestimate.

5. Obtaining K-Values for Low-Dose Exposure

The Key Assumption, and Overview of the Method :

In Chapters 14 and 29, it was demonstrated that (A)
the dose-response relationship in the A-Bomb Study --
for both cities, both sexes, and all five age-bands
combined -- is concave-downward in shape
(supra-linear), and (B) the best fit to the data is obtained
by using Dose^0.75 in the equation of cancer
death-rate versus dose. Indeed, the fit is excellent, with
R-Squared values of 0.9831 for the T65DR dosimetry
(Table 29-B) and 0.9825 for the DS86 dosimetry (Table
29-C).

Since the ten age-sex subsets examined here, by
the Cancer-Rate Ratio Method, represent the entire
substrate which generated that dose-exponent, it is a
reasonable expectation that approximately the same
dose-exponent characterizes the ten age-sex groups
individually.

Because of the small-numbers problem, this
expectation cannot yet be tested; another decade or
more of follow-up will perhaps produce adequate
numbers to do curvilinear regression analysis for the ten
groups separately. Meanwhile, the assumption that they
DO share a similar dose-response curve seems far
more reasonable than a speculative claim that they do
NOT. Therefore, we will make the approximation that
the dose-exponent of 0.75, which characterizes
dose-response for the overall population, also applies
individually to each of the population's ten subsets.

With this single assumption, we can write individual
equations of best fit for each subset, based on the
real-world observations belonging to that particular
age-sex group (from Tables 15-B through 15-K), and
then we can use the equations to determine the
corresponding LOW-DOSE K-values for each age-sex
group.

Before demonstrating the two-step procedure, first
we will show the origin of the additional equations to be
used. In the end, we also use Equation (7) again.

Equations (8) Through (12) :

With our combined dose-groups, we can refer to
two categories:

The "L" Group is the Lower Group
        (Dose-Groups 1 + 2 + 3).

===

The "H" Group is the Higher Group
            (Dose-Groups 4 + 5 + 6 + 7 + 8).
In Group L, we have a dose, D1, where the
            observed cancer-rate is R1.
In Group H, we have a dose, D2, where the
            observed cancer-rate is R2.

Equation (8) below states the general dose-response relationship which, as noted in Chapter 29, is an equation which produces a straight line if dose is plotted in units of cSv^0.75 instead of cSv:

● -- Equation (8) :
     Cancer-Rate
           = (Coefficient)(Dose^0.75) + (Constant)

Readers will recognize that the format of Equation (8) is the analytic expression of a straight line: y = mx + b. Since b is the line's y-intercept, the Constant in Equation (8) is the cancer-rate when dose is zero (the spontaneous cancer-rate).

We can write Equation (9) for Group L, and Equation (10) for Group H.

● -- Equation (9) :
     R1 = (Coefficient)(D1^0.75) + (Constant)

● -- Equation (10) :
     R2 = (Coefficient)(D2^0.75) + (Constant)

   Since these linear equations necessarily share the same Coefficient and Constant, and since Tables 15-B through 15-K provide the values of R1, R2, D1, and D2, we will be able to solve these two equations for both the Coefficient and the Constant. Solving for the Coefficient first, we subtract Equation (9) from Equation (10), to obtain:

R2-R1 = (Coefficient)(D2^0.75 - D1^0.75) , and then

● -- Equation (11) :
     (Coefficient) = (R2-R1) / (D2^0.75 - D1^0.75)

     For the Constant, we re-arrange Equation (9).

● -- Equation (12) :
     Constant = (R1) - (Coefficient)(D1^0.75)

   Since we evaluated the Coefficient in Equation (11), and since R1 and D1^0.75 are knowns, we now have the value of the Constant -- or would, if we had been using actual observations. In Step 1 below, we shall apply these equations to some real numbers from the tables.

Step 1 -- ●
Obtaining the Equation of Best Fit

   The procedure to be demonstrated is general, and has been applied to all ten age-sex groups under study here. It will be illustrated below by using the input from Table 15-B for the males age 0-9 years ATB, in the T65DR dosimetry. Any other set of data (Tables 15-C through 15-K) would serve just as well. The results become entries in Table 15-L.

D1 = 2.90 cSv
D2 = 96.64 cSv
R1 = 31.08 cancers per 10,000 persons, 1950-82
R2 = 105.26 cancers per 10,000 persons, 1950-82

        D1^0.75 =   (2.9)^0.75 = 2.2222
        D2^0.75 =   (96.64)^0.75 = 30.822

Applying Equation (11), we solve for Coefficient:

Coefficient = (R2-R1) / (D2^0.75 - D1^0.75)
Coefficient = (105.26-31.08) / (30.82248-2.222278)
Coefficient = 2.593687

Applying Equation (12), we solve for Constant:
        Constant = R1 - (Coefficient)(D1^0.75)
        Constant = 31.08 - (2.593687)(2.222278)
        Constant = 25.31610

   And now, with Equation (8) as the model, we can write the entire Equation of Best Fit for this particular age- and sex-group:

   Cancer-Rate = (2.5937)(Dose^0.75) + (25.3161)

   Precisely this entry is to be found in Table 15-L for the Equation of Best Fit for males, 0-9 years of age ATB, in the T65DR dosimetry.

Step 2 -- ●
Obtaining (R2/R1) & Solving for Low-Dose K :

   In order to calculate the appropriate K-value for a total dose up to 5 cSv, we now need to use this Equation of Best Fit to obtain the predicted cancer-rates at zero-dose and at 5 cSv.

For 5 cSv :
Cancer-rate = (2.5937)(5^0.75) + (25.3161)
        Since 5^0.75 = 3.343701
Cancer-rate = (2.5937)(3.343701) + (25.3161)
        = 33.98865

For Zero cSv :
Cancer-rate = (2.5937)(0^0.75) + (25.3161)
        Since 0^0.75 = 0,
Cancer-rate = 25.3161

        Thus, for these two doses and cancer-rates :
            D1 = 0 cSv
            D2 = 5 cSv
            R1 = 25.3161
            R2 = 33.98865
            R2/R1 = 33.98865 / 25.3161 = 1.3425

Now, going back to Equation (7) and making the approximation that dose-response is linear between 0 and 5 cSv, we can calculate the K-value which is appropriate for low-dose exposure:

● -- Equation (7) :

$$K = \frac{(R2/R1) - 1}{(D2) - (R2/R1)(D1)}$$

Substituting our values, we have for the average K-value up to 5 cSv of total dose:

$$K = \frac{1.34257 - 1}{5 - (1.34257)(0)}$$

$$K = 0.34257 / 5 = 0.06851$$

In Table 15-L of low-dose K-values, exactly this K-value of 0.06851 is entered for males 0-9 years of age ATB, in the T65DR dosimetry. All twenty low-dose K-values in Table 15-L are derived in the same way.

6. Discussion of Low-Dose K-Values

There are two checks which confirm that the method is correct for obtaining low-dose K-values from the evidence at hand.

Checking the Constants :

First, since the constants in the Equations of Best Fit in Table 15-L are the predicted spontaneous cancer-rates when the dose is zero, those constants should be consistent with the rates observed in the Reference Group, whose exposure was not far above zero. Since Tables 15-B through 15-K include the cancer-rate per 10,000 initial persons in the Reference Group, such comparisons are easily made with the constants in Table 15-L. The correspondence between predicted and observed rates is very good, especially for the older age-bands where the number of cancer-cases is statistically the most stable.

Checking the Ratio (Low-Dose K / Raw K) :

Second, the ratio between the low-dose K-values and the raw K-values for each of the ten subsets should be about the same magnitude as it would be, if the comparable ratio were determined for the COMBINATION of all age-bands and both sexes. We made this check by using Equation (7) with appropriate entries from Tables 14-A and 14-B.

Because raw K-values for the subsets were calculated with D2 equal to about 85 cSv, and D1 equal to about 3 cSv, in making a calculation of the corresponding K-value with all ages and both sexes combined, we chose the closest values available in Tables 14-A and 14-B. We used D2 = 80 cSv and D1 = 2 cSv. For the low-dose K-value, of course we used D2 = 5 cSv and D1 = 0 cSv. The resulting ratios are below:

T65DR without age-sex subdivision:
        RATIO, LOW-DOSE K TO RAW K = 2.104 .

DS86 without age-sex subdivision:
        RATIO, LOW-DOSE K TO RAW K = 2.103 .

This assures us that the overall ratio is, indeed, about the same magnitude as the individual ratios shown in the tabulations which follow. Moreover, everything here is consistent with the ratios of low-dose and higher-dose Minimum Fatal Cancer-Yields in Table 13-B, Row 1.

Tabulations follow on next page.

===

| ------------------ T65DR ------------------ | | ------------------ DS86 ------------------ |
Sex & Age ATB (Years)	Raw K-Value	Low-Dose K-Value	Ratio, Low-Dose K over Raw K		Sex & Age ATB (Years)	Raw K-Value	Low-Dose K-Value	Ratio, Low-Dose K over Raw K
M 0-9	0.02749	0.068510	2.49		M 0-9	0.02565	0.066170	2.58
M 10-19	0.00677	0.015190	2.24		M 10-19	0.00647	0.014840	2.29
M 20-34	0.00157	0.003426	2.18		M 20-34	0.00150	0.003344	2.23
M 35-49	0.00228	0.004936	2.16		M 35-49	0.00207	0.004634	2.24
M 50+	0.00162	0.003454	2.13		M 50+	0.00140	0.003114	2.22
F 0-9	0.01922	0.046150	2.40		F 0-9	0.01771	0.043880	2.48
F 10-19	0.01097	0.024570	2.24		F 10-19	0.01081	0.024700	2.28
F 20-34	0.00492	0.010730	2.18		F 20-34	0.00442	0.010000	2.26
F 35-49	0.00289	0.006152	2.13		F 35-49	0.00250	0.005565	2.23
F 50+	0.00288	0.005945	2.06		F 50+	0.00252	0.005425	2.15

It deserves emphasis, however, that correctness of method and computation can never overcome inherent sampling variation and the small-numbers problem in a set of observations. It is self-evident from the raw data in Tables 15-B through 15-K that every analyst who subdivides A-bomb data is dealing with some small and unstable numbers. Even if K-values are biologically constant for the lifespan which follows irradiation, future follow-ups may cause a K-value to rise or fall due to the random variation of sampling. (However, the values for the oldest age-band ATB are as stable as they will ever become, since almost all of this age-band had died before the end of the 1950-1982 follow-up.)

Effect of Extrapolation from High Doses :

The ratios between low-dose K-values, and their corresponding raw K-values, range from 2.1 to 2.5. Like Tables 13-B, 14-A, and 14-B, this indicates that failure to appreciate the supra-linearity of the dose-response relationship accounts for more than a 2-fold underestimate of fatal cancer-risk when high doses and the linear dose-response are used to evaluate the hazard from low-dose exposure.

This finding is in great contrast to the "old refrain" that extrapolation from high doses would exaggerate the cancer-risk at low doses from ionizing radiation. However, we repeat that it is not necessary for anyone to extrapolate at all. One should use the findings which are based DIRECTLY upon human exposure in the low dose-range.

Free from Speculation :

Low-dose K-values, like the raw K-values, are "in-the-box." Readers have seen for themselves that low-dose K-values are derived from the actual observations (1950-1982) of D1, R1, D2, R2, in Tables 15-B through 15-K, without any reliance on speculation, hypotheses, or models of radiation carcinogenesis. As shown in Chapter 14, the dose-exponent of 0.75 (used in Steps 1 and 2) ALSO

comes from the evidence itself, not from speculation, hypothesis, or pre-judgment.

Low-dose K-values vary with age ATB, as do the raw K-values. Comments in Part 4 of this chapter regarding age and sex apply equally to raw and low-dose K-values.

7. Some Ties between K-Values, Supra-Linearity, Duration

K-Values and Supra-Linearity :

For the sake of exploration, we are going to use the RAW K-values at the bottom of Table 15-L, to predict the consequences of radiation exposure, regardless of dose-level.

Let us say that the raw K-values at the bottom of Table 15-L, for the children who were age 0-9 years old ATB, are "good" -- by which we mean, if there were a billion such children in the study instead of 18402 children, we would still observe a raw K-value of about 0.02, or 2 % per rem, from the 1950-1982 follow-up. In other words, suppose there is no basis for thinking 0.02 is spuriously high or low, due to sampling variation.

If we use the approximation for this exploration that, in populations with a long lifespan, some 20 % of people die from SPONTANEOUS cancer, and if we make the presumption that the magnitude of the raw K-value neither rises nor falls with further follow-up, then what would we expect for children irradiated between 0-9 years of age?

SCENARIO 1 : Among every 10,000 children who receive one rem (cSv) of whole-body internal organ-dose, we would expect that 2,000 would die eventually from spontaneous cancer, and from the definition of K -- which is the fractional increase in the spontaneous rate per rem -- we would also expect (2000 spontaneous cancers x 0.02 per rem x 1 rem), or 40 radiation-induced cancers. Combined lifelong cancer-deaths expected for this group = 2,040 per 10,000 initial persons.

SCENARIO 2 : Among every 10,000 children who receive 25 rems (cSv) of whole-body internal organ-dose, we would expect that 2,000 would die eventually from spontaneous cancer, and from using the raw K-value of 0.02, we would also expect (2000 spontaneous cancers x 0.02 per rem x 25 rems), or 1,000 radiation-induced cancers. Combined lifelong cancer-deaths expected for this group = 3,000 per 10,000 initial persons.

SCENARIO 3 : Among every 10,000 children who receive 200 rems of whole-body internal organ-dose, we would expect that 2,000 would die eventually from spontaneous cancer, and still using the raw K-value of 0.02, we would also expect (2000 spontaneous cancers x 0.02 per rem x 200 rems), or 8,000 radiation-induced cancers. Combined lifelong cancer-deaths expected for this group = 10,000 per 10,000 initial persons.

Thus, use of the same K-value at high doses and low doses would, in certain circumstances, lead to absurd predictions at HIGH doses.

In the A-Bomb Study, there are about 200 children who survived the acute effects of 200 rems or more of whole-body internal organ-dose (see Dose-Groups 7 and 8, in Tables 15-B and 15-G). If a single raw K-value were applicable at every dose-level and if it persisted lifelong, then all of these 200 persons would be expected to die of cancer. (The expectation would be 40 spontaneous fatal cancers, plus 160 radiation-induced cases.)

But in reality, it would NOT happen that way, because non-cancer causes of death would "compete" with cancer in this group. As a result, the ultimate observation would be fewer than 200 cancers per 200 initial persons. Therefore, under these circumstances, the single raw K-value of 0.02 could NOT characterize all dose-levels. The K-value at 200 rems would have to be LOWER than 0.02 -- and that would be consistent with SUPRA-linearity of dose-response.

A recurrent finding in this field is that K-values are high for children. Unless dose-response is supra-linear (meaning lower K-values at high doses than at low doses), predictions based on high doses and on high, lifelong K-values will "require" lifetime cancer death-rates which exceed 100 percent. In contrast to such an absurdity, high and lifelong K-values at LOW

doses are consistent with predictions which are credible.

K-Values and Duration of Magnitude :

Absurd predictions for high-dose consequences, illustrated in Scenario 3 above, could be avoided by acceptance of different K-values for different dose-levels (in accordance with the current evidence from the A-bomb survivors), but there is also another route to credible high-dose estimates. One could speculate that K-values, though truly observed and reported for a given follow-up period, will not remain constant for the full remainder of a lifespan follow-up.

For instance, if one observed a very high K-value like 0.5 per rem (not 0.05 or 0.005 per rem) in some sample of irradiated children during an incomplete lifespan follow-up, then K = 0.5 per rem would mean that a dose of only 8 rems would cause everyone in that sample to die from cancer, if the K-value remained at the SAME magnitude of 0.5 for the remaining lifespan:

(2,000 spontaneous cancers per 10,000 initial persons) x (0.5 per rem) x (8 rems) = 8,000 radiation-induced cancers. When the expected 2,000 spontaneous cancer-deaths are added, cancer would claim 10,000 out of every 10,000 initial persons in such a sample.

Nonetheless, the observation of K = 0.5 may be exactly right for the time-period which has passed. One cannot presently rule out the possibility that K-values vary with time -- as well as with dose-level. On the other hand, one cannot rule out predictions which come fairly close to 100 % cancer-mortality either. For instance, among persons with chronic hepatitis-B infection, the lifetime incidence of a SINGLE TYPE of cancer alone (hepatocellular carcinoma) has been reported as high as 50 % (Ober89).

Supra-Linearity
in the Absence of High K-Values :

Table 4-B is a reminder that the supra-linearity presently observed in the A-bomb survivors is overwhelmingly generated by the cancer-response of those who were already adults at the time of bombing, because fully 92.7 percent of all the cancers observed during the 1950-1982 follow-up have come from the three oldest age-bands ATB. Yet these three oldest age-bands are the LEAST sensitive to radiation carcinogenesis. If we do an exploration with their highest raw K-value, which is near 0.005, we do not "run out of people" for the expected cancers, even at a very high dose:

Among every 10,000 adults who receive 200 rems of whole-body internal organ-dose, we would expect that 2,000 would die eventually from spontaneous cancer, and under the specified K-value, we would also expect (2000 spontaneous cancers x 0.005 per rem x 200 rems), or 2,000 radiation-induced cancers. Combined lifelong cancers expected for this group would be 4,000 per 10,000 initial persons.

Therefore we can rule out pressure from competing causes of death as the main CAUSE of the supra-linearity observed in the 1950-1982 dose-response of the adult A-bomb survivors.

8. The Bottom Line on Radiation Risk, by Age and Sex

1. K is defined as the fractional increase in the spontaneous cancer death-rate per centi-sievert of whole-body internal organ-dose. A K-value measures the size of an observed cancer-response, and is independent from any particular hypotheses and models of radiation carcinogenesis itself.

2. The main part of Table 15-L presents the low-dose K-values for each of RERF's five age-bands and both sexes. Separate sets of K-values have been calculated for the T65DR dosimetry and the current version of the DS86 dosimetry. These K-values come from observation of the A-bomb survivors from 1950-1982. No follow-up years -- and no Dose-Groups -- have been thrown out of our analysis (see Chapter 14, Part 2). All the available observations were included in finding the equation of best fit, for each of the ten groups.

3. The low-dose K-values from Table 15-L will be used in the next chapter to estimate the Minimum and Lifetime Fatal Cancer-Yields from low-dose exposure, not only for the A-bomb survivors, but also for a population with an age-sex distribution like the one of the United States.

Table 15–A
Correction of Dose–Data for Small Body–Size: Ages 0–9 at Time of Bombing.

MALES AGE 0-9 ATB: T65DR Dosimetry, Neutron RBE = 2.0 || **MALES: DS86 Dosimetry, Neutron RBE = 20.**

Col. A Dose- Group MALES	Col. B Uncorrected Dose in cSv	Col. C Correction Factor MALES	Col. D Corrected Dose in cSv	Persons MALES		Col. E Dose- Group MALES	Col. F Uncorrected Dose in cSv	Col. G Correction Factor MALES	Col. H Corrected Dose in cSv
Group 1	0	1.000	0.000	3787	||	Group 1	0.081943	1.074	0.088
Group 2	1.450	1.171	1.698	3031	||	Group 2	1.593	1.128	1.797
Group 3	10.49	1.179	12.368	1547	||	Group 3	13.32	1.138	15.158
Group 4	34.78	1.175	40.867	359	||	Group 4	39.79	1.162	46.236
Group 5	71.64	1.173	84.034	189	||	Group 5	72.79	1.169	85.092
Group 6	120.19	1.172	140.863	105	||	Group 6	116.90	1.179	137.825
Group 7	170.63	1.186	202.367	43	||	Group 7	175.39	1.192	209.065
Group 8	256.45	1.182	303.124	64	||	Group 8	305.99	1.203	368.106
SUM				9125					

FEMALES AGE 0-9 ATB: T65DR Dosimetry, Neutron RBE = 2. || **FEMALES: DS86 Dosimetry, Neutron RBE = 20.**

Col. A Dose- Group FEMALES	Col. B Uncorrected Dose in cSv	Col. C Correction Factor FEMALES	Col. D Corrected Dose in cSv	Persons FEMALES		Col. E Dose- Group FEMALES	Col. F Uncorrected Dose in cSv	Col. G Correction Factor FEMALES	Col. H Corrected Dose in cSv
Group 1	0	1.000	0.000	3842	||	Group 1	0.081863	1.074	0.088
Group 2	1.429	1.173	1.676	3093	||	Group 2	1.581	1.128	1.783
Group 3	10.700	1.178	12.605	1547	||	Group 3	13.55	1.138	15.420
Group 4	34.65	1.173	40.644	372	||	Group 4	39.23	1.161	45.546
Group 5	70.31	1.181	83.036	213	||	Group 5	74.07	1.173	86.884
Group 6	122.17	1.177	143.794	99	||	Group 6	122.06	1.183	144.397
Group 7	175.91	1.189	209.157	41	||	Group 7	182.27	1.194	217.630
Group 8	267.01	1.176	314.004	70	||	Group 8	313.59	1.199	375.994
SUM				9277					

NOTES: -----

Average age of the 0-9 year-old children ATB was 4.1 years (Table 26-E).

Entries in Col.B and Col.F are calculated from Master Table 26-A,B,C,D.

Entries in Col.C and Col.G come from Tables 31-A and 31-B.

Entries in Col.D = (Col.B) x (Col.C).

Entries in Col.H = (Col.F) x (Col.G).

Cols. D and H provide the organ-doses for Tables 15-B and 15-G.

Table 15-B
Calculation of Raw K-Values for Males 0-9 Years of Age ATB.

T65DR DOSIMETRY, NEUTRON RBE = 2.0

The Basic Data for 0-9 year-old Males ATB
(Hiroshima plus Nagasaki combined)
from Tables 15-A, 11-B, and 26-A,B.

Dose-Group	Organ-Dose in cSv	Total Cancers for 1950-82	MALES Entered into Study	Cancers per Initial 10,000
Group 1+2	0.75	25	6818	36.67
Group 3	12.37	1	1547	6.46
Group 4	40.87	0	359	0.00
Group 5	84.03	2	189	105.82
Group 6	140.86	5	105	476.19
Group 7	202.37	0	43	0.00
Group 8	303.12	1	64	156.25

Combining the dose-classes, we have

Dose-Groups Combined	Organ-Dose in cSv	Total Cancers for 1950-82	Persons Entered into Study	Cancers/10,000 persons (R value)
1+2+3	2.90	26	8365	31.08
4+5+6+7+8	96.64	8	760	105.26

For application of Equation (7) to these data,

D_1 = 2.90 centi-Sieverts (rems)
D_2 = 96.64 centi-Sieverts (rems)
R_1 = 31.08 cancers per 10,000 persons, 1950-82
R_2 = 105.26 cancers per 10,000 persons, 1950-82
R_2/R_1 = 3.39

The numerator for Equation (7) is :
$$(R_2/R_1) - 1 = 2.39$$

The denominator for Equation (7) is :
$$(D_2) - (R_2/R_1)(D_1) = (96.64) - (3.39)(2.90)$$
$$= 86.81$$

The quotient, the K value = 0.02749

DS86 DOSIMETRY, NEUTRON RBE = 20

The Basic Data for 0-9 year-old Males ATB
(Hiroshima plus Nagasaki combined)
from Tables 15-A,11-B, and 26-A,B.

Dose-Group	Organ Dose in cSv	Total Cancers for 1950-82	MALES Entered into Study	Cancers per Initial 10,000
Group 1+2	0.85	25	6818	36.67
Group 3	15.16	1	1547	6.46
Group 4	46.24	0	359	0.00
Group 5	85.09	2	189	105.82
Group 6	137.83	5	105	476.19
Group 7	209.07	0	43	0.00
Group 8	368.11	1	64	156.25

Combining the dose-classes we have,

Dose-Groups Combined	Organ Dose in cSv	Total Cancers for 1950-82	Persons Entered into Study	Cancers/10,000 persons (R value)
1+2+3	3.49	26	8365	31.08
4+5+6+7+8	104.87	8	760	105.26

For application of Equation (7) to these data,

D_1 = 3.49 centi-Sieverts (rems)
D_2 = 104.87 centi-Sieverts (rems)
R_1 = 31.08 cancers per 10,000 persons, 1950-82
R_2 = 105.26 cancers per 10,000 persons, 1950-82
R_2/R_1 = 3.39

The numerator for Equation (7) is:
$$(R_2/R_1) - 1 = 2.39$$

The denominator for Equation (7) is :
$$(D_2) - (R_2/R_1)(D_1) = (104.87) - (3.39)(3.49)$$
$$= 93.04$$

The quotient, the K value = 0.02565

Table 15-C
Calculation of Raw K-Values for Males 10-19 Years of Age ATB.

T65DR DOSIMETRY, NEUTRON RBE = 2.0

The Basic Data for 10-19 year-old Males ATB
(Hiroshima plus Nagasaki combined)
from Tables 11-B and 26-A,B.

Dose-Group	Organ-Dose in cSv	Total Cancers for 1950-82	MALES Entered into Study	Cancers per Initial 10,000
Group 1+2	0.83	113	6378	177.17
Group 3	11.11	19	1112	170.86
Group 4	35.24	9	342	263.16
Group 5	71.79	5	371	134.77
Group 6	124.73	7	167	419.16
Group 7	172.18	4	70	571.43
Group 8	265.93	6	126	476.19

Combining the dose-classes, we have

Dose-Groups Combined	Organ-Dose in cSv	Total Cancers for 1950-82	Persons Entered into Study	Cancers/ 10,000 persons (R value)
1+2+3	2.36	132	7490	176.23
4+5+6+7+8	97.65	31	1076	288.10

For application of Equation (7) to these data,

D_1 =   2.36 centi-Sieverts (rems)

D_2 =   97.65 centi-Sieverts (rems)

R_1 =   176.23 cancers per 10,000 persons, 1950-82

R_2 =   288.10 cancers per 10,000 persons, 1950-82

R_2/R_1 =   1.63

The numerator for Equation (7) is :
$$(R_2/R_1) - 1 =   0.63$$

The denominator for Equation (7) is :
$$(D_2) - (R_2/R_1)(D_1) =   (97.65) - (1.63)(2.36)$$
$$=   93.80$$

The quotient, the K value   =   0.00677

DS86 DOSIMETRY, NEUTRON RBE = 20

The Basic Data for 10-19 year-old Males ATB
(Hiroshima plus Nagasaki combined)
from Tables 11-B and 26-A,B.

Dose-Group	Organ Dose in cSv	Total Cancers for 1950-82	MALES Entered into Study	Cancers per Initial 10,000
Group 1+2	1.11	113	6378	177.17
Group 3	13.92	19	1112	170.86
Group 4	36.53	9	342	263.16
Group 5	67.75	5	371	134.77
Group 6	117.37	7	167	419.16
Group 7	180.64	4	70	571.43
Group 8	325.58	6	126	476.19

Combining the dose-classes we have,

Dose-Groups Combined	Organ Dose in cSv	Total Cancers for 1950-82	Persons Entered into Study	Cancers/ 10,000 persons (R value)
1+2+3	3.01	132	7490	176.23
4+5+6+7+8	103.06	31	1076	288.10

For application of Equation (7) to these data,

D_1 =   3.01 centi-Sieverts (rems)

D_2 = 103.06 centi-Sieverts (rems)

R_1 = 176.23 cancers per 10,000 persons, 1950-82

R_2 = 288.10 cancers per 10,000 persons, 1950-82

R_2/R_1 =   1.63

The numerator for Equation (7) is:
$$(R_2/R_1) - 1 =   0.63$$

The denominator for Equation (7) is :
$$(D_2) - (R_2/R_1)(D_1) = (103.06) - (1.63)(3.01)$$
$$=   98.14$$

The quotient, the K value   =   0.00647

Table 15-D
Calculation of Raw K-Values for Males 20-34 Years of Age ATB.

T65DR DOSIMETRY, NEUTRON RBE = 2.0

The Basic Data for 20-34 year-old Males ATB
(Hiroshima plus Nagasaki combined)
from Tables 11-B and 26-A,B.

Dose-Group	Organ-Dose in cSv	Total Cancers for 1950-82	MALES Entered into Study	Cancers per Initial 10,000
Group 1+2	0.67	224	3293	680.23
Group 3	11.57	54	703	768.14
Group 4	35.54	11	237	464.14
Group 5	71.15	22	224	982.14
Group 6	123.33	17	122	1393.44
Group 7	171.24	2	53	377.36
Group 8	273.22	3	57	526.32

Combining the dose-classes, we have

Dose-Groups Combined	Organ-Dose in cSv	Total Cancers for 1950-82	Persons Entered into Study	Cancers/10,000 persons (R value)
1+2+3	2.59	278	3996	695.70
4+5+6+7+8	92.43	55	693	793.65

For application of Equation (7) to these data,

D1 =   2.59 centi-Sieverts (rems)
D2 =   92.43 centi-Sieverts (rems)
R1 =   695.70 cancers per 10,000 persons, 1950-82
R2 =   793.65 cancers per 10,000 persons, 1950-82
R2/R1 =   1.14

The numerator for Equation (7) is :
$$(R2/R1) - 1 = 0.14$$

The denominator for Equation (7) is :
$$(D2) - (R2/R1)(D1) = (92.43) - (1.14)(2.59)$$
$$= 89.48$$

The quotient, the K value = 0.00157

DS86 DOSIMETRY, NEUTRON RBE = 20

The Basic Data for 20-34 year-old Males ATB
(Hiroshima plus Nagasaki combined)
from Tables 11-B and 26-A,B.

Dose-Group	Organ-Dose in cSv	Total Cancers for 1950-82	MALES Entered into Study	Cancers per Initial 10,000
Group 1+2	0.99	224	3293	680.23
Group 3	15.34	54	703	768.14
Group 4	38.01	11	237	464.14
Group 5	70.73	22	224	982.14
Group 6	116.33	17	122	1393.44
Group 7	174.19	2	53	377.36
Group 8	340.73	3	57	526.32

Combining the dose-classes we have,

Dose-Groups Combined	Organ-Dose in cSv	Total Cancers for 1950-82	Persons Entered into Study	Cancers/10,000 persons (R value)
1+2+3	3.51	278	3996	695.70
4+5+6+7+8	97.69	55	693	793.65

For application of Equation (7) to these data,

D1 =   3.51 centi-Sieverts (rems)
D2 = 97.69 centi-Sieverts (rems)
R1 = 695.70 cancers per 10,000 persons, 1950-82
R2 = 793.65 cancers per 10,000 persons, 1950-82
R2/R1 = 1.14

The numerator for Equation (7) is:
$$(R2/R1) - 1 = 0.14$$

The denominator for Equation (7) is :
$$(D2) - (R2/R1)(D1) = (97.69) - (1.14)(3.51)$$
$$= 93.68$$

The quotient, the K value = 0.00150

Table 15-E
Calculation of Raw K-Values for Males 35-49 Years of Age ATB.

T65DR DOSIMETRY, NEUTRON RBE = 2.0

The Basic Data for 35-49 year-old Males ATB
(Hiroshima plus Nagasaki combined)
from Tables 11-B and 26-A,B.

Dose-Group	Organ-Dose in cSv	Total Cancers for 1950-82	MALES Entered into Study	Cancers per Initial 10,000
Group 1+2	0.65	963	5999	1605.27
Group 3	11.47	240	1381	1737.87
Group 4	35.66	82	438	1872.15
Group 5	69.45	72	368	1956.52
Group 6	120.43	24	133	1804.51
Group 7	171.23	12	70	1714.29
Group 8	266.80	28	111	2522.52

Combining the dose-classes, we have

Dose-Groups Combined	Organ-Dose in cSv	Total Cancers for 1950-82	Persons Entered into Study	Cancers/10,000 persons (R value)
1+2+3	2.67	1203	7380	1630.08
4+5+6+7+8	88.21	218	1120	1946.43

For application of Equation (7) to these data,

D_1 =   2.67 centi-Sieverts (rems)
D_2 =   88.21 centi-Sieverts (rems)
R_1 =   1630.08 cancers per 10,000 persons, 1950-82
R_2 =   1946.43 cancers per 10,000 persons, 1950-82
R_2/R_1 =   1.19

The numerator for Equation (7) is :
$(R_2/R_1) - 1$ = 0.19

The denominator for Equation (7) is :
$(D_2) - (R_2/R_1)(D_1)$ = (88.21)-(1.19)(2.67)
= 85.02

The quotient, the K value = 0.00228

DS86 DOSIMETRY, NEUTRON RBE = 20

The Basic Data for 35-49 year-old Males ATB
(Hiroshima plus Nagasaki combined)
from Tables 11-B and 26-A,B.

Dose-Group	Organ Dose in cSv	Total Cancers for 1950-82	MALES Entered into Study	Cancers per Initial 10,000
Group 1+2	0.95	963	5999	1605.27
Group 3	15.47	240	1381	1737.87
Group 4	40.56	82	438	1872.15
Group 5	74.85	72	368	1956.52
Group 6	121.05	24	133	1804.51
Group 7	175.05	12	70	1714.29
Group 8	326.23	28	111	2522.52

Combining the dose-classes we have,

Dose-Groups Combined	Organ Dose in cSv	Total Cancers for 1950-82	Persons Entered into Study	Cancers/10,000 persons (R value)
1+2+3	3.67	1203	7380	1630.08
4+5+6+7+8	98.10	218	1120	1946.43

For application of Equation (7) to these data,

D_1 = 3.67 centi-Sieverts (rems)
D_2 = 98.10 centi-Sieverts (rems)
R_1 = 1630.08 cancers per 10,000 persons, 1950-82
R_2 = 1946.43 cancers per 10,000 persons, 1950-82
R_2/R_1 = 1.19

The numerator for Equation (7) is:
$(R_2/R_1) - 1$ =   0.19

The denominator for Equation (7) is :
$(D_2) - (R_2/R_1)(D_1)$ = (98.10)-(1.19)(3.67)
= 93.72

The quotient, the K value = 0.00207

Table 15-F
Calculation of Raw K-Values for Males 50+ Years of Age ATB.

T65DR DOSIMETRY, NEUTRON RBE = 2.0

The Basic Data for 50+ year-old Males ATB
(Hiroshima plus Nagasaki combined)
from Tables 11-B and 26A,B.

Dose-Group	Organ-Dose in cSv	Total Cancers for 1950-82	MALES Entered into Study	Cancers per Initial 10,000
Group 1+2	0.63	747	5097	1465.57
Group 3	11.05	155	1145	1353.71
Group 4	35.67	51	308	1655.84
Group 5	72.24	40	234	1709.40
Group 6	122.73	15	74	2027.03
Group 7	177.14	3	34	882.35
Group 8	269.80	8	65	1230.77

Combining the dose-classes, we have

Dose-Groups Combined	Organ-Dose in cSv	Total Cancers for 1950-82	Persons Entered into Study	Cancers/ 10,000 persons (R value)
1+2+3	2.54	902	6242	1445.05
4+5+6+7+8	84.66	117	715	1636.36

For application of Equation (7) to these data,

D1 =   2.54 centi-Sieverts (rems)
D2 =   84.66 centi-Sieverts (rems)
R1 =   1445.05 cancers per 10,000 persons, 1950-82
R2 =   1636.36 cancers per 10,000 persons, 1950-82
R2/R1 =   1.13

The numerator for Equation (7) is :
        (R2/R1) - 1 = 0.13

The denominator for Equation (7) is :
  (D2) - (R2/R1)(D1) = (84.66)-(1.13)(2.54)
                      = 81.78

The quotient, the K value = 0.00162

DS86 DOSIMETRY, NEUTRON RBE = 20

The Basic Data for 50+ year-old Males ATB
(Hiroshima plus Nagasaki combined)
from Tables 11-B and 26A,B.

Dose-Group	Organ-Dose in cSv	Total Cancers for 1950-82	MALES Entered into Study	Cancers per Initial 10,000
Group 1+2	0.90	747	5097	1465.57
Group 3	14.81	155	1145	1353.71
Group 4	42.64	51	308	1655.84
Group 5	81.51	40	234	1709.40
Group 6	129.76	15	74	2027.03
Group 7	195.16	3	34	882.35
Group 8	339.69	8	65	1230.77

Combining the dose-classes we have,

Dose-Groups Combined	Organ-Dose in cSv	Total Cancers for 1950-82	Persons Entered into Study	Cancers/ 10,000 persons (R value)
1+2+3	3.45	902	6242	1445.05
4+5+6+7+8	98.63	117	715	1636.36

For application of Equation (7) to these data,

D1 = 3.45 centi-Sieverts (rems)
D2 = 98.63 centi-Sieverts (rems)
R1 = 1445.05 cancers per 10,000 persons, 1950-82
R2 = 1636.36 cancers per 10,000 persons, 1950-82
R2/R1 = 1.13

The numerator for Equation (7) is:
        (R2/R1) - 1 = 0.13

The denominator for Equation (7) is :
  (D2) - (R2/R1)(D1) = (98.63)-(1.13)(3.45)
                     = 94.73

The quotient, the K value = 0.00140

Table 15-G
Calculation of Raw K-Values for Females 0-9 Years of Age ATB.

T65DR DOSIMETRY, NEUTRON RBE = 2.0

The Basic Data for 0-9 year-old Females ATB
(Hiroshima plus Nagasaki combined)
from Tables 15-A, 11-D, and 26-C,D.

Dose-Group	Organ-Dose in cSv	Total Cancers for 1950-82	FEMALES Entered into Study	Cancers per Initial 10,000
Group 1+2	0.75	38	6935	54.79
Group 3	12.61	9	1547	58.18
Group 4	40.64	3	372	80.65
Group 5	83.04	3	213	140.85
Group 6	143.79	4	99	404.04
Group 7	209.16	1	41	243.90
Group 8	314.00	1	70	142.86

Combining the dose-classes, we have

Dose-Groups Combined	Organ-Dose in cSv	Total Cancers for 1950-82	Persons Entered into Study	Cancers/10,000 persons (R value)
1+2+3	2.91	47	8482	55.41
4+5+6+7+8	97.61	12	795	150.94

For application of Equation (7) to these data,

D1 = 2.91 centi-Sieverts (rems)
D2 = 97.61 centi-Sieverts (rems)
R1 = 55.41 cancers per 10,000 persons, 1950-82
R2 = 150.94 cancers per 10,000 persons, 1950-82
R2/R1 = 2.72

The numerator for Equation (7) is :
$$(R2/R1) - 1 = 1.72$$

The denominator for Equation (7) is :
$$(D2) - (R2/R1)(D1) = (97.61)-(2.72)(2.91)$$
$$= 89.68$$

The quotient, the K value = 0.01922

DS86 DOSIMETRY, NEUTRON RBE = 20

The Basic Data for 0-9 year-old Females ATB
(Hiroshima plus Nagasaki combined)
from Tables 15-A, 11-D, and 26-C,D.

Dose-Group	Organ-Dose in cSv	Total Cancers for 1950-82	FEMALES Entered into Study	Cancers per Initial 10,000
Group 1+2	0.84	38	6935	54.79
Group 3	15.42	9	1547	58.18
Group 4	45.55	3	372	80.65
Group 5	86.88	3	213	140.85
Group 6	144.40	4	99	404.04
Group 7	217.63	1	41	243.90
Group 8	375.99	1	70	142.86

Combining the dose-classes we have,

Dose-Groups Combined	Organ-Dose in cSv	Total Cancers for 1950-82	Persons Entered into Study	Cancers/10,000 persons (R value)
1+2+3	3.50	47	8482	55.41
4+5+6+7+8	106.90	12	795	150.94

For application of Equation (7) to these data,

D1 = 3.50 centi-Sieverts (rems)
D2 = 106.90 centi-Sieverts (rems)
R1 = 55.41 cancers per 10,000 persons, 1950-82
R2 = 150.94 cancers per 10,000 persons, 1950-82
R2/R1 = 2.72

The numerator for Equation (7) is:
$$(R2/R1) - 1 = 1.72$$

The denominator for Equation (7) is :
$$(D2) - (R2/R1)(D1) = (106.90)-(2.72)(3.50)$$
$$= 97.36$$

The quotient, the K value = 0.01771

Table 15-H
Calculation of Raw K-Values for Females 10-19 Years of Age ATB.

T65DR DOSIMETRY, NEUTRON RBE = 2.0

The Basic Data for 10-19 year-old Females ATB
(Hiroshima plus Nagasaki combined)
from Tables 11-D and 26C,D.

Dose-Group	Organ-Dose in cSv	Total Cancers for 1950-82	FEMALES Entered into Study	Cancers per Initial 10,000
Group 1+2	0.65	116	7403	156.69
Group 3	10.71	23	1663	138.30
Group 4	36.46	7	543	128.91
Group 5	72.44	18	556	323.74
Group 6	122.62	8	264	303.03
Group 7	172.26	8	118	677.97
Group 8	263.31	6	111	540.54

Combining the dose-classes, we have

Dose-Groups Combined	Organ-Dose in cSv	Total Cancers for 1950-82	Persons Entered into Study	Cancers/10,000 persons (R value)
1+2+3	2.50	139	9066	153.32
4+5+6+7+8	89.20	47	1592	295.23

For application of Equation (7) to these data,

D1 =   2.50 centi-Sieverts (rems)
D2 = 89.20 centi-Sieverts (rems)
R1 = 153.32 cancers per 10,000 persons, 1950-82
R2 = 295.23 cancers per 10,000 persons, 1950-82
R2/R1 = 1.93

The numerator for Equation (7) is :
      (R2/R1) - 1 = 0.93

The denominator for Equation (7) is :
  (D2) - (R2/R1)(D1)   = (89.20)-(1.93)(2.50)
                       = 84.39

The quotient, the K value = 0.01097

DS86 DOSIMETRY, NEUTRON RBE = 20

The Basic Data for 10-19 year-old Females ATB
(Hiroshima plus Nagasaki combined)
from Tables 11-D and 26C,D.

Dose-Group	Organ Dose in cSv	Total Cancers for 1950-82	FEMALES Entered into Study	Cancers per Initial 10,000
Group 1+2	0.80	116	7403	156.69
Group 3	13.79	23	1663	138.30
Group 4	39.15	7	543	128.91
Group 5	68.10	18	556	323.74
Group 6	110.72	8	264	303.03
Group 7	183.68	8	118	677.97
Group 8	324.60	6	111	540.54

Combining the dose-classes we have,

Dose-Groups Combined	Organ Dose in cSv	Total Cancers for 1950-82	Persons Entered into Study	Cancers/10,000 persons (R value)
1+2+3	3.18	139	9066	153.32
4+5+6+7+8	91.74	47	1592	295.23

For application of Equation (7) to these data,

D1 =   3.18 centi-Sieverts (rems)
D2 = 91.74 centi-Sieverts (rems)
R1 = 153.32 cancers per 10,000 persons, 1950-82
R2 = 295.23 cancers per 10,000 persons, 1950-82
R2/R1 = 1.93

The numerator for Equation (7) is:
      (R2/R1) - 1 = 0.93

The denominator for Equation (7) is :
  (D2) - (R2/R1)(D1) = (91.74)-(1.93)(3.18)
                     = 85.62

The quotient, the K value = 0.01081

Table 15-(Eye)
Calculation of Raw K-Values for Females 20-34 Years of Age ATB.

T65DR DOSIMETRY, NEUTRON RBE = 2.0

The Basic Data for 20-34 year-old Females ATB
(Hiroshima plus Nagasaki combined)
from Tables 11-D and 26-C,D.

Dose-Group	Organ-Dose in cSv	Total Cancers for 1950-82	FEMALES Entered into Study	Cancers per Initial 10,000
Group 1+2	0.66	396	9260	427.65
Group 3	10.98	121	2189	552.76
Group 4	35.61	36	670	537.31
Group 5	72.59	22	436	504.59
Group 6	122.38	22	192	1145.83
Group 7	172.35	6	103	582.52
Group 8	256.22	13	152	855.26

Combining the dose-classes, we have

Dose-Groups Combined	Organ-Dose in cSv	Total Cancers for 1950-82	Persons Entered into Study	Cancers/10,000 persons (R value)
1+2+3	2.63	517	11449	451.57
4+5+6+7+8	87.38	99	1553	637.48

For application of Equation (7) to these data,

$D1$ = 2.63 centi-Sieverts (rems)

$D2$ = 87.38 centi-Sieverts (rems)

$R1$ = 451.57 cancers per 10,000 persons, 1950-82

$R2$ = 637.48 cancers per 10,000 persons, 1950-82

$R2/R1$ = 1.41

The numerator for Equation (7) is :

$(R2/R1) - 1 = 0.41$

The denominator for Equation (7) is :

$(D2) - (R2/R1)(D1) = (87.38)-(1.41)(2.63)$

$= 83.66$

The quotient, the K value = 0.00492

DS86 DOSIMETRY, NEUTRON RBE = 20

The Basic Data for 20-34 year-old Females ATB
(Hiroshima plus Nagasaki combined)
from Tables 11-D and 26-C,D.

Dose-Group	Organ Dose in cSv	Total Cancers for 1950-82	FEMALES Entered into Study	Cancers per Initial 10,000
Group 1+2	0.89	396	9260	427.65
Group 3	14.85	121	2189	552.76
Group 4	42.38	36	670	537.31
Group 5	75.91	22	436	504.59
Group 6	121.79	22	192	1145.83
Group 7	182.47	6	103	582.52
Group 8	320.87	13	152	855.26

Combining the dose-classes we have,

Dose-Groups Combined	Organ Dose in cSv	Total Cancers for 1950-82	Persons Entered into Study	Cancers/10,000 persons (R value)
1+2+3	3.56	517	11449	451.57
4+5+6+7+8	98.16	99	1553	637.48

For application of Equation (7) to these data,

$D1$ = 3.56 centi-Sieverts (rems)

$D2$ = 98.16 centi-Sieverts (rems)

$R1$ = 451.57 cancers per 10,000 persons, 1950-82

$R2$ = 637.48 cancers per 10,000 persons, 1950-82

$R2/R1$ = 1.41

The numerator for Equation (7) is:

$(R2/R1) - 1 = 0.41$

The denominator for Equation (7) is :

$(D2) - (R2/R1)(D1) = (98.16)-(1.41)(3.56)$

$= 93.14$

The quotient, the K value = 0.00442

Table 15-J
Calculation of Raw K-Values for Females 35-49 Years of Age ATB.

T65DR DOSIMETRY, NEUTRON RBE = 2.0

The Basic Data for 35-49 year-old Females ATB
(Hiroshima plus Nagasaki combined)
from Tables 11-D and 26-C,D.

Dose-Group	Organ-Dose in cSv	Total Cancers for 1950-82	FEMALES Entered into Study	Cancers per Initial 10,000
Group 1+2	0.63	925	8838	1046.62
Group 3	10.99	274	2291	1195.98
Group 4	34.65	76	582	1305.84
Group 5	70.01	42	366	1147.54
Group 6	120.80	20	155	1290.32
Group 7	176.89	12	74	1621.62
Group 8	262.14	18	97	1855.67

Combining the dose-classes, we have

Dose-Groups Combined	Organ-Dose in cSv	Total Cancers for 1950-82	Persons Entered into Study	Cancers/10,000 persons (R value)
1+2+3	2.76	1199	11129	1077.37
4+5+6+7+8	80.87	168	1274	1318.68

For application of Equation (7) to these data,

D1 = 2.76 centi-Sieverts (rems)
D2 = 80.87 centi-Sieverts (rems)
R1 = 1077.37 cancers per 10,000 persons, 1950-82
R2 = 1318.68 cancers per 10,000 persons, 1950-82
R2/R1 = 1.22

The numerator for Equation (7) is :
$$(R2/R1) - 1 = 0.22$$

The denominator for Equation (7) is :
$$(D2) - (R2/R1)(D1) = (80.87)-(1.22)(2.76)$$
$$= 77.49$$

The quotient, the K value = 0.00289

DS86 DOSIMETRY, NEUTRON RBE = 20

The Basic Data for 35-49 year-old Females ATB
(Hiroshima plus Nagasaki combined)
from Tables 11-D and 26-C,D.

Dose-Group	Organ Dose in cSv	Total Cancers for 1950-82	FEMALES Entered into Study	Cancers per Initial 10,000
Group 1+2	0.84	925	8838	1046.62
Group 3	15.22	274	2291	1195.98
Group 4	43.00	76	582	1305.84
Group 5	78.94	42	366	1147.54
Group 6	127.99	20	155	1290.32
Group 7	195.39	12	74	1621.62
Group 8	328.33	18	97	1855.67

Combining the dose-classes we have,

Dose-Groups Combined	Organ Dose in cSv	Total Cancers for 1950-82	Persons Entered into Study	Cancers/10,000 persons (R value)
1+2+3	3.80	1199	11129	1077.37
4+5+6+7+8	94.24	168	1274	1318.68

For application of Equation (7) to these data,

D1 = 3.80 centi-Sieverts (rems)
D2 = 94.24 centi-Sieverts (rems)
R1 = 1077.37 cancers per 10,000 persons, 1950-82
R2 = 1318.68 cancers per 10,000 persons, 1950-82
R2/R1 = 1.22

The numerator for Equation (7) is:
$$(R2/R1) - 1 = 0.22$$

The denominator for Equation (7) is :
$$(D2) - (R2/R1)(D1) = (94.24)-(1.22)(3.80)$$
$$= 89.59$$

The quotient, the K value = 0.00250

Table 15-K
Calculation of Raw K-Values for Females 50+ Years of Age ATB.

T65DR DOSIMETRY, NEUTRON RBE = 2.0

The Basic Data for 50+ year-old Females ATB
(Hiroshima plus Nagasaki combined)
from Tables 11-D and 26-C,D.

Dose-Group	Organ-Dose in cSv	Total Cancers for 1950-82	FEMALES Entered into Study	Cancers per Initial 10,000
Group 1+2	0.62	608	6007	1012.15
Group 3	10.82	159	1365	1164.84
Group 4	35.35	39	374	1042.78
Group 5	71.74	27	171	1578.95
Group 6	119.04	9	70	1285.71
Group 7	175.10	3	33	909.09
Group 8	274.06	7	34	2058.82

Combining the dose-classes, we have

Dose-Groups Combined	Organ-Dose in cSv	Total Cancers for 1950-82	Persons Entered into Study	Cancers/ 10,000 persons (R value)
1+2+3	2.51	767	7372	1040.42
4+5+6+7+8	71.73	85	682	1246.33

For application of Equation (7) to these data,

$D1 = $ 2.51 centi-Sieverts (rems)
$D2 = $ 71.73 centi-Sieverts (rems)
$R1 = $ 1040.42 cancers per 10,000 persons, 1950-82
$R2 = $ 1246.33 cancers per 10,000 persons, 1950-82
$R2/R1 = $ 1.20

The numerator for Equation (7) is :
$(R2/R1) - 1 = 0.20$

The denominator for Equation (7) is :
$(D2) - (R2/R1)(D1) = (71.73)-(1.20)(2.51)$
$= 68.72$

The quotient, the K value $= 0.00288$

DS86 DOSIMETRY, NEUTRON RBE = 20

The Basic Data for 50+ year-old Females ATB
(Hiroshima plus Nagasaki combined)
from Tables 11-D and 26-C,D.

Dose-Group	Organ Dose in cSv	Total Cancers for 1950-82	FEMALES Entered into Study	Cancers per Initial 10,000
Group 1+2	0.82	608	6007	1012.15
Group 3	14.90	159	1365	1164.84
Group 4	43.68	39	374	1042.78
Group 5	77.44	27	171	1578.95
Group 6	125.23	9	70	1285.71
Group 7	192.27	3	33	909.09
Group 8	343.56	7	34	2058.82

Combining the dose-classes we have,

Dose-Groups Combined	Organ Dose in cSv	Total Cancers for 1950-82	Persons Entered into Study	Cancers/ 10,000 persons (R value)
1+2+3	3.43	767	7372	1040.42
4+5+6+7+8	82.65	85	682	1246.33

For application of Equation (7) to these data,

$D1 = $ 3.43 centi-Sieverts (rems)
$D2 = $ 82.65 centi-Sieverts (rems)
$R1 = $ 1040.42 cancers per 10,000 persons, 1950-82
$R2 = $ 1246.33 cancers per 10,000 persons, 1950-82
$R2/R1 = $ 1.20

The numerator for Equation (7) is:
$(R2/R1) - 1 = 0.20$

The denominator for Equation (7) is :
$(D2) - (R2/R1)(D1) = (82.65)-(1.20)(3.43)$
$= 78.55$

The quotient, the K value $= 0.00252$

Table 15–L   T65DR

K-Values for Low-Dose Exposure, up to 5 Centi-Sieverts.
K is the fractional increase in the spontaneous cancer death-rate per cSv of whole-body organ-dose.

T65DR DOSIMETRY, NEUTRON RBE = 2.0

AGE ATB	MALES EQUATION OF BEST FIT	Low-Dose K Per cSv
0–9	Ca-Rate = (2.5937)(Dose^0.75)+(25.3161)	0.06851
10–19	Ca-Rate = (3.8365)(Dose^0.75)+(168.925)	0.01519
20–34	Ca-Rate = (3.5274)(Dose^0.75)+(688.498)	0.003426
35–49	Ca-Rate = (11.8508)(Dose^0.75)+(1605.326)	0.004936
50+	Ca-Rate = (7.3871)(Dose^0.75)+(1430.187)	0.003454

AGE ATB	FEMALES EQUATION OF BEST FIT	Low-Dose K Per cSv
0–9	Ca-Rate = (3.3140)(Dose^0.75)+(48.0263)	0.04615
10–19	Ca-Rate = (5.2487)(Dose^0.75)+(142.885)	0.02457
20–34	Ca-Rate = (7.0116)(Dose^0.75)+(437.0894)	0.01073
35–49	Ca-Rate = (9.7200)(Dose^0.75)+(1056.556)	0.006152
50+	Ca-Rate = (9.0896)(Dose^0.75)+(1022.294)	0.005945

1. The two-step method for obtaining the Equation of Best Fit and the low-dose K-value for each age-sex group is explained by the text in detail.

---

2. The raw K-values (assembled below from Tables 15-B through 15-K) were calculated for the purpose of comparison with the low-dose K-values above. The low-dose K-values are larger -- due to the supra-linearity of dose-response -- by a factor of about 2.2 (details in text). Therefore the raw K-values will underestimate cancer-risk from low-dose exposure by more than 2-fold, and should not be used for such exposures.

T65DR

Age-Band ATB	Males Raw K	Females Raw K
0–9	0.02749	0.01922
10–19	0.00677	0.01097
20–34	0.00157	0.00492
35–49	0.00228	0.00289
50+	0.00162	0.00288

Table 15–L <u>DS86</u>

K-Values for Low-Dose Exposure, up to 5 Centi-Sieverts.
K is the fractional increase in the spontaneous cancer death-rate per cSv of whole-body organ-dose.

DS86 DOSIMETRY, NEUTRON RBE = 20

AGE ATB	MALES EQUATION OF BEST FIT	Low-Dose K Per cSv
0–9	Ca-rate = $(2.4549)(Dose^{0.75})+(24.8117)$	0.06617
10–19	Ca-Rate = $(3.7215)(Dose^{0.75})+(167.7256)$	0.01484
20–34	Ca-Rate = $(3.4358)(Dose^{0.75})+(686.8894)$	0.003344
35–49	Ca-Rate = $(11.0924)(Dose^{0.75})+(1600.667)$	0.004634
50+	Ca-Rate = $(6.6506)(Dose^{0.75})+(1428.214)$	0.003114

AGE ATB	FEMALES EQUATION OF BEST FIT	Low-Dose K Per cSv
0–9	Ca-Rate = $(3.1131)(Dose^{0.75})+(47.4440)$	0.04388
10–19	Ca-Rate = $(5.2055)(Dose^{0.75})+(140.9239)$	0.02470
20–34	Ca-Rate = $(6.5018)(Dose^{0.75})+(434.7191)$	0.01000
35–49	Ca-Rate = $(8.7670)(Dose^{0.75})+(1053.509)$	0.005565
50+	Ca Rate = $(8.2725)(Dose^{0.75})+(1019.570)$	0.005425

1. The two-step method for obtaining the Equation of Best Fit and the low-dose K-value for each age-sex group is explained by the text in detail.

----

2. The raw K-values (assembled below from Tables 15-B through 15-K) were calculated for the purpose of comparison with the low-dose K-values above. The low-dose K-values are larger -- due to the supra-linearity of dose-response -- by a factor of about 2.2 (details in text). Therefore the raw K-values will underestimate cancer-risk from low-dose exposure by more than 2-fold, and should not be used for such exposures.

T65DR

Age-Band ATB	Males Raw K	Females Raw K
0–9	0.02565	0.01771
10–19	0.00647	0.01081
20–34	0.00150	0.00442
35–49	0.00207	0.00250
50+	0.00140	0.00252

Low–Dose Cancer–Yields by the Cancer–Rate Ratio Method, for the A–Bomb Survivors and for a United States' Population

This chapter is arranged in six parts:

Then tables.

1. Minimum Fatal Cancer–Yield for the A–Bomb Survivors

The K-values provided by the A-Bomb Study represent the fractional increase in the spontaneous cancer death-rate per centi-sievert (or per rem) of whole-body internal organ-dose -- for a specific period of observation. Our "in-the-box" low-dose K-values come from observations in the 1950-1982 period. As usual, the Reference Group (1+2) is regarded as unexposed, and cancer death-rates are the cumulative rates among a set of initial persons.

To illustrate how the low-dose K-values in Table 15-L convert into Minimum Fatal Cancer-Yields, we can ask this question, which uses numbers from Table 11-E, Entries F72 and N72:

If 38 cancers occurred spontaneously in the time-period 1950-1982 among a set of 6,935 unexposed children at Hiroshima and Nagasaki, how many radiation-induced cancers must have occurred during the same period in a comparable group of 6,935 children exposed to 1 cSv of whole-body organ-dose? The low-dose K-value from Table 15-L enables us to calculate directly what that number of radiation-induced cancers must have been.

$$\text{Persons} = 6935$$
$$\text{Cancers} = 38$$

K-Value, T65DR Dosimetry = 0.04615

If 38 cancers occurred without radiation exposure, and if K is 0.04615 per centi-sievert (rem) of exposure, we multiply (38) by (0.04615) to ascertain the radiation-induced increment in cancers for 1950-1982 per centi-sievert. This yields 1.7537 cancers among 6,935 initial persons each exposed to one cSv (rem).

And 1.75 is the entry found in Table 16-B, Column G, for the youngest age-band of females. Table 16-A provides the customary details about Table 16-B (where space was insufficient).

Calculations comparable to the one just illustrated provide the additional entries in Column G, for the other 9 age-sex subsets. For the period 1950-1982, the sum from all ten subsets is 29.59 radiation-induced cancers per 66,028 initial persons each exposed to an average whole-body organ-dose of 1 cSv (rem). When this rate is converted (in the next row) to the equivalent rate per 10,000 persons, it becomes the Minimum Fatal Cancer-Yield, prior to the adjustment for under-ascertainment of cancer-deaths -- which is shown on the next row.

The final Minimum Fatal Cancer-Yield in the T65DR dosimetry, by the Cancer-Rate Ratio Method, is 5.51 "in-the-box." The corresponding value from a "constant-cohort, dual-dosimetry" analysis yields 5.17 in the current version of the DS86 dosimetry.

2. Lifetime Fatal Cancer–Yield for the A–Bomb Survivors

The Necessity of Making Assumptions :

Every estimate of a Lifetime Fatal Cancer-Yield incorporates assumptions, by one analyst or another (or by some committee), about what future follow-ups will show in the A-Bomb Study. Estimates which we make by the Cancer-Rate Ratio Method incorporate two assumptions.

Spontaneous Rate: We are assuming that the lifetime follow-up will show a spontaneous cancer-rate in the Reference Group which is close to our estimate of 14.5 percent (from Table 28-D, entry G13).

Constant K-Values: We are assuming that the low-dose K-values observed from the 1950-1982 evidence will persist at about their same magnitude in the additional observations beyond 1982. The best available evidence on duration would justify no OTHER assumption at this time, in my opinion (Chapter 17). Indeed, RERF analysts seem to have reached the same conclusion, for they project their own current risk-coefficients into the remainder of the follow-up when they make their lifetime estimates (TR-9-87, p.34, and TR-5-88, p.50+53; current risk-coefficients in the latter report explicitly exclude the 1950-1955 data, p.50).

In assuming constant K-values, all of us realize, of course, that the best available evidence is just the best AVAILABLE evidence in science, and that subsequent observations are "entitled" to change the story.

The Method for
Obtaining Lifetime Fatal Cancer-Yields :

Table 16-A, Note 7 onward, explains the method step-by-step. We just apply the low-dose K-values, which are valid for 1950-1982, to the estimated number of spontaneous cancers expected to occur ULTIMATELY in each subset of the Reference Group, and then sum those contributions. The result is adjusted to the denominator of 10,000 persons, and then adjusted by the BEIR-RERF underascertainment factor, and "that is that."

The final best estimate is 31.65 in the T65DR dosimetry, and 30.43 in the current version of the DS86 dosimetry.

The Role of the Youngest Age-Band :

Inspection of Table 16-B, Columns G and J, shows what a trivial contribution is made by the youngest age-band to the MINIMUM Fatal Cancer-Yield. In the T65DR dosimetry, for instance, the share is only (1.25 from the males + 1.75 from the females), or 3 out of the total of 29.59 (Column G). This low contribution, in spite of the higher K-values in this age-band, comes from the very low spontaneous rates in the youngest age-band during the 1950-1982 follow-up period, compared with every other age-band (Column D).

By contrast, inspection of Columns H and K shows what a very big contribution is made by the youngest

age-band to the estimated LIFETIME Fatal Cancer-Yield. In the T65DR dosimetry, for instance, the share is (54.79 from the males + 39.21 from the females), or 94 out of the total of 169.91 (Column H). This result comes not from an extraordinarily high lifetime spontaneous rate (indeed, Column E shows a somewhat lower estimate for the ultimate lifetime spontaneous rate in this age-band). This shift from a trivial role to a dominant role comes from the combination of a SPONTANEOUS cancer "story" which has hardly even begun for this age-band during the 1950-1982 follow-up period, with the relatively high K-values for this same age-band.

Cancer-Yield as Percent Increase per Rad :

A Lifetime Fatal Cancer-Yield can be easily converted to "percent increase in the spontaneous cancer death-rate per cSv."

For instance, our estimates in Table 16-B are based on the estimate that 14.47 % of the LSS mixed-age population sample will die of spontaneous cancer (Table 29-D, entry G13). Out of each 10,000 initial persons, the estimated spontaneous cancer deaths will be 1,447. Table 16-B estimates that about 31 additional cases will occur per cSv of whole-body internal organ-dose, per 10,000 initial persons.

Thus, for this particular mixed-age group of persons, the percent increase in the lifetime spontaneous rate is (31 / 1,447) x (100), or 2.14 % per cSv.

In principle, the conversion is clearly easy. In reality, it is often hard to ascertain the post-irradiation lifetime spontaneous rate which was assumed in someone else's analysis. For some limited purposes, a "ball-park" spontaneous rate for a mixed-age population may suffice.

3. Lifetime Fatal Cancer-Yield for
a USA Population

The Cancer-Rate Ratio Method makes it self-evident that the relative distribution of ages and sexes in an irradiated population will affect the population's Minimum and Lifetime Fatal Cancer-Yields. The minimum (or interim) values will come predominantly from the older and less sensitive age-bands, and increments to the minimum values will come predominantly from the younger and MORE sensitive age-bands.

There is no reason to assume that the age-sex distribution in the Reference Group of the A-Bomb

Study is comparable to the age-sex distribution in the current United States population; indeed, we know that the distributions differ. Therefore, we want to provide a Cancer-Yield which is appropriate for the United States.

We can provide a LIFETIME Fatal Cancer-Yield for the U.S. population if we make just one reasonable approximation. We will say that the FRACTIONAL INCREASE in the spontaneous cancer death-rate will be the same for humans here as for humans there, per centi-sievert of exposure.

Table 16-C provides both the input and output for the estimate.

The best lifetime estimate is 26.64 in the T65DR dosimetry, and 25.56 in the current version of the DS86 dosimetry. These lifetime estimates are somewhat LOWER for the U.S. population than the A-bomb survivors, even though we have estimated that the A-bomb survivors will have the lower ultimate SPONTANEOUS cancer-rate (see Note 3, Table 16-C).

The explanation is no mystery, however. Table 28-D, Column E, shows that in the normalized Reference Group, 24626.32 out of 66028.01 initial persons are in the two youngest and most radio-sensitive age-bands at the time of exposure. This share is 37.3 percent. By contrast, Table 16-C, Column C, shows a lower percentage in the United States' population: 3,169 out of 10,000 persons, or 31.7 percent. In addition, the USA population has a higher percentage of males than the normalized Reference Group -- 49 percent versus 42 percent -- and males have generally lower K-values than females (so far).

The estimates in Table 16-C are not new iterations, revisions, or replacements of my earlier estimate of 37.71. See Table 16-C, Note 7.

4. Comparison of Results, This Method vs. Cancer Difference Method

Minimum Fatal Cancer-Yields :

How do the Minimum Fatal Cancer-Yields derived by the Cancer-Rate Ratio Method compare with the values derived by the Cancer Difference Method with the best-fit curve? The values below come from Table 14-A, Row 2, and from Table 16-B:

```
T65DR: Cancer Difference = 5.80 fatal cancers/cSv
T65DR: Cancer-Rate Ratio = 5.51 fatal cancers/cSv
```

```
DS86: Cancer Difference  = 5.41 fatal cancers/cSv
DS86: Cancer-Rate Ratio  = 5.17 fatal cancers/ cSv
```

The two methods produce closely similar answers, although the methods appear to be quite different.

One method kept the observations combined for all ages and sexes, subtracted the best-fit cancer-rates at zero-dose from the best-fit cancer-rates at 5 cSv, and divided the answer by five.

The other method subdivided the same observations into ten age-sex subsets, and for each subset of observations, derived an equation of best fit, based on observations exclusively from that subset together with the common dose-exponent of 0.75. Then it used the equation to predict best-fit points at zero-dose and 5 cSv, used those two points to derive a low-dose K-value (fractional increase in the spontaneous cancer-rate per cSv), applied the K-value to the corresponding number of spontaneous cancers in the subdivided Reference Group to obtain the radiation-induced increment from a dose of one cSv, and obtained the Minimum Fatal Cancer-Yield by adding up the increments expected from each of the ten subsets.

In spite of the difference in method, if computational errors are absent, one should EXPECT good agreement when two valid but different approaches are made to exactly the same set of observations. When the observations are "in-the-box," the residual uncertainty lies in sampling variation, which could work in either direction -- either to underestimate or to overestimate the true value.

Lifetime Fatal Cancer-Yields :

How do the findings for LIFETIME Fatal Cancer-Yields compare in the two methods?

```
T65DR: Cancer Difference = 12.90 fatal cancers/cSv
T65DR: Cancer-Rate Ratio = 31.65 fatal cancers/cSv
```

```
DS86: Cancer Difference = 12.03 fatal cancers/cSv
DS86: Cancer-Rate Ratio = 30.43 fatal cancers/cSv
```

It was predictable that the Cancer Difference Method would give much lower values for the LIFETIME Cancer-Yields than does the Cancer-Rate Ratio Method. The reason is that every estimate of lifetime values necessarily uses assumptions and approximations to fill in for the missing observations, and the two methods use one crucially different approximation.

The Cancer Difference Method, with its conversion-factor of 2.223 from minimum to lifetime values, is using the approximation that the cancers which will occur beyond 1982 will be arising from a population with the same age-distribution and radiation-sensitivity as the population which produced the cancers observed between 1950-1982. This approximation is simply unrealistic, as already noted in Chapter 13.

For the 1950-82 period, the cancer deaths are coming predominantly from the older and less sensitive groups ATB, whereas in the post-1982 period, the cancer deaths will be coming predominantly from the younger and much more sensitive groups ATB. The Cancer-Rate Ratio Method takes this into account, whereas the Cancer Difference Method does not.

5. Merits and Pitfalls of the Methods

The comparisons in Part 4 above show that two methods, which produce nearly identical estimates for the Minimum "in-the-box" Fatal Cancer-Yields, produce LIFETIME estimates which differ by 2.5-fold. The factor of 2.5 is a measure of the potential error one would make by ignoring the fact that the residual population-sample beyond 1982 is NOT like the sample which generated the 1950-1982 observations. In other words, the Cancer-Rate Ratio Method is more realistic in its underlying assumptions about the LIFETIME risk than is the Cancer Difference Method. That is its great merit.

But this does not necessarily mean that the estimates of 30 or 32 fatal cancers per 10,000 persons per rem will match the ultimate estimate for low-dose exposure, when the full lifespan study is complete. We have made it clear how much depends on the future "behavior" of the youngest age-band, and also on the ultimate spontaneous cancer death-rate in the Reference Group. These unknowns are the biggest "pitfalls" in any such estimate.

● -- The true Lifetime Fatal Cancer-Yield for low-dose exposure could turn out considerably LOWER than 30 or 32 :

(A) If the ultimate spontaneous cancer death-rates in the Reference Group have been OVERestimated in our analysis;

(B) If the observed K-values in the youngest age-band "droop" or "melt down" during additional years of observation; this could happen due to sampling variation in the presently sparse observations, or due to

a true (biological) reduction of effect beyond 40 years post-irradiation, or due to a reduced degree of supra-linearity in all age-bands after additional observations, or due to a less supra-linear dose-response in children than in adults.

● -- The true Lifetime Fatal Cancer-Yield for low-dose exposure could turn out considerably HIGHER than 30 or 32 :

(A) If the ultimate spontaneous cancer death-rates in the Reference Group have been UNDERestimated in our analysis;

(B) If the observed K-values in the youngest age-band increase during additional years of observation; this could happen due to sampling variation in the presently sparse observations, or due to an increased degree of supra-linearity in all age-bands after additional observations, or due to a greater supra-linear dose-response in children than adults. This would be very serious, since our estimate of 30-32 has ignored supra-linearity between 0 and 5 cSv, and has used the linear approximation in that dose-region.

Conclusion regarding Uncertainties :

These uncertainties are simply unavoidable. But they do not make it reasonable to accept the UNREALISTIC premise of the Cancer Difference Method with respect to lifetime estimates -- namely, that the population which will generate the cancers beyond 1982 is like the population which generated the cancers between 1950-1982.

Moreover, since the uncertainties in the Cancer-Rate Ratio Method could readily operate toward UNDERestimating the risk, which may turn out much HIGHER than 30-32, it would be a sign of bias if I "preferred" using lifetime estimates which are 2.5-fold lower (from the Cancer Difference Method).

As a physician, I might add that information does not always need to be exact, in order to be extremely useful for human health.

6. The Bottom-Line from the Cancer-Rate Ratio Method

1. The Cancer-Rate Ratio Method produces about the same MINIMUM Fatal Cancer-Yields for low-dose exposure as the Cancer Difference Method, in both dosimetries (text, Part 4). With their close agreement, the two analyses are excellent confirmation of each other with respect to evidence "in-the-box." By both

methods, the Minimum Fatal Cancer-Yield is about 5.5 fatal radiation-induced cancers among 10,000 persons per cSv (rem) of whole-body organ-dose.

2. The Cancer-Rate Ratio Method produces estimates of LIFETIME Fatal Cancer-Yields for low-dose exposure which are predictably higher, and inherently more realistic, than the estimates produced -- for comparison -- by the Cancer Difference Method (text, Part 5). The Lifetime Fatal Cancer-Yields produced by the Cancer-Rate Ratio Method are 30-32 fatal radiation-induced cancers among 10,000 A-bomb survivors per cSv (rem) of whole-body organ-dose (Table 16-B). When the estimates are adjusted for a United States' population, they are 26-27 fatal radiation-induced cancers among 10,000 persons per cSv (rem) of whole-body organ-dose (Table 16-C). These values apply directly to low-dose exposure, acute or slow, between 0 and 5 cSv (rems).

3. Lifetime values in the range of 26 (USA) to 30 (A-bomb survivors) are very much higher than the values of 1-2 which are routinely used by the radiation community. Nonetheless, values like 26-30 may underestimate the cancer-hazard from X-ray exposure by about two-fold (see Chapter 13, Part 4).

4. Unlike some other analyses, our work does not throw away any of the evidence (follow-up years, or Dose-Groups) in the A-Bomb Study. It is based on the whole story, 1950-1982, and its legitimate prospective structure. We look forward to the time when the data become available to do a "constant-cohort, dual dosimetry" analysis with the additional observations through 1985.

Table 16-A
Notes for Table 16-B, Cancer-Yields by the Cancer-Rate Ratio Method, for the A-Bomb Survivors.

1. In Col.A, "H+N" abbreviates Hiroshima plus Nagasaki.

2. In Col.B, mean age ATB for RERF's five age-bands is calculated for the Reference Group from Master Table 26-A,B,C,D, in excellent agreement with Tables 11-C,E.

3. Col.C and Col.D entries are the normalized values from Tables 11-C and 11-E. These entries can also be found in Table 28-D, Columns E and H. Persons are those enrolled for the study in RERF Dose-Groups 1+2 (the Reference Class) in 1950. Spontaneous cancers are those cancer-deaths already observed (1950-1982) in this cohort.

4. Col.E entries for LIFETIME spontaneous cancers are from Table 28-D, Col.F. They are the estimated spontaneous cancer-deaths which will have accumulated among this cohort during the post-irradiation period, beginning in 1950 through the time when the last member of this cohort has died of one cause or another. These numbers may be underestimated (see Chapter 13, Part 6).

5. Col.F entries for low-dose K-values come from the body of Table 15-L, for the T65DR dosimetry. K is defined as the fractional increase in the spontaneous cancer death-rate per cSv of average whole-body organ-dose. Low-dose K-values apply to a total dose up to 5 cSv. Because the dose-response relationship is supra-linear (concave-downward), different dose-ranges have different K-values.

6. Col.G entries for radiation-induced cancer-deaths 1950-1982 per cSv are (Col.F x Col.D). Entries represent the number of radiation-induced cancers which would occur among an identical EXPOSED group of comparable size during 1950-1982, per cSv of average whole-body organ-dose.

7. Col.H entries for LIFETIME radiation-induced cancer-deaths per cSv are (Col.F x Col.E). This step incorporates the approximation that the low-dose K-values observed during the first 32 years of follow-up will remain at about the same magnitude for the cohort's remaining lifespan. The evidence at hand justifies no OTHER presumption at this time (Chapter 17).

8. Cols.I, J, and K represent the appropriate entries based on the current version of the DS86 dosimetry.

9. The row of sums apply to the 66,028 persons in the Reference Group, not to 10,000 persons. Therefore the values are reduced by the factor (10,000 / 66,028) in the next row.

10. The values must then be increased by the RERF-BEIR factor of 1.23 for underascertainment of cancer (see Chapter 11.)

11. The box at the foot of Table 16-B presents the final MINIMUM FATAL CANCER-YIELD BY THE CANCER-RATE RATIO METHOD:

    5.51   by T65DR, or 5.51 cancers x 10^{-4} persons x rem^{-1}.
    5.17   by DS86, or 5.17 cancers x 10^{-4} persons x rem^{-1}.

12. The box presents the final estimated LIFETIME FATAL CANCER-YIELD BY THE CANCER-RATE RATIO METHOD:

    31.65 by T65DR, or 31.65 cancers x 10^{-4} persons x rem^{-1}.
    30.43 by DS86, or 30.43 cancers x 10^{-4} persons x rem^{-1}.

13. Cancer-hazard from X-rays may be underestimated by the A-Bomb Study (see Chapter 13, Part 4).

Table 16-B
Estimation of Minimum and Lifetime Fatal Cancer-Yields for Hiroshima + Nagasaki A-Bomb Survivors.
By the Cancer-Rate Ratio Method, for Low-Dose Whole-Body Exposure per cSv, up to 5 cSv.   Leukemia Excluded.

Initial persons and spontaneous cancer-deaths are from the Reference Group (Dose-Groups 1+2).

Col.A Population Sample (Ref Grp)	Col.B Mean Age ATB	Col.C Initial Persons	Col.D Spontaneous Cancers 1950-82	Col.E Spontaneous Cancers LIFETIME	Col.F K per cSv T65DR	Col.G Rad'n-Induced Cancers 1950-82 per cSv T65DR	Col.H Rad'n Induced Cancers LIFETIME per cSv T65DR	Col.I K per cSv DS86	Col.J Rad'n-Induced Cancers 1950-82 per cSv DS86	Col.K Rad'n Induced Cancers LIFETIME per cSv DS86
Males, H+N	4.16	4976.25	18.25	799.7347	0.06851	1.25	54.79	0.06617	1.21	52.92
Males, H+N	13.95	5312.07	94.11	920.2082	0.01519	1.43	13.98	0.01484	1.40	13.66
Males, H+N	28.04	6644.57	451.98	1124.797	0.00343	1.55	3.85	0.00334	1.51	3.76
Males. H+N	42.60	6341.76	1018.02	1125.653	0.00494	5.02	5.56	0.00463	4.72	5.22
Males, H+N	58.14	4310.36	631.71	637.6347	0.00345	2.18	2.20	0.00311	1.97	1.99
Females. H+N	4.08	6935	38	849.648	0.04615	1.75	39.21	0.04388	1.67	37.28
Females, H+N	14.90	7403	116	1064.396	0.02457	2.85	26.15	0.02470	2.87	26.29
Females, H+N	26.69	9260	396	1234.162	0.01073	4.25	13.24	0.01000	3.96	12.34
Females, H+N	41.71	8838	925	1169.435	0.00615	5.69	7.19	0.00557	5.15	6.51
Females, H+N	59.05	6007	608	627.055	0.00595	3.61	3.73	0.00543	3.30	3.40
SUM OF ALL		66028	4297.07	9552.724		29.59	169.91		27.74	163.36
Cancers/10,000 persons			650.80			4.48	25.73		4.20	24.74
RERF-BEIR Correction Factor of 1.23 for Underascertainment of Cancer						5.51	31.65		5.17	30.43

FATAL CANCER-YIELD =

NUMBER OF FATAL RADIATION-INDUCED CANCERS AMONG 10,000 PERSONS PER cSv OF AVERAGE WHOLE-BODY ORGAN-DOSE.

SUMMARY OF FATAL CANCER-YIELDS BY THE CANCER-RATE RATIO METHOD
After correction for underascertainment of cancer.

	T65DR	DS86
MINIMUM "IN-THE-BOX"	5.51	5.17
LIFETIME	31.65	30.43

Cancer-hazard from X-rays may be underestimated by the A-Bomb Study. See Chapter 13, Part 4.

NOTES: See Table 16-A.

Table 16-C
Estimation of Lifetime Fatal Cancer-Yield for the United States' Population.
By the Cancer-Rate Ratio Method, for Low-Dose Whole-Body Exposure per cSv, up to 5 cSv. Leukemia Excluded.

Col.A Age-Band (Years)	Col.B Sex	Col.C Persons	Col.D Remaining Lifespan: Fraction Dying of Cancer	Col.E Remaining Lifespan: Number of Spontaneous Ca-Deaths	T65DR Dosimetry Col.F K per cSv	T65DR Dosimetry Col.G Lifetime Rad'n-Induced Fatal Cancers per cSv	DS86 Dosimetry Col.H K per cSv	DS86 Dosimetry Col.I Lifetime Rad'n-Induced Fatal Cancers per cSv
0-9	Males	721.95	0.185	133.56	0.06851	9.15	0.06617	8.84
10-19	Males	896.45	0.185	165.84	0.01519	2.52	0.01484	2.46
20-34	Males	1238.98	0.188	232.93	0.00343	0.80	0.00334	0.78
35-49	Males	814.4	0.190	154.74	0.00494	0.76	0.00463	0.72
50+	Males	1206.59	0.183	220.81	0.00345	0.76	0.00311	0.69
0-9	Females	687.71	0.160	110.03	0.04615	5.08	0.04388	4.83
10-19	Females	863.27	0.160	138.12	0.02457	3.39	0.02470	3.41
20-34	Females	1233.53	0.161	198.60	0.01073	2.13	0.01000	1.99
35-49	Females	841.38	0.159	133.78	0.00615	0.82	0.00557	0.74
50+	Females	1495.75	0.137	204.92	0.00594	1.22	0.00543	1.11
Totals		10000		1693.33		26.64		25.56

LIFETIME FATAL CANCER-YIELD =
NUMBER OF FATAL RADIATION-INDUCED CANCERS AMONG 10,000 PERSONS PER cSv OF AVERAGE WHOLE-BODY ORGAN-DOSE.

```
        U.S. POPULATION (1978 COMPOSITION):
   LIFETIME FATAL CANCER-YIELD BY THE CANCER-RATE RATIO METHOD
      Based on T65DR                  Based on DS86

           26.64                          25.56
```

NOTES:
  1. Col.A has grouped the U.S. population into the same age-bands used by RERF for the A-Bomb Study.
----
  2. Col.C gives the age-sex distribution for 1978 in the U.S., for a sample of 10,000 persons (calculated from data in Nrc85, p.I-78, Table A.6). When the distributions change in the future, so will the estimated Lifetime Fatal Cancer-Yield.
----
  3. Col.D gives the estimated fraction of persons in Col.C who will die of cancer spontaneously -- without extra radiation-exposure -- over the entire remaining lifespan of the cohort (from Go81, Tables 31 and 32); these fractions are higher than the fractions used for the A-bomb survivors (Table 28-D, Col.G).
----
  4. Col.E = (Col.C x Col.D).
  5. Col.F and Col.H are the low-dose K-values from Table 15-L for the two dosimetries.
  6. By K's definition, lifetime radiation-induced fatal cancers per cSv = (K-value) x (Lifetime Spontaneous Cancers). Therefore, Col.G = (Col.F x Col.E). Likewise, Col.I = (Col.H x Col.E).
----
  7. The estimate of 26-27 above is not an iteration or revision of my earlier estimate of 37.71 (Go81, p.314). The estimate above is a new entity. The 1981 estimate and this one come out of very different input in terms of approximations and data (for instance, the 1981 estimate used some 20 different studies, not just the A-Bomb Study).
----
  8. Cancer-hazard from X-rays may be underestimated by the A-Bomb Study. See Chapter 13, Part 4.

CHAPTER 17

The Duration of Radiation's Carcinogenic Effect

This chapter is arranged in five parts:

Then tables.

Introduction :

====================

In Chapters 13 and 16, we emphasized that a most crucial determinant of realistic Lifetime Fatal Cancer-Yields is the DURATION of the radiation's effect in producing cancers, additional to those occurring spontaneously.

In making our estimates of Lifetime Fatal Cancer-Yield in Chapter 16, we made the approximation that the K-values determined for the period 1950-1982 will continue to operate beyond 1982, for the remainder of the lifespan of the residual survivors. (K is defined as the fractional increase in the spontaneous cancer death-rate per centi-sievert of exposure. Multiplied by 100, K becomes the percent increase in the spontaneous rate, per cSv.)

In this chapter, we shall examine the basis for our approximation about duration. First, we shall quantify and evaluate the trends within the A-Bomb Study itself. Then we shall consider some of the other data reported in the literature. Radiation studies having over forty years of follow-up beyond the time of radiation exposure are very rare indeed. Studies with insufficient quantitative information, and anecdotal reports, are not considered in our evaluation.

There are two ways in which we shall analyse the A-bomb data. First, we shall compare the behavior of cancer-risk -- with the passage of time -- in all the exposed survivors combined, versus the unexposed survivors. Second, we shall make the same comparisons for each of the five age-bands separately. (As always, we will make the approximation that the Reference Group is an unexposed group.)

1. A-Bomb : The Evidence from Combined Age-Bands

Table 17-A provides the analysis for all ages combined, both cities, both sexes, for the study of cancer-induction by radiation, over the period 1950-1982. In this table, the initial sample of 91,231 persons has been divided into two groups: The 25,203 exposed survivors (Dose-Groups 3, 4, 5, 6, 7, and 8), and the 66,028 virtually UNexposed survivors (Dose-Groups 1+2, our familiar reference group).

During 8 four-year follow-ups, the 91,231 persons have accumulated 6,050 cancer-deaths (Column B plus Column C of Row 9). Rows 1 through 8 show WHEN the 6,050 cancer-deaths occurred. This detailed information comes from the diskette R10ALL (R-Ten-All) provided by RERF; see Chapter 7. These are the "raw" numbers. There is no need for age-normalization here, for we will look at the age- bands separately in Part 2.

Within any specified time-period after the bombing, some new cancer-deaths occur in each of the two groups (exposed and reference). In Columns D and E, the cancer death-rates per 10,000 initial persons apply to the rates of NEW cases which occurred during a particular period (Note 4, Table 17-A). This chapter is the only one in which we are NOT dealing with the aggregate observations for all eight follow-up periods combined.

The ratio of the cancer death-rates (rate in exposed / rate in reference), or R2/R1 -- during a specified set of years -- is provided in Column F.

Because the difference in mean dose received by the

two groups, from the bombings, was fixed forever in August 1945, the dose-difference is the same in all successive follow-ups. Therefore, we can compare the ratios in Column F directly, as indicators of how radiation's carcinogenic effect behaves over time.

In Column G, we also provide the indicator commonly called "excess relative risk." The quantity (R2/R1)-1 is equivalent in this case to (O-E) / E, or (O/E)-1, because R2 designates cancer-rate in the exposed group, or the "Observed" (O) value, while in this case R1 designates the cancer-rate in the virtually unexposed group, or the spontaneous "Expected" (E) value.

It should be noted that the quantity (R2/R1)-1 is also the numerator of the equation from which we derive K-values in Chapter 15, namely Equation (7). It is an excellent indicator with which to compare the carcinogenic potency of radiation, during one set of years versus another set of years.

Findings from Our Analysis :

With respect to predicting the duration of the radiation effect beyond 1982, Table 17-A incorporates an important confounding variable. We shall discuss it after examining what the table does show, and what a similar analysis by RERF analysts shows.

Readers who inspect Table 17-A, Column F, Rows 1-14, can see for themselves that a consistent picture emerges from the successive follow-ups, in spite of fluctuations.

1. In Rows 1 through 8, the Cancer-Rate Ratios and the excess relative risks are in a general rising trend, with some recent entries notably higher than the overall value (Row 9) for the 1950-1982 follow-up as a unit. For specific four-year periods, there are some deviations which are almost surely the result of sampling variation.

2. The rising trend is confirmed when we divide the entire 32 years of observation into two equal intervals of 16 years (Rows 10 and 11). The Cancer-Rate Ratio rises from 1.104 to 1.263. The term, (R2/R1)-1, rises from 0.104 to 0.263. This 2.53-fold increase describes the increase in effective K-value over the two halves of the follow-up, or the increase in excess relative risk.

3. If we divide the observations at 25 years post-bombing (Rows 13 and 14), the excess relative risk beyond 25 years does not vanish, fall, or even level out. On the contrary, it rises by the factor of (0.266 / 0.139), or 1.91. This is a striking contrast with reports (which we will examine in Part 3 of this chapter) that the

radiation effect is finished after 25 years, in the Ankylosing Spondylitis Study.

4. The most recent four-year follow-up period, 1979-1982, shows the highest Cancer-Rate Ratio of any interval of the first 32 years, 1.308, and the highest value of (R2/R1)-1, namely 0.308. However, the findings from any isolated four-year follow-up are unstable relative to values from eight-year, twelve-year, or sixteen-year periods. A four-year follow-up deserves noting, but not too much weight.

Findings by RERF Analysts :

The findings in our Table 17-A are confirmed in a totally separate study by RERF analysts, Shimizu and co-workers (TR-5-88). Although they are looking at RERF's DS86 "sub-cohort" of 75,991 persons (not the full 91,231 sample), and although RERF has moved many persons into and out of the unexposed sample (see our Tables 10-A and 10-B), their results and ours should be in general agreement, and they are.

Shimizu and co-workers present the following data, for excess relative risk as a function of follow-up time in the A-Bomb survivors (Shi88, Table 2-4). The data are for all cancers combined, leukemia omitted.

Follow-Up Interval	Excess Relative Risk per Gray
1950-55	0.2372
1956-60	0.1230
1961-65	0.2264
1966-70	0.2576
1971-75	0.2900
1976-80	0.3958
1981-85	0.4301
1983-85	0.4717

Their results are in very close agreement with those in our Table 17-A. Shimizu and co-workers also show an "aberrant" point at 1956-60, and also show the highest excess relative risk occurring in the most recent follow-up -- which means through the 40th post-bombing year (1985) in their DS86 "sub-cohort."

In both their study and ours, a strong trend exists over a 32-35 year period toward an increasing excess relative risk, and there is no sign of a downturn in the trend. The trend for the combined age-groups is still upward at 1985.

Because both the Shimizu analysis and our Table 17-A examine all five age-bands combined, the results are exactly what we would expect to see if we assume that the individual K-value for each age-band remains CONSTANT through time. The expectation, of rising Cancer-Rate Ratio and rising excess relative risk, rests on two observations.

(1) Our study of K-values (Table 15-L) shows that the highest K-values occur for those who were young ATB. K-values decrease progressively (with negligible exceptions) for persons of successively older age ATB. And K-values are directly related to the term (R2/R1)-1.

(2) From the very beginning of the follow-up in 1950, some people in every age-band die during each follow-up period, but obviously, people die off fastest from the oldest age-band (50+ years of age ATB). In the oldest age-band, the mean age ATB in 1945 was 58.5 years.

By late 1982, Table 4-B shows that only 4.8 % of the oldest age-band ATB was still alive, whereas 96 % of the youngest age-band ATB was still alive. The effect of this general selective mortality, according to age itself, means that the effective age ATB of the residual survivors keeps decreasing with each passing year of follow-up. (Note that age ATB is a very different number than age ATTAINED at some particular year of the follow-up.)

With lower age ATB, we know that we find greater cancer-induction by radiation (higher K-values). And so the rising values in Columns F and G of Table 17-A are what we would expect, if K-values for each age-band do not change with time but the average age ATB of the residual survivors is constantly shifting downward between 1950-1982.

The steady "replacement" of the study-sample by one with an ever younger effective age ATB -- and thus an ever rising effective K-value -- is the confounding variable which we mentioned at the beginning, with respect to the duration of the effect.

Although both Table 17-A and the Shimizu analysis can tell us directly that the radiation effect on cancer-induction is certainly NOT finished at 25, 30, 35, or 40 years after the bombing, neither study can tell us whether the K-values for INDIVIDUAL age-bands are showing any increase or decrease, with the passage of time, which might help predict the duration and magnitude of the radiation effect for the ages separately. Therefore, we will explore the issue further in Part 2.

2. A-Bomb: The Evidence from Separate Age-Bands

The data and findings for the study's five separate age-bands ATB are in Table 17-B (cities and sexes combined).

The Small-Numbers Problem:

As usual whenever analysts subdivide these data, we face the small-numbers problem to a serious degree.

The problem is particularly bad when we isolate a single four-year time-period, such as the most recent one (1979 through 1982). Nonetheless, in order to make Tables 17-A and 17-B comparable, we do isolate the most recent follow-up period.

The instability of small numbers, in ANY of the isolated four-year periods, needs to be recognized. Readers inspecting such entries, above the dotted line in each age-band, will see how their irregular progression results in irregular progression ("bounciness") of the Cancer-Rate Ratio. It would be preposterous and misleading to "interpret" each wiggle as anything other than sampling variation, in data which have been excessively subdivided. To look for believable trends in the current data, one must re-combine some intervals -- as shown.

The 3 Groups in the Middle of the Age-Range :

In the middle of the age-range are three age-bands: 10-19, 20-34, and 35-49 years of age ATB. In all three of these age-bands, the Cancer- Rate Ratio in Column F is well above 1.0 in the follow-up period 1971-1982, which shows that the radiation effect was NOT finished by 25 years after the bombing. Also in all three, the Cancer-Rate Ratio is higher in the second 16-year period than in the first 16-year period.

"Relative" versus "Absolute" Risk-Models :

It might be noted that, in the Reference Group of all three of these age-bands, the spontaneous cancer death-rate per 10,000 initial persons (Column E) increases with each four-year follow-up. In other words, the spontaneous frequency grows as age advances. (In the 35-49 year group, this trend ends in the 1979-1982 follow-up, when the YOUNGEST member of that cohort was about 70 years old.)

Yet even while the spontaneous risk (R1) is tripling or more within these age-bands, the ratio R2/R1 (which is equivalent to Observed/Expected) is approximately constant or even growing, when one divides the observations into two equal intervals.

These observations are consistent with the so-called "relative risk" model of radiation carcinogenesis, and inconsistent with the so-called "absolute risk" model.

Oldest and Youngest Age-Bands ATB :

The remaining two-age bands are represented by those very young ATB (average age ATB = 4.1 years) and those in the oldest age-band ATB (average age ATB = 58.5 years).

The Oldest Age-Band :

For the oldest group, Table 17-B shows that the radiation effect appears to have declined in the second half of the study (1.103 falling to 1.038). During the most recent follow-up, 1979-82, the ratio fell below 1.0. The ratio of 0.669 is based on rapidly dwindling numbers of cases. The total cancer-deaths (exposed plus reference) were 63 in the years 1979-1982, and by late 1982, Table 4-B shows that only 720 persons out of the original 15,011 persons were still alive (the YOUNGEST would be 87 years old).

It just does not matter whether or not the ratio in this age-band ever climbs above 1.0 again, in terms of properly estimating a Lifetime Fatal Cancer-Yield. The K-value for this age-band, used in Table 16-B, is based on all the observations through 1982, and is valid for the 1950-1982 period. The presumption in Table 16-B, that the same K-value will persist beyond 1982, adds almost nothing to the Lifetime Fatal Cancer-Yields. Readers can see this for themselves in Table 16-B by comparing Columns G and H in the two rows (male and female) for the oldest age-band.

The Youngest Age-Band :

What does matter a great deal, in estimating Lifetime Fatal Cancer-Yield, is what will happen beyond 1982 in the youngest age-band ATB (0-9 years).

By late 1982, the OLDEST member of this cohort would be about 46 years old (9 years ATB + 37 years since the bombing). The youngest would be only 37. In Table 17-B, Column E, the LOW spontaneous cancer death-rates in this age-band's Reference Group confirm that the decades of high spontaneous cancer-mortality are still ahead for this age-band.

What, if anything, can Table 17-B tell us about the likely behavior of the Cancer-Rate Ratio in this age-band, during the decades ahead?

For the age-band 0-9 years ATB, the total number of cancers (exposed plus reference classes) in the first half of the follow-up period, 1950-66, was only six. There were five cancer-deaths in the Exposed Group, and one in the Reference Group. The problem of statistical instability for this first half of the whole follow-up is self-evident. Sampling variation in the early period is such that a comparison of the early versus late follow-up periods cannot be taken seriously.

For the entire period beyond 1970 (the period more than 25 years post-irradiation), with 75 total cancer-deaths, the Cancer-Rate Ratio is 1.228, which suggests that the carcinogenic effect of radiation did NOT cease by 25 years after exposure.

It can be noted that the highest Cancer-Rate Ratio of any follow-up period occurs in the most recent period (1979-82), where the ratio of 1.690 is based on a total of 33 cancer-deaths. Our statement knowingly ignores the ratio of 5.917, observed in the 1959-62 period, because it was based on a total of THREE cancer-deaths.

Although in the 1979-82 period, the numbers are still small and unstable, the observed ratio of 1.690 is very different indeed from the three preceding periods. On the other hand, when the data are so very bouncy, no one should be surprised if the ratio is appreciably LOWER than 1.690 in the next follow-up period.

Summary on the Separate Age-Bands :

Examination of the five age-bands, separately, leads us to two statements.

(1) With the one exception of the oldest age-band ATB, the carcinogenic effect did not cease 25 years after the exposure. In the two age-bands (20-34 ATB, 35-49 ATB) which are currently contributing most heavily to the cases, there was not even any detectable DECLINE in the effect after 25 years.

(2) The evidence at hand provides no basis for assuming that the average K-values, which will characterize the post-1982 period, will be either higher or lower than the K-values which characterize the 1950-82 period as a whole. Within the data, the reasonable assumption is that average K-values will be about the same in the future as in the past -- approximately constant K-values.

3. Evidence from other Human Studies

The Ankylosing Spondylitis Study

REFERENCE: DARBY, 1987 (Dar87).

TITLE: "Long Term Mortality after a Single Treatment Course with X-Rays in Patients Treated for Ankylosing Spondylitis."

To begin, we will cite the summary of conclusions from the study of the ankylosing spondylitis patients (Dar87, p.179):

"Mortality up to 1 January 1983 has been studied in 14,106 patients with ankylosing spondylitis given a single course of X-ray treatment during 1935-1954. For neoplasms other than leukemia or colon cancer, mortality was 28 % greater than that of members of the general population of England and Wales, and this increase is likely to have been a direct consequence of the treatment. The proportional increase reached a maximum of 71 % between 10.0 and 12.4 years after irradiation and then declined. There was only a 7 % increase in mortality from these tumours more than 25.0 years after irradiation and only for cancer of the esophagus was the relative risk significantly raised in this period. Neither the magnitude of the relative risk, nor its temporal pattern following treatment, were [sic] greatly influenced by the age of the patient at first treatment."

Before continuing, we would like to correct the impression that this study is a study of 14,000 patients. It is really a study of half that number. While it is true that some 14,000 persons entered the study, the authors reveal that "By 1 January 1983 just over half the patients had been re-treated ..." After 18 months following re-treatment, the re-treated patients were deleted from further follow-up study of cancer. Since the re-treatment constitutes a possible confounding variable, it is not clear why the authors include these patients at all in the results.

Readers may wonder why Darby and co-workers exclude colon-cancer in the statement above. They report on colon-cancer separately (Dar87, p.179): "For colon cancer, which is associated with spondylitis through a common association with ulcerative colitis, mortality was increased by 30 %." For this reason, they treat it separately. Among the ankylosing spondylitics, the mortality- rate from ulcerative colitis was 12.8 times the rate in the general population (Dar87, Table 10).

(People with ulcerative colitis are said to have an elevated rate of fatal colon-cancer. It is my opinion that analysts and physicians need to consider the possibility that an elevated rate of fatal colon-cancer in such people may result, partly or even largely, from the many diagnostic X-ray exams invoked by the presence of ulcerative colitis.)

Duration of the Effect from Radiation :

On the issue of duration of carcinogenic effect, from the X-ray exposure, Darby and co- workers state (Dar87, p.188):

"This is the first large study to suggest an apparent end to the effects of exposure to radiation for neoplasms other than leukemia and the possibility must be considered that the findings are spurious ..."

We shall try to evaluate the possibility in this chapter, Parts 3 and 4.

Division of Results at 25 Years :

From Table 5 of the Darby paper, we extract the summary values for observed and expected deaths from neoplasms, other than leukemia or colon cancer, occurring before age 85 years. Darby and co-workers obtained their expected values from population statistics for England and Wales. The data below are for all ages at first treatment.

```
Time since First Treatment, in Years.
=====================================================
5 to 24.9 Years          | 25 Years or More
-----------------------------------------------------
Observed Expected  O/E  | Observed Expected   O/E
  385     279.39  1.38  |   178    166.56    1.07
```

We should note here that Darby and co-workers report that approximately 40% of the cancer-deaths in each of the time periods were from lung-cancer. We shall return to this point, in Part 4 of this chapter.

Darby and co-workers state that the value 1.38, for O/E in the earlier period, is significantly different from the value 1.07, for O/E in the later period, and that neither in males nor females was the O/E value significantly elevated in the later period.

The data summarized above are the data which lead to the suggestion that the radiation-induction of cancer is at "an apparent end" by the 25th year post-irradiation.

==

Contrast with the A-Bomb Study :

With respect to the duration of radiation's carcinogenic effect, this report from the Ankylosing Spondylitis Study is clearly at variance with the A-Bomb Study.

Other Studies on the Duration Question
=======================================

In view of the apparent conflict between the A-Bomb Study and the Spondylitis Study, analysts have to consider which data are more reliable.

One approach to the question is to examine other studies in the literature. While such studies will be much less comprehensive than the A-bomb or the spondylitis studies, some of them are capable of addressing the particular question at hand here: Is the carcinogenic effect finished at 25 years, or is it appreciable beyond 25 years?

(1) --
REFERENCE: BOICE, 1985 (Boice85).
Irradiation: X-ray Therapy for Cervical Cancer.
  Cancers Evaluated:
Cancers arising in sites (in or near the radiation field) which "likely" received over 100 rads, including stomach, small intestine, colon, rectum, gallbladder, pancreas, uterine corpus, ovary, other genital organs, kidney, bladder, bone, and connective tissue. O/E was measured for all these sites as a function of time after irradiation. The comparison was made between those cervical cancer cases exposed to radiation and those cervical cancer cases not exposed to radiation.

  Effect Beyond 25 Years:
Radiation-induction of cancer showed no diminution of risk even after 30 years of observation. The authors' exact statement: "Apparently, after a period of about 10 years, the risk of radiation- induced solid tumors following exposure in adult life will persist, if not increase further, for at least 30 years and possibly throughout the remainder of life."

Consistent with A-Bomb Study.
Inconsistent with Spondylitis Study.

(2) ---
REFERENCE: HILDRETH, 1983, 1985, 1989 (Hild83, Hild85, Hild89).
Irradiation: Thymus Irradiation in Infancy.
  Cancers Evaluated: Breast-Cancer.
This is a study of females whose breast irradiation occurred in early infancy. Excess cancer has been ob-served in adulthood, as predicted elsewhere(Go81,p.260).

Effect beyond 25 Years:
The earliest effect was observed 28 years post-irradiation. In the exposed group, the median age at diagnosis is 39 years. The excess relative risk is 2.60, and has been essentially constant since the effect was first observed (Hild89, p.1283).

Consistent with A-Bomb Study.
Inconsistent with Spondylitis Study.

(3) ---
REFERENCE: HOWE, 1984 (Howe84). Also MILLER, 1989 (Mi89).
Irradiation: Fluoroscopic exposure of patients being treated for tuberculosis.
Cancers Evaluated: Breast-Cancer.
  Effect Beyond 25 Years:
Howe reported (Howe84) that "All age at first exposure groups continue to show increased risk of breast cancer mortality up to 40 years after first exposure, the data beyond 40 years being too sparse for for meaningful interpretation." Miller and co-workers report (Mi89, Table 4) the temporal distribution of risk as follows:

```
    5-14 years post-irradiation :  1.47
   15-24 years post-irradiation :  1.40
   25-34 years post-irradiation :  1.48
=> 35    years post-irradiation :  1.24
```

Consistent with A-Bomb Study.
Inconsistent with Spondylitis Study.

(4) ---
REFERENCE: MARTIN, 1970 (Mart70).
Irradiation: X-ray therapy for benign skin disorders.
Cancers evaluated: Skin-cancers in or adjacent to irradiated sites.
  Effect beyond 25 Years:
Definite persistence of effect well beyond 25 years post-irradiation. In 73 of total observed 368 cases, the skin-cancers appeared after latent periods of 31 to 50 years post-irradiation.

Consistent with A-Bomb Study.
Inconsistent with Spondylitis Study.

(5) ---
REFERENCE: MODAN, 1989 (Modan89).
Irradiation: X-ray Therapy for Tinea Capitis (Ringworm of the Scalp). Israel Series.
Cancers Evaluated: Breast-Cancer.
  Effect Beyond 25 Years:
The exposure occurred between 1949 and 1959, so 1954 was the midpoint. The follow-up recently accomplished is 1982 through 1986, so 1984 was its midpoint. Thus, about 30 years have passed since exposure. During the 1982-1986 follow-up, a total of

==

22 cases of breast-cancer occurred (exposed plus unexposed) and the relative risk of breast-cancer for the exposed versus the controls was 2.11, for an average dose of 1.6 rads to the breast.

Consistent with A-Bomb Study.
Inconsistent with Spondylitis Study.

(6) --
REFERENCE: RON, 1988 (Ron88).
Irradiation: X-ray Therapy for Tinea Capitis
    (Ringworm of the Scalp). Israel Series.
Cancers Evaluated: "Head and Neck Tumors" -- a
    conglomerate of many separate sites.
    Effect Beyond 25 Years:
Cannot demonstrate excess of head and neck tumors beyond 25 years. Total cancers observed beyond 25 years = 7 cases, including both exposed and unexposed.

Inconsistent with A-Bomb Study.
Consistent with Spondylitis Study.

(7) --
REFERENCE: SHORE, 1984 (Sho84).
Irradiation: Treatment of Tinea Capitis in Children.
Cancers Evaluated: Skin.
Effect Beyond 25 years: O/E still rising at 35 years
post-irradiation.
Consistent with A-Bomb Study.
Inconsistent with Spondylitis Study.

(8) --
REFERENCE: SHORE, 1985 (Sho85).
Irradiation: Thymus Irradiation in Infancy.
Cancers Evaluated: Malignant & Benign Thyroid Tumors.
Effect Beyond 25 Years:
    Thyroid carcinoma: Excess cancer persists at least out to 40 years.
    Thyroid adenoma: Excess benign tumors at least out to 45 years.
Consistent with A-Bomb Study.
Inconsistent with Spondylitis Study.

(9) --
REFERENCE: SHORE, 1986 (Sho86).
Irradiation: X-ray Therapy for Post-Partum Mastitis.
Cancers Evaluated: Breast-Cancer.
Effect Beyond 25 Years: Excess breast-cancer
occurring beyond 30 years.
Consistent with A-Bomb Study.
Inconsistent with Spondylitis Study.

Conclusion, from the Survey Above
==

With only one exception (entry 6 above), the evidence from these other studies, of irradiation for medical reasons, is consistent with the A-bomb evidence and not consistent with the spondylitis evidence. On the duration issue, our survey confirms that the warning from Darby and co-workers was certainly appropriate: "... the possibility must be considered that the findings are spurious ..." (Dar87, p.188).

4. A-Bomb Study
versus Spondylitis Study

Both the A-Bomb Study and the Ankylosing Spondylitis Study are studies of reasonably large size, in terms of numbers of observations, and both are of reasonably long duration. The question is, "Which is the more reliable study, with respect to the duration of radiation's carcinogenic effect?"

In my judgment, the credibility of the A-Bomb Study is clearly superior to that of the Spondylitis Study on this issue. Not only is the A-Bomb Study supported by, and the Spondylitis Study at variance with, almost all other human evidence, but there are at least two possibly serious confounding variables in the Spondylitis Series, and they raise real questions about studying temporal behavior of radiation in that series.

In addition, confidence in any database is necessarily undermined severely, when its original input disappears from the on-going analysis. The dosimetry of the Ankylosing Spondylitis Study has been retroactively altered more than once -- in Beir72, again in Beir80, and now it is undergoing yet another retroactive alteration. According to Darby and co-workers (Dar87, p.181), for "many organs previously classed as lightly irradiated" (including liver, kidney, bladder, uterus), the new revised doses will be high enough to re-classify them as HEAVILY irradiated. In a study with two classes of dose -- heavy and light -- it is no minor matter when the distinction is retroactively obliterated for many organs. Yet for this study, I am unaware of any effort to maintain continuity with a "constant-cohort, dual-dosimetry" approach -- an approach which we have demonstrated for the A-Bomb Study through its 1982 follow-up.

(1) Health of Exposed versus Controls
======================================

For the A-bomb survivors, the exposed and reference groups are matched except for the variable, radiation. And in Table 11-H, Column S, we have positive evidence that the non-cancer mortality rate is the same for exposed and reference groups. Thus, there is no force of mortality that might alter the temporal response of radiation-induced cancer.

For the spondylitics, the exposed and reference groups are far from alike. The reference group is the general population. The exposed group is a patient-group suffering from a severe chronic malady associated with a 51 % excess non-neoplastic mortality-rate (Dar87, p179). And this excess mortality-rate covers a wide range of diseases, in addition to a small number previously expected to be associated with ankylosing spondylitis.

Can anyone be confident that the presence of a serious increase in force of mortality (evidenced by the 51 % increase in non-malignancy death-rate) has no effect in altering the temporal course of radiation-induced cancer-mortality in the spondylitics? If the temporal course were shifted, then the use of national rates for the "expected" cancer-rates may be totally unwarranted.

It would seem rational that any challenge, to the temporal course of radiation-induction of cancer observed in the A-bomb survivors, should NOT be made from a series of persons with a serious increase in mortality-rate from a wide assortment of non-malignant diseases.

(2) Smoking among Exposed versus Controls
======================================

In the spondylitic data, the case for a drastic decline in radiation-induced cancer, beyond the 25th year after exposure, rests very heavily on the lung-cancer rates for the early and late periods.

In the early period, (5.0-24.9 years post- therapy), 155 out of a total of 385 cancer-deaths are lung-cancer deaths, with an O/E of 1.37. In the late period (25.0 years or more post-therapy), 69 out of a total of 178 cancer-deaths are lung-cancer deaths, with an O/E of 0.97. The data on lung-cancer, below, are from Table 4 of the 1987 Darby paper.

Cancer of the Lung
==

Follow-Up Period	Observed	Expected	O/E
5 - 24.9 Years	155	113.08	1.37
25 or more Yrs	69	71.41	0.97

Darby et al acknowledge that the exclusion of lung-cancer makes it impossible to prove any significant difference in O/E for the early period versus the late period. And of course, analysts should never be excluding data frivolously in any case. We simply point out that, for the reason which follows, there must necessarily be some serious reservations about the heavy dependence on lung-cancer, for their finding about duration. There may be a reasonable alternate explanation for the change (above) in the O/E ratio.

It is an interesting fact that the spondylitis cases had been treated with X-rays at some time between 1935 and 1954. It so happens that approximately 1954 is the time that the worldwide recognition of the relationship between cigarette-smoking and bronchogenic (lung) cancer occurred.

During the latter (and still large) part of the follow-up beyond 1954, it is extremely likely that patients with spondylitis -- who fare badly from a variety of respiratory ailments -- were placed under special pressure to stop smoking cigarettes. It is reasonable to consider the possibility that lung-cancer may have been cut down as a result of less smoking among the spondylitics, during the latter part of the follow-up period.

But among the general population (the control group), the pressures to stop smoking in the population-at-large would have been less. Thus, if the spondylitics reduced their smoking more than did the general population, the result expected in the latter part of the follow-up would be a decline in the O/E value for lung-cancer -- a decline wholly unrelated to radiation exposure.

Obviously, we do not know that the spondylitics of the British series were in fact reducing their cigarette-use after 1954. All we say is that it is reasonable to worry about smoking as a possible confounding variable, and that it might explain the anomalous results on duration.

Conclusion on Reliability
==

For all the reasons given above, we think analysts

==

should place far more credence in the A-Bomb Study (1950-1982) on the issue of duration, than in the Ankylosing Spondylitis Study. We have shown several grounds for heeding the warning about the Spondylitis Study that "... the possibility must be considered that the findings [on duration] are spurious ..." (Dar87, p.188).

Nonetheless, the Spondylitis Study is sure to be cited by some as if it were the scientifically weighty evidence on duration. In fact, Robin Mole (a former member of the ICRP) has already done so in LANCET. The parenthesis is his own:

"The data from the X-rayed spondylitics suggested that the risk of excess cancer other than leukemia was possibly not continued to the end of life (as commonly assumed for purposes of radiological protection) but may be limited to 2-3 decades after exposure. Direct observation on man is more to be relied upon than hypotheses based on extrapolation from the bomb survivors' experience" (Mole87).

We cannot understand why Mole characterizes the Spondylitic Study as "direct observation on man," and then dismisses direct observations on the A-bomb survivors -- of comparable duration -- as merely the basis for "hypotheses" about duration. Nor can we understand Mole's failure to mention findings from the other studies cited in Part 3 of this chapter.

By contrast, we think the issue is too important for casual treatment.

Having examined the available evidence in Parts 1,2,3, and 4 of this chapter, we think it would be scientifically indefensible to estimate Lifetime Fatal Cancer-Yields on the basis of an end to the carcinogenic effect two to three decades after exposure, or to drop the presumption of lifelong duration on the basis of the Spondylitis Study. Virtually all the non-spondylitic evidence (1) is overwhelmingly against an end to the effect by 25 years post-irradiation, and (2) is pointing to a lifelong effect.

Within the A-Bomb Study, which merits far more credence than the Spondylitic Study on this issue, the evidence to date not only supports the presumption of a lifelong effect out to the age of about 80 years, but the evidence for most age-bands does not even show any

meaningful DECLINE in the average intensity of the effect, when the periods before and after 25 years post-irradiation are compared. Indeed, in some age-bands, the data show the intensity INCREASING in the period beyond 25 years (Table 17-B).

5. The Bottom Line

1. For reasons given in detail above, evidence from the A-bomb survivors is inherently more reliable on the issue of duration of effect, than evidence from the ankylosing spondylitic patients. Moreover, evidence from other studies is -- almost without exception -- consistent with the A-Bomb Study and inconsistent with the Spondylitic Study.

2. In the A-Bomb Study, we have demonstrated (Tables 17-A, 17-B) that the induction of cancer by radiation is clearly NOT over by 25 years after the irradiation. In some age-bands, the average effect appears to be even greater in the period BEYOND 25 years after exposure, than in the period BEFORE the 25th year.

3. Therefore, the only reasonable presumption from the evidence at hand is that the radiation effect in cancer-induction will be lifelong, and that its intensity will remain approximately constant, at the average level observed so far in the A-Bomb Study. (As noted in Chapter 13, Part 6, and Chapter 16, Part 2, RERF analysts are using the same presumption in estimating their Lifetime Fatal Cancer-Yields.)

4. Only time, and preservation of the A-Bomb Study as a legitimate prospective study, can validate or invalidate the presumption. Meanwhile, if we were to use any other presumption, unsupported by the available evidence, it would be a clear sign of some sort of bias.

Table 17-A
Change in Cancer-Rate Ratio, and in Excess Relative Risk, with Time after Exposure.

	Col.A	Col.B	Col.C	Col.D	Col.E	Col.F	Col.G
	Follow-Up Interval	Exposed Group 25,203 Persons	Reference Group 66,028 Persons	Exposed Group	Reference Group	Cancer-Rate Ratio	Excess Rel. Risk
	--------	-- CANCER-DEATHS, RAW ---		--- CANCER-RATES --		--------	--------- (R2 / R1)
				(R2)	(R1)	R2 / R1	Minus 1.0
Row 1	1950-54	150	353	59.517	53.462	1.113	0.113
Row 2	1955-58	150	423	59.517	64.064	0.929	-0.071
Row 3	1959-62	216	478	85.704	72.394	1.184	0.184
Row 4	1963-66	236	531	93.640	80.420	1.164	0.164
Row 5	1967-70	257	536	101.972	81.178	1.256	0.256
Row 6	1971-74	268	588	106.337	89.053	1.194	0.194
Row 7	1975-78	311	631	123.398	95.566	1.291	0.291
Row 8	1979-82	307	615	121.811	93.142	1.308	0.308
Row 9	1950-82	1895	4155	751.895	629.278	1.195	0.195

==

Division of Follow-Up into Two Equal Parts :

	Col.A	Col.B	Col.C	Col.D	Col.E	Col.F	Col.G
Row 10	1950-66	752	1785	298.377	270.340	1.104	0.104
Row 11	1967-82	1143	2370	453.517	358.939	1.263	0.263

==

Most Recent Follow-Up Period :

	Col.A	Col.B	Col.C	Col.D	Col.E	Col.F	Col.G
Row 12	1979-82	307	615	121.811	93.142	1.308	0.308

==

Division of Follow-Up at 25 Years Post-Bombing :

	Col.A	Col.B	Col.C	Col.D	Col.E	Col.F	Col.G
Row 13	1950-70	1009	2321	400.349	351.518	1.139	0.139
Row 14	1971-82	886	1834	351.545	277.761	1.266	0.266

==

NOTES: 1. The exposed group, in Columns B and D, represents all individuals for both cities in Dose-Groups 3 through 8. In this combined group, 25,203 persons have been followed-up since 1950.

----

2. The reference group, in Columns C and E, represents all individuals for both cities in Dose-Groups 1 + 2. In this nearly UNexposed group, 66,028 persons have been followed-up since 1950.

----

3. The entries in Columns B and C, for each four-year follow-up period separately, are obtained from RERF's diskette "R10ALL" (R-Ten-All); see Chapter 7. Cumulative cancer-deaths, 1950-1982, amount to 6,050 cases; Columns B and C show WHEN they occurred.

----

4. In Columns D and E, all cancer-rates per 10,000 initial persons apply to the rate produced by the new cancer-deaths which occurred during the particular time-interval indicated in Column A. Thus the rate from 1950-1966 (Row 10), in the exposed group, is (752 cases / 25203 persons) times (10000 persons) = 298.377 .

----

5. (Column F) = (Column D entry) / (Column E entry).

----

6. (Column G) = (Column F minus 1.0). As noted in the text, Part 1, entries in Col. G are commonly called "excess relative risk" when R1 is the rate observed in the unexposed group. The quantity (R2/R1)-1 is also the numerator of Equation (7) in Chapter 15, for calculating K-values. In this table, it provides a direct basis for comparing strength of cancer-risk, during one set of follow-up years, with strength of cancer-risk during any other set of years.

Table 17-B
The Time-Course of Cancer-Rate Ratios, for the Individual Age-Bands.

AGE-GROUP = 0-9 years ATB.
Exposed Persons = 4649. Reference = 13753.

Follow-up Interval (A)	CANCER-DEATHS Exposed Group (B)	Reference Group (C)	CANCER-RATES Exposed Group (D)	Reference Group (E)	Cancer Rate-Ratio (F)
1950-54	0	0	0	0	Ind.
1955-58	1	0	2.151	0	Ind.
1959-62	2	1	4.302	0.727	5.917
1963-66	2	0	4.302	0	Ind.
1967-70	3	9	6.453	6.544	0.986
1971-74	4	11	8.604	7.998	1.076
1975-78	6	21	12.906	15.269	0.845
1979-82	12	21	25.812	15.269	1.690

Division of Follow-Up into Two Equal Parts

1950-66	5	1	10.755	0.727	14.791
1967-82	25	62	53.775	45.081	1.193

Most recent Follow-Up Period

1979-82	12	21	25.812	15.269	1.690

Division of Follow-Up at 25 Years after Exposure

1950-70	8	10	17.208	7.271	2.367
1971-82	22	53	47.322	38.537	1.228

AGE-GROUP = 10-19 years ATB.
Exposed Persons = 5443. Reference = 13781.

Follow-up Interval (A)	CANCER-DEATHS Exposed Group (B)	Reference Group (C)	CANCER-RATES Exposed Group (D)	Reference Group (E)	Cancer Rate-Ratio (F)
1950-54	1	1	1.837	0.726	2.532
1955-58	2	9	3.674	6.531	0.563
1959-62	3	8	5.512	5.805	0.949
1963-66	6	12	11.023	8.708	1.266
1967-70	17	24	31.233	17.415	1.793
1971-74	19	37	34.907	26.849	1.300
1975-78	43	61	79.001	44.264	1.785
1979-82	29	77	53.279	55.874	0.954

Division of Follow-Up into Two Equal Parts

1950-66	12	30	22.047	21.769	1.013
1967-82	108	199	198.420	144.402	1.374

Most recent Follow-Up Period

1979-82	29	77	53.279	55.874	0.954

Division of Follow-Up at 25 Years after Exposure

1950-70	29	54	53.279	39.184	1.360
1971-82	91	175	167.187	126.986	1.317

AGE-GROUP = 20-34 years ATB.
Exposed Persons = 5138. Reference = 12553.

Follow-up Interval (A)	CANCER-DEATHS Exposed Group (B)	Reference Group (C)	CANCER-RATES Exposed Group (D)	Reference Group (E)	Cancer Rate-Ratio (F)
1950-54	8	24	15.570	19.119	0.814
1955-58	10	28	19.463	22.305	0.873
1959-62	15	42	29.194	33.458	0.873
1963-66	31	71	60.335	56.560	1.067
1967-70	47	69	91.475	54.967	1.664
1971-74	58	97	112.884	77.272	1.461
1975-78	77	133	149.864	105.951	1.414
1979-82	83	156	161.541	124.273	1.300

Division of Follow-Up into Two Equal Parts

1950-66	64	165	124.562	131.443	0.948
1967-82	265	455	515.765	362.463	1.423

Most recent Follow-Up Period

1979-82	83	156	161.541	124.273	1.300

Division of Follow-Up at 25 Years after Exposure

1950-70	111	234	216.037	186.410	1.159
1971-82	218	386	424.290	307.496	1.380

AGE-GROUP = 35-49 years ATB.
Exposed Persons = 6066. Reference = 14837.

Follow-up Interval (A)	CANCER-DEATHS Exposed Group (B)	Reference Group (C)	CANCER-RATES Exposed Group (D)	Reference Group (E)	Cancer Rate-Ratio (F)
1950-54	57	107	93.966	72.117	1.303
1955-58	59	153	97.263	103.121	0.943
1959-62	98	186	161.556	125.362	1.289
1963-66	101	226	166.502	152.322	1.093
1967-70	126	276	207.715	186.021	1.117
1971-74	134	300	220.903	202.197	1.093
1975-78	154	330	253.874	222.417	1.141
1979-82	171	310	281.899	208.937	1.349

Division of Follow-Up into Two Equal Parts

1950-66	315	672	519.288	452.922	1.147
1967-82	585	1216	964.392	819.573	1.177

Most recent Follow-Up Period

1979-82	171	310	281.899	208.937	1.349

Division of Follow-Up at 25 Years after Exposure

1950-70	441	948	727.003	638.943	1.138
1971-82	459	940	756.677	633.551	1.194

AGE-GROUP = 50+ years ATB.
Exposed Persons = 3907. Reference = 11104.

Follow-up Interval (A)	CANCER-DEATHS Exposed Group (B)	Reference Group (C)	CANCER-RATES Exposed Group (D)	Reference Group (E)	Cancer Rate-Ratio (F)
1950-54	84	221	214.999	199.027	1.080
1955-58	78	233	199.642	209.834	0.951
1959-62	98	241	250.832	217.039	1.156
1963-66	96	222	245.713	199.928	1.229
1967-70	64	158	163.809	142.291	1.151
1971-74	53	143	135.654	128.782	1.053
1975-78	31	86	79.345	77.450	1.024
1979-82	12	51	30.714	45.929	0.669

Division of Follow-Up into Two Equal Parts

1950-66	356	917	911.185	825.829	1.103
1967-82	160	438	409.521	394.452	1.038

Most recent Follow-Up Period

1979-82	12	51	30.714	45.929	0.669

Division of Follow-Up at 25 Years after Exposure

1950-70	420	1075	1074.994	968.120	1.110
1971-82	96	280	245.713	252.161	0.974

Notes 1 through 5 of Table 17-A apply here, too.
   Total persons = 91,231.
   Total cancer-deaths = 6,050. These are the "raw"
      values from Tables 11-B and 11-D.
Each age-band includes both sexes in both cities.
"Exposed" class includes all Dose-Groups 3 through 8.
"Reference" class includes Dose-Groups 1 + 2.

Initial persons in each class are stated, near the top
   of each age-band.
Cancer Death-Rates, per 10,000 persons initially in a
   class, are for the specified interval.
Cancer Death-Rates are (number of deaths
   from Col.B or Col.C / initial persons) x (10,000).
"Ind." abbreviates "indeterminate."

COMMENTS ON THIS TABLE ARE IN TEXT, PART 2.

17-empty, after tables.

Disproof of Any Safe Dose or Dose-Rate of Ionizing Radiation, with Respect to Induction of Cancer in Humans

This chapter is arranged in eight parts:

1. Overview -- with a Five-Point Summary

Probably the most important issue in this field is whether or not there exists SOME low dose, or dose-rate, of low-LET ionizing radiation which produces no cancer at all in exposed populations. In short, is there a SAFE region below some threshold of danger?

If the idea of a safe dose or dose-rate prevails -- and the idea has some very influential backing (see Chapters 24, 34, 35) -- then both voluntary and involuntary human exposures are bound to increase dramatically above their current levels. If the idea prevails and is FALSE, it could ultimately result in a hundred million or more unnecessary, premature cancers over time, worldwide. Thus, the stakes of the threshold issue are high indeed. And this book does not even open the issue of HERITABLE genetic injuries.

Meaning of "Safe Dose or Dose-Rate" :

Because not all readers of this book will be epidemiologists, we want to be explicit about the meaning of "safe dose or dose-rate." Confusion can arise from two different meanings of safe: (1) free from danger; secure, and (2) having escaped danger or injury; unharmed. For instance, NOT everyone exposed to battle gets killed. As the battle begins, no one is safe. After the battle, some are dead and some are safe.

With respect to ionizing radiation, the meaning of a SAFE dose or dose-rate is a dose or dose-rate at which

all exposed persons are safe as the exposure occurs, and all are safe afterwards. NO fraction will be killed later by radiation-induced cancer. In sharp contrast, "no safe dose or dose-rate" means that no one is safe as the exposure occurs, and afterwards, some FRACTION of the exposed persons will die from radiation-induced cancer, and the rest will be safe from it.

Our Approach to the Subject :

Elsewhere (Chapters 24 and 34), we have assembled statements from various members of the radiation community to the effect that (A) there is a reasonable chance that safe doses and dose-rates DO exist for low-LET radiation, and (B) it is impossible to resolve the threshold issue from the existing evidence.

By contrast, we think human evidence and logic combine to make a case which is already CONCLUSIVE -- by any reasonable standard of proof -- AGAINST the existence of any safe dose or dose-rate of ionizing radiation, with respect to cancer-induction.

The disproof of any safe dose or dose-rate, presented in this book, represents an expansion and closer examination of the case presented in Go81 (pp.404-411) and in Go86 (Section 2 and Technical Appendix 1). Our analysis ignores high-LET radiation, because almost everyone admits that there is no safe dose or dose-rate from alpha particles and other high-LET radiations.

We will summarize the case in a single chapter (this one), and will place the supporting evidence, calculations, and "what if" materials, into auxiliary chapters of their own. Some readers will prefer to read Chapters 19, 20, and 21 BEFORE this summary chapter, and other readers will prefer to read this chapter first.

For curious readers, we have also provided an overview (Chapter 35) of the kinds of evidence cited by various authors who have been speculating that perhaps, someday, a net benefit will be discovered for human health, from low-dose exposure to ionizing radiation. Readers will see for themselves that this is sheer speculation, centering largely around possible stimulation of repair and immune responses.

In contrast with such conjecture is the real-world human epidemiological evidence, discussed in Chapter 21, which shows fatal cancer-induction even at minimal doses and dose-rates of ionizing radiation. When excess fatal cancer is observed in humans after such exposures, the excess has occurred DESPITE any possible stimulation of the repair- and immune-responses by low-doses. The NET result is injury, not benefit. I wish it were otherwise.

A Five-Point Summary
=============================

The argument against any safe dose or dose-rate is summarized below. For the sake of brevity, various statements are necessarily omitted.

● -- 1. The dose from low-LET ionizing radiation is delivered by high-speed electrons, traveling through human cells and creating primary ionization tracks. One track is the least possible disturbance which can occur at the cellular level. "High dose" means many tracks per cell; "low dose" means few tracks per cell; "low dose-rate" means few tracks per cell per unit time. Whenever there is any dose at all, it means some cells and cell-nuclei are being traversed by tracks (see Chapter 19).

● -- 2. Single, primary ionization-tracks, acting independently from each other, are never innocuous with respect to creating carcinogenic injuries in the cells which they traverse. Every track -- without help from any other track -- has a chance of inducing cancer by creating such injuries (see Chapter 19, including "The Yalow Model").

● -- 3. This implies that there can never be any safe dose or dose-rate. However, if every carcinogenic alteration induced by tracks were successfully and invariably "un-done" by repair processes, then there WOULD be an inherently safe dose or dose-rate. The key question is: Does repair of carcinogenic injuries

operate flawlessly, when dose is sufficiently low and slow?

● -- 4. Human epidemiological evidence shows that repair FAILS to prevent radiation-induced cancer, even at doses where the repair-system has to deal with only one or a few tracks at a time, and even at dose-rates which allow ample time for repair before arrival of additional tracks. See Chapter 21, and this one. Such evidence is proof, by any reasonable standard, that there is no dose or dose-rate which is safe ... unless we can find some wholly additional cancer-prevention mechanism which is perfect whenever the REPAIR-mechanism at low doses fails.

● -- 5. The radiation-induced cancers arising from the unrepaired lesions at low doses do not wear a little flag identifying them as any different from cancers induced by higher doses of radiation, or induced by causes entirely unrelated to radiation. Therefore, threshold proponents cannot argue that the cancers arising from the lowest conceivable doses of radiation will somehow be eliminated by the immune system or any other bodily defenses against cancer. Such an argument would require the elimination of cancer in general by such defenses. Instead, we observe that cancer is a major killer (roughly 15-20% of many populations). So the proposition would lead to a non-credible consequence, and must be rejected. This means that repair is the key, and that Point 4 stands: There is no dose or dose-rate which is safe with respect to human carcinogenesis.

The Heart of the Issue :

Points 1 and 2 above are explained in detail in auxiliary chapters, and are not controversial. We regard Point 5 above as self-evident. Therefore, this chapter will focus on discussing Points 3 and 4. "Repair" is at the heart of the threshold issue.

2. A Troublesome Trio :
Unrepaired ...
Unrepairable ...
Misrepaired Injuries

In 1914, Theodore Boveri suggested the hypothesis that imbalance of chromosomal information is a central feature of carcinogenesis (Bov14). Imbalance could include missing genetic information, erroneous genetic information, excess genetic information, and genetic information in the wrong locations. In other words, the idea that carcinogenesis is tied to defective or inappropriate genetic information, in the cell nucleus, is an idea which goes back many decades. With advances

==

in research techniques and tools, the evidence in favor of the idea is rapidly increasing.

Today, in our field, the underlying presumption is that the carcinogenic lesions caused by ionizing radiation are occurring in genetic material -- namely, in the DNA or chromosomes of cell nuclei. UNSCEAR uses this presumption in its 1986 report, after making the following comments (Un86, pp.12-13):

"Cancer initiation is believed to be a uni-cellular process occurring at random in single cells. This is ... a working hypothesis that has not yet definitely been proved." In speaking of radiation effects on cells, UNSCEAR adds: "These effects involve the cells' genetic material, which is also thought to be the primary target for cancer initiation."

While not everyone accepts these premises, most do -- and I am emphatically one of those who do, for many reasons which do not need discussion in this particular book.

The remarkable scientific work on DNA of the past few decades has established convincingly that biological repair of injury to DNA molecules undoubtedly takes place. There is a large literature on the subject, and the knowledge and detail are quite sophisticated. Some repair of chromosomes also occurs, although here the evidence is not so certain about the details.

No one welcomed the findings about DNA and chromosome repair more than did many segments of the radiation community, for the prospect seemed newly bright that people could be irradiated with no cancer-consequences. It was -- and still is -- widely suggested that repair could certainly take care of low doses of radiation or low dose-rates. But while hope springs eternal, there is the nasty problem of scientific reality: "Does repair always succeed?"

And this is why we call attention to three warnings from the literature.

● -- Brackenbush and Braby (Brack88, p.256) state the following: "Since most cells repair radiation damage with a characteristic time ranging from a few minutes to a few hours, it is evident that irreparable or misrepaired damage must dominate the low-LET radiation effect at low dose-rates."

● -- UNSCEAR (Un86, p.179) comments as follows on repaired, unrepaired, and misrepaired carcinogenic lesions induced by radiation: "The error-free repair of the DNA, which is the most likely target involved, leaves some fraction of the damage unrepaired and the error-prone repair may produce misrepaired sequences in the DNA structure."

● -- Albrecht Kellerer (Kelle87, p.346) describes a type of radiation-induced lesion which would be difficult to repair: "A simple example would be two neighboring single-strand breaks on opposing strands of DNA, which interfere with excision repair." Kellerer's warning is confirmed by Feinendegen and co-workers (Fein88, p.29) who, reporting on irradiated cells, say "not all double-strand breaks are fully repaired."

Important cause for concern is contained in these statements, with their reference to "unrepaired," "misrepaired," and "irreparable" lesions inducible by radiation.

And there is no basis for limiting the concern to DNA, when it belongs to chromosomes too. Although we undoubtedly see chromosomes with apparent repair (for instance, we sometimes see the rejoining of breaks in the strands), it is far from clear that all the pre-injury links have been restored perfectly to their original state. Some apparent repairs may really be incomplete or functionally incorrect, even if residual damage cannot be visualized microscopically. It is appropriate to suggest that some portion of "repair" is really misrepair.

No matter how great the capacity and speed may be of genetic repair mechanisms in a cell nucleus, there are no laws stating that EVERY type of injury is repairable, and that misrepair can never happen. Indeed, imperfect repair is the potential "Achilles Heel" for any concept of a safe dose or dose-rate with respect to radiation-induced cancer. This should have been evident for a long time, as we shall see.

3. Evidence on the Capacity and Speed of Repair Systems

In auxiliary Chapter 20, Table 20-M, readers will find tables which estimate the average number of primary ionization tracks which traverse a cell-nucleus at a specified dose. Of course, the derivation of those tables is also shown, step-by-step. The results of the work are used in several parts of this chapter, including this part.

For disproof of any safe dose or dose-rate, it is more important to establish the dose in terms of the average number of tracks per nucleus, than to establish it in terms of rads. The reason is that the lowest conceivable dose or dose-rate with respect to repair is not a millionth or any other tiny fraction of a rad or centi-gray. The lowest conceivable dose or dose-rate is one track per nucleus plus sufficient time to repair it. (For more about dose-RATE, see Chapter 20, Part 3.)

Below, in this chapter, we will be citing studies of repair conducted on human cell-cultures following X-irradiation, typically from a 250 kilovolt machine. In such studies, reported doses are often "a few Grays" -- a few hundred rads. In the next chapter, Table 20-"O" tells us that, at a dose of 3 Grays or 300 rads, each cell-nucleus is feeling the disturbance from about (2.3 tracks / rad) x (300 rads), or some 690 tracks on the average. If the dose is an acute one, the tracks are virtually simultaneous, of course.

Our purpose in citing the studies which follow is to establish (A) whether or not human cells are running short of repair-capacity at doses where radiation-induced cancer has been epidemiologically demonstrated, and (B) how much time the cells take to finish all the repair of which they are capable.

Repair-Capacity -- Undiminished at Doses of Several Grays :

============================

Kellerer, who is a leading expert in the field of microdosimetry, has reported:

"... there is little or no evidence for an impairment of enzymatic repair processes at doses of a few grays. Studies, for example, by Virsik et al. [Vir82] on chromosome aberrations, have established characteristic repair times that are substantially constant up to 10 Gy, that is, up to the highest doses investigated. Similar observations have been obtained in various cell survival studies. Most of the enzymatic DNA repair processes that are known are of the catalytic type. The enzymes are not used up in the repair process, and under usual conditions it is safe to assume that the concentration of enzymes is sufficient to maintain constant repair efficiency at the concentration of lesions produced by several grays ..." (Kelle87, p.358-359).

Writing about studies of human cells irradiated with doses up to ten Grays (1,000 rads), Kellerer emphasizes that reduced success of repair at high doses is not the result of insufficient repair-capacity (but rather, the greater frequency of injuries which are very close to each other):

"... there is, at present, no experimental evidence for a reduction of the repair capacity or the rate of repair at doses of a few gray which are relevant to cellular radiation effects. Reduced efficiency of repair or enhanced misrepair are apparent at elevated doses of sparsely ionizing radiations and at all doses of densely ionizing radiations, but they can be understood in terms of the greater proximity of sublesions of DNA and the resultant failure of DNA repair. A simple example would be two neighboring single-strand breaks on opposing strands of DNA, which interfere with excision repair. Such interference with repair due to spatial proximity is, in a somewhat loose terminology, included in the general notion of the 'interaction' of sublesions" (Kelle87, p.346).

(Our auxiliary Chapter 19, Part 4, points out, however, that such interactions do not REQUIRE the presence of two separate tracks -- they can also occur between lesions along a single track.)

The key point is that Kellerer, who has looked closely at the evidence on repair, concludes as recently as 1987 that "... it is safe to assume that the concentration of enzymes is sufficient to maintain constant repair efficiency at the concentration of lesions produced by several grays ..." (see above).

Keeping Order in the Genetic Library :

With respect to natural doses of ionizing radiation, such massive repair-capacity would never be needed today. But it exists nonetheless. One can speculate that, during the epoch when DNA was evolving, the natural doses were much higher than now, or that there were viral "vandals" in the "library" of genetic information, and a system with great capacity was necessary to restore order. Whatever the history, what we observe today in the cell-studies is that ionizing radiation tears "books" from their shelves in the genetic library, but massive squads of vigilant librarians very rapidly restore order -- with only an occasional book overlooked or misplaced.

Activation of Repair-Capacity :

No one is implying that repair-enzymes are always present in a cell-nucleus at a constant concentration, whether the menace is one track or 700 tracks. The concentration of the enzymes probably varies with the stimulus. It has been suggested by Goodhead and others that possibly the repair-system needs a "kick" to get started. For instance: "... it is also conceivable that the cell would repair relatively more efficiently if there were more damage to stimulate its repair processes" (Good88, p.234-5). If the suggestion is someday confirmed, it would seem to imply difficulties for the safe-dose proponents. At doses or dose-rates too low to provide adequate stimulation, repair of carcinogenic injuries might operate the least efficiently of all, or even

==

be entirely absent. Presently, such matters remain in the realm of speculation.

Repair-Times
of 8 Hours and Much Less :
==============================

Studies of human cells in vitro, following X-irradiation, indicate that whatever repair is achieved, is complete within 6 hours or less after irradiation, even at doses of 100 and 200 rads (for instance, in Ben82; Nata82; Pres80). Indeed, in the references cited, all the repair occurs within the first two hours after irradiation, and by three hours, the repair curve is flat.

Other sources of evidence are in good agreement on the issue of the time required for a variety of repair functions following radiation injury.

We already cited Brackenbush and Braby (Brack88, p.252) who stated: "Since most cells repair radiation damage with a characteristic time ranging from a few minutes to a few hours, it is evident that irreparable or misrepaired damage must dominate the low-LET radiation effects at low dose-rates."

Upton (Up88, p.606, in his Figure 1) shows that,

a. Repair of sublethal damage is such that the surviving fraction of cells has reached as high a value as it ever will, by between 4 and 6 hours post-irradiation following, doses of 400 rads in vitro for C3H10T1/2 cells.

b. For chromosome aberrations in the same cell system and at 400 rads, repair has reduced the number of chromosome aberrations to as low a value as it would ever achieve, somewhere between 4 and 6 hours after irradiation.

Bender, discussing repair of chromosome breaks, reports repair half-times which are "typically of the order of 1 or 2 hr" (Ben84, p.286).

Bond , in a discussion of single-hit and multi-hit phenomena in irradiated cells, refers to the half-time for repair as "frequently in the range of hours or less" (Bon84, p.393).

Feinendegen and co-workers report, "Whereas the majority of single-strand breaks and base changes are very efficiently and quickly repaired with half-times less than 1 h, the reconstitution of a double-strand break probably lasts much longer, perhaps up to several hours, and not all double-strand breaks are fully repaired" (Fein88, p.29).

Rat Experiments at 1200 Rads :
Burns and Sargent have presented data concerning DNA repair times in rat epidermis (Burns81). These studies involve whole-animal irradiation of rat epidermis with 0.8 MeV electrons. It was found that single-strand breaks in DNA were removed after irradiation with a half-time of 21 minutes in vivo. Concerning the period within 60 minutes post-irradiation with 1200 rads, the authors state:

"By 60 min [their abbreviation] after irradiation, the breaks had returned approximately to the value in unirradiated controls, indicating essentially complete repair."

Reporting on some separate studies of radiation carcinogenesis in rat skin, the authors state that split-dose experiments indicated the half-time for repair of carcinogenically-related events was between 110 and 240 minutes.

4. Two Implications from the Repair Studies

Speed -- An Implication :

The cell studies indicate that repair systems finish their work within about 3 to 6 hours, even after acute doses up to 400 rads (about 900 simultaneous tracks per cell-nucleus). The in vivo study with rats indicates half-time for repair is about 2 to 4 hours, which means that essentially all possible repair-work is completed in less than 24 hours, in spite of very high doses indeed.

The dazzling speed of repair has an extremely important implication for settling the threshold issue. It means that certain HIGH-dose evidence can reveal a great deal, as we will explain.

If a radiation dose is received within the time-frame required for repair, and if repair operates FLAWLESSLY and leaves no carcinogenic damage, then the net effect of that radiation-dose toward cancer-production is obviously ZERO, by definition.

Opportunity to Prove a Safe Dose :
So we can describe a scenario in which repair is flawless at a specified low dose, and in this scenario, individuals receive their first exposure to this dose on Monday. Repair is flawless and complete within hours. The individuals have no cancer-risk due to the first exposure. On Tuesday, these individuals receive their second dose of the same size. Since repair is perfect, there is still no risk of radiation-induced cancer from the

combined exposures, Monday and Tuesday.

Under these circumstances, such individuals could gradually accumulate a very high dose from dozens or hundreds of low-dose exposure-sessions, and yet the group would show no excess (radiation- induced) cancer when followed-up post-irradiation.

If the same very high dose, received all at once, is known to cause cancer, and if the studies of very high doses accumulated through a series of low doses were large enough and long enough to show a cancer-excess, and if such studies typically FAILED to show any excess cancer, we would conclude: Division of the very high total dose into low doses and dose-rates permitted repair to produce a SAFE dose and dose-rate -- even though repair was overwhelmed and flawed when the same number of ionization tracks was received all at once. The weight of such evidence would be persuasive in FAVOR of a threshold.

Opportunity to Disprove a Safe Dose, Too :
High-dose studies of this same type could also provide proof that repair is NOT flawless at the low doses and dose-rates tested. If the follow-up studies typically revealed excess cancer in SPITE of the fact that the high total dose had been received in a series of low doses, we would necessarily conclude that repair had NOT worked perfectly at low doses.

Indeed, our disproof of any safe dose or dose-rate includes four studies which are ostensibly high-dose studies, but really tell "all" about minimal doses and dose-rates. We are not alone in recognizing their implication. Upton refers to "... the dose-dependent excess of breast-cancer, which is of similar magnitude per unit dose in a) women exposed to A-bomb radiation, b) women given therapeutic irradiation for postpartum mastitis, c) women subjected to multiple fluoroscopic examinations of the chest during the treatment of pulmonary tuberculosis with artificial pneumothorax, and d) women exposed occupationally to external gamma radiation in the painting of luminous clock and instrument dials" (Up87, p.300-301). In groups (c) and (d), serial exposures to low doses accumulated into high doses.

Upton echoes the NIH Report (Nih85, p.26) when he concludes: "The similarity of the dose-incidence relationships in all four groups of women, in spite of marked differences among the groups in the duration of exposure, implies that the carcinogenic effect of a small dose on the breast is largely irreparable and that the effects of successive doses are additive" (Up87, p.301).

Upton appropriately regards the results from successive small doses as "... support for the hypothesis that there may be no threshold in the dose-incidence relationship" (Up87, p.300; full context provided in our Chapter 34).

Capacity -- An Implication :

The abilities demonstrated by nuclear DNA repair-mechanisms might, at first, appear very helpful to proponents of a safe dose with respect to cancer-induction. "Just observe! Repair takes only minutes to hours, and repair can handle 400 rads, even 1000 rads, without evidence of inadequate capacity. A system which can take care of 500 rads delivered acutely (some 1,150 simultaneous tracks per nucleus) is surely going to have no difficulty coping with 10-20-50 tracks in the low-dose region!" I know that such a repair-capacity gladdened a few hearts within the nuclear enterprise ... and mine, too.

One can look with awe, humility, and gratitude at a system of repair with the capacities demonstrated by the DNA repair-system. But an independent analyst, or a realist of any stripe, does not casually dismiss the troublesome trio:

Unrepaired lesions.
Unrepairable lesions.
Misrepaired lesions.

Many physiological systems are amazing and awesome without being perfect: Reproduction, immune defenses, digestion, temperature control, and on and on. Imperfection is the rule rather than the exception. One cannot fault the repair-system in cell-nuclei for leaving a relatively small number of injuries unrepaired, or misrepaired, or for having some inherent inability to repair every conceivable type of injury inflicted at random by the tracks of high-speed electrons.

One could look at all the epidemiological studies (the A-bomb survivors and numerous others) which have demonstrated radiation-induced human cancer at doses between 10 and 400 rems. Those are doses where -- if cell-studies mean anything at all -- we should not anticipate any shortage of repair capacity, and yet excess cancer did occur. If CAPACITY of the repair-system were the issue, we would not even be discussing radiation carcinogenesis today, since it looks as if repair has enough CAPACITY to handle all the carcinogenic damage between 10-400 rems.

Moreover, the human epidemiological evidence on dose versus cancer-response provides no support for the speculation that repair makes each rad less carcinogenic as dose falls. If that were the net result of

==

repair, the shape of dose-response would be concave-UPWARD. But what is seen in the A-Bomb Study and in others (see Chapter 22) is NOT concavity-upward. The finding is either supra-linearity or linearity -- both of which are inconsistent with the speculation that repair processes make each rad less carcinogenic as dose and dose-rate fall.

Our entire experience with human radiation carcinogenesis should have made it evident that the problem we might be facing is that -- regardless of dose-level -- some fraction of radiation injury to nuclei is unrepaired ... some fraction is unrepairable ... and some fraction is misrepaired.

If this is the problem, and if the fraction is about the same over the entire dose-range, we can never expect any safe dose or dose-rate.

5. Conclusive Human Evidence
below 10 Rads

In the five-point outline in Part 1, the fourth point deserves repeating here: Human evidence shows that repair is FAILING to prevent radiation-induced cancer, even at doses where cells have to deal with only one or a few tracks at a time, and even at dose-rates which allow ample time for repair before arrival of additional tracks. See Chapter 21. Such evidence is proof that there can be no conceivable dose or dose-rate which is safe ... unless we invoke a cancer-prevention mechanism wholly additional to repair mechanisms (a reference to the summary's fifth point).

From Chapter 21, we have brought Table 21-A forward, onto the next page. Table 21-A provides the bottom line from nine separate epidemiological studies in which radiation-induced cancer has been observed in the human following dose-rates which delivered twelve tracks or FEWER, on the average, to cell-nuclei. In the four high-dose studies where multiple low-dose exposures occurred, there was ample time between exposure-sessions for repair to be completed before the arrival of additional tracks.

Because epidemiology is inherently inexact, it is inevitable that some analysts may challenge the goodness of one study or another, but the case against any safe dose or dose-rate does not rely on a single study. Far from it. We are presenting nine studies, which reinforce each other.

There may be additional human studies, now or in the future, suitable for this type of analysis. It is very probable that, among 20 suitable studies, there will be

at least one (5 percent) which will NOT confirm the finding of no safe dose or dose-rate. In epidemiology -- as in so many other fields -- it is reasonable to have confidence in the weight of the evidence, and to regard it as proof. If I were to have any OTHER attitude toward the evidence here, I would have to question my own objectivity.

It should be noted that the case against any safe dose or dose-rate does not depend upon exactitude in the estimate of tracks per nucleus in Table 21-A. If one accepts the presumption of genetic molecules as the site of radiation injury for carcinogenesis, then there is clearly a vast amount of excess repair-capacity in all nine studies of Table 21-A. Thus, even if the number of tracks per nucleus were higher, the disproof of any safe dose or dose-rate would not be undermined. (In Chapter 20, we show exactly how our track-estimates were derived, and in Chapter 33, we compare them with estimates made by others.)

The nine studies entered in Table 21-A demonstrate that the following doses are NOT safe, with respect to cancer-induction: 9.0 rads, 7.5 rads, 4.6 rads, 1.6 rads, 1.0 rad, 0.9 rad, 0.5 rad, and 0.1 rad. Claims abound that epidemiological evidence for human cancer-induction is absent at low doses, but such claims are clearly mistaken.

Many proponents of a safe dose and dose-rate will immediately say, about the evidence in Table 21-A: "But the table omits all the medical, occupational, and natural-background studies which show NO excess cancer from low-dose exposure at slow dose-rates! You cannot just ignore them!"

And we do NOT ignore them. Studies of that type are examined in Chapter 21, Part 2.

Such studies -- which are potentially infinite in number -- are simply irrelevant to settling the threshold issue, as explained in Chapter 21, and as usually admitted by their authors, and as admitted by the BEIR-3 Committee. Irrelevant material does not BELONG in Table 21-A.

The relevant studies are those which are CAPABLE of settling the issue. For instance, as we explained in Part 4 of this chapter, the ostensibly HIGH-dose studies included in our disproof of any safe dose or dose-rate, are CAPABLE of helping to settle the issue. Those studies had their opportunity to provide powerful evidence in FAVOR of a safe dose and dose-rate, and they failed. Instead, they contribute powerful evidence AGAINST any threshold.

Table 21-A
Average Tracks per Nucleus, from Each Exposure in Nine Human Studies.

Number Assigned in the Text		Col.A Rads per Exposure	Col.B Tracks-per-Nucleus at 1 Rad	(Col.A times Col.B) Average Number of Tracks-per-Nucleus from Each Exposure	
1.	Nova Scotia Fluoroscopy	7.5	1.3378	10.0335	10 Rounded
2.	Israeli Scalp-Irradiation	7.5	1.3378	10.0335	10 Rounded
	(Authors' revised est.)	9.0	1.3378	12.0402	12 Rounded
3.	Massachusetts Fluoroscopy	4.6	1.3378	6.1539	6 Rounded
4.	Canadian Fluoroscopy (Excludes Nova Scotia)	4.6	1.3378	6.1539	6 Rounded
5.	Stewart In-Utero Series	0.5	1.3378	0.6689	< One 51 % with no track.
6.	MacMahon In-Utero Series	0.9	1.3378	1.2040	~ One
7.	British Luminizers	0.1	2.9370	0.2937	< One 75 % with no track.
8.	Harvey Twins In-Utero Series	1.0	1.3378	1.3378	~ One
9.	Israeli Breast-Cancer in Scalp-Irradiation Study	1.6	1.3378	2.140	~ 2

Entries in Column A come from the text of Chapter 21. Where more than one
   exposure occurred (Studies 1, 3, 4, 7), these entries are the average
   doses or delivery-rates at which higher total doses accumulated.
   See Chapter 18, Part 4 and Chapter 21, Part 1.
Entries in Column B come from Chapter 20, Table 20-K.
Entries on the righthand side are (Col.A times Col.B). For Studies 5 and 7, percents
   (of unhit nuclei) come from Tables 21-B and 21-C.

In the nine studies tabulated in Table 21-A, the observation of radiation-induced cancer means that repair is FAILING to become flawless even when it has to cope with average track-frequencies per nucleus of only 12 tracks, only 10, only 6, only 2 tracks, only 1 track, only 0.67 track, and only 0.29 track. If repair had been flawless, it would have successfully un-done every carcinogenic lesion, and so there would have been no excess cancer at all, in any of the nine studies. Yet LARGE excesses were observed (see Chapter 21, Part 1).

The evidence suggests operation of the troublesome trio: The persistence of some unrepaired, unrepairable, or misrepaired carcinogenic injuries which occur at low doses in proportion to tracks, right down to the lowest conceivable dose and dose-rate.

By any reasonable standard of proof, the combined evidence in Table 21-A is conclusive that there is no safe dose or dose-rate of ionizing radiation with respect to cancer-induction. Given the redundancy of repair "equipment" which is implied by the cell studies (and by analogous physiological responses), it would not be reasonable to exclude any of the nine studies on the ground that repair of the carcinogenic injuries might have been flawless, "if only there had been fewer tracks at once."

From the evidence tabulated in Table 21-A, it would be overwhelmingly more reasonable to conclude that there is no safe dose or dose-rate.

6. A Supplemental Approach --
Also via Epidemiological Evidence

We expect every sort of effort will be made to deny that the threshold issue is already settled by existing human evidence. (See Chapters 24, 34, 35.) Therefore, we are going to explore an additional piece of evidence and line of reasoning below. We do not regard this Part 6 as essential to disproof of any safe dose or dose-rate, which has been done in Part 5 by any reasonable standard of proof. We regard Part 6 as a supplemental approach. On an issue of such enormous importance to human health, we think every reasonable, alternative approach is worthwhile.

The approach to be demonstrated in Part 6 uses Baverstock's British Luminizer Series (Bav81), a series recognized as important evidence in this field by the radiation community (for instance, Nih85, p.26, and Up87, p.301).

We recognize, of course, that only about 20 % of the study-population has died of any cause, so far,

and that further follow-up of the women could either weaken or strengthen the observations of excess breast-cancer mortality. (On the other hand, even zero as a LIFESPAN excess would not alter the interim observation of an EARLY excess -- which is a very serious radiation-effect in itself; see Chapter 12, Part 3.) Further follow-up of the UK Radium Luminizer Survey is planned. See our Chapter 21, Part 1.

Meanwhile, it is reasonable to use the existing data -- and in so doing, we will demonstrate a general method which could be applied to any other suitable data which may develop in the future.

The "Above Average" Rate of Tracks :

A line of resistance which we anticipate, to the disproof already presented, can be stated as a question: "Is it not POSSIBLE that all the excess cancer in the nine studies above arose only from the cell-nuclei which experienced the 'above average' rate of tracks -- and that there might have been NO excess cancer if 1, 2, 6, 10, or 12 tracks per nucleus had been the MAXIMUM number instead of the AVERAGE number?"

Let us consider the five studies where the average frequency of tracks per nucleus ranged from less than 1 track, to 2 tracks at once. By definition, some nuclei experience an "above average" frequency -- say 10 tracks at once. In view of the repair-capacity demonstrated in cell-studies, we regard it as self-evident that the repair-system could NOT be overloaded by the stress of 10, 20, 50 tracks at once. But as we stated at the outset, supplemental ways of settling the threshold issue deserve consideration.

The Essence of Flawless Repair :

The essence of perfect repair of carcinogenic damage from a track is that the carcinogenic damage DISAPPEARS. Repair completely "un-does" it. With respect to any extra cancer-risk from the track, it is as if the track never traversed the nucleus at all.

It follows that, if repair were routinely and invariably perfect in every nucleus which received 4 tracks or fewer, and if the dose or dose-rate were such that no nucleus ever received MORE than 4 tracks (with sufficient time for flawless repair before arrival of additional tracks), then all doses and dose-rates which never deliver more than 4 tracks per nucleus would be SAFE.

If repair could "deliver" a threshold, everyone --

ourselves included -- would like it to occur at as high a dose as possible (to enlarge the range of SAFE doses). Since dose is proportional to tracks, we will explore flawless repair of damage from as MANY tracks, per nucleus, as the evidence might conceivably allow. Therefore, when we are referring to this supplemental approach to the threshold issue, we can call it "Max Trax."

Readers who have already studied Chapter 20, Part N, have seen how the Poisson equation can tell us -- when the AVERAGE frequency of tracks per nucleus is, say, 1.0 -- how many nuclei per million receive no track, 1 track, 2 tracks, 3 tracks, 4 tracks, 5 tracks, etc. Either a nucleus is traversed somewhere by a track, or it is not. In that sense, there are no fractional tracks; fractional tracks are just an artifact from averaging the experience of many nuclei (including, of course, the nuclei which completely escape traversal).

Frequency of Multiple Nuclear Tracks in the Luminizer Study :

In the study of the British Luminizers, the average dose per exposure-session (work-day) was 0.1 rad and the average number of tracks per nucleus was 0.2937 during each exposure-session. In Chapter 20, Part N, we demonstrated how to use the Poisson equation to find out the distribution of tracks when the AVERAGE frequency per nucleus has been determined. In Chapter 21 (Table 21-C), we used the Poisson equation to show the following:

Poisson Distribution of Tracks, Luminizers :
Mean number of tracks = 0.2937 per cell-nucleus.
How many nuclei will get 0,1,2,3,4,5 tracks?

0.745500 = chance of exactly 0 track per nucleus.
0.218953 = chance of exactly 1 track per nucleus.
0.032153 = chance of exactly 2 tracks per nucleus.
0.003147 = chance of exactly 3 tracks per nucleus.
0.000231 = chance of exactly 4 tracks per nucleus.
0.000013 = chance of exactly 5 tracks per nucleus.

0.035545 = chance of 2 or more tracks per nucleus.
(Since the probability of MORE than five tracks per nucleus is so low, it is reasonable to refer to two-to-five tracks as "two or more.")

We anticipate that threshold defenders will say, looking at the Poisson calculations, "Ah ha! In the Luminizer Study, 13 out of every million nuclei received five tracks per nucleus. So the excess cancer in this study does not absolutely rule out a safe dose when NO nucleus receives 5 tracks at once! Maybe repair works flawlessly and provides a safe dose when there are up

through four tracks per cell-nucleus, but above four tracks per nucleus, it fails to be flawless. The fifth track is the overload where trouble begins for repair. And in the Luminizer Series, there are 13 nuclei per million which have a fifth track per nucleus, and so those nuclei remained capable of causing the radiation-induced cancers observed in the Luminizer Study."

Before we can examine such a speculation, a few additional statements and definitions will be needed.

Exposures Which Increase Breast-Cancer by 50 % :

The Max Trax analysis which follows is based on comparison of the British Luminizer Study with the A-Bomb Study.

Since the conclusions do not depend upon on exactitude of input, readers are urged to accept the following approximation, which we borrow from Upton (Up87, pp.300-301). Upton states that the observed excess of breast-cancer is "of similar magnitude per unit dose" in "women exposed to A-bomb radiation" and in "women exposed occupationally to external gamma radiation in the painting of luminous clock and instrument dials" (Upton specifically includes the Baverstock study of British Luminizers, 1981).

Recently, Baverstock has reported a relative risk for breast-cancer of 1.5 in the luminizers who, at a mean age of 20, received a total dose of 40 breast-rads, at the rate of about 0.1 rad per day (see Chapter 21, Part 1). We will make the approximation that 1.5 is also the relative risk for breast-cancer in the A-Bomb Study for 20-year-old women ATB who received 40 breast-rads. This is the same as an excess relative risk of 0.5 from 40 rads, a doubling dose of 80 rads, and a K-value of 0.0125 per rem (or rad).

We insert the following interruption, however, to avert any possible misunderstanding. We recognize full well that the appropriate K-value in the A-Bomb Study might be lower than 0.0125. Nonetheless, since it does not matter here exactly what risk-coefficient we use for the A-bomb women (as we shall demonstrate shortly), we will just use Upton's generalization that the risk-coefficients are "of similar magnitude."

At 40 Rads, Number of Tracks per Nucleus :

A-Bomb Women: From Table 20-L, we will use the estimate that there were about 5.41 tracks per nucleus, on the average, from a rad of A-bomb radiation. So,

(5.41 tracks per nucleus / rad) x (40 rads) = 216.4 tracks per nucleus. Since A-bomb exposure was acute, a nucleus felt all 216.4 tracks at about the same time.

British Luminizers: From Table 21-A, which is reproduced in Part 5 above, we will use the estimate that there are about 2.937 tracks per nucleus, on the average, from a rad of radium-226 gamma-rays. So, (2.937 tracks per nucleus / rad) x (40 rads) = 117.48 total tracks per nucleus. This total was spread over about 400 exposure-sessions (work-days), each delivering about 0.1 rad or 0.2937 track per nucleus, on the average.

Definition of "L" and "Effective Track" :

Meaning of "L" : For the explanation which follows, we define the symbol "L" to be whatever number of carcinogenic lesions happens to occur along one primary ionization track, as it traverses a nucleus.

Meaning of "Effective Track": Within a nucleus, this means any primary track which MAY remain effective in producing cancer because its carcinogenic lesions (L) receive no guarantee of perfect repair. Its carcinogenic lesions may, or may not, be perfectly repaired by attempted repairs. This nuclear track has no repair-warranty.

When five nuclear tracks are present and we say that the carcinogenic lesions from four nuclear tracks are perfectly repaired, we mean that NO FEWER than (4 x L) or at LEAST (4 x L) carcinogenic lesions are perfectly repaired -- regardless of which track actually produced them.

Does Repair Work Perfectly on 4 Nuclear Tracks, but Not on 5 ?

====================================

Now the foundation has been laid for answering the original question: Is it possible that repair is invariably flawless in every nucleus where it has to deal with a maximum of only four tracks at once?

We can handle the analysis by discussing the exposure of a million breast-cells by each type of radiation: A-bomb and radium-226.

We know from the Poisson calculation above that, when a million breast-cells were exposed in the Luminizer Study, only 13 nuclei per million experienced 5 tracks per exposure-session (per work-day). Since there were 400 exposure-sessions, a total of (13 x 400), or 5,200 nuclei per million experienced 5 tracks per work-day.

We are testing the proposition that all carcinogenic injury from FOUR tracks is flawlessly repaired within the nucleus. Perfect repair makes the carcinogenic lesions from four tracks DISAPPEAR from the nucleus. Therefore, in these 5,200 nuclei which received five tracks each, the equivalent of only one effective track is left per nucleus. Thus, this scenario has a total of only 5,200 effective tracks per million breast-cells -- or 5,200 nuclear tracks which are potentially effective toward cancer-production.

Since we are considering a million breast-cells at risk, we need to account now for (1,000,000 minus 5,200), or the other 994,800 nuclei. The Poisson table above shows that all of them received four tracks or even fewer. Indeed, 74.55 % of them received no track at all. Since we are testing the proposition here that repair is flawless when it is challenged by only four tracks or fewer, it means that there are NO tracks left potentially effective toward cancer-production in these 994,800 nuclei.

It follows that all the excess breast-cancer in the Luminizer Study arose from a total of 5,200 nuclear tracks (per million breast-cells at risk). And it must be emphasized that "a total of 5,200 nuclear tracks" has a totally different meaning from "5,200 tracks per nucleus."

By contrast, the A-bomb women received 216.4 tracks per nucleus, all in one acute dose. Since the proposition is that 4 were flawlessly repaired, this left 212.4 effective tracks in every nucleus. With a million breast-cells at risk, this means that the the excess breast-cancer arose from 212,400,000 effective tracks. So:

● -- A-Bomb Women (Acute Exposure) :
212,400,000 effective tracks per million breast-cells provoked a 50 % increase in breast-cancer.

● -- British Luminizers (Slow Exposure) :
5,200 effective tracks per million breast-cells provoked a 50 % increase in breast-cancer.

Guaranteed perfect repair of 4 tracks "un-did" so many of the tracks, during slow delivery, that the Luminizers had to cope with (212.4 million / 5,200), or 40,846-fold fewer effective tracks than the A-bomb women. And since both groups of women showed an equal cancer-effect, we would have to conclude that each effective ("no warranty") track was 40,846 times more potent (more likely to result in cancer) in the Luminizer Study than in the A-Bomb Study. Now we will adjust for the "built-in" part of this finding. Per rad of dose,

A-bomb radiation delivers 5.41 tracks per nucleus, on the average, while radium-226 delivers 2.937. So if an equal cancer-effect comes from an equal dose (40 rads), it must mean that each nuclear track from radium-226 is more potent by a factor of (5.41 / 2.937), or 1.84. So we divide the 40,846-fold disparity by the initial 1.84, and thus reduce it to 22,199.

Conclusion about
Flawless Repair at 4 Tracks per Nucleus :

It is not credible that each effective Luminizer track is 22,199-times more likely to lead to cancer than each effective A-bomb track. A proposition which leads to a non-credible conclusion must be false, and so we conclude that repair does NOT operate flawlessly upon all carcinogenic injuries from four tracks per nucleus -- does NOT invariably make all carcinogenic damage from at least 4 tracks per nucleus "disappear." In other words, doses and dose-rates which deliver a MAXIMUM of only 4 tracks per nucleus are NOT safe doses or dose-rates. But we can still hope that repair operates perfectly at THREE tracks per nucleus.

Why the Exact Risk-Value Does Not Matter :

Before testing the next proposition, we will show the same result even if 80 rads (not 40 rads) were needed to provoke a 50 % increase in breast-cancer in the A-Bomb Study. Delivery of 2-fold more energy requires 2-fold more tracks: 432.8 tracks per nucleus instead of 216.4 . (The subtraction of 4 tracks -- whose carcinogenic damage is perfectly repaired -- is negligible.) In the luminizers, cumulative tracks per nucleus would remain 117.48, total. So, the relative potency of each effective track in the luminizers would appear to rise by 2-fold. But the correction-factor by which we divide at the end would also rise by 2-fold. It was (5.41 x 40) / (2.937 x 40), or 1.84. It would become (5.41 x 80) / (2.937 x 40), or 3.684 -- which is 2-fold greater than 1.84. When the factor of 2.0 operates once in each direction, it cancels itself out.

Does Repair Work Perfectly
on 3 Nuclear Tracks, but Not on More ?

=======================================

One should explore the implications of speculating that repair can work flawlessly up through three tracks per nucleus, but becomes flawed beyond three. Again, we can calculate the relative track-potency under such a proposition.

British Luminizers: Out of a million breast-cells, the Poisson tabulation tells us that 231 nuclei will feel 4 tracks per exposure-session (meaning per work-day). We are testing the proposition that the carcinogenic

alterations along three tracks are flawlessly repaired, which leaves one effective track in each of these 231 nuclei per exposure session, times 400 exposure-sessions, or 92,400 effective tracks per million breast-cells at risk.

In addition, there are 13 nuclei per million breast-cells which receive 5 tracks per nucleus in each session. Since damage from three tracks in each nucleus is flawlessly repaired, this leaves 13 nuclei with 2 effective tracks in each, or 26 effective tracks per exposure-session, times 400 exposure-sessions, or 10,400 additional effective tracks per million breast-cells at risk.

Total effective tracks per million breast-cells at risk = 92,400 + 10,400 = 102,800 effective tracks. In all the other nuclei, the proposition is that repair is flawless because it is not strained by an overload and it can repair the lesions along 3 tracks perfectly. Thus, in all the other nuclei, there could be no tracks left potentially effective toward cancer-production.

The A-Bomb Women: These women received 216.4 tracks per nucleus. Since the proposition is that all carcinogenic alterations inflicted by 3 tracks are flawlessly repaired, there are 213.4 effective tracks left in every nucleus. Per million breast-cells at risk, there are 213,400,000 effective tracks left.

● -- _A-Bomb Women (Acute Exposure) :_
213,400,000 effective tracks per million breast-cells induced a 50 % increase in breast-cancer for the A-bomb women.

● -- _British Luminizers (Slow Exposure) :_
102,800 effective tracks per million breast-cells induced a 50 % increase in breast-cancer for the British Luminizers.

Conclusion: Each effective track in the Luminizer Study must be 2,076 times more potent in inducing cancer than each effective track in the A-Bomb Study. Then we adjust the ratio by the 1.84 correction factor, and reduce the disparity in track-potency to 1,128-fold.

Conclusion about
Flawless Repair at 3 Tracks per Nucleus :

It is not credible that each effective track in the Luminizer Study is 1,128 times more potent, in terms of carcinogenesis, than each effective track in the A-Bomb Study.

A proposition which leads to a non-credible conclusion must be false, and so we rule out the speculation that repair operates flawlessly up through three tracks per nucleus. In other words, doses and dose-rates which deliver a MAXIMUM of only 3 tracks per nucleus are NOT SAFE doses or dose-rates.

Does Repair Work Perfectly on 2 Nuclear Tracks, but Not on More?

Now that readers are familiar with the necessary steps in testing the various propositions, we will abbreviate as we test the proposition that repair is flawless up through two tracks per nucleus, but becomes flawed beyond two.

British Luminizers: Out of a million breast-cells, the Poisson tabulation tells us that 3,147 nuclei will feel exactly 3 tracks per exposure-session. We are testing the proposition that the carcinogenic alterations along two tracks are flawlessly repaired, which means:

3147 nuclei / million will have one effective track left. For 400 sessions, we have (400 x 3147 x 1), or 1,258,800 effective tracks.

231 nuclei / million will have 2 effective tracks left. For 400 sessions, we have (400 x 231 x 2), or 184,800 effective tracks.

13 nuclei / million will have 3 effective tracks left. For 400 sessions, we have (400 x 13 x 3), or 15,600 effective tracks.

Total effective tracks per million breast cells in the Luminizer Series : 1,258,800 + 184,800 + 15,600 = 1,459,200 effective tracks.

The A-Bomb Women: These women received 216.4 tracks per nucleus. Since the proposition is that all carcinogenic alterations inflicted by 2 tracks are flawlessly repaired, there are 214.4 effective tracks left in every nucleus. Per million breast-cells at risk, there are 214,400,000 effective tracks left.

● -- A-Bomb Women (Acute Exposure) :
214,400,000 effective tracks per million breast-cells induced a 50 % increase in breast-cancer for the A-bomb women.

● -- British Luminizers (Slow Exposure) :
1,459,200 effective tracks per million breast-cells induced a 50 % increase in breast-cancer for the British Luminizers.

Conclusion: Each effective track in the Luminizer Study must be 147 times more potent in inducing cancer

than each effective track in the A-Bomb Study. Then we adjust the ratio by the 1.84 correction factor, and reduce the disparity in track-potency to 78-fold.

Conclusion about Flawless Repair at 2 Tracks per Nucleus :

It is not credible, in our opinion, that each effective track in the Luminizer Study is 78 times more potent, in terms of carcinogenesis, than each effective track in the A-Bomb Study.

A proposition which leads to a non-credible conclusion must be false, and so we reject the speculation that repair operates flawlessly upon two tracks per nucleus. In other words, doses and dose-rates which deliver a MAXIMUM of only 2 tracks per nucleus are NOT SAFE doses or dose-rates.

Does Repair Work Perfectly upon 1 Nuclear Track, but Not upon More?

Using the same steps which we used in the previous tests, we will test the proposition that repair of carcinogenic injuries is flawless on one track per nucleus, but becomes flawed beyond one.

British Luminizers: Out of a million breast-cells, the Poisson tabulation tells us that 32,153 nuclei will feel exactly 2 tracks per exposure-session. We are testing the proposition that the carcinogenic alterations along one track are flawlessly repaired, which means:

32,153 nuclei / million will have one effective track left. For 400 sessions, we have (400 x 32,153 x 1), or 12,861,200 effective tracks.

3147 nuclei / million will have 2 effective tracks left. For 400 sessions, we have (400 x 3147 x 2), or 2,517,600 effective tracks.

231 nuclei / million will have 3 effective tracks left. For 400 sessions, we have (400 x 231 x 3), or 277,200 effective tracks.

13 nuclei / million will have 4 effective tracks left. For 400 sessions, we have (400 x 13 x 4), or 20,800 effective tracks.

Total effective tracks per million breast-cells in the Luminizer Series : 12,861,200 + 2,517,600 + 277,200 + 20,800 = 15,676,800

The A-Bomb Women: These women received 216.4 tracks per nucleus. Since the proposition is that all carcinogenic alterations inflicted by 1 track are flawlessly repaired, there are 215.4 effective tracks left in every nucleus. Per million breast-cells at risk, there are 215,400,000 effective tracks left.

● -- A-Bomb Women (Acute Exposure) :

215,400,000 effective tracks per million breast-cells induced a 50 % increase in breast-cancer for the A-bomb women.

● -- British Luminizers (Slow Exposure) :

15,676,800 effective tracks per million breast-cells induced a 50 % increase in breast-cancer for the British Luminizers.

Conclusion: Each effective track in the Luminizer Study must be 13.74 times more potent in inducing cancer than each effective track in the A-Bomb Study. Then we adjust the ratio by the 1.84 correction factor, and reduce the disparity in track-potency to 7.47-fold.

Conclusion about
Flawless Repair at 1 Track per Nucleus :

This finding (of a 7.47-fold disparity) is plausible enough. When we "ask" repair to work perfectly on the carcinogenic lesions from only ONE track per nucleus, the scenario leaves SO MANY effective tracks that no absurd disparity develops in "track-potency." In other words, when we push the analysis to the most extreme possible speculation, it simply becomes inconclusive -- given the epidemiological evidence which is available.

However, this TYPE of analysis is capable of addressing even the the "one track perfectly, but not two" question, if studies come along in which 40 rads are accumulated at a SLOWER rate than 0.1 rad per exposure-session, and if the studies have enough persons and follow-up so that radiation-induced cancer could be epidemiologically detectable. If exposure extends over 10, 20, or 30 years, the radio-sensitivity of the exposed persons will gradually decline DURING the exposure, of course, and this decline will somewhat reduce the final radiation-induced excess cancer, in comparison with exposure to the same total dose received over a shorter period.

If the British Luminizers had happened to accumulate their 40 rads at a dose-rate of 0.02937 track per nucleus on the average -- instead of 0.2937 track -- the ultimate disparity in track-potency would have risen from 7.47-fold to 68.7-fold, if we disregard a gradual decline in radio-sensitivity. (The bottom of Table 20-N provides the Poisson distribution needed by readers who may want to do the other calculations.)

It would not be credible for each effective track in the Luminizer Study to be 69-fold more potent, in terms of carcinogenesis, than each effective track in the A-Bomb Study. So if the luminizers' dose-rate had been ten-fold slower, the Luminizer Study might have addressed even the most extreme scenario, and might have ended possible speculation that repair might handle a maximum of ONE nuclear track flawlessly, but not TWO.

Conclusion from
the Entire Supplemental Approach :
=============================

For convenience, we shall summarize the findings here from the comparisons made above:

Perfectly Repairable Tracks per Nucleus	Relative Carcinogenic Potency of Effective Tracks (Luminizer / A-Bomb)
4 yes, but not 5 or more	22,199
3 yes, but not 4 or more	1,128
2 yes, but not 3 or more	78
1 yes, but not 2 or more	7

The supplemental evidence provides strong, additional confirmation of the conclusion reached in Part 5 of this chapter: Repair of carcinogenic alterations does NOT become invariably perfect in every injured nucleus, even when the MAXIMUM strain per nucleus falls to MINIMUM levels. Strain, in this context, means the number of primary ionization tracks per nucleus, per exposure-session.

The distinction between MAXIMUM strain and AVERAGE strain per nucleus is crucial. In the British Luminizer Study, when the average strain was 0.2937 track per nucleus per exposure-session, strain was absent (no track at all) in about 75.55 percent of the nuclei, the MAXIMUM strain in 22 percent of the nuclei was one track, and the MAXIMUM strain in about 3.5 percent of the nuclei was two to five tracks, per exposure-session (work-day).

The supplemental approach to the threshold issue, demonstrated here in Part 6, shows that speculation about "perfect repair" leads to non-credible consequences, even when the repair-system is tested for perfection in handling a maximum of only 4 tracks, 3 tracks, or 2 tracks per nucleus. In other words, the supplemental approach says that doses and dose-rates which deliver a MAXIMUM of only 4, 3, or 2 tracks per nucleus are NOT SAFE doses or dose-rates. With respect to a MAXIMUM rate of one track per nucleus,

==

the British Luminizer data are incapable of shedding additional light, one way or the other.

We conclude Part 6 with a reminder. Disproof of any safe dose or dose-rate was achieved in Part 5, by any reasonable standard of proof. It did not depend on the British Luminizers. Far from it. Part 6 has been a supplemental approach, presently tied to the British Luminizer Series. However, the general Max Trax method demonstrated above is applicable to ANY suitable studies which might become available in the future.

7. Comparison of Two Explanations for the Observations

Although the Max Trax approach was inconclusive with respect to perfect repair when we tested the available evidence for a maximum strain of ONE track per nucleus, there are overwhelming reasons to rule out any proposition that doses or dose-rates which inflict a maximum strain of one track per nucleus are SAFE.

For instance, such a safe-dose proposition would have to be plausibly reconciled with the indication by Max Trax that repair is NOT perfect when the maximum strain per nucleus is only four, three, or two simultaneous tracks per nucleus. To achieve reconciliation, safe-dose proponents might have to propose that the repair-system runs SHORT of some necessary enzyme or other necessity, as the strain on the system rises from one track up to two, three, or four tracks per nucleus, per work-day.

However, this proposition would lead to a non-credible consequence, namely gross incompatibility with the evidence from cell-studies that -- even in the presence of HUNDREDS of simultaneous tracks -- there is no shortage of repair-capacity for DNA and chromosome injuries.

(On the other hand, if repair is especially poor at low doses because of insufficient stimulation, then safe-dose proponents are in real difficulty, too. Perhaps one track per nucleus stimulates the LEAST repair-capacity per track.)

Rescue for the Safe-Dose Hypothesis ?

Altogether, the findings in this chapter would seem to require that threshold supporters develop a drastically revised defense for their safe-dose hypothesis. Their casual references to "repair" -- as if "repair" would automatically assure some safe dose -- have become

at variance with the actual epidemiologic evidence. Some supporters may propose a chain of new speculations, along the following line.

A. They might deny that carcinogenesis is related to injury of DNA or chromosomes at all. They might dismiss the huge and growing body of evidence which suggests that it is. Then they could deny that evidence from cell-studies, about DNA and chromosome repair, is RELEVANT to radiation carcinogenesis.

B. But this would amount to their proposing that cancer induced by ionizing radiation, in the nine studies of Table 21-A and in all the higher-dose studies too, results from some wholly unknown mechanism at some wholly unknown site.

C. Then -- in order to suggest the possibility of a safe dose -- they would need to propose that this wholly unknown process also has its own wholly unknown repair-system.

D. But, because it is clear (from the failure of dose-response to be concave-upward) that this wholly unknown repair-system is not reducing the cancer-risk per rad as dose approaches zero, and because it is clear (from the nine studies) that this wholly unknown repair-system is not perfect even when track-frequency is very low, they would need to propose that this repair-system becomes saturated at very low doses and that saturation accounts for repair's failure in the nine studies.

E. And lastly, in order to rescue the safe-dose hypothesis, they would need to propose that there is SOME frequency of ionization tracks per cell -- an average frequency even lower than in the nine studies -- at which this wholly unknown repair-system is un-depleted and also FLAWLESS.

Although this chain of speculations may seem far-fetched to some readers, points A and B have already been proposed as a response to our disproof of any safe dose or dose-rate. Points C, D, and E would seem to follow from A and B, since threshold proponents have an obligation to take account of the real-world human epidemiological evidence in SOME way, if NOT in our way.

Denial of the premise (about the role of DNA and chromosomes in radiation's carcinogenic action) cannot restore plausibility to the safe-dose hypothesis. It can only change the number of tracks per exposure, somewhat, by postulating that the cytoplasm, not the nucleus, is the site of carcinogenic injury.

Even so, if there is any radiation dose at all, primary ionization tracks occur and inflict injury in random fashion. So unless FLAWLESS repair suddenly were to occur at track-rates below the very low rates of the nine studies, there would be unrepaired, unrepairable, or misrepaired carcinogenic injuries (located in the cytoplasm), right down to the lowest conceivable dose or dose-rate.

A Competing Explanation of the Evidence :

Scientists worldwide are familiar with the great principle of economy in logic known as "Ockham's Razor," enunciated (in Latin) by the 14th century English philosopher, William of Ockham. The principle warns against fabricating many explanations when one is sufficient: "Entities [explanations] should not be multiplied beyond what is needed."

Instead of fabricating a series of speculations like paragraphs A through E above, and instead of dismissing without any basis a whole body of evidence (which links genetic information with cancer), we think it is far more reasonable for us to suggest a highly plausible -- virtually obvious -- explanation of all the observations which relate to the threshold issue:

Whenever an ionization track traverses a nucleus, there is always a chance that it will cause a carcinogenic lesion and that the lesion will be unrepaired, inherently unrepairable, or misrepaired. In short, there is an inherent failure-rate in the repair-system.

This hypothesis requires no denial of all the evidence linking genetic information with cancer. Moreover, it is consistent with the observation of imperfect operations in other physiological systems. And it would explain all sorts of the specific observations in this field.

For instance, this hypothesis would explain why radiation-induced cancer is found in a host of human studies between 10-400 rems -- a dose-range where cell-studies indicate no shortage of genetic repair-CAPACITY.

For instance, this hypothesis would explain the observation (in several human studies) of radiation-induced chromosome aberrations persisting in persons who received their doses at MINIMAL dose-rates -- from weapons-fallout, elevated background doses, and routine occupational exposures.

For instance, this hypothesis would explain the observation of radiation-induced cancer in the nine studies (Table 21-A) where repair was challenged by so very few tracks per nucleus, on the average.

And this hypothesis would explain the supplemental Max Trax results, which indicate that the repair-process is NOT routinely and invariably flawless even when it has to cope with a MAXIMUM track-rate per nucleus of only four, three, or two tracks.

This hypothesis is, of course, incompatible with any safe dose or dose-rate of ionizing radiation. If there is any dose at all, tracks occur and inflict injuries in a random fashion. So if there is some inherent chance of failure in the repair of carcinogenic damage whenever there are ionization tracks, then this chance will be present right down to the lowest conceivable dose or dose-rate.

8. The Bottom Line

No one denies anymore that low-LET ionizing radiation is a human carcinogen. The threshold question is: Does it STOP being a human carcinogen when the dose or dose-rate is sufficiently low?

There are a multitude of low-dose human studies which are inherently incapable of helping to settle the threshold issue (discussion in Chapter 21, Part 2). However, we have assembled nine human epidemiological studies which ARE capable.

Together, they amount to proof that repair of radiation-induced carcinogenic lesions, at the cellular level, fails to "deliver" a safe dose or dose-rate of ionizing radiation with respect to human cancer-induction, even when the strain on the repair-system is minimal. Indeed, in five of the nine studies, the strain per cell-nucleus is an average of only one or two simultaneous tracks ... with an average even below 1.0 in some studies.

The nine studies are supplemented by an analysis which also relies on epidemiological observations. The supplemental analysis indicates that the hypothesis of perfect repair leads to non-credible conclusions, and that there is a failure-rate in the repair-system for carcinogenic lesions -- even when a nucleus has to cope with a MAXIMUM of only 4, 3, or 2 primary tracks per nucleus, per exposure-session.

And so the human epidemiological evidence establishes -- by any reasonable standard of proof -- that there is no safe dose or dose-rate ... unless there exists some wholly separate, post-repair system in the body which also needs consideration.

===

The Immune System, or
Other Post-Repair Defense Mechanisms :

We all know the common refrain that the body has surveillance systems which are constantly rejecting cancers which are constantly being formed in the body, and "without the immune surveillance system, EVERYONE would die of cancer."

So we will consider the proposition that, if the immune or other surveillance system has such prowess in preventing cancer, such a system must be easily able to "take care of" the residual problem left by repair's small failure-rate.

How we wish this attractive proposition were true. But clearly it is not. The reality is that, in countries like the United States, about twenty percent of the population dies of cancer. The percentage of persons with cancers -- not prevented by immune or other defense mechanisms -- is even larger if the non-fatal cancers are included. Obviously, the immune or other surveillance mechanisms are failing to prevent huge numbers of cancers, since they are failing to prevent about one in five persons from being killed by this disease.

Is it possible to reconcile this reality with the hope that, somehow, the same flawed defense mechanisms "take care of" every potential radiation-induced cancer missed by repair, provided the carcinogenic injury occurred along a track received at a very low dose? Reconciliation would require some pure fantasies.

For instance, potential cancers induced by IONIZING RADIATION would have to look different from other potential cancers which are watched by the surveillance systems. Otherwise, the surveillance systems would be unable to select them out for special (perfect) treatment.

In addition, in order for this last line of defense to work perfectly for LOW-dose radiation when it obviously does not work perfectly at higher doses, the potential cancers induced by tracks at low doses would have to sprout a little flag identifying themselves as LOW-dose products.

Since such fantasies would strain even the greatest credulity, we must discard this last hope for a safe dose or dose-rate.

The Initial Five Points, Condensed :

Below, we shall condense the five-point summary (from Part 1 of this chapter) even further:

1. One primary ionization track is the least possible disturbance which can occur at the cellular level from ionizing radiation. Without a track, there is no dose at all.

2. Every primary ionization track has a chance of inducing cancer by inducing carcinogenic injuries; it needs no help from any other track.

3. This means that there is no conceivable dose or dose-rate which can be safe, unless (A) the repair-system always successfully un-does every carcinogenic lesion, when the dose or dose-rate is sufficiently low, or (B) every failure of the repair-system, at low doses, is always successfully eliminated by some post-repair defense-system.

4. Human epidemiological evidence shows that the repair-system for radiation-induced carcinogenic lesions has a failure-rate even under minimal strain.

5. Observation and logic show that post-repair defense-systems (for instance, the immune system) cannot possibly be perfect with respect to providing a safe dose or dose-rate of ionizing radiation.

It follows that there is no safe dose or dose-rate of ionizing radiation, with respect to induction of human cancer. The risk is related to dose, right down to zero dose.

Beyond A Reasonable Doubt :

The existing human evidence shows, beyond a reasonable doubt, that there is no conceivable dose or dose-rate of low-LET ionizing radiation which is safe, with respect to producing fatal cancer in humans.

From 9 rads right down to 0.1 rad, the epidemiological evidence speaks for itself, without reliance on any hypothesis or presumption at all. The evidence includes adults, children, high-energy gamma rays, diagnostic X-rays, acute delivery and very slow delivery. And between zero dose, and the doses tested directly by the nine studies, the calculations which disprove any safe dose or dose-rate rely on only one extremely reasonable assumption -- namely, that radiation-induced cancer originates from events in the nucleus.

In the face of the evidence, I could not possibly suggest in this book that the safe-dose question cannot be answered at all or that it could readily go in either direction.

==

One might watch out for inconsistent attitudes toward what constitutes proof. Chapter 22 shows that, without any proof of correctness whatsoever and in the face of CONTRARY human evidence of good quality, much of the radiation community has routinely divided observed per-rad cancer-risks by numbers like 2 to 10 when estimating per-rad risk at LOW doses and dose rates. Now, when it comes to settling the safe-dose issue, it would appear inconsistent if similar segments of the radiation community were to demand unreasonably large amounts of human evidence, or were to become "ultra-careful" about acceptable levels of proof.

Real vs. Imaginary Radiation-Casualties :

By reasonable standards of proof, the safe-dose hypothesis is not merely implausible -- it is disproven.

Disproof of any safe dose or dose-rate invalidates suggestions that, whenever an analyst calculates a NUMBER of radiation-induced cancers to be caused by very low-dose exposure, the cancers are just "hypothetical," "speculative," "theoretical," "non-existent," or "imaginary."

It is true, of course, that radiation-induced cancers in a population from very low doses will rarely if ever be detectable epidemiologically, because of the signal-to-noise ratio (see Chapter 21). But it does NOT follow (from the lack of direct observation) that the cancers are therefore unreal, hypothetical, speculative, theoretical, non-existent, or imaginary. No rational person will deny that one of the most commonplace (and important) functions of science is to let people know what is REALLY HAPPENING when direct observation is impossible.

We conclude with a warning: Disproof of any safe dose or dose-rate means that fatal cancers from minimal doses and dose-rates of ionizing radiation are not imaginary. They are really occurring in exposed populations. Proposals, to declare that they need not be considered, have health implications extending far beyond the radiation issue, as pointed out in Chapter 24, Part 10 and Chapter 25, Part 5.

==========================

CHAPTER 19

The Special Interaction of Ionizing Radiation with Living Tissue

This chapter is arranged in four parts:

This chapter and the two other "auxiliary chapters" (Chapters 20 and 21) provide the support for certain points used in the proof that no safe dose of low-LET ionizing radiation exists -- either for acute exposure or for slow exposure -- with respect to human carcinogenesis.

1. Distinctive Characteristics of Ionizing Radiation

With respect to ionizing radiation, "dose" is a macroscopic concept describing the total energy deposited in tissue, and tissue-doses are expressed in energy-units per gram of irradiated tissue.

The biologically important characteristics of low-LET radiation are that its energy is carried through tissue by high-speed electrons, and that the transfers of this energy occur along paths (tracks) in extremely localized or concentrated fashion.

One need only consider the common fever in order to ponder the very high probability that the biological potency of ionizing radiation is related to its spatial concentration along tracks, rather than to its meager addition of energy to cells (Go81, pp.52-53). A dose of 400 cGy (400 rads) is equivalent in heat to only 4.184×10^{-3} joules per gram of tissue -- enough to provoke a mini-fever of 0.001 degree Centigrade -- yet 400 cGy of ionizing radiation to the whole body, acutely delivered, will kill about half the humans exposed to it.

Ionizing radiation as a toxic agent differs fundamentally from toxic substances, which can be introduced to a solution slowly and diluted to a lower and lower uniform concentration. By contrast, for low-LET radiations such as X-rays and beta particles, the minimal unit is the primary ionization track left by a single high-speed electron. The electron cannot be subdivided, and it cannot make its delivery of energy more gentle by diluting it evenly throughout the whole cell; the initial transfer of energy occurs very abruptly and very close to the primary track, as we shall see in detail in Part 2 of this chapter.

Definition of "Particle Track":

Here it is useful to define "Particle Track," well-described by Kellerer, as follows (Kelle87, p.360):

"A particle track is the random configuration of energy transfers produced by a charged particle and / or its secondaries." Kellerer adds the important information that the individual energy deposits may be either ionizations or excitations of molecules or atoms, and that the term "particle track" denotes the set of ALL transfers of energy produced by a charged particle and its secondaries, the secondaries being primarily electrons set in motion by the original charged particle. In the case of low-LET radiation, the initial charged particle creating the track is the electron itself.

Definition of the "Least Possible Disturbance":

Because the minimal event in dose-delivery of ionizing radiation is a single track, we can define the least possible disturbance to a single cell-nucleus: It is the traversal of the nucleus by just one primary ionization track.

This is not the same as an AVERAGE of one primary ionization track per cell-nucleus. That average can be achieved by some nuclei in irradiated tissue having NO tracks through them, others having one track through them, and some having multiple tracks through them. At very low doses, when a gram of tissue is irradiated, not every nucleus is "hit" by a track. The nuclei which receive no track at all actually receive no dose at all, even though the tissue as a whole is called "exposed" at the macroscopic level. At the "microdosimetric level," however, wherever there is no track, there is no dose.

Although we can, and will, speak of doses which

correspond with fractional tracks -- say, 2.937 primary ionization tracks per nucleus, on the average -- fractional tracks exist only because an average has been computed. Fractional tracks do not exist. Either a track traverses a nucleus somewhere (one nuclear track) or it does not (zero nuclear track). We shall discuss the "off-center" traversals in Part 2.

As we examine what is going on at the cellular level when tissue is exposed to low-LET exposure, it will become evident that the biologically important question for settling the threshold issue is not "What human studies exist at the lowest conceivable doses?", but rather, "What human studies exist which can address carcinogenesis (or its absence) when cell nuclei experience the least possible disturbance by ionizing radiation?"

2. Primary and Secondary Electrons

Gamma rays and X-rays are photons which injure cells and cell-nuclei by ejecting an electron from a molecule or atom and putting it into high-speed motion; in Chapter 20, we will take account of the three ways in which such photons transfer their radiant energy to high-speed electrons. Beta particles, of course, are already high-speed electrons.

The Primary Electrons :

Electrons in motion travel primarily in straight lines through human tissue, although occasionally one will suffer a major deflection and then travel in another straight line.

The distance traveled (range) depends, of course, on an electron's initial energy; ranges are tabulated in Chapter 20, Table 20-FG. At the energies which characterize the nine epidemiological studies in Table 21-A, the high-speed electron travels through more than one cell. The diameter of a typical human cell is about 14.2 micrometers or microns (Chapter 20).

The key issue is that the interaction between ionizing radiation and living tissue occurs along the track of the electron, as described nicely by Freeman below (Free87b, p.278-279). Although Freeman is discussing effects of irradiating hydrocarbon liquids (instead of human tissue), the interactions will be very similar, since the interactions of electrons with matter are overwhelmingly determined by the average atomic number of the matter being traversed -- and the atomic numbers which characterize tissue and hydrocarbons are "in the same ballpark." We quote Freeman, with only the minor change of expressing all energies in MeV or eV:

"The collision of a 0.6 MeV photon with a molecule usually causes an electron to be ejected with about half the initial photon energy. The ~0.3 MeV electron moves through the liquid losing energy in small bits (a few tens of electron-volts) and ionizes about 10^4 other molecules along its path. Thus, nearly all of the physical and chemical changes in the system are produced by the energetic electron and not by the initial photon. The kinetics of reactions induced by high-energy photons are therefore similar to those obtained if high-energy electrons are used as the primary radiation."

As the primary electron transfers its energy bit by bit, of course it loses speed. When it is slower, the average distance decreases between consecutive transfers of energy, and the amount of energy transferred per unit of distance increases, on the average. In other words, its LET (Linear Energy Transfer, or amount of energy transferred per unit of path traveled) is constantly rising until its energy is too low for further ionization events.

In both the low-LET and high-LET regions of a single primary electron track, RANDOM variations occur in the distance between consecutive energy-transfers and in the amount of energy imparted during consecutive transfers.

All along its track, the primary electron is setting secondary electrons into motion, and they have their own tracks known as delta rays. Most delta rays are only a few nanometers long -- extremely short compared with the track of the primary electron. (There are 1,000 nanometers per micrometer.)

The fate of the primary electron in creating further secondaries is a matter of statistical probabilities -- and independent of what has just happened before. The result is that the distribution of energy-transfer events is hardly ever the same for one primary electron as it is for another of the same initial energy. Therefore, when describing the various excited molecules, secondary electrons, and ions which result, analysts deal with the variation from one region to another by speaking in terms of probabilities.

Microzones and the Secondary Electrons :

As the primary electron is creating its ionization track, it is setting secondary electrons into motion at irregular intervals. For example, a primary electron with an initial energy of about 300 KeV is producing secondary electrons at irregular intervals of a few hundred nanometers on the average (a few tenths of a micrometer). Freeman has described the energy-deposition events very carefully (Free87b, pp.278-281). Of course, the energy-deposition events creating the secondary electrons, with some several tens of electron volts of energy-loss for each deposition-event, reduce the energy of the primary electron.

The amount of disturbance caused by a secondary electron depends on how much energy it acquired when it was ejected from its molecule by the primary electron. Freeman has suggested the following energy distributions per secondary-electron creation.

About 75% of secondary electrons along a primary ionization track acquire enough energy to move away from their sibling ions, but not enough energy to remove an electron from another molecule. Where a single secondary electron is produced, the region is called a microzone of reactivity (Free87b, p.280). Secondary electrons of this class lose their excess energy by colliding with other molecules until they acquire the average energy of molecules in the vicinity; they become "thermalized." Paretzke reports that the time-interval between ejection of the secondary electron to the time it is thermalized is of the order of 10^{-11} to 10^{-13} seconds (Par87, p.92, Fig.3.2).

About 15% of secondary electrons acquire enough energy (~40 electron-volts) to remove an electron from one additional molecule. This second ionization occurs at an average distance of only 0.4 nanometer from the first ion. The two electrons scatter more or less randomly and become thermalized a few nanometers from the positive ions. When there are two such pairs of electrons and positive ions, the region is called a two-pair microzone.

About 10% of secondary electrons acquire enough energy to remove electrons from two or more additional molecules -- sometimes from 10 or more other molecules. In a five-pair microzone, all the pairs would be produced within about one nanometer of each other, and within a time-interval of pico-seconds (trillionths of a second).

"Off-Center" Nuclear Traversals :

When the Least Possible Disturbance to a cell-nucleus was defined in Part 1 as traversal by just one primary ionization track, the location of the track was deliberately left unspecified.

Obviously, not all primary tracks which traverse a cell-nucleus go right through its full diameter. Although most tracks will be "off-center" (short chords, in the language of microdosimetry), one cannot assume that

short chords menace a nucleus with fewer energy-transfers and with a lower chance of carcinogenic injury than do longer chords. When the primary electron is slow near the end of its track, and its LET has become high, an off-center track can pack more transfers of energy (more microzones of reactivity) into a nucleus than can a full-length chord when the electron's LET is still low. Thus, it would be biologically meaningless to introduce a distinction between off-center and central tracks, in the concept of the Least Possible Disturbance.

3. Some Chemical Consequences: Free Radicals, Scavengers, and Altered Genetic Molecules

Freeman remarks: "The time scales of the reactions in an irradiated liquid divide naturally into two regimes: those that occur quickly within the individual reactive microzones and those of the species that diffuse away from the microzones, which occur at later times" (Free87b, p.281).

Paretzke (Par87, p.92) refers to the first of these two regimes as the "physical stage," and the second regime as the "chemical stage." The times at which the various events in the "physical stage" occur are provided in his Figure 3.2 and are summarized below.

Events of the "Physical Stage" :

A. The energy transfer to molecules in the irradiated medium occurs in times of the order of 10^{-17} to 10^{-16} seconds. Short times indeed.

B. The energy transfer produces excited atoms or molecules -- with a large increment in energy -- which means these excited species are capable of undergoing a variety of unusual further reactions. The time scales for production of these excited molecules are between 10^{-16} and 10^{-11} seconds after the energy transfer has occurred.

C. Dissociation, which represents break-up of excited molecules to produce a variety of species still possessing excess energy, occurs in time scales of the order of 10^{-13} to 10^{-11} seconds. Some of the dissociations are actually ionizations, productive of a positive atom-ion or molecule-ion plus an electron.

D. Electrons produced in the ionizations of Step C interact by collision with atoms and molecules, with final reduction in energy of the electrons to the average energy of the species in the medium. This process is known as "thermalization", and occurs in time scales of the order of 10^-13 to 10^-11 seconds.

E. The various events described in (A) through (D) are considered to be over by 10^-10 seconds after the initial energy transfer. Paretzke describes this time as the end of the physical stage and as the initial condition for the chemical stage of reactions. This is a time of one ten-billionth of a second.

Events of the "Chemical Stage" :

Magee and Chatterjee provide a well-stated overview of the chemical stage (Magee87, p.171):

"Radiation chemistry must always be considered in terms of track reactions. Energy is deposited by radiation in tracks and then follows a sequence of nonhomogeneous processes that create and transform reactive intermediates until final radiation chemical products are formed."

Magee and Chatterjee (Magee87, pp.210-211) emphasize that the track reactions of the radiation's chemical stage are nonhomogeneous, because the reactive species which form the radiation's chemical products are created in tracks, rather than in a homogeneous solution. They state that the structure of the tracks is actually quite complicated, and that a large part of their effort involves the devising of reasonable track models.

Their statement that the problem is quite complicated can be regarded as a massive understatement, especially for tissues, where we have nonhomogeneity of the cellular or nuclear medium itself, with structures such as chromosomes being present -- all over and above the nonhomeogeneity of the radiation tracks themselves.

They confirm Paretzke's estimates of time scales with their statement (Magee87, pp.210-211) that "Our treatment of the track reactions begins at about 3 ps [three pico-seconds, or three trillionths of a second], at which time the chemical species are more or less thermalized following the initial deposition of energy at about 10^-16 s" [s = seconds].

Production of Free Radicals :

Now we can examine the nature of some of those reactive intermediates and some of the final products, together with inspection of the time scales of the reactions which occur in an aqueous phase (cellular material is fundamentally based on an aqueous phase). Water itself is attacked in the earliest phase of the chemical reactions which develop. The transfer of

energy to the water molecule excites the electrons of that molecule, to produce an excited water molecule, with much excess energy compared to its normal energy. The most probable event is an ionization, as follows:

- (A) :

$$H_2O \longrightarrow H_2O^+ \text{ plus } e,$$

where e = electron. The extremely reactive H_2O^+ molecule-ion undergoes further reactions as follows:

- (B) :

$$H_2O^+ \text{ plus } H_2O \longrightarrow H_3O^+ \text{ plus } OH$$

Both H_2O^+ and OH have an unpaired electron, so both species are "free radicals" and are themselves extremely reactive.

Magee and Chatterjee estimate that reaction (B) occurs in about 10^{-14} seconds, and converts all the H_2O^+ to H_3O^+ and OH, on this time scale.

The free "dry" electron reacts with water to produce a hydrated electron, designated as e^- (aqueous), on a time scale of the order of 4×10^{-13} seconds.

Above we stated that ionization is the "most probable" event following energy-deposition from radiation, but other reactions also occur, such as:

- (C) :

$$H_2O \text{ (excited) } \longrightarrow H \text{ plus } OH, \text{ and,}$$

- (D) :

$$H_2O \text{ (excited) } \longrightarrow H_2 \text{ plus } O$$

===

Note that H (hydrogen atoms), and OH (hydroxyl radicals), and O (oxygen atoms) are all themselves "free radicals," possessing an unpaired electron, and they are extremely reactive species which will interact with a variety of chemicals in the aqueous medium. For example:

● (E) :
H_2O plus O ----> H_2O_2 , which is
    hydrogen peroxide.

These various reactions account for the production of what Magee and Chatterjee regard as the major chemical entities produced, and these reactions are over well before "thermalization." So they are over well before 10^{-11} seconds, following energy-deposition.

Magee and Chatterjee suggest that by 10^{-10} seconds after passage of a charged particle through a solution, we have the various highly reactive chemical species (described above) present in thermal equilibrium but far from chemical equilibrium, and they are present in a nonhomogeneous spatial distribution. These reactive species react with each other or diffuse away from each other. It is their suggestion that the reactive intermediate chemical species formed in one track react completely with each other AND with constituents of the aqueous medium before they can diffuse far enough to encounter intermediates from another track.

Since the reactive intermediates not only react with each other, but also react with constituents of the medium, it follows that the ultimate products depend upon what else is present in the medium. For example, in biological tissues oxygen is present, and hence reactions such as (F) and (G) occur:

● (F) :
e^- (aqueous) plus O_2 --> O_2^- plus H_2O
    In this reaction, the hydrated electron converts oxygen molecules to the superoxide ion (which is O_2^-).

● (G) :
H plus O_2 ----> HO_2

The product, HO_2, is a free radical not previously mentioned above.

Magee and Chatterjee suggest that the host of reactions, between the initial radicals themselves and between the radicals and constituents of the solution, are pretty well completed to yield final products by times of the order of 10^{-5} seconds following the initial energy-deposition event.

Action by "Scavengers" :

The word "scavenger," which means any person, creature, or thing which removes impurities, refuse, or rubbish, is enormously useful in chemistry -- including radiation chemistry.

Biological tissue is a water-based medium, in which are present numerous small molecules as well as large molecules (e.g., proteins), PLUS the structures such as chromosomes, which themselves contain DNA molecules, ribose-nucleic acids, and proteins. Any and all of these entities can act as scavengers for the various highly reactive radical intermediates which were formed in the early radiation reactions. Some products of such scavenging may be involved in the ultimate production of cancer.

Direct Action on Genetic Molecules :

It would be a grave mistake for anyone to overlook the fact that genetic molecules (DNA, chromosomes) can suffer injury from DIRECT interaction with a primary ionization track.

Goodhead has pointed out that a variety of biochemical and other data would imply that diffusion-distances of radicals in cells are very small (less than a few nanometers) and, therefore, "that the only reasonable probability of multiple adjacent damage to DNA arises when a cluster [of radiation damage] is produced directly in, or very near the DNA" (Good88, p.238). Goodhead states further (p.238):

"For low-LET radiations, approximately one-third of the energy deposition is via very low energy, < ~ 2 KeV electrons, which are known to have a relatively high RBE and a relatively high probability of producing localized clusters (of, say, >~100 eV in the DNA), so this may well be the critical component of low-LET radiations."

Such considerations echo the opening theme of this

chapter: In ways which no one yet fully fathoms, the spatial arrangement of energy-transfers along a track is important. Kellerer, one of the leading figures in the microdosimetry of ionizing radiation, points out that the effectiveness or menace of ionizing radiation is not "a mere function of the specific energy in the nucleus; it depends in an insufficiently understood way on the spatial microdistribution of energy" (Kelle87, p.347).

Other sources (see, for instance, Sies85 and Bav89) are also reporting that the specific geometry of the initial injury-site is crucial to the final outcome of subsequent molecular alterations. In other words, when microzones of energy-transfer (from the primary ionization track) occur directly upon or within the genetic molecules, the geometry of the particular site, the particular juxtaposition of components, the reduced mobility of reactive intermediates, possible transfers of energy along the molecule, and other such considerations (including altered chance of repair), can put such events into a very different class from interactions between genetic molecules and external free radicals in the medium.

Some proponents of the safe-dose idea suggest a benign analogy between normal metabolism and ionizing radiation, by saying only that both of them produce free radicals in the medium. The comparison is misleading, if the important differences -- such as direct interaction of an ionization track with a genetic molecule -- are not mentioned.

"The Yalow Model" :

Dr. Rosalyn Yalow (see Chapter 34) features free radicals in an article about "radiation phobia." She writes (Ya89, p.160-161):

"The question as to whether there exists a threshold below which radiation effects in man do not occur should continue to be addressed. One can develop a tenable model that would be consistent with such a threshold. Since human beings are more than 75 % water, low-LET ionizing radiation is largely absorbed in the water resulting in the production of free radicals. Thus, many of the potential biochemical changes initiated in the cell and, in particular, damage to cellular DNA are probably a consequence of the action of the products of water radiolysis. If molecules which scavenge radicals and which are normally present in tissue greatly exceed in concentration the free radicals generated at low dose rates, there may well be no initiating event, i.e., damage to DNA. The threshold could be the dose rate at which the radiation-induced free radicals exceed the scavengers."

We do not find the "Yalow Model" to be tenable or plausible as a safe-dose model:

Not even a shoulder-to-shoulder "army" of other scavengers in the aqueous medium can protect the genetic molecules against DIRECT interaction with an ionization track -- regardless of dose. The chance of direct interaction will be proportional to the number of tracks (that is, to the dose) right down to the lowest conceivable dose or dose-rate.

Moreover, direct interactions may well be the IMPORTANT events in causing permanent alterations of genetic molecules (as pointed out by Goodhead above).

No Track, No Products :

All of the events which occur because of the primary ionization track -- from the secondary electrons to all of their consequent products -- must be treated with the primary track itself as a single unit. If there were no primary track passing through a cell or cell-nucleus, none of the secondary events would occur. No track, no products.

As we analyze the threshold issue, we must disregard any leakage of radiolytic products into an un-hit nucleus from the cytoplasm -- if such leakage occurs at all. No matter how low the dose or dose-rate, some nuclei necessarily experience direct hits and not just leakage. High-speed electrons traveling through tissue in straight lines do not know how to avoid the nuclei. Some nuclei necessarily continue to experience one primary ionization track until there is no tissue-dose at all.

A Reminder about Time Scales :

We close this section on "the chemical stage" of radiation injury with a reminder: While the damaging events from ionizing radiation do indeed occur in very short time-spans (small fractions of a second) and in close physical proximity to the initial energy-deposition events, there are very important events which follow. For example, DNA and chromosomal repairs -- and misrepairs -- go on for periods of the order of minutes to several hours after radiation damage (Chapter 18).

4. Intra-Track and Inter-Track Carcinogenesis

We can think of all the energy-transfers and consequent products along a single primary track as "intra-track" phenomena, to distinguish them from

===

similar events which would occur elsewhere in the same cell or cell-nucleus as a result of the passage of a wholly separate primary electron.

If there is any interaction of the products of one primary track with the products of another primary track, we would speak of "inter-track" phenomena.

It is self-evident, from the nature of radiation tracks, that if track-phenomena are going to interact with each other, what matters is the nature of the interacting phenomena -- and it does not matter which track happened to produce them.

Single-Site and Multi-Site Lesions :

Now let us examine the following premise: A fully competent carcinogenic lesion may consist of an alteration at only one site in the nucleus, or it may also consist of alterations which occur at two (or more) separate sites in the nucleus and then interact to become carcinogenic. Let us call the first type of fully competent carcinogenic lesion 'A'. For the second type, we will consider alterations at two sites, and call this type of lesion 'B + C'. In terms of the diagrams:

The A1 Lesion :

A1 illustrates the A type of lesion; by itself, this single-site alteration, created by a single track, would be a fully competent carcinogenic lesion of the INTRA-track variety. The frequency with which A type lesions occur would be related to the number of tracks, or $Dose^1$.

The B1 + C1 Lesion :

B1 + C1 illustrates a fully competent carcinogenic lesion, of the type which requires the interaction of sub-lesions B1 and C1. This lesion, B1 + C1, is an INTRA-track lesion, because the B1 and C1 sub-lesions are both created by a single primary ionization track. The diagram shows that no other track is involved. Like the A type of lesion, the B1 + C1 lesion is the result of single-track action, and therefore its frequency would be related to the number of tracks, or $Dose^1$.

The diagram does not indicate whether B1 and C1 are sub-lesions within the same molecule, or sub-lesions within two different molecules. (Both situations are possible.) The purpose of the diagram is to indicate that B1 and C1 are two lesions caused by the same primary TRACK.

The B1 + C2 Lesion :

B1 + C2 illustrates a fully competent carcinogenic lesion of the INTER-track variety, because the B1 and C2 sub-lesions are created by different tracks. The frequency with which B1 + C2 lesions occur would be related to $Tracks^2$, or $Dose^2$.

Comparison of the Multi-Site Lesions :

The orientation of a track relative to a genetic molecule is determined by chance -- the molecules are not stationary in the nucleus, the person is not stationary during occupational and environmental irradiation, and the tracks themselves are rarely coming from a single direction.

Therefore, despite the visual suggestion by the diagrams that such orientation might differ between the two multi-site lesions (B1 + C1, versus B1 + C2), in fact the orientations AND EVERYTHING ELSE about these two lesions can be identical -- except for the fact that one is an intra-track lesion and the other is an inter-track lesion.

If these intra-track and inter-track multi-site lesions can be IDENTICAL, it would be preposterous for anyone to suggest that only one could be carcinogenic and the

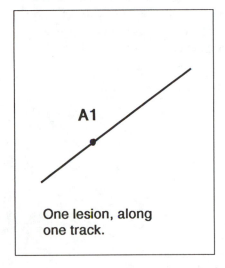

One lesion, along one track.

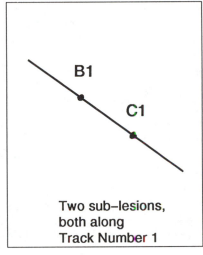

Two sub-lesions, both along Track Number 1

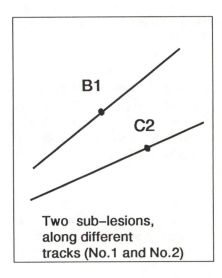

Two sub-lesions, along different tracks (No.1 and No.2)

other could be innocuous.

Now, we return to the premise with which we started. Our purpose was to emphasize that -- even if interaction between multiple sites is sometimes or always involved in radiation carcinogenesis (which is by no means certain) -- intra-track carcinogenesis as well as inter-track carcinogenesis would occur.

The Capability of Single-Track Action:

Before leaving the topic of intra-track carcinogenesis, it needs to be said that any lesion which can be inflicted in a nucleus by a PAIR of tracks, can also be inflicted by a single track acting ALONE.

For instance, it is obvious that breaking a chromosome requires that two strands of DNA be broken. But this result does not require two separate ionization tracks. Events occurring along the SAME track can do it.

A single track is also capable of inflicting damage on more than one chromosome. There is just no doubt that a single track can interact with more than one chromosome, as the track passes through the nucleus. Indeed, if a DOZEN chromosomes were ever in the same plane as the track and if they were lying across its trajectory, a single track could injure all twelve of them, in principle. Or if a single chromosome happened to be folded across the track's trajectory, a single track could interact with the SAME chromosome several times.

Another example of capabilities involves the multi-pair microzone. It is true that a single track cannot intersect with itself and cannot superimpose two microzones upon each other, whereas a pair of tracks may sometimes intersect and produce (say) a 2-pair microzone and a 3-pair microzone in the same place. The result would be a 5-pair microzone -- and this is something which a single track produces on its own from time to time (see Part 2), without any help from another track.

Lastly, we should mention again the possibility that sometimes carcinogenesis may be associated with multiple genetic injuries. And if so, such injuries can be inflicted by a single track. The earlier parts of this chapter leave no doubt that events at multiple, separate sites are certainly producible by a single track, acting alone.

The bottom line from this discussion was stated in Chapter 18, Part 1: "Single, primary ionization tracks, acting independently from each other, are never innocuous with respect to creating carcinogenic injuries in the cells which they traverse. Every track -- without help from any other track -- has a chance of inducing cancer by creating such injuries."

Linear-Quadratic Model of Dose-Response :

In Chapter 18, we said that the statement quoted above is not controversial. Agreement about intra-track carcinogenesis is reflected in the Linear-Quadratic (LQ) model of dose-response which is almost universally used by the radiation community (see Chapter 22). In that model, the linear term (the L term) represents the relationship of intra-track events with Dose^1, and the quadratic term (the Q term) represents the relationship of inter-track events with Dose^2.

It should be noted that the LQ model is fully consistent with our disproof of any safe dose or dose-rate. Indeed, the LQ model acknowledges that -- in the studies which we used in the disproof -- the probability is very high that the excess cancer which was observed all arose from SINGLE-track action (intra-track events). In the LQ model, intra-track events are overwhelmingly dominant at low doses and dose-rates. This is true when the LQ model has a concave-upward shape, and also when it has a concave-downward, supra-linear shape.

The linear-quadratic model is examined in detail in Chapter 23.

Meaning of "Fully Competent Lesion" :

The statement that intra-track lesions can be fully competent carcinogenic lesions should not be interpreted as a statement that every carcinogenic lesion becomes a clinically manifest cancer.

A potential cancer may need assistance from promotional agents in order to reach a clinical stage, and may also have to evade a series of defenses by the body. But as far as radiation itself is concerned, a single primary ionization track has all the properties which make ionizing radiation a human carcinogen.

===================

Number of Primary Electron–Tracks per Cell–Nucleus, per Rad of Dose Received from Various Sources of Radiation

This chapter is arranged in three parts:

1. List of the Information Needed to Calculate the Number of Tracks per Nucleus, p.1
2. Provision of the Input, the Calculations, and the Answer, p.2
3. The Fallacy of Slow Delivery of Very Low Doses, p.6
Then tables.

Readers of Chapter 18 already know how the disproof of any safe dose or dose–rate is related to the approximate number of primary ionization tracks occurring in cell–nuclei.

In this chapter, we will show step–by–step how we determined the number of tracks per nucleus which are occurring at any particular dose (for instance, one rad or centi–gray), from a particular radiation source. Separately, in Chapter 33, we will show that our method and the methods of other analysts must be in good agreement, because they produce closely similar results.

1. List of the Requisite Information

In order to find out how many primary electron tracks traverse a nucleus at a tissue–dose of one rad, (and how many rads correspond with an average of one track per nucleus), we will need the pieces of information described below. Although the average number of tracks per nucleus, at one rad, comes from Item I (Eye) divided by Item J, we cannot skip the earlier items because each of them is required in order to obtain the value for Item Eye.

● -- (A) Definition of a rad (or centi–gray). A dose of 1 centi–gray (1 rad) of low–LET radiation is, by definition, the deposition of 10^{-5} joules, or 6.24×10^{10} KeV, per gram of tissue.

● -- (B) Average KeV per photon. We will consider photons from medical X–rays, radium–226 (and daughters), cesium–137, and A–bomb gamma rays.

● -- (C) Number of photons whose energy must be totally absorbed in one gram of tissue to produce a dose of one centi–gray (cGy).

● -- (D) Number and energy of the high–speed electrons produced per photon. The term "electron–packet" will be defined.

● -- (E) Distance across a typical human cell.

● -- (F) Distance traveled by each high–speed electron. Relationship to range (see Chapter 33, p.10).

● -- (G) Number of cells traversed by each electron in an electron– packet.

● -- (H) The total number of CELL–traversals made by all the primary electrons required to deliver a tissue–dose of 1 centi–gray to 1 gram. Photo–electrons and Compton electrons are both "primary" electrons, in contrast to secondary electrons produced along a primary electron track.

● -- (Eye) The total number of NUCLEAR–traversals made by all the primary electrons required to deliver a dose of 1 cGy to 1 gram of tissue.

● -- (J) The total number of cell–nuclei which are available to be traversed in a gram of tissue.

● -- (K) The average number of primary ionization tracks through each nucleus at a tissue–dose of 1 cGy (1 rad). This item is (Eye / J).

● -- (L) The tissue–dose when the average track–rate per nucleus = 1.0.

● -- (M) An "If...Then" table showing correspondences between tracks and various doses. When we have the rate of tracks per nucleus at 1 cGy, we can readily tabulate the average number of tracks per nucleus at any dose above or below 1 cGy, since the number of tracks is proportional to dose^1 for a specific

==

radiation source. In addition, we can start with an average of one track (or any other number of tracks) per nucleus, and calculate the tissue-dose associated with that number of tracks.

● -- (N) The Poisson distribution of tracks. When the average number of tracks per nucleus is 1.0, some nuclei will have no tracks at all, and some will have more than one track. We shall examine the distribution of tracks by using the Poisson equation. Readers have already seen (Chapter 18, Part 6) that, after the AVERAGE number of tracks per nucleus has been determined for a specified dose, the Poisson equation tells the probability of various numbers of tracks per nucleus.

2. Provision of the Input, the Calculations, and the Answer

We shall take up the topics in the alphabetical order above. Items F and G are handled together. Because Topics A, B, E, and J require no tables, the reader will find no Tables 20-A, 20-B, 20-E, or 20-J at the end.

● -- (A) Definition of a Rad or Centi-Gray (cGy) :
=======================================

One rad or cGy means 6.24 x 10^10 KeV of energy per gram of tissue.

● -- (B) Average KeV per Photon :
=======================================

This analysis will consider photons of four different energy regions.

(1) 30 KeV X-Rays :
These X-rays are the most likely ones to characterize the medical exposures in eight of the nine epidemiological studies summarized in Chapter 21 (and in Table 21-A). When peak kilovoltage across an X-ray tube is 90, the average energy per photon is about 30 KeV.

(2) Radium-226 and Its Daughters :
These gamma rays are the source of exposure in one of the nine studies in Table 21-A (the British Luminizers). The estimated energy per average photon is 596 KeV.

(3) Cesium-137 Gamma Rays :
Cesium-137 is the principal source of population-exposure from the Chernobyl nuclear power accident; the gamma ray is actually from barium-137m decaying to barium-137, and the estimated energy is 662 KeV per photon. Although Chernobyl is not part of our disproof of any safe dose or dose-rate, some readers may wish to know how cesium-137 compares with radium-226 and medical X-rays, so it is evaluated here for reference.

(4) Atomic-Bomb Gamma Rays at Hiroshima :
Radiation from the Hiroshima and Nagasaki atomic bombs included quite a mixture of energies. Since the study of A-bomb survivors is not one of our nine studies in Chapter 21, we need only a "ballpark" estimate of the KeV per average photon. I have done a very simplified estimate based on Hiroshima data in the DS86 system. The value we shall use is 1608 KeV per average photon. (See Chapter 32 for calculation of this value.)

From Photons to Primary Electrons :

In order to determine values for Item D below, we will have to take account of the three ways in which high-energy photons deliver energy to the molecules of cellular tissue.

PHOTO-ELECTRIC EFFECT. The photo-electric effect means that the photon disappears and a single electron is set into high-speed motion. The electron carries off all the energy of the photon minus a much smaller amount of energy required to lift the electron out of the atom (Par87, p.93). We will disregard the latter. The photo-electric effect is dominant for photon energies below about 40 KeV, in materials of low atomic number such as cellular tissue (Par87, p.93).

COMPTON EFFECT. In the Compton effect, which dominates at energies above those where the photo-electric effect dominates, only part of the energy of the photon is transferred to set an electron into high-speed motion, and the remainder of the energy is carried off by a new photon. This new photon, if its energy is sufficient, can then again participate in what is commonly called a Compton process: Setting an electron in motion and again creating a new photon of further reduced energy. Finally, when these reduced-energy photons have energies where the photo-electric effect dominates, the remaining energy is transferred in toto to an electron.

PAIR PRODUCTION. If the photon's energy is above 1.02 MeV, another type of interaction is possible, namely disappearance of the original photon, its energy being distributed as follows: 1.02 MeV is converted into two particles, an electron and a positron, and the remaining energy goes into energy of motion of the electron and the positron. Since photons cannot create the positron-electron pair at any energy below 1.02 MeV, pair production is irrelevant for the gamma rays of radium-226, cesium-137, and for the low energy X-rays, which are of major interest in this analysis. For part of our analysis, which deals with the gamma rays from A-bomb radiation where pair production is possible, we shall make the approximation of neglecting pair production in comparison with the other processes described above. Paretzke agrees that for gamma energies below 2 MeV, pair production can be neglected compared with the Compton process (Par87, p.95).

COHERENT SCATTERING. There is a fourth process of interaction of photons with tissue, known as coherent (Rayleigh) scattering. No energy is delivered to tissue, but the direction of the photon is changed. This process becomes prominent at energies below about 0.1 MeV. Because there is no energy transferred, we will not need to consider coherent scattering in our analyses.

● -- (C) Number of Photons Required
   to Deliver 1 Rad to 1 Gram :
==

In this analysis, we are not at all concerned with photons which pass right through a tissue without converting to high-speed electrons. Such photons contribute no dose to the tissue. We are concerned with the question: When a tissue receives a dose of one rad (one centi-gray), how many photons did convert to high-speed electrons in order to deliver that dose to a single gram of tissue?

The answer comes from dividing the energy-deposition required (Item A), by the average energy supplied by each photon (Item B). Table 20-C provides the answers for the four types of radiation which we are evaluating.

While we are considering large-area radiation with essentially total absorption of the energy of the initial photon (if it interacts at all), we have given attention to the implication for our results if some post-Compton photons are lost from tissue. See Chapter 33 for these considerations.

● -- (D) Electrons per Photon, and
   "Packets" Defined :
==

For the medical X-rays, the photo-electric effect is overwhelmingly dominant, so we are fully justified in stating that there will be one high-speed electron produced per 30-KeV photon, and that it carries all of the photon's energy (except for the very small binding

energy of the electron).

For the radium, cesium, and A-bomb gamma rays, no such simplification would be realistic because each photon produces several high-speed electrons of successively lower energy by Compton processes. We shall call the whole set, produced from a single photon, its "packet" of high-speed or primary electrons. Since each electron in a packet produces its own primary ionization track, we must take account of each electron.

The calculations are presented in Chapter 32; the results have been transferred forward into Table 20-D.

● -- (E) Distance across a
   Typical Human Cell, Cuboid Model :
==

The choice of appropriate cell-size is based on measurements from 38 electron micrographs of normal human cells (Elias78; Gar76; Ham85; Jo85). The mean nuclear diameter was 5.9 micrometers for 29 non-fetal human cells; 6.1 micrometers for 6 fetal cells; 5.7 micrometers for one non-fetal thyroid cell; 6.9 micrometers for one fetal thyroid cell; and 5.5 micrometers for one non-fetal breast cell.

To the weighted average of 5.9 micrometers, two corrections were made. Because it was impossible to know that the nuclei pictured were cut exactly through the maximum dimension, a factor of 1.1 increase was applied. Because it was possible that fixation of the tissue may have caused some shrinkage of cells, another factor of 1.1 increase was applied. With these corrections to the observations, the diameter of nuclei taken for this analysis is 7.1 micrometers -- as it was in Go86.

A very reasonable estimate, from examination of numerous histology texts, is that cell diameter is twice the nuclear diameter, or 14.2 micrometers.

With regard to our nuclear diameter of 7.1 micrometers, it is interesting to note that others are now using similar values for similar purposes. For instance, Brackenbush and Braby use a nuclear diameter of 7.0 micrometers. In a recent discussion of the microdosimetric basis for exposure limits, they state:

"Since most biological effects appear to be the consequence of the autonomous response of individual cells, the frequency and magnitude of the events in cells is pertinent. If we consider a 7 micrometer-diameter sphere as typical of a cell nucleus, we can estimate this frequency" (Brack88, p.252). Readers may note that Brack88 goes directly to the nucleus as the relevant site in the cell.

Goodhead (Good88, p.237) uses a value of 7.5 micrometers for the typical nuclear diameter. Neither Brack88 nor Good88 provides the basis for the value chosen.

Adjusted Values for a Cuboidal Model :

For simplification of this analysis, we are going to treat the cells and their nuclei as though they are cuboidal rather than spherical. This treatment will not result in any major changes in our expectations of cells traversed by tracks, and the mathematics are grossly simplified.

A spherical nucleus with a diameter of 7.1 micrometers has the same volume as a cuboidal nucleus of 5.7 micrometers per edge of the cube. A spherical cell with a diameter of 14.2 micrometers has the same volume as a cuboidal cell of 11.4 micrometers per edge.

For further simplification, we are going to treat the radiation source as one which is normal (perpendicular) to one face of the cuboidal cells. With the data for cuboidal cells and the approximation that all the photo-electrons and Compton electrons come in perpendicular to one face of all the cuboidal cells, we can proceed to the analysis of the tracks per cell and tracks per nucleus from the various radiations of interest.

● –– (F) Distance Traveled by
    Each High–Speed Electron (Range),
    and
● –– (G) Number of Cells Traversed by
    Each Electron in a Packet :
====================================

The derivation of the ranges for all primary electrons is shown in detail in Chapter 33. The answers from Chapter 33 have been brought forward here into Table 20-FG, as Item F.

Item G, the number of cells traversed by each electron, is obviously the electron's range in micrometers, divided by 11.4 micrometers (the depth of the cuboidal cell).

● –– (H) Total Cell–Traversals
    by Tracks Delivering 1 Rad to 1 Gram :
====================================

The next step is the determination of the total number of cell-traversals (by primary electrons) which occur when 1 rad is delivered to 1 gram of tissue. In Table 20-H, the total number of cell-traversals per rad of tissue-dose is presented for each type of radiation. This is, of course, the number of photons required to deliver one rad to one gram (Item C), times the total cells traversed by all the primary electrons produced by such photons (Item G, sum).

Total number of cell-traversals does not mean number of DIFFERENT cells traversed. Some cells experience multiple traversals.

As stated in Item C (text), our treatment is based on the approximation, which we consider reasonable for large-area irradiation, that for each original photon which undergoes the Compton process, all the energy of the post-Compton photon is also converted to electron energy by successive processes in the tissue.

● –– (Eye) Total Nuclear-Traversals
    by Tracks Delivering 1 Rad to 1 Gram :
==

In our model of the cuboidal cells and cuboidal nuclei, the area of one face of the nucleus is 1/4 of the area of the one face of the whole cell, since the edge length of the nucleus is 1/2 of that of the whole cell. Thus, for electrons normal to the cells, the nuclear area "seen" by the electrons is 1/4 of the cellular area "seen." Therefore the nuclear traversals are going to be the cellular traversals (Item H) times (0.25). These values are presented in Table 20-Eye.

Total number of nuclear-traversals does not mean number of DIFFERENT nuclei traversed. Some nuclei experience multiple traversals.

● –– (J) Number of Nuclei Available
    for Traversal in 1 Gram of Tissue :
==

We need to know how many nuclei are present and available for traversal, in one gram of tissue. Number of nuclei = number of cells. We will know the number of cells present in one gram of tissue if we divide (volume of one gram of cells) / (volume of a single cell).

Volume of One Gram of Cells: At an approximate density of 1.0 gram per cm^3, the volume of one gram of cells is 1.0 cm^3 (one cubic centimeter). And one cm^3 represents 10^12 micrometers^3 (one trillion cubic microns).

Volume of a Single Cell: For a cuboidal cell, 11.4 micrometers on an edge, the volume is (11.4 micrometers)^3, or 1481.544 micrometers^3.

==

So, number of nuclei per gram of cells = (10^12 / 1481.544) = 6.75E+08 nuclei per gram of cells, or about 675 million.

● -- (K) Average Number of Primary Tracks Traversing a Nucleus at 1 Rad :

======================================

We need only divide the total number of nuclear-traversals which are occurring (Item Eye), by the total number of nuclei which are available for traversal in a gram of tissue (Item J), in order to determine how many tracks are traversing each nucleus, on the average, at a tissue-dose of 1 rad (cGy). The results are provided in Table 20-K.

Comparison with Other Estimates: Is there a disparity between our estimates in Table 20-K, and estimates recently made by some other analysts? The short answer is, "no." What may seem like differences are reconciled in Chapter 33. It looks, perhaps, as if not everyone is taking the Compton process into account yet.

Variation in Tissues: When we did this type of analysis earlier (Go86), we had to ask ourselves a question which some readers may be asking themselves, too: "Are the values in Table 20-K valid even where the number of nuclei per gram might vary, due to the presence of connective tissue, nerves, interstitial fluid, and such things?" The short answer is, "yes."

The ratio (tracks per nucleus at 1 cGy or rad) would not be altered if there were fewer nuclei per gram of tissue, due to the presence of connective tissue, interstitial fluid, and so forth. Likewise, the ratio is not altered when cells which do not produce cancer -- such as nerve and muscle cells -- are part of the irradiated gram of tissue. The volume so occupied can be regarded as if it were all occupied by cells containing no relevant nuclei. For instance, if there are 25 % fewer nuclei in a gram, then Item J would become (0.75) x (nuclei present). Likewise, Item Eye would become (0.75) x (nuclear traversals). When Item Eye is divided by Item J, the effect cancels out, and the ratio of average tracks per nucleus remains the same.

● -- (L) Tissue-Dose When the Average Track-Rate per Nucleus Is One :

======================================

Because we know, from Table 20-K, the rate of nuclear tracks per rad, it follows that we also know the rate of rads per nuclear track. As a convenience, Table 20-L provides the computed values for each of the four types of radiation which we have examined.

● -- (M) "If ... Then" Table, Showing Corresondence between Tracks & Doses :

======================================

As a convenient reference, Table 20-L uses the basic ratios (of average tracks per nucleus) from Table 20-K to compute, "If the total tissue-dose is X, then the average number of tracks per nucleus is Y." And in reverse, "If the average number of tracks per nucleus is Y, then the tissue-dose is X."

Readers who compare the entries for 30 KeV X-rays, with the entries for A-bomb gamma rays, will notice that the A-bomb electron-tracks have to traverse about four-fold more nuclei in order to deliver the SAME amount of dose (for instance, 1 rad). In other words, electron-tracks from the medical X-rays deliver the same amount of energy in a shorter linear range. They pack the energy-transfers more densely, on the whole.

This observation is related to our warning, that the cancer-hazard from medical X-rays may be underestimated by the A-Bomb Study (Chapter 13, Part 4). It is widely thought that the biological menace of ionizing radiation (its RBE, or Relative Biological Effectiveness) rises with the density of its energy-depositions. Indeed, in Chapter 13, we cite estimates that the RBE of 250 kVp X-rays may be two, compared with high-energy gamma rays.

● -- (N) Poisson Distribution of Tracks

======================================

In an irradiated tissue, either a nucleus is "hit" by one or more tracks, or it is not hit at all.

When events occur independently of each other, as tracks do, we can use Poisson statistics to determine the chance of getting zero, 1, 2, 3, 4, 5, etc., events (tracks) per nucleus when we know that the AVERAGE is one track per nucleus -- or any other average. The equation which describes the distribution of probabilities is:

$$p(V) = \{EXP(-N)\} \times \{N^V / V!\}$$

Where:
   ● -- V is the number of tracks for which we want the probability calculated. (Compare Column A versus Column B in the tabulation.)
   ● -- p(V) is the probability of exactly "V" events occurring.
   ● -- N is the average number of events: Tracks per nucleus.

● -- V! is "V factorial," which means the product of all numbers starting with 1 and going up through "V" -- for all V greater than zero. For instance, for V = 5, V! = 1x2x3x4x5.

    ● -- An important reminder: 0! = 1, NOT zero.

    ● -- {EXP(-N)} means raising the value e (base of natural logarithms) to the power, (-N). The value of e is 2.718281828.

Exp(N) is a widely used device (perhaps not in all countries, however) which avoids superscripts when stating that the value "e" is raised to the power "N." Of course, Exp(-N) is the same as 1/Exp(N).

The tabulation illustrates the use of the Poisson equation to estimate the probability of getting zero events and getting 5 events when the average number of events is 1 track per nucleus. For simplicity of calculations, it is useful to set up a tabular format. The desired information, p(V), is in Column G. Readers will see that Column G = (Column C x Column F) -- in harmony with the original equation with which we started.

```
========================================================
Col.   Col.   Col.   Col.  Col.  Col.     Col.
A      B      C      D     E     F        G

       V =                               p(V) =
       Number of                         Probability
N =    Tracks for                        of
Avg.   Which the                         Exactly
Number Probability                       V
of     Is Desired                        Tracks
Tracks

N      V      EXP(-N) N^V   V!    N^V/V!   p(V)
-------------------------------------------------------
1.00   0      0.367879 1    1     1        0.367879
1.00   5      0.367879 1    120   0.008333 0.003065
========================================================
```

The entries in Column D are the value of N raised to the power, V. Thus, 1^0 = 1, and 1^5 = 1 also.

The entries in Column E are V!. Thus, 0! = 1, and 5! = 1x2x3x4x5 = 120.

We can use the equation to construct tables, like the three in Table 20-N. Each line, of each table, requires one use of the equation. Of course, the equation can be set up on a computer, with the entire calculation done in one step.

3. The Fallacy of Slow Delivery of Very Low Doses

The previous chapter made it clear why the Least Possible Disturbance to a single nucleus is traversal by one primary electron-track. However, there is no tissue-dose at which disturbance occurs UNIFORMLY in cell-nuclei. The top section of Table 20-N has used the Poisson equation to find out what the actual distribution of tracks per nucleus is, when the AVERAGE frequency from a tissue-dose is one track per nucleus.

It turns out (Table 20-N) that, at a tissue-dose where the average track-frequency is one per nucleus, only 26.4 % of the nuclei in the exposed tissue "feel" more than the Least Possible Disturbance (one track). The distribution is:

```
36.8 % of the nuclei receive no track at all.
36.8 % of the nuclei receive exactly one track.
26.4 % of the nuclei receive two or more tracks.
-------
100.0 %
```

In other words, for many purposes, it would be reasonable to regard an acute tissue-dose which delivers one primary electron per nucleus, on the average, as the lowest conceivable dose and dose-rate AT THE LEVEL OF THE NUCLEUS. What is that dose? Both Tables 20-L and 20-M provide the information, for the four types of radiation examined in this chapter.

Of course, the average number of tracks is directly proportional to dose (Items C and D). As dose falls below the level where 1.0 is the average number of tracks per nucleus, the track-average falls accordingly. With each change in the average, the distribution of tracks has to be newly calculated with the Poisson equation. The mid-section of Table 20-N shows the distribution for tissue-doses where the average is 0.05 track per nucleus:

```
95.1 % of the nuclei receive no track at all.
 4.8 % of the nuclei receive exactly one track.
 0.1 % of the nuclei receive two or more tracks.
-------
100.0 %
```

Correct Perception of Dose-Rate :

The two lists of percentages above can help improve the perception of dose-RATE. We will use 30 KeV X-rays to illustrate what is, and is not, meant by "a

==

lower dose-rate."

We will compare the dose-rate of 0.7475 rad per exposure with the dose-rate of 0.0374 rad per exposure. These tissue-doses are chosen because 0.7475 rad (747.5 millirads) corresponds with an average of 1.0 primary track per nucleus (Table 20-L), and because we want, for comparison, a dose which gives an average of only 0.05 track per nucleus -- which will be a dose 20-fold lower than 0.7475 rad (tracks are proportional to dose) :

(0.7475 rad / nuclear track) x (0.05 track) = 0.0374 rad.

When the track-average = 0.05 , we can see from the percentages above that 95 % of the nuclei are completely escaping irradiation even though the tissue-dose is 0.0374 rad (37.4 millirads) per exposure.

Now let us consider the particular nuclei which do get hit by one or two tracks at the tissue-dose of 37.4 millirads. Each nucleus which is traversed receives the entire energy-transfer in a tiny fraction of a second (Chapter 19).

There is no slower transfer of the energy.

These nuclei feel just as much damage as the nuclei which receive one or two tracks at the higher tissue-dose of 0.7475 rads (747.5 millirads). For the nuclei which are hit, the 20-fold reduction in tissue-dose makes no difference. None at all.

Brackenbush and Braby (Brack88, p.252) make a similar point in a discussion of neutrons. We quote: "For a neutron exposure of 3 mGy (30 mSv), only 1.5% of the cell nuclei in the irradiated tissue receive any damage, but they get the same amount as cells exposed to 200 mGy in a dose-response study."

In our comparison of 37.4 versus 747.5 millirads from the 30 KeV X-rays, in spite of the 20-fold reduction in dose-rate (tissue-dose per exposure), 99.9 % of the nuclei exposed at the lower rate have EXACTLY the same experience as most of the nuclei exposed at the higher dose-rate -- namely, either 1.0 track or no track. The only difference between 747.5 millirads per exposure, and 37.4 millirads per exposure, is the FRACTION of nuclei which experiences two tracks or more.

Further reduction of the dose-rate can only reduce the fraction -- a point now widely recognized (see, for instance, Fein88, p.27). Suppose the 37.4 millirads were delivered evenly over a year. We can regard this as 365

exposures, with each daily exposure about 0.1 millirad. Of course, the same number of primary electron tracks are required to deliver the total dose of 37.4 millirads, regardless of delivery-rate. However, we have just reduced the average frequency of tracks PER EXPOSURE by a factor of 365. If the Poisson equation were applied to this reduced AVERAGE, it would show the number of nuclei which ever experience two tracks simultaneously to be tiny, indeed.

Slow Delivery and the Repair-System :

In the region of very low doses, the change in this fraction is the only meaning of "lower dose-rate." Is there any biological meaning to changing this fraction? Let us consider the repair-system. The challenge on the repair-system, within a nucleus, can be reduced for a very few nuclei from two simultaneous tracks to one track, and for the overwhelming percentage of nuclei, the challenge to the repair system cannot be reduced by a lower dose-rate at all. Not at all.

Barendsen, commenting on a report of Hill, Han, and Elkind (Hi84), has also felt compelled to point this out: "Before analysing the interpretations of the dose rate effect suggested by the authors, it should be pointed out that at extremely low doses no difference can possibly exist between high and low dose rates, because at doses where the probability of more than one ionizing particle passing through a cell nucleus is vanishingly small, effects can only be caused by single particle tracks. The concept of dose rate loses its meaning at these very low doses because it depends only on the time in which a single particle traverses a cell" (Bar85).

Table 20-C
Photons Required to Deliver a Dose of 1 Centi-Gray (1 Rad) to 1 Gram of Tissue.

(Item A): 6.24 x 10^10 KeV required to deliver 1 centi-gray (cGy) to 1 gram of tissue.

PHOTON SOURCE	Item B INITIAL PHOTON ENERGY	(Item A / Item B) ENERGY REQUIRED, DIVIDED BY PHOTON ENERGY	Item C NUMBER of PHOTONS REQUIRED TO DELIVER 1 RAD TO 1 GRAM
Medical X-rays	30 KeV	6.24 x 10^10 / 30	2.08E+09 or 2.08 x 10^9 photons or 2.08 billion photons or 2,080,000,000 photons
Radium-226 and daughters	596 KeV	6.24 x 10^10 / 596	1.05E+08 or 1.05 x 10^8 photons or 105 million photons or 105,000,000 photons
Cesium-137	662 KeV	6.24 x 10^10 / 662	9.43E+07 or 9.43 x 10^7 photons or 94.3 million photons or 94,300,000 photons
A-Bomb Gammas	1608 KeV	6.24 x 10^10 / 1608	3.88E+07 or 3.88 x 10^7 photons or 38.8 million photons or 38,800,000 photons

NOTES -----

Item C is the number of photons whose energy must be totally absorbed in one gram of tissue to produce a tissue-dose of one centi-gray (one rad) in that gram.

For readers who are not yet familiar with the exponential format for numbers, we have used the space available in this table to express these rather large numbers in additional ways.

There are no Tables 20-A,B,E, or J. See text, Part 2.

Table 20-D
Energies of Electrons in the "Packets" Associated with Various Photons.

Data are brought forward from Tables 32–A, 32–B, and 32–C.
(Energies are given in both KeV and MeV)

PHOTON SOURCE	TYPE OF ELECTRON	Item D ELECTRON ENERGY (Kev)	ELECTRON ENERGY (MeV)
30 KeV Photons Medical X-rays			
	Photo-electron	30	0.030
596 KeV Photons Radium-226 and daughters			
	Compton	208.583	0.2086
	Compton	116.728	0.1167
	Compton	69.626	0.0696
	Compton	44.273	0.0443
	Compton	29.813	0.0298
	Compton	21.078	0.0211
	Compton	15.516	0.0155
	Photo-electron	90.384	0.0904
662 KeV Photons Cesium-137			
	Compton	238.825	0.2388
	Compton	131.931	0.1319
	Compton	77.571	0.0776
	Compton	48.656	0.0487
	Compton	32.377	0.0324
	Compton	22.663	0.0227
	Compton	16.546	0.0165
	Photo-electron	93.429	0.0934
1608 KeV Photons A-Bomb Gammas			
	Compton	693.765	0.6938
	Compton	357.271	0.3573
	Compton	190.906	0.1909
	Compton	107.792	0.1078
	Compton	64.914	0.0649
	Compton	41.645	0.0416
	Compton	28.259	0.0283
	Compton	20.107	0.0201
	Compton	14.880	0.0149
	Photo-electron	88.460	0.0885

These tabulations are based on the assumption that all of the energy of the
original photon is absorbed in the tissue, for those photons which interact
at all with the tissue. See text (C) and (D).

Table 20-FG
Ranges and Cell-Traversals for Various Primary Electrons. (Micrometer = Micron.)

PHOTON SOURCE	Item D ELECTRON ENERGY (KeV)	Item F ELECTRON RANGE (microns)	Item E CUBOIDAL CELL DEPTH (microns)	Item G NUMBER OF CELLS TRAVERSED	Item G (sum) CELLS TRAVERSED PER ELECTRON, OR PER ELECTRON-PACKET
30 KeV Photons Medical X-rays	30	19.779	11.4	1.735	1.735
596 KeV Photons Radium-226 + daughters	208.582	462.635	11.4	40.582	
	116.727	150.107	11.4	13.167	
	69.626	73.866	11.4	6.479	
	44.273	38.353	11.4	3.364	
	29.813	19.543	11.4	1.714	
	21.078	8.687	11.4	0.762	
	15.516	1.975	11.4	0.173	
	90.384	105.343	11.4	9.241	
				Sum =	75.483
662 KeV Photons Cesium-137	238.825	566.577	11.4	49.700	
	131.931	185.777	11.4	16.296	
	77.571	85.659	11.4	7.514	
	48.656	44.262	11.4	3.883	
	32.377	22.802	11.4	2.000	
	22.663	10.629	11.4	0.932	
	16.546	3.206	11.4	0.281	
	93.429	110.143	11.4	9.662	
				Sum =	90.268
1608 KeV Photons A-Bomb Gammas	693.765	2517.482	11.4	220.832	
	357.271	1031.762	11.4	90.505	
	190.906	384.423	11.4	33.721	
	107.792	132.116	11.4	11.589	
	64.914	67.022	11.4	5.879	
	41.645	34.857	11.4	3.058	
	28.259	17.583	11.4	1.542	
	20.107	7.504	11.4	0.658	
	14.880	1.217	11.4	0.107	
	88.460	102.335	11.4	8.977	
				Sum =	376.869

Item D entries come from Table 20-D.

Item F entries are brought forward from Chapter 33. For 30 KeV photons, there are only photo-electrons, all of the same energy. For all other classes, all entries except the lowest row are for Compton electrons. The lowest row is for photo-electrons.

Item E entry, depth of a cuboidal cell, is from the text. Micron = Micrometer.

Item G entries, number of cell-traversals per electron, are calculated:
(Range of the Electron / Depth of Cell), or (Item F / Item E).

Table 20–H
Total Cell–Traversals for 1 Rad (cGy) of Dose Delivered to 1 Gram of Cellular Tissue.

	Item C	Item G (sum)	Item H	
Origin of Electron Packets	Packets Required to Deliver One Rad (cGy)	Cell-Traversals by Electrons of a Single Packet	Total Cell-Traversals in Delivery of 1 Rad to 1 Gram	
30 KeV X-Rays	2.08E+09	1.735	3.61E+09	or 3.61 billion
596 KeV gammas Source: Radium-226	1.05E+08	75.483	7.93E+09	or 7.93 billion
662 KeV gammas Source: Cesium-137	9.43E+07	90.268	8.51E+09	or 8.51 billion
1608 KeV gammas Source: A-bomb	3.88E+07	376.869	1.46E+10	or 14.6 billion

Item C entries are from Table 20-C.
Item G entries are from Table 20-FG.
Item H entries are calculated: (Packets x Cell-Traversals per Packet), or (Item C x Item G, sum).
"Cell-traversals" does NOT mean separate cells traversed. Some cells experience multiple traversals.

Table 20–(Eye)
Total Nuclear–Traversals for 1 Rad (cGy) of Dose Delivered to 1 Gram of Cellular Tissue.

	Item H	Item I (Eye)	
Origin of Electron Packets	Total Cell Traversals in Delivery of One cGy (Rad)	Total Nuclear-Traversals by Primary Tracks in Delivery of 1 cGy (Rad) to 1 Gram	
30 KeV X-Rays	3.61E+09	9.03E+08	or 903 million
596 KeV gammas Source: Radium-226	7.93E+09	1.98E+09	or 1.98 billion
662 KeV gammas Source: Cesium-137	8.51E+09	2.13E+09	or 2.13 billion
1608 KeV gammas Source: A-bomb	1.46E+10	3.65E+09	or 3.65 billion

Item I (Eye) entries are (Item H) x (0.25). This follows from the model in which cells and
cell-nuclei are cuboidal, and electrons come in normal to one face. See text, parts (E) and (I, or Eye).

Table 20-K
Average Number of Primary Electron Tracks per Nucleus at a Dose of 1 Rad (1 cGy).

ORIGIN OF ELECTRON PACKETS	Item I (Eye) TOTAL NUCLEAR-TRAVERSALS FOR DELIVERY OF 1 cGy	Item J NUMBER OF NUCLEI PER GRAM OF TISSUE	Item K AVERAGE NUMBER OF NUCLEAR TRAVERSALS PER NUCLEUS, AT A TISSUE-DOSE OF 1 cGy
30 KeV X-rays	9.03E+08	6.75E+08	1.3378
596 KeV gammas Source: Radium-226	1.98E+09	6.75E+08	2.9370
662 KeV gammas Source: Cesium-137	2.13E+09	6.75E+08	3.1556
1608 KeV gammas Source: A-bomb	3.65E+09	6.75E+08	5.4074

Item J entry comes from the text, part (J).

Item K entries are calculated: (Total nuclear-traversals / number of nuclei available to be traversed), or (Item I / Item J). The "average number of nuclear traversals per nucleus at 1 rad" is the same as "average number of primary ionization tracks per nucleus at one rad."

It will be exceedingly rare for a nucleus to be traversed by two high-speed electrons originating from the SAME initial photon. Each time the Compton process occurs, it creates only one high speed electron plus a new photon of reduced energy. The new photon, traveling at the speed of light, is in a different location when the next Compton electron is produced.

Table 20-L
Tissue-Dose in Centi-Gray When the Average Track-Rate per Nucleus Is ONE.

ORIGIN OF ELECTRON PACKETS	Item K AVERAGE NUCLEAR-TRAVERSALS PER NUCLEUS IN DELIVERY OF 1 cGy (1 RAD) [Tracks / Nucleus / cGy]	Item L DOSE IN CENTI-GRAY WHEN AVERAGE TRACK-RATE PER NUCLEUS IS ONE [cGy / Track / Nucleus]
30 KeV X-rays	1.3378	0.7475 cGy, or 747.5 millirads
596 KeV gammas Source: Radium-226	2.937	0.3405 cGy, or 340.5 millirads
662 KeV gammas Source: Cesium-137	3.156	0.3169 cGy, or 316.9 millirads
1608 KeV gammas Source: A-bomb	5.4074	0.18493 cGy, or 184.9 millirads

Item L entries are calculated: (1 / Item K).

Table 20-M
"If ... Then" : Relationship between Tissue-Doses and Average Tracks per Nucleus.
Tracks refer to primary ionization tracks, or primary electron tracks.

For 30 KeV X-Rays

If Total Tissue-Dose Is This (in Rads) (or cGy)	Then the Average Number of Tracks / Nucleus Is	If Average Number of Tracks / Nucleus Is	Then the Tissue-Dose in Rads (or cGy) Is
0.001	0.0013	1	0.7475
0.010	0.0134	2	1.4950
0.050	0.0669	3	2.2425
0.100	0.1338	4	2.9900
0.500	0.6689	5	3.7375
0.7475	1.0000	6	4.4850
1.000	1.3378	7	5.2325
5.000	6.6890	8	5.9800
10.000	13.3779	9	6.7275
50.000	66.8896	10	7.4750
100.000	133.7793	20	14.9500
200.000	267.5585	50	37.3750
		100	74.7500

For 596 KeV Gamma Rays (Ra-226)

If Total Tissue-Dose Is This (in Rads) (or cGy)	Then the Average Number of Tracks / Nucleus Is	If Average Number of Tracks / Nucleus Is	Then the Tissue-Dose in Rads (or cGy) Is
0.001	0.0029	1	0.3405
0.010	0.0294	2	0.6810
0.050	0.1468	3	1.0215
0.100	0.2937	4	1.3620
0.3405	1.0000	5	1.7025
0.500	1.4684	6	2.0430
1.000	2.9370	7	2.3835
5.000	14.6843	8	2.7240
10.000	29.3686	9	3.0645
50.000	146.8429	10	3.4050
100.000	293.6858	20	6.8100
200.000	587.3715	50	17.0250
		100	34.0500

For 662 KeV Gamma Rays (Cs-137)

If Total Tissue-Dose Is This (in Rads) (or cGy)	Then the Average Number of Tracks / Nucleus Is	If Average Number of Tracks / Nucleus Is	Then the Tissue-Dose in Rads (or cGy) Is
0.001	0.0032	1	0.3169
0.010	0.0316	2	0.6338
0.050	0.1578	3	0.9507
0.100	0.3156	4	1.2676
0.3169	1.0000	5	1.5845
0.500	1.5778	6	1.9014
1.000	3.1556	7	2.2183
5.000	15.7778	8	2.5352
10.000	31.5557	9	2.8521
50.000	157.7785	10	3.1690
100.000	315.5570	20	6.3380
200.000	631.1139	50	15.8450
		100	31.6900

For 1608 KeV Gamma Rays (A-Bomb)

If Total Tissue-Dose Is This (in Rads) (or cGy)	Then the Average Number of Tracks / Nucleus Is	If Average Number of Tracks / Nucleus Is	Then the Tissue-Dose in Rads (or cGy) Is
0.001	0.0054	1	0.1849
0.010	0.0541	2	0.3698
0.050	0.2704	3	0.5547
0.100	0.5407	4	0.7396
0.1849	1.0000	5	0.9245
0.500	2.7042	6	1.1094
1.000	5.4074	7	1.2943
5.000	27.0416	8	1.4792
10.000	54.0833	9	1.6641
50.000	270.4164	10	1.8490
100.000	540.8329	20	3.6980
200.000	1081.666	50	9.2450
		100	18.4900

Table 20-N
Poisson Distribution of Events (Nuclear Tracks). Equation Is in the Text, Part (N).
Event means a primary ionization track somewhere through a cell–nucleus.

Probability (or Chance) of Exactly V Primary Tracks per Nucleus When Average Number of Tracks (N) Equals 1.0

Mean number of tracks = 1.0 track per nucleus.
Question: How many nuclei will receive exactly 0, 1, 2, 3, 4, 5, etc. tracks?

==

0.367879	chance of zero events	if average = 1.0
0.367879	chance of 1 event	if average = 1.0
0.183940	chance of 2 events	if average = 1.0
0.061313	chance of 3 events	if average = 1.0
0.015328	chance of 4 events	if average = 1.0
0.003066	chance of 5 events	if average = 1.0
0.000511	chance of 6 events	if average = 1.0
0.000073	chance of 7 events	if average = 1.0
0.000009	chance of 8 events	if average = 1.0
0.000001	chance of 9 events	if average = 1.0

The sum of probabilities must add up to 1.0000. By the time we reach 9 events per nucleus, the sum is exceedingly close to 1.0000: Sum of probabilities of zero or more events = 0.999999

Sum of probabilities of 2 or more events when average is one: 0.264241 (26.4 per 100 nuclei).

Probability (or Chance) of Exactly V Primary Tracks per Nucleus When Average Number of Tracks (N) Equals 0.05

Mean number of tracks = 0.05 track per nucleus.
Question: How many nuclei will receive exactly 0, 1, 2, 3, etc. tracks?

Probability of zero track	=	0.951229
Probability of exactly 1 track	=	0.047561
Probability of exactly 2 tracks	=	0.001189
Probability of 3 or more tracks	=	0.000021

Probability (or Chance) of Exactly V Primary Tracks per Nucleus When Average Number of Tracks (N) Equals 0.02937

Mean number of tracks = 0.02937 track per nucleus.
Question: How many nuclei will receive exactly 0, 1, 2, 3, etc. tracks?

Probability of zero track	=	0.971057	(97.1 percent)
Probability of exactly 1 track	=	0.028519	(2.85 percent)
Probability of exactly 2 tracks	=	0.000418	(418 per million nuclei)
Probability of exactly 3 tracks	=	0.000004	(4 per million nuclei)
Probability of exactly 4 tracks	=	3.01E-08	(3 per 100 million nuclei)
Probability of exactly 5 tracks	=	1.77E-10	(2 per 10 billion nuclei)

In Chapter 21, tables also provide Poisson distributions when average is 0.2937 and 0.6689 track.

Table 20-"O"
83.3 and 100 KeV Photo-Electrons :
Estimated Number of Primary Electron Tracks per Nucleus, at a Dose of 1 Rad (cGy).

Experimental irradiation of cells in the laboratory often involves X-irradiation from a 250 kilovolt machine -- which means that the average energy of the photons in the resulting X-ray beam is about one-third of the maximum 250 KeV. So the average photon energy is about 83.3 KeV.

We have used the approximation that, at 100 KeV or less, the photon's energy is transferred entirely to a single photo-electron, although the Compton process will occur sometimes too (Chapter 32 text, and Table 32-A, Note 6).

In this table, we will derive an estimate of the average number of tracks per cell-nucleus, at a dose of one rad (cGy) delivered by 83.3 KeV photo-electrons. We include the corresponding estimate for 100 KeV photo-electrons too.

===

Photons Required to Deliver a Dose of 1 Rad (6.24 x 10^10 KeV) to 1 Gram of Tissue (Item C) :
Number of photons required = (Total energy needed) / (Energy per photon).

Total energy needed	Energy per photon	Photons required for 1 rad to one gram.
6.24 x 10^10 KeV	83.3 KeV	7.49E+08 photons, which all become electrons.
6.24 x 10^10 KeV	100 KeV	6.24E+08 photons, which all become electrons.

===

Estimated Range of 83.3 KeV Photo-Electrons (Item F) :
In Table 20-FG, we have two values between which we can interpolate:

	Energy (KeV)	Range (microns)
Cs-137	77.571	85.659
Cs-137	93.429	110.143
Difference	15.858	24.484

But we are going from 77.571 to 83.3, or 5.429 KeV.
So we pick up (5.429 / 15.858) of the difference: (5.429 / 15.858) x (24.484) microns,
    which is 8.38212 microns.
Total range for 83.3 KeV photo-electrons = 85.659 microns + 8.382 microns = 94.041 microns.

Estimated Range of 100 KeV Photo-ElectronsS (Item F) :
In Table 20-FG, we have two values between which we can interpolate:

	Energy (KeV)	Range (microns)
Cs-137	93.429	110.143
A-bomb	107.792	132.116
Difference	14.363	21.973

But we are going from 93.429 to 100, or 6.571 KeV.
So we pick up (6.571 / 14.363) of the difference: (6.571 / 14.363) x (21.973) microns,
    which is 10.05253 microns.
Total range for 100 KeV photo-electrons = 110.143 microns + 10.053 microns = 120.196 microns.

===

Total Cell Traversals in Delivery of 1 Rad to 1 Gram (Item H) :
Cell traversals per electron = (Range per electron in microns) / (11.4 microns per cell -- Item E).
Total cell traversals = (Cell traverals per electron) x (Number of electrons required for 1 rad).

Photo-electrons	Cell traversals per electron	Total cell traversals (Item H):
83.3 KeV	94.041 / 11.4 = 8.249	8.249 x 7.49E+08 = 6.18E+09
100 KeV	120.196 / 11.4 = 10.544	10.544 x 6.24E+08 = 6.58E+09

===

Estimated Number of Primary Electron Tracks per Nucleus, at a Dose of 1 Rad (cGy).
Total nuclear traversals in delivery of 1 rad = (Total cell traversals) x (0.25; see Table 20-Eye).
Tracks = (Total nuclear traversals) / (Number of nuclei available, or 6.75E+08 nuclei per gram).

Photo-electrons	Total nuclear traversals	Nuclear traversals / nuclei available
83.3 KeV	(0.25 x 6.18E+09) = 1.54E+09	(1.54E+09 / 6.75E+08) = 2.28 tracks
100 KeV	(0.25 x 6.58E+09) = 1.64E+09	(1.64E+09 / 6.75E+08) = 2.43 tracks

20-empty, after tables.
==

Decisive Epidemiological Evidence from Humans

This chapter is arranged in three parts:

Then tables.

1. The Nine Human Epidemiological Studies Used in Chapter 18

Our earlier presentation of the case against existence of any threshold, for induction of human cancer by ionizing radiation (Go86), included five studies of cancer-induction at very low doses or dose-rates. This expanded analysis considers a total of nine human epidemiological investigations, generally recognized to be well done and valid, which show radiation-induction of cancer at very low doses and dose-rates. Readers are acquainted only with the "bottom line" of these studies, from Chapter 18. Below, we describe the nature of each study.

It is the coupling of these critical studies at very low radiation doses and dose-rates, with the information from Chapter 20 concerning the frequency of radiation tracks in cell-nuclei, which makes it possible to refute speculation that there is a safe dose or dose-rate with respect to induction of human cancer. (See Chapter 18.)

● -- Study 1, Nova Scotia Fluoroscopy Study :

====================================

In the Nova Scotia Fluoroscopy Study, Myrden and Hiltz (My69) studied 243 women who (in the course of tuberculosis treatment) had chest fluoroscopies with the beam traveling from front to back. According to Boice et al, "... all the Nova Scotia women faced the X-ray tube during the fluoroscopy examination ..." (Boice78, p.389).

The estimated absorbed breast-dose was 7.5 rads per fluoroscopy (Beir80, p.276). Time between fluoroscopies was days or weeks. The total breast-dose accumulated per woman was about 1,221 rads when the pneumothorax therapy was bilateral, and about 741 rads when it was unilateral. The average breast-dose in this series of women was about 850 rads

(Go81, pp.242-243).

Breast-cancer was observed at more than six times the expected rate during a limited follow-up period (My69; Boice78, p.388, Table 11).

The Implication of Serial Doses :

Here at the outset, we will briefly review the explanation in Chapter 18 of why a study with such a high total dose is appropriately included in a series of low-dose, low-dose-rate epidemiological studies.

Whenever there is any dose at all, some cell-nuclei are being traversed by tracks.

Every track, acting alone, has a chance of inducing fully competent carcinogenic lesions.

It follows that there can never be any safe dose or dose-rate ... unless every carcinogenic alteration is successfully and invariably "un-done" by repair processes, whenever exposures are sufficiently low and slow.

"Sufficiently low and slow" refers not to the TOTAL dose of radiation accumulated, but rather, to the dose per exposure and the time between exposures. If there were some low dose whose carcinogenic damage could always be flawlessly un-done within a certain time-interval, then people could receive such a dose once every interval, SAFELY, because they would never have any cancer-risk left from the previous exposure when they received the subsequent exposure. If this were true, the TOTAL dose would not be of any importance, and people would be able to accumulate HUGE doses without any cancer-risk at all, if the huge doses were delivered by a series of small doses -- each of which were safe.

Although the Nova Scotia Fluoroscopy Study looks as if it were a high-dose study, it is able to reveal whether or not a low dose -- 7.5 rads -- is safe, when accompanied by ample time for repair to do everything of which repair is capable. In Chapter 18, it was shown that repair certainly has ample opportunity to do the best it can, in periods of well under 24 hours, likely under 12 hours. In the Nova Scotia Fluoroscopy Study, the radiation doses were far more widely separated, by periods of days or more. Hence, there can be no question that the repair-systems had every possible opportunity to perform flawless repair -- if that is indeed possible.

If carcinogenic injury was produced in the irradiated women at their first fluoroscopy exposure-session, but if repair-systems were able to perform flawless repair afterwards, then that particular exposure-session would have left no residual harm, in terms of any increased risk of future breast-cancer.

Similar carcinogenic injury inflicted at EVERY subsequent fluoroscopy session would also have been without residual harm, if a flawless repair-system operated at a total dose per exposure-session of 7.5 rads. And thus, after accumulating 850 rads in this fashion, the irradiated women would have had NO radiation-induced breast-cancer.

The Dose-Entry in Table 21-A :
The Nova Scotia Fluoroscopy Study by itself is an important test of whether or not it is reasonable even to consider flawless repair as a hypothesis. Readers are reminded that 7.5 rads from 30 KeV X-rays is a tissue-dose which corresponds with an average of only about 10 primary ionization tracks per nucleus (Table 21-A).

The Nova Scotia Study is certainly not a high-dose study; at every critical step along the way, it is a test of how perfectly the repair-system can un-do carcinogenic injury produced by 7.5 rads, or 10 nuclear tracks on the average -- a LOW dose and dose-rate.

The test supplies strong evidence that the flawless-repair hypothesis fails -- at least for single doses of 7.5 rads, or an average track-rate of only 10 tracks per nucleus. A greater than six-fold increase in the breast-cancer rate, among those women who were in the exposed group, is far from a small increase. It is large and definitive.

In this study, carcinogenic damage -- inflicted by the individual low-dose exposure-sessions -- accumulated in the women from each exposure, by unrepaired, unrepairable, or misrepaired injury. This is not the behavior of a flawless repair-system for low radiation doses.

● -- Study 2, Israeli Scalp-Irradiation Study (Thyroid-Cancer Endpoint) :

In the Israeli Scalp-Irradiation Study, Modan and co-workers (Modan77) reported on the excess of thyroid-cancers observed among over 10,000 children in Israel who received X-irradiation for ringworm of the scalp. The estimated thyroid dose per child was 7.5 rads, total.

Thyroid-cancer was observed at five times the expected rate during a limited follow-up period.

In a later publication (Modan89), the dose was stated to have been 9 rads, rather than the 7.5 rads reported earlier. Also, the thyroid-cancer rate was given as four times that of the children who were not irradiated. Neither of the changes materially alters the study for our present considerations. The control group in this study appears to be carefully matched by age, sex, and demographics, and a second control group of unirradiated siblings is also part of the study (Un86, p.228, Para.388).

This is totally a low-dose study, since there was only a single exposure, from a dose of 7.5 or 9 rads to the thyroid gland.

This study by itself is another crucial test of the hypothesis that the repair system, given sufficient time to operate, will flawlessly un-do carcinogenic injury from low-dose radiation injury (in this case, a total dose of 7.5 to 9.0 rads). The hypothetical flawless repair-system failed the test, and a four-fold increase in the incidence of thyroid-cancer was the result -- surely the result of unrepaired, unrepairable, or misrepaired injury -- even at a dose-level corresponding with only 10 or 12 primary ionization tracks per nucleus, on the average (Table 21-A).

Modan on the Pituitary Dose :
In their most recent follow-up study (Modan89), Modan and co-workers mention that one might wish to consider the possibility that radiation delivered to the pituitary, in the course of scalp-irradiation, might have been an indirect basis for the development of thyroid-cancer, perhaps in addition to the direct effect of radiation on the thyroid. The authors stated that the dose to the pituitary was between 4.8 and 6.6 rads.

Modan's suggestion, if accepted, would not be helpful to a safe-dose proposition. The suggestion implies that a few primary ionization tracks per cell-nucleus in the pituitary gland may contribute to a multi-fold increase in cancer at sites affected by pituitary hormones (and such sites are numerous).

However, we wonder if Modan et al may have erroneously stated the pituitary dose in Modan89, because in UNSCEAR 1986 (p.228, para.391), the pituitary dose is referred to as perhaps of the order of 50 rads (not 5). Modan et al will surely address this question of which pituitary dose is correct.

UNSCEAR 1986, citing the work of Lee et al (Lee82) with rats, comments: "The role of pituitary irradiation in the induction of thyroid cancer was ... explored by delivering doses of 4.1 Gy of x rays to the pituitary alone, or to the thyroid and the pituitary together: findings were negative in this respect" (Un86, p.208, para.253). Un86 is not commenting in para.253 specifically on the Modan Study.

● -- Study 3,
   Massachusetts Fluoroscopy Study :
=====================================

In the Massachusetts Fluoroscopy Study, Boice and Monson (Boice77) also studied women who had received repeated chest fluoroscopy during tuberculosis treatment (see STUDY 1).

In the Massachusetts series, the beam was usually from back to front. Boice and co-workers make the approximation that in 75 % of the exams, patients had their backs to the X-ray tube, and in 25 % of exams, patients were facing the tube (Boice78, Table 10). Overall, the estimated average absorbed breast-dose per single exam was 1.5 rads (Boice77; Boice 78, p.385).

The accumulated breast-dose was about 150 rems, total. Among the women whose average age was 20 years at the time of irradiation, breast-cancer was observed at more than twice the expected rate during a limited follow-up period. "For the exposed women, the onset of the period of risk for breast cancer development was assumed to be the date of the first fluoroscopic examination, and, for the non-irradiated controls, the date of admission to the sanitorium" (Un86, p.225, para.370).

What was stated above concerning STUDY 1, the Nova Scotia Fluoroscopy Study, applies here too. This is another study of repeated, or serial, low-dose exposures separated by sufficient time for repair to un-do whatever carcinogenic injuries it was ever capable of un-doing. The Massachusetts series is another test of the speculation that the repair-system may operate flawlessly for low-dose damage. And the

study represents another failure for perfect repair.

The Dose-Entry in Table 21-A :
Just HOW low was the dose, in the terms which matter -- namely, average number of tracks per nucleus, per exam?

In this study, unlike the Nova Scotia Study, the answer is not self-evident. For diagnostic X-rays, tracks per nucleus at one rad are about 1.3378 (from Table 20-K), so tracks per nucleus from 1.5 rad would be 2.0067 tracks on the average. But (unlike Go86), we have decided that two tracks would not be the appropriate track-rate to use under the conditions described above.

In this chapter, we are investigating the hypothesis of perfect repair. We start with the premise that, for a given type of radiation, injury per cell-nucleus is proportional to the number of primary ionization tracks which traverse ("disturb") the nucleus. This premise is explained by the nature of the interaction of ionizing radiation with living tissue (Chapter 19). For a given type of radiation, the number of tracks is an index of the strain on the repair-system.

If we want a realistic measure of strain, we have to take account of the fact that there is a substantial difference in breast-dose caused by orientation with respect to the X-ray beam. For instance, in Go85 at p.404, we estimate that the absorbed breast dose is about 19 times higher when the woman is facing the beam than when she has her back to the beam. UNSCEAR 88, discussing the Canadian Fluoroscopy Study (Study 4 in this chapter), refers to a 20-fold difference too (Un88, p.456, para.367).

So, even though the average breast-dose per exam was only 1.5 rad, almost all of the rads received had to be rads which were received while the woman was facing the beam. Indeed, we will show below that 87 % of the rads were received while facing the beam.

The estimate of 1.5 rad per exam sets an upper-limit on the dose from exams done facing the beam. To simplify, we can imagine that in 3 out of 4 exams or 75 % of exams, when the women were told to face AWAY from the beam, their breasts received no dose at all. We can imagine that in 1 out of 4 exams or 25 % of exams, when the women were told to face the beam, their breasts received 6 rads. Then the weighted average dose per exam would be (0.75 x 0 rads) + (0.25 x 6 rads) = 1.5 rad.

But the dose facing AWAY from the beam was not zero rads, so we must calculate what it was. We will call

the low dose (while facing AWAY from the beam) "d".
Then 20d = the higher dose (while FACING the beam).
The lower dose, d, was received during 75 % of the
exams. The higher dose, 20d, was received during 25
% of the exams. Their weighted average = 1.5 rads.
Thus:

```
(0.75d) + (0.25 x 20d) = 1.5
(0.75d) + (5d) = 1.5
(5.75d) = 1.5
d = 0.261
20d = 5.22
```

For every four exams performed, 6 rads were
received, since we are told that the average dose per
exam was 1.5 rads. The six rads per four exams were
delivered as follows: 3 exams (each 0.261 rad)
contributed 0.783 rad, and 1 exam (delivering 5.22 rads)
contributed 5.22 rads. And (5.22 rads / 6 rads) x (100) =
87 %. In other words, 87 % of the rads received in this
study were received at a rate of 5.22 rads per delivery or
exposure-session, not 1.5 rad per exposure.

Therefore, we think we are not entitled to regard this
study as a test of the flawless-repair hypothesis at the
average rate of two tracks per nucleus (from 1.5 rads).
The weighted average rate of tracks will be higher.
Some 87 % of tracks will arrive at the rate set by 5.22
rads per exam. This rate is (1.3378 tracks per nucleus
at 1 rad) x (5.22 rads), or 6.9833 tracks per nucleus per
exam. Some 13 % of tracks will arrive at the rate set by
0.261 rad per exam. This rate is (1.3378 tracks per
nucleus at 1 rad) x (0.261 rad), or 0.3492 track per
nucleus per exam. So the weighted average
delivery-rate which we will use for this study is as
follows:

```
(0.87 x 6.9833 tracks) + (0.13 x 0.3492 track)
    = 6.1209 tracks per nucleus, on the average.
```

We will check this answer by obtaining the weighted
average delivery-rate for rads, and then converting it to
tracks per nucleus. Some 87 % of the rads are
delivered at the rate of 5.22 rads per exam, and 13 %
are delivered at the rate of 0.261 rad per exam. So the
weighted average delivery rate is:

```
(0.87 x 5.22) + (0.13 x 0.261) = 4.575 rads per
    delivery, or per exposure-session.
```

```
(l.3378 tracks per nucleus at 1 rad) x (4.575 rads)
    = 6.1204 tracks per nucleus, on the average.
```

Before making an entry into Table 21-A, we will
round the dose to 4.6 rads per exposure-session, and
adjust the tracks to 6.1539 .

Readers who have followed this presentation will
understand that we are not changing the facts as
reported at all. The average dose per exam remains 1.5
rads. But for a test of the flawless-repair hypothesis, it
is more appropriate to consider the average
delivery-rate of the rads, and we have shown this to be
4.6 rads at one time.

● -- Study 4,
Canadian Fluoroscopy Study :
===

This is a very large on-going study in Canada based
upon patients with a history of hospitalization for
pulmonary tuberculosis (Howe84; Mi89).

Originally, the plan was to incorporate the Nova
Scotia fluoroscopy cases with the larger Canadian
series. However, because the Nova Scotia patients
were fluoroscoped with the beam entering the front of
the body -- with consequently a much larger radiation
dose to the breasts than was the case for all other parts
of the Canadian study, where the fluoroscopy was
conducted primarily with beam-entry from the back -- it
was decided to keep the study in two separate parts.
We have therefore considered the total Canadian
experience as two separate large studies, one labeled
Canadian Fluoroscopy Study, and the other labeled
Nova Scotia Fluoroscopy Study (STUDY 1, above).

According to Miller and co-workers, who released
another interim report on this study in November 1989,
"The principal difference among sanatoriums was that
in Nova Scotia the patients usually faced the x-ray
source, whereas in other provinces they usually faced
away from it" (Mi89, p.1286).

We cannot find any estimate of dose PER EXAM in
the Howe or Miller reports. However, since irradiation
conditions in the Canadian Study were closest to those
of the Massachusetts Fluoroscopy Study, and since the
authors say that they used data from Boice78 to help
themselves estimate dose per patient (Mi89, p.1286),
we will use the approximation that the average absorbed
dose in the Canadian Study was also 1.5 rads to the
breast for each fluoroscopic examination. Thus, we will
say that the weighted average rate at which these rads
were delivered was 4.6 rads per exam, as we did in
Study 3. This means, per exam, an average of only
about 6 primary ionization tracks per nucleus.

Like the Nova Scotia and Massachusetts Studies, the
Canadian Study must be regarded as a very low-dose
study, since it involved single low-dose exposures,
given serially and separated by ample time for the
repair-system to operate flawlessly, if it can. The result

was that the hypothesis of flawless repair failed, again. For instance, for breast tissue-doses in the range 200-499 rads, the breast-cancer mortality was 2.2 times that for the unexposed persons, in a limited follow-up (Howe84). The later paper (Mi89) does not give relative risk for the non-Nova-Scotia segment separately. (Additional discussion of this study will be found in Chapter 22.)

**● -- Study 5,
Stewart In-Utero Studies :**

In the In-Utero Series, Stewart and co-workers compared the X-ray history (maternal) for children who died of cancer or leukemia, with the X-ray history for matched controls who had no malignant disease (Stew56; Stew58; Stew70). Stewart and co-workers demonstrated that diagnostic X-rays during pregnancy, irradiating the fetus-in-utero, provoked about a 50 % increase in the frequency of childhood cancer and leukemia. This study, widely known as the "Oxford Study," is the original work of this type on in-utero irradiation.

The results of this long-term study have recently been up-dated in three publications (Knea87 at p.215; Knox87; and Gilm88). Two features are to be noted. First, all three papers are in agreement that for obstetric radiography, which Gilman and co-workers take to be synonymous with third-trimester X-rays, the best estimate for mean dose to the fetus was 0.5 rad per obstetric examination. They suggest a best estimate per film to have been 0.3 rad. Second, the estimated relative risk of cancer associated with obstetric radiography is now estimated to be about 1.94, which is appreciably higher than the earlier estimates for the Oxford Studies. Knox (Knox87, p.11) explains this as follows:

"The radiation-RR [RR= relative risk] was larger than previously suspected. The confounding factors had masked rather than exaggerated its true extent. Over the whole period it was about 1.94, reducing from greater values in the earlier years to a lower value in the later years."

The Dose-Entry in Table 21-A :
On the basis of the papers cited above, we shall use the dose-estimate of 0.5 rads to the fetus for obstetric radiography in the Stewart In-Utero Studies.

This dose corresponds with an average rate of only 0.67 track per nucleus (Table 21-A). The Poisson equation shows that, when the average is 0.67, only 14.5 % of the cell-nuclei receive two or more tracks

(Table 21-B). The overwhelming percentage of nuclei is either receiving the Least Possible Disturbance (a single primary ionization track per nucleus) or no disturbance at all.

The Stewart In-Utero Studies provide powerful additional evidence for failure of the hypothesis that, if dose were just sufficiently low and slow, then repair of carcinogenic injury would be flawless. If repair had been flawless, no radiation-induced malignancies would have occurred from the in-utero irradiation by only 0.5 rad.

The Causality Issue :
The number of persons who doubt the Stewart findings seems to decline steadily. The observations themselves are not questioned, but the causal nature of the relationship is sometimes challenged.

A few persons still suggest that some "third factor" leads some women to "need" to have obstetric radiography and the same "third factor" leads them to have children with cancer or leukemia, so that radiation is exonerated. No such third factor has ever been identified. One can say that, with all the evidence relating radiation to cancer and leukemia under all sorts of different circumstances, it is really a violation of the law of minimum hypotheses to invoke some "third factor" as the cause of the excess malignancies in this series.

Of course, confidence in the causal relationship, between in-utero irradiation and excess childhood malignancies, rises appropriately when the same result is found among a wholly different set of children in a wholly different set of circumstances by a wholly different set of investigators. The Stewart In-Utero Studies have been confirmed in this manner, and more than once (Studies 6 and 8, below).

Nonetheless, the 1988 UNSCEAR Committee (Un88, pp.427-429, para.157,162,163,169) -- challenges all these findings by pointing repeatedly to the failure to find a comparable result in the A-bomb in-utero series -- a series where the total expectation of childhood cancer was a maximum of only SIX CASES (two cases were observed).

However, I have shown elsewhere (Go81, pp.753-756) that undue weight has been given to this "failure." Those who emphasize it are ignoring the presence of undeniable bias-problems in diagnosis during the early post-bombing period within the A-bomb in-utero series, and later, probable diagnostic error associated with an excess rate of severe mental retardation in this in-utero series. Such problems (shown in detail in Go81) can distort conclusions badly in the A-bomb in-utero series, where so very few cases of childhood cancer were expected at all.

UNSCEAR 1988 neither mentions these specific bias-problems nor rebuts their significance.

At the end of its discussion, however, UNSCEAR says that "... it would be prudent to assume that pre-natal irradiation does have an effect, especially with regard to leukaemogenesis" (Un88, p.429, para.170).

It might be noted that RERF is now beginning to report an excess of ADULT-type cancers occurring in the A-bomb in-utero series (Yoshi88). In this current phase of the follow-up, diagnostic bias is still a concern.

It has long been my opinion that the case in favor of causality in the Stewart In-Utero Studies is very strong indeed. I note that Dr. Robin H. Mole, a former member of the ICRP, has explicitly gone on record as follows (Mole88): "A clear statistical association between excess childhood cancer and prenatal abdominal radiography of the mother was established by Dr. Alice Stewart some time ago. The scientific issue was whether this meant causation. If so, the no-threshold hypothesis for cancer induction would be virtually unassailable, instead of being merely a prudent assumption by ICRP. Good scientific reasons exist (Mole74) for accepting that the small dose involved in the radiography did cause the cancer."

● -- Study 6,
    MacMahon In-Utero Study :

=======================================

In a totally separate study of in-utero irradiation, MacMahon (Mac62) carried through a study of childhood mortality from neoplastic diseases (leukemia and other malignancies) in relation to diagnostic X-ray examinations during the relevant pregnancy. His population sample was a 1 % sample of 734,243 children born in and discharged alive from any of 37 large maternity hospitals in the Northeast United States in the years 1947-1954.

A highly significant increase in mortality from malignant disease was found in children whose mothers received diagnostic X-rays to the abdominal or pelvic region during the relevant pregnancy. The majority of the X-rays were performed in the third trimester. In this study, hospital records were examined to ascertain X-ray exposure, whereas the original Stewart Study was based on mothers stating whether or not they had had X-rays in the pregnancy. No study is perfect in this

regard, since neither hospital records nor memories are flawless.

The careful study by MacMahon included correction for possible confounding variables, and concluded, in MacMahon's direct words, that:

"The higher frequency of prenatal X ray in the cancer cases than in the sample was statistically significant. After correction for birth order and other complicating variables, it was estimated that cancer mortality [including leukemia mortality] was about 40% higher in the X-rayed than in the unX-rayed members of the study population. This relationship held for each of the three major diagnostic categories -- leukemia, neoplasms of the central nervous system, and other neoplasms."

While no estimates of X-ray exposure-dose were made by MacMahon, he provided the following information which we will use to make a dose-estimate. The X-rayed cases were ranked into three categories in order of probable dose (adapted from MacMahon's Table 8):

X-Ray Exposure :	Number of Exams
Abdominal flat plate, often for diagnosis of twins; usually 1-film or 2-films per woman.	183
Pelvimetry; usually 3 films per woman.	520
Multiple procedures; these combinations included flat plates with pelvimetry; repeated pelvimetry; additional exams of kidneys, intestines, etc.	67
Total Exams	770

With the overwhelming representation of pelvimetries, and with the greater frequency of "abdominal flat plate" than "multiple procedures," it is reasonable to assign an average of 3 films for the X-ray exposures experienced during these pregnancies. And since "repair time" was most uncommon between films, these exams were acute exposures.

The Dose-Entry for Table 21-A :
Since MacMahon did not provide an average dose per film, we shall use the central estimate of Knox and co-workers (STUDY 5), which is 0.3 rad per film. Using this estimate of dose per film, and the estimate above of three films per examination in the MacMahon series, we

==

arrive at an average exposure of 0.9 rad to the fetus. This dose increased the rate of childhood cancer or leukemia among the exposed children to 1.4 times the rate observed for children who were not exposed during gestation.

The MacMahon study is still another instance in which the hypothesis of flawless repair of carcinogenic injury has failed, despite very low dose. In this case, flawless repair failed after a single exposure-session with a dose of 0.9 rad (0.9 cGy), which corresponds with an average number of tracks of only 1.2 per cell-nucleus (Table 21-A).

The question of causality between the X-ray exposure and the childhood malignancies has, of course, been raised for this study just as it was for the Stewart Study. My opinion is that the grounds for questioning causality in either study are very poor indeed. STUDY 8 (below) is another study, undertaken by Harvey and co-workers to address the speculation that some unidentified "third factor" could be causing occurrence of the X-rays as well as occurrence of the excess childhood malignancies.

● -- Study 7,
   British Luminizer Study :

=======================================

Baverstock and co-workers studied the experience of British workers involved in the preparation of instrument-dials made luminous with radium (Bav81, Bav83). They reported highly significant proof of breast-cancer induction by gamma radiation in young female workers who applied the radium-226 to the instruments. These investigators were able to rule out internal radiation by alpha particles as the cause, and identified external gamma radiation as the source of the breast exposure. The total breast-dose accumulated by the young women was 40 rads (centi-grays).

The dose-rate of external gammas to the breasts was, by measurement, 0.5 rad (cGy) per week or less. For a 40-hour week, this represents a dose of 0.1 rad per 8 hours (per work-day). In Table 21-A, we treat each work-day as one exposure. Of course, the "repair time" available with each exposure-session was a minimum of 16 hours (between the end of one work-day and the beginning of the next). After we consider the Poisson distribution of tracks (below), we will see that the average repair-time was actually greater than 24 hours.

Among the women whose average age was 20 years at the time of first employment, breast-cancer was observed at twice the expected rate during a limited

follow-up period. Follow-up will continue in this UK Radium Luminizer Survey, as noted in Chapter 18, Part 6.

Like the fluoroscopy studies cited above, the British Luminizer Study also converts an apparent "high-dose" study into what should appropriately be considered a low-dose radiation study. The true dose with which repair-systems had to cope in this study was 0.1 rad per exposure -- which corresponds with an average of approximately 0.2937 track per cell-nucleus (Table 21-A). This is certainly far down on the scale of low-doses.

And repair-time between exposures was ample. The time is affected by the Poisson distribution of tracks. The Poisson equation shows that, when the average is 0.2937 track per nucleus, about 75 % of the nuclei are receiving no primary ionization track at all (Table 21-C). Because the tracks received during one work-day cannot be targeted upon the 25 % of nuclei which were hit by tracks during the previous work-day, in reality, most nuclei had MORE than a work-day between any disturbance at all, in the British Luminizer Study.

It should be noted, from Table 21-C, that only 3.6 % of nuclei receive two or more tracks per exposure. About 96.4 % of cell-nuclei either experience the Least Possible Disturbance per exposure (a single primary ionization track, with ample time for repair to operate) or no disturbance at all per exposure.

The British Luminizer Study, with an exceedingly low dose and dose-rate per exposure-session, constitutes still another failure of the hypothesis that flawless repair of carcinogenic injury occurs at minimal doses and dose-rates.

British Luminizers -- An Up-Date :

=======================================

After our initial use (Go86) of this study, Baverstock and Papworth issued an interim up-date report which brings ascertainment of deaths up to January 1986 (Bav87). There are now 243 total deaths from all causes, up from 89 in the initial report. About 80 % of the study population is still living.

Our use of this study is limited to the women who were younger than age 30 at the start of luminizing. Due to declining radio-sensitivity with advancing age, one does not expect to find a provable excess of breast-cancer in such a study among the luminizers who began their luminizing work beyond age 30 (total breast-cancer deaths equals 7). For the group under age 30 at first exposure, the up-dated report by

Baverstock and Papworth provides the following data in their recent interim report:

	------ Exposure Category --------		
Breast Cancers	<0.2 Gy	=>0.2 Gy	Total Group
Observed	5	16	21
Expected	3.00	10.62	13.62
O / E	1.67	1.51	1.54
p-value (1-tailed)	0.18	0.074	0.04
Significance	N.S.	Suggestive	Significant
Mean Absorbed Dose			
(in rads)	8.5	51	40
Person-years	8,569	27,299	35,868
Persons at risk	255	678	933

When p-values are between 0.05 and 0.1, the significance is often called "Suggestive."

The O / E value (relative risk) of 1.54 for breast-cancer deaths is significantly elevated in the study population compared with expectation, which is based on the general population. This result is for a total mean absorbed dose of 40 breast-rads, accumulated gradually by the luminizer women.

For these women, the O / E value is reduced from about 2.0 in the early interim report (Bav81) to about 1.5 in the follow-up to January 1986. However, the precise value of O / E is of no concern for the purpose of assessing flawless repair of carcinogenic lesions. Any significant radiation-induced elevation of O / E above 1.0 means that repair is not operating flawlessly. Thus, the up-dated interim report alters nothing about our use of this study in analyzing the threshold issue.

In neither the initial report nor the recent up-date are the data strong enough to permit a meaningful test for internal dose-response relationship among the luminizer women. A positive dose-response trend (a rising relative risk with rising dose) would be a powerful indication of causality in this study between the irradiation and the excess mortality from breast cancer.

Meanwhile, the presumption is reasonable that radiation is indeed the cause of the observed excess. It would seem unreasonable to attribute the excess breast-cancer deaths to a more efficient ascertainment of total deaths or cancer deaths in the study population. All causes of death (omitting cancer) show an O / E

value of 0.81, when all the luminizers are contrasted with the general population. And all cancer-deaths (breast-cancer excluded) show an O / E value of 1.02, so a more diligent search for cancer-deaths in particular does not seem like a reasonable suspicion. By contrast, the O / E for breast-cancer deaths is 1.37 when all the luminizers (regardless of age at exposure) are compared with the general population.

The nature of the radiation exposure makes it extremely reasonable to expect that the radiation dose to the breasts was higher than dose to other organs. And this is consistent with the observation that breast-cancer deaths are provably in excess whereas other cancers are not. Nonetheless, pending a positive dose-response it remains possible that some unidentified variable, other than radiation, accounts for the excess.

The British Luminizer Study once again illustrates the "small-numbers" problem which manifests itself most severely when a single type of cancer is under study in a population of limited size. Even in the A-Bomb Study, despite combining all cancer-sites and despite much higher cancer expectations than in the Baverstock study, considerable sampling variation occurred from one follow-up interval to the next, as plainly seen in Chapter 17, Table 17-B. In the British Luminizers, Baverstock and Papworth find a decline in relative risk from about 2.0 to about 1.5 from one follow-up to the next. Whether this decline is the result of sampling variation alone or is a meaningful time-trend cannot be ascertained within the data.

Like Baverstock and Papworth, we will be highly interested in whatever is shown by future follow-ups in the Luminizer Study.

● -- Study 8, Harvey In-Utero Twins Study :

====================================

Because of suggestions that some underlying medical status led women to being X-rayed during pregnancy and also led to giving birth to children likely to develop cancer or leukemia, Harvey and co-workers (Har85) elected to do a case-control study in twins. The reasoning was that the likelihood of medical selection bias would be reduced in the study of twins. Harvey and co-workers stated:

"Twins were exposed to prenatal x-rays more frequently than singletons to confirm their twin status or to determine the fetal position before birth and not necessarily because of any medical condition of the mother or child that could conceivably predispose to cancer. It is generally believed that the demonstration of excess childhood cancer in twins would be the best evidence that prenatal x-ray exposure is truly causal and not merely correlated indirectly with an increase in cancer frequency."

The records of over 32,000 twins born in Connecticut from 1930 to 1969 were used. These were linked to the Connecticut Tumor Registry with the result that 31 incident cases of cancer were identifed. These were each matched with four twin controls, according to sex, year of birth, and race. A twin was considered exposed if the mother had been exposed to X-rays in the abdominal region during the twin pregnancy -- e,g., pelvimetry or plain films of the abdomen.

Radiation dose to the fetus was estimated to have had an average value of 1.0 rad.

Analysis showed a significant excess of X-rays in the twins who developed childhood cancer, contrasted with the controls. The final estimated overall relative risk associated with prenatal X-ray exposure was 2.4, adjusted only for twin birth-weight.

The authors point out: "The observed 2.4-fold risk of childhood cancer associated with prenatal x-ray exposure in twins is consistent with the results of two major investigations from England and the northeastern United States [reference to Stew58 and Mac62] and with a reanalysis of the twin segment from the English series" [reference to Mole74].

While it would have been helpful if the entire series of cases in the Harvey Twins Study were larger, the 95 % confidence limits on the relative risk were 1.0 to 5.9. We consider that this study is a valid addition to the seven studies already considered here.

The Harvey Twin Study indicates that repair was not able to un-do all the carcinogenic injury from a single, acute dose of only 1.0 rad, which corresponds with a track-average of 1.3 per cell-nucleus.

● -- Study 9, Breast-Cancer in the Israeli Scalp–Irradiation Study

Very recently, Modan and co-workers (Modan89) have published an update of some aspects of the same scalp-irradiation study described as STUDY 2 above. In this update, the incidence of breast-cancer was examined for the 1982-1986 period, as part of an on-going evaluation of various cancers occurring in the children irradiated between 1949 and 1959 in the Israeli tinea capitis series.

Their finding is that the relative risk of breast-cancer in the period 1982-1986 is 2.11 for the irradiated female children contrasted with unirradiated controls. The 90 % confidence-limits are 1.05 and 4.24. Modan and co-workers point out that they used 90 % confidence-limits "... since we did not expect a protective anti-carcinogenic effect of radiation."

The radiation dose estimated for the breasts of the female children is given as 1.6 rads. The authors of the paper were themselves surprised by the magnitude of the effect for this dose-level. They explored possible underestimates of dose to the breast as a result of movement of some of the children during the scalp-irradiation, but did not reach any definitive conclusions on this point. Also they explored the possibility that the dose received by the pituitary might have indirectly been involved in producing the breast-cancer.

It is my opinion that retroactive re-evaluation of radiation dose, simply because findings surprise the investigator, leaves much to be desired and can lead to bias. The appropriate use of these data is to take the observations as they were made.

This study, taken at face value, would represent another failure of repair in un-doing carcinogenic injury, from a single acute dose of only 1.6 rads, which corresponds with an average of 2.1 tracks per cell-nucleus (Table 21-A). Even if one were to double the estimated radiation dose to the breast, this would still be a study with only 4.2 tracks per cell-nucleus, on the average.

Summary and a Key Question :

With respect to all nine studies described above, Table 21-A summarizes the crucial information which demonstrates failure of the hypothesis that very LOW-dose carcinogenic injury is flawlessly repaired. It should be noted that the same evidence is perfectly consistent with the hypothesis of an approximately constant fraction of unrepaired, unrepairable, and misrepaired damage throughout the dose-range, right down to the complete disappearance of dose.

Five of the nine epidemiological studies have their TOTAL doses evaluated in Table 21-A. Four studies in the table have dose-entries which are very low per exposure, even though many repetitions of the exposure finally added up to large doses. Large total doses may be required in order to DETECT an excess of a few types of cancer when a limited sample of adults is exposed and followed-up for a limited time-period, but this statement is certainly not a suggestion that large doses of radiation are required to CAUSE any excess cancer. The two statements are very different, as every epidemiologist knows. With respect to the hypothesis that repair can flawlessly un-do all carcinogenic damage from tracks, provided dose is sufficiently low and slow, these four studies of successive small doses qualify as highly relevant evidence.

Readers may note that Arthur Upton, chairman of the BEIR-5 radiation committee, explicitly selects the fluoroscopy studies, the Baverstock Luminizer Study, the Modan tinea capitis study, and the in-utero studies, when he states: "Several lines of epidemiological evidence support the hypothesis that there may be no threshold in the dose-incidence relationship ..." (Up87. p.300; full context provided in our Chapter 34).

Regrettably, Upton makes no attempt to analyse the extremely low rate of tracks per nucleus in these studies -- an analysis which is the crucial step in showing that the combined evidence amounts to PROOF that there is no threshold.

In Table 21-A, the doses per exposure range from 9 rads right down to 0.1 rad per exposure, and in five of the nine studies, the average number of tracks per nucleus was between 2.14 and 0.2937. Since the Least Possible Disturbance is one primary track per nucleus, plus time for repair to un-do it, these studies are most certainly studies of VERY low radiation doses and dose-rates.

In Chapter 18, we have asserted that -- by any reasonable standard -- repair's failure to prevent excess cancer in these studies is proof that there is no dose or dose-rate where repair is flawless with respect to carcinogenic injuries. And in the title of Chapter 21, we have referred to "decisive" epidemiological evidence on the threshold issue.

The question which many readers will have, of course, is: "Why should I believe the studies which DO show excess cancer at such low doses and dose-rates, instead of the more numerous studies which FAIL to show any excess at such doses?" Part 2 will address that question.

2. Inconclusive Evidence on a Threshold: Types and Supply

An inconclusive study with respect to the threshold issue is, of course, any study which is incapable of helping to resolve it. Below, we will provide some examples of such studies from influential journals. A study whose results are consistent with opposites (safe dose, no safe dose) is obviously inconclusive with respect to the safe-dose issue.

The abstracts of many such studies feature the phrase "no significant risk was found." Unfortunately, even some people in medicine mistakenly interpret the phrase to mean, "If radiation were carcinogenic, an elevated cancer-risk SHOULD have been found," and so they mistakenly treat the study as evidence in favor of a safe dose. If they looked hard enough in such papers, however, they would usually find that the authors warned them SOMEWHERE, directly or indirectly, against this mistake. (We include one example, however, where the authors do otherwise.)

Here at the outset of this section, it should be stressed that observations, reported in studies which are inconclusive on the threshold issue, can be fully correct data which are valuable with respect to OTHER issues. A classic example is the A-Bomb Study itself. Dose-Groups 1 and 2 are separated by a total dose less than 2 rems (Table 11-H) -- and even this small difference is not so certain (see Chapter 8, Part 4). A provable excess of cancer in Dose-Group 2 does NOT lie within expectation. Thus the A-Bomb Study cannot possibly address the threshold issue directly. Yet the A-Bomb Study is by far the most valuable study on many OTHER issues -- issues which cannot be addressed by the nine studies of Table 21-A.

Although inconclusive studies are commonly treated as if they were evidence supporting a safe dose and dose-rate, they are not. Such "no-effect-found" studies are merely studies which are consistent with both the existence and non-existence of a threshold.

This is a very different status from a study where a cancer-effect from radiation clearly SHOULD have been found, but was not. By definition, such a study would NOT be consistent with the thesis of no safe dose or dose-rate.

It is still difficult, however, for analysts to KNOW when radiogenic cancer should have been found in a particular study, or should not have been found. The radiogenic expectation depends critically on knowing in advance the MAGNITUDE of the radiation's carcinogenicity. It is self-evident that the accuracy of radiogenic risk-values for specific cancer-sites and for limited classes of cancer (e.g., "childhood cancers") is far lower than that for cancers overall. (See discussion in Chapter 22, Part 5.)

What threshold proponents need is a collection of

==

mutually reinforcing human studies in which the magnitude of radiogenic risk is firm enough to say, with reasonable certainty, that an excess of cancer should have been found and was NOT found.

However, an accumulation of INAPPROPRIATE evidence would be worse than worthless -- it would be a misleading distortion. When scientists speak of "the weight of the evidence" in any field, they mean the weight of APPROPRIATE evidence.

The human studies commonly cited as supporting a safe dose or dose-rate do NOT qualify as studies where an excess of cancer clearly should have been found, but was not found, as we will illustrate here in Part 2.

We are not suggesting that readers disbelieve the DATA reported in those studies, but we are emphatically pointing out that such data cannot be believed to represent evidence for a safe dose or dose-rate of ionizing radiation.

● -- *Occupational Exposure :*
==

In 1985, in the BRITISH MEDICAL JOURNAL, Beral and co-workers reported on a follow-up of 39,546 atomic power workers in Britain (Ber85). Of these, 20,382 with a radiation record received a mean whole-body exposure of 3.24 cSv (rems), and 19,164 had no record of radiation exposure. The average follow-up time was 16 years for both groups of workers. (These data come from Table 1 and p.441 of Ber85.) We must comment here that 16 years is a rather short follow-up period.

Beral and co-workers clearly acknowledged that their study was inconclusive with respect to excess cancer when they said, in a later version (Ber87, p105): "The findings so far are consistent with there being no increased cancer risk at all, and at the same time, with a risk ten to fifteen times the ICRP figures."

A study which is compatible both with a safe dose, and with no safe dose, is simply incapable of helping to resolve the threshold issue. It would be a real mistake to regard it as relevant evidence.

In an additional report on the UK atomic workers, these investigators add a comment which is highly pertinent to our topic of inconclusive negative studies (Ins87, p.87): "In conclusion, the data presented here illustrate some of the problems encountered in relating the mortality of a workforce to different levels of occupational radiation exposure when the exposures themselves are low, cannot be measured accurately,

and have been assessed in different ways over time."

Their statement needs recognition as an appropriate warning that there are some severe limits to what such studies can ever reveal. It is a warning against exaggerated expectations. My own analysis of radiation-induced cancer in the Hanford atomic workers also pointed up some difficulties and inherent limitations of such studies (Go79).

● -- *Medical Exposure :*
==

The Linos Study :

In 1980, in the NEW ENGLAND JOURNAL OF MEDICINE, Linos and co-workers at the Mayo Clinic authored the report "Low Dose Radiation and Leukemia" (Lin80). They say at the beginning: "No statistically significant increase was found in the risk of developing leukemia after radiation doses of 0 to 300 rads (3 Gy) to the bone marrow when these amounts were administered in small doses over long periods of time, as in routine medical care."

However, in the conclusion of the SAME paper they write: "Consequently, we maintain that low levels of exposure to medical radiation most probably did not increase the risk of leukemia in this community, but that if it did, the factor of increase is almost surely less than 2.0."

Linos and colleagues are saying, in short, that the size of their sample and their procedure were of such a design that, even if low-dose medical exposures were nearly doubling the leukemia-rate in a community, their study could have missed the effect. Thus the study is inherently inconclusive on the threshold issue because it is compatible with opposite conclusions (safe dose, no safe dose). Specifics of the paper are discussed in detail elsewhere (Go81, pp. 699-706; Go85, pp.290-291).

The Spengler Study :

Another typical example of an inconclusive negative study, with respect to medical irradiation, appeared in the journal PEDIATRICS in 1983. By Spengler and co-workers, the paper is "Cancer Mortality Following Cardiac Catheterization: A Preliminary Follow-Up Study of 4,891 Irradiated Children" (Spen83). Its abstract reports that "The preliminary findings did not demonstrate a significant leukemia risk arising from diagnostic catheterization."

Later, near the conclusion, the authors state: "In essence, the size of our cohort is not sufficient to detect accurately a low-dose radiation effect." That is true.

When we checked this out independently, by using our own risk estimates (Go85, p.291-296), we found that the expectation of leukemia without irradiation was 1.88 case, and the expectation with irradiation was 2.07 cases. The observation of leukemia in the irradiated group was 3.0 cases.

Even though the observation slightly exceeded expectations, the difference between 1.88 and 3.0 was not statistically significant under the circumstances. Therefore the Spengler study is a negative study -- "no-effect-found" -- or as its abstract announces, "The preliminary findings did not demonstrate a significant leukemia risk arising from diagnostic catheterization." And none SHOULD have been found, unless low-dose radiogenic risk is GREATER than our own estimates. In terms of the perfect-repair hypothesis, the Spengler Study is just inconclusive.

The Davis Study vs. the Hrubec Study :

In 1987, in the JOURNAL OF THE NATIONAL CANCER INSTITUTE (USA), Davis, Boice, Kelsey, and Monson authored the report "Cancer Mortality after Multiple Fluoroscopic Examinations of the Chest" (Davis87). Their paper reports on a previously unstudied group of Massachusetts tuberculosis patients who experienced multiple chest fluoroscopies during pneumothorax therapy between 1930 and 1954.

This study has the potential, if extended, to study fractionated radiation doses for lung cancer and for breast cancer, but in its current state, it can only be regarded as an inconclusive study, compatible either with no safe dose or a safe dose.

We are not going to discuss the lung-cancer aspect of this study at all, due to severe confounding variables. For instance, the authors report only 1/3 of the cancer cases were verifiable, in part because some hospitals were no longer in existence, and records are gone. A real hazard exists for under-diagnosis of lung-cancer in patients with a history of tuberculosis of the lung. Additionally, the authors themselves report their study has a "large number of subjects with incomplete smoking data" and that "it is possible that greater consumption [of cigarettes] among unexposed relative to exposed may have masked any radiation effect for smoking-related cancer sites "(Davis87, p.651).

The results for breast cancer are quite

inconclusive for several reasons. Davis et al state: "The SRR [standardized relative risk] for breast cancer mortality was 1.1 (95% C.I. = 0.6-2.1) when we compared the exposed to unexposed groups and controlled for time since exposure and age at exposure" (Davis87, p.649). In other words, the observed excess was not provably significant.

Defects of Davis study as of this time: (a) Only mortality cases are available -- 24 in all for exposed group (only 1/3 verifiable); (b) mortality studies are clearly inferior to incidence studies early in a follow-up (see discussion below) -- even for histologically-verified cases, and (c) average breast-dose is much lower in Davis study than in our Study 3 (this chapter).

We expect that the Davis study will be amplified, that incidence cases will be sought, and that some definitive conclusions will become possible following such additional follow-up research.

In great contrast, in 1989 Hrubec, Boice, Monson, and Rosenstein have reported an extended follow-up of this chapter's Study 3 (to 30.2 years): "Breast Cancer after Multiple Chest Fluoroscopies. Second Follow-Up of Masachusetts Women with Tuberculosis" (Hru89). The search for cases, by incidence and mortality is very much more exhaustive, both in exposed and unexposed women. By now, a total of 74 histologically-verified cases of breast cancer are available for analysis (56 among exposed, and 18 among unexposed, women).

The findings are that the relative risk of breast cancer induction from multiple fluoroscopic exams is even greater than observed in the earlier follow-up (our Study 3). The findings are statistically stronger than before. And over 97% of the individuals have been located, with 63% still living.

The Hrubec study not only confirms and strengthens the excess breast-cancer findings of Study 3, but it is also now showing that the dose-response is supra-linear (a significantly NEGATIVE coefficient of the quadratic term in an L-Q analysis, p.232).

We are not at all critical of the Davis study. Both the Davis and the Hrubec studies emanate from the investigations of the Boice-Monson group. What is clear is that the Hrubec study is much further along than is the Davis study. Further the Hrubec study has a complement of younger women than does the Davis study, and it is clear that the radiation-sensitivity for breast-cancer is greater in the younger women.

Another point: In the earlier follow-up of the Hrubec

cohort (our Study 3) -- in which all 56 cases were histologically confirmed -- those breast-cancers ascertained by incidence showed a strikingly higher association with radiation (Relative Risk) than did those ascertained from mortality, We have calculated the following for those earlier cases (data from Boice81):

Mortality cases:
Relative risk = (16/9.4) / (8/5.5) = 1.17.
Incidence cases:
Relative risk = (25/13.9) / (7/8.6) = 2.21.

The lesson is that in the early years of follow-up, the radiation-excess is not nearly so manifest in mortalities as in incidence for breast-cancer in exposed young women. Therefore, we should not be surprised that the Davis Study of mortalities only (and poorly verified at that) provides no conclusive results for breast-cancer.

In terms of the flawless repair hypothesis, the Davis Study is simply another inconclusive study, with confidence limits of 0.6 to 2.1 on the relative risk (Davis87, p.649). Thus it is consistent with both the existence and non-existence of a threshold.

Patients Receiving Diagnostic Radio-Iodine :

We have examined a number of studies in the medical literature which report finding no excess cancer in patients who received radio-iodine (Go81, pp.642-658). We have used our own risk-per-rad estimates to find out how many excess (radiation-induced) cancers should be EXPECTED in those negative studies. It turned out that the studies were so small and the follow-up periods were so short that the expectation was a very low fraction of one extra case per study -- a surely undetectable excess.

Instead of being studies where excess cancer SHOULD have been detected but was not, these studies turned out to be studies where excess cancer should NOT have been detected (unless the risk-per-rad were much higher than our own estimates). In other words, the results of the studies were bound to be negative before the studies were ever undertaken.

There is no limit to the number of such studies which can be performed. Even a HUGE collection of such studies would contribute no weight at all to the argument for a safe dose or dose-rate.

The Holm Study in Sweden :

In Chapter 22, Part 5, a Swedish study of over 35,000 patients who received radio-iodine (Holm88) is examined by us in detail. This study is commonly cited as a study (A) showing no excess thyroid-cancer from the radio-iodine, and (B) showing that slow dose-delivery is less carcinogenic in humans than acute delivery. In reality, this is a study in which a very large excess of thyroid-cancer occurred (relative risk of about 3.9), and from which no conclusions in any direction should be drawn -- for the many reasons shown in Chapter 22, Part 5.

● -- Natural Background Radiation :

There have been many studies comparing cancer mortality in regions which have different background doses of natural radiation. We call such studies "Denver-Type" studies because so many Americans must have heard threshold advocates using the refrain, "If there is no safe dose of radiation, why isn't the cancer-rate higher in Denver (Colorado), since Denver has a higher natural background dose than most other places?"

This section will show why one cannot EXPECT high background doses to correlate with high cancer mortality, and low background doses to correlate with low cancer mortality, with any regularity.

Rule 1 -- Signal-to-Noise Ratio :
To test whether or not a study is inherently capable of detecting a cancer-effect from a difference in background radiation, the first thing to check is whether other variables are important enough to confound the results, to conceal the radiation-effect which is supposedly tested.

The cardinal rule is that we should never look for a relatively small carcinogenic effect from low-dose radiation in the presence of massively larger variation in non-radiation effects. Land has appropriately described the essence of this type of problem as a low "signal-to-noise" ratio (Land88, p.269). In a related context, Upton has spoken of "trying to listen to one violin when the whole orchestra is playing. You can't hear it" (Up89, p.418). Failure to detect the signal and the violin does not mean that they are absent.

Non-radon background doses, which vary with altitude and other factors, are roughly in the "ballpark" of 100 millirads per year of whole-body dose, mostly low-LET. Elsewhere I have estimated that, for a U.S. population of mixed ages, one should expect about a 16 % increment in cancer mortality-rate from doubling such exposure (Go81, p.307, pp.566-567; also pp.232-233). The estimate used 1976 age-specific cancer mortality-rates, and would likely be only slightly different if it used the 1986 age-specific rates -- even though the fraction of all deaths which are cancer-deaths has risen, from about 17 % in 1976, to about 22 % in 1986 (Silver90, p.12).

In terms of the signal-to-noise problem, one can regard the estimated 16 % elevation in cancer mortality per additional 100 millirads as the signal. The question is: Should this signal be detectable, despite the noise of variations in cancer mortality which are unrelated to low-LET radiation? Later in this part, we will demonstrate that this signal is fully compatible with the observation of BELOW-normal cancer mortality, normal cancer mortality, and ABOVE-normal cancer mortality.

Rule 2 -- Comparability of Populations :

Another cardinal rule, directly related to the first one, has been discussed already in connection with the A-Bomb Study: One should be very careful about drawing conclusions about radiation carcinogenesis from comparisons of cancer-rates in various groups, unless there is a good basis for confidence that the underlying NON-radiation cancer-rates -- the so-called spontaneous rates -- are alike (Chapters 11 and 12). Unless groups are equivalent, or can be rendered equivalent, in all the important variables which determine the non-radiation-induced cancer-rate, such groups certainly cannot be used to study the effect of small radiation doses on cancer-rate. Moreover, until better ways develop to quantify radon exposure and its carcinogenicity, radon alone is sufficient to confound "Denver-Type" studies. In what follows, we used measured exposures from the literature, but we know that ostensibly equal doses may really be different. This would not alter the point.

Two "Denver-Type" Studies :

In 1976, Frigerio and co-workers compared the average natural background dose in all 50 states of the USA with the Vital Statistics on cancer death-rates per state (Frig76). One of their findings was that the cancer death-rate was lowest in the fourteen states with the HIGHEST natural background radiation. However, the fourteen states with the LOWEST natural background radiation did not have the highest cancer death-rate. The twenty-two states with the intermediate background doses had the highest cancer death-rate. In other words, the relationship was irregular (Go81, 567-70).

This should surprise no one. Data in their Figure 1 demonstrate that in 10 states where Frigerio and Stowe report the SAME average yearly background dose of

135 millirems / year, the annual cancer mortality ranged from 125 up to 170 per 100,000. Thus the highest cancer-rate is some 36 % higher than the lowest rate, without there being any difference at all in average background dose. This very large variation in the non-radiation cancer-rate is the "noise" in the signal-to-noise ratio. I concluded that such a study is inherently incapable of testing whether or not background doses affect cancer death-rates in the general population, in either direction. The BEIR-3 Committee also reached the same conclusion (Beir80, pp.469-471).

In 1981, in HEALTH PHYSICS, a similar study appeared by Hickey and co-workers (Hic81). The authors claim in their abstract (Hic81, p.625) that their work "suggests that models implying important long-term deleterious effects of low-levels of ionizing radiation on humans may be invalid," and they claim again in their conclusions (Hic81, p.635) that their negative bi-variate correlations -- the two variables being cancer-rate and background dose of radiation -- "are not compatible with models that assert that all levels of radiation, no matter how low, are damaging." We will demonstrate, in the section entitled "Demonstration," that such findings are FULLY compatible with there being no safe dose. But first, we have other observations to make.

The statistical work in the Hickey paper confirms what can be shown far more directly below: The background dose of radiation is a small signal, compared with the noise from other factors which cause variation in the cancer-rate. In the Hickey study, 43 metropolitan areas of the USA were included, of which ten are southern (lying below the latitude of 36 degrees) and ten are in the northeast. When Hickey's data are tabulated by regions, as they are below, we discover immediately that confounding variables are having the dominant impact on cancer-rates:

	South	South & All Areas except Northeast	North- East
NATURAL BACKGROUND DOSE (Millirems per year)	85.10	87.17	87.29
ANNUAL CANCER DEATH-RATE PER 100,000 (1961-1964)	131.54	150.86	185.04

What is obvious from the tabulation is that cancer death-rates vary enormously at the SAME average background dose -- the Frigerio "story" all over again. Cancer-rates for those years were 41 % higher in the ten northeastern areas than in the ten southern areas even though the background radiation exposures were almost identical.

==

The Frigerio and Hickey studies, and others like them, are not capable of addressing the threshold question because it is evident that something other than background exposure is causing big differences in cancer-mortality. When cancer-mortality varies by 36 % or 41 % at the SAME background dose, whatever the non-radiation causes of the variation may be, those non-radiation causes are clearly important enough to confound a much smaller radiation effect (see "Demonstration" section).

Comparison of "Denver-Type" Studies with the A-Bomb Study :

In the A-Bomb Study, after normalization for age and sex differences across the Dose-Groups, we were able to have confidence that all Dose-Groups shared a closely similar underlying rate of spontaneous cancer, unrelated to their exposures to bomb radiation. In Chapter 4, we mentioned the fact that one of the study's most important scientific virtues is the fact that it provides its own internal reference group.

In sharp contrast with the A-Bomb Study, the "Denver-Type" studies are looking for an effect of small differences in radiation dose upon groups of people, in different regions, who are NOT alike in variables other than radiation dose. Indeed, by comparing cancer-rates in groups in different regions who receive the SAME background doses, we ascertain that the underlying non-radiation-induced cancer-rates are FAR from uniform in all regions.

So the fatal flaw of the "Denver-Type" studies is that they lack any way to know or to achieve the crucial comparability of the non-radiation cancer-rates across dose-groups (the dose-groups being the populations in different regions with different background doses), and yet because of their very low signal-to-noise ratio, they need to be SUPERIOR to other studies on matching those underlying rates.

A Demonstration with Realistic Numbers :

Notwithstanding the fallacy of addressing the threshold issue with "Denver-Type" studies, such studies are often mentioned as evidence in favor of a safe dose or dose-rate (for instance, see Webs87, p.425; Alex88b, p.592-593; Sag89, p.574).

Therefore, we think it is worthwhile to use some realistic numbers to DEMONSTRATE exactly how an elevated natural background dose -- actively inducing extra cancer in the population -- is fully compatible with observation of cancer-rates which are BELOW expectation, normal, and ABOVE expectation.

First, we have already shown with Hickey's own data that great variation exists from one region to another in cancer mortality, with rates 41 % greater in one region than in another region, when the background radiation dose is the SAME.

Second, we need to remember that cancer mortality consists of two parts: Non-radiation-induced, and radiation-induced. As stated above, my estimate is that a yearly dose of 0.1 rad per year (100 millirads per year) is expected to increase cancer-mortality by approximately 16 % over the NON-radiation rate.

Third, we can use the approximation that about 17 % of all deaths were cancer-deaths in the United States, when the Frigerio and Hickey studies were done.

We can let x = the non-radiation-induced part of the cancer death-rate, and we can let the average background dose be 0.1 rad per year.

Then, total cancer-rate = $x + (0.16)(x)$ = 17 percent.

Or, we can say $(1.16)(x)$ = 17 percent, and x = 14.7 percent.

But we showed above that some places have non-radiation cancer death-rates much above normal, and some have such rates well below normal -- all occurring at the same average natural dose of ionizing radiation. Let us consider three possible regions, where the non-radiation-induced cancer-rates are as follows, instead of the normal 14.7 % :

Region Considered	Non-Radiogenic Cancer-Rate
A	11.7 %
B	12.7 %
C	16.7 %

Let us also suppose that measurements show background radiation to be twice the average of 0.1 rad per year, namely 0.2 rad per year, in all three regions. The numbers below demonstrate that under these circumstances, despite the doubled background dose -- alike in all three regions -- analysts will observe one cancer-rate BELOW normal, one rate NORMAL, and one rate ABOVE normal.

If the elevated natural background dose of 0.2 rad is actively inducing extra cancer in the population, with an increment of 16 % for each 0.1 rad, we would have the following radiation-induced cancer death-rates (0.32 times the non-radiation cancer-rate):

Region Considered	Radiation-Induced Ca-Rate (%)
A	0.32 x 11.7 % = 3.74 %
B	0.32 x 12.7 % = 4.06 %
C	0.32 x 16.7 % = 5.34 %

And the OBSERVED cancer death-rates would be as follows:

Region Considered	OBSERVED Ca-Rate (%) (Spontaneous + Radiogenic)
A	11.7 % + 3.74 % = 15.44 %
B	12.7 % + 4.06 % = 16.76 %
C	16.7 % + 5.34 % = 22.04 %

It is self-evident that Region A would have a cancer mortality rate BELOW the normal 17 percent. Region B's rate would look normal. Region C's rate would be ABOVE normal. Using a risk-increment per 0.1 rad (100 millirads) which we think is realistic, we have just demonstrated (in Regions A and B) how carcinogenesis at very low doses is fully compatible with finding cancer-rates below normal, or not above normal, in "Denver-Type" studies. Such findings lie WITHIN expectations, in our scenario, because of differences in the underlying NON-radiation-induced cancer-rates.

In our scenario, if people failed to consider the fact that NON-radiation cancer-rates differ markedly from one region to another, and if they carelessly assumed that such rates were the same everywhere, then some of them might even "interpret" the observed cancer-rate in Region A as evidence that an extra dose of 100 millirads per year is "protective" against cancer if you live in Region A ... although the same dose is "without any effect" in Region B ... notwithstanding the observation that the same dose is "extremely carcinogenic" if you live in Region C.

This would be nonsense. No one would be entitled to draw any of those conclusions from such a study. The assumption, that the underlying NON-radiation-induced cancer-rates are the same in all three regions, is unjustified. Yet no one would have a believable way of FINDING OUT the three non-radiation rates which were associated with each of the three observed rates. (We "know" the underlying non-radiation-induced cancer-rates in Regions A, B, and C only because we WROTE the scenario.) Therefore, no one could evaluate the possible contribution from the radiation to the observed rates.

And that is the fatal flaw, in "Denver-Type" studies. Such studies are just inconclusive, and will remain so.

The Proper Exclusion of Inconclusive Studies :

=======================================

Our Table 21-A included none of the "no-effect-found" studies described above. The purpose of Part 2 has been to show why they are PROPERLY excluded from any true effort to resolve the safe-dose issue.

We pointed out that studies which are consistent with BOTH the existence and non-existence of a threshold are irrelevant. They cannot contribute to the weight of the evidence, in either direction.

For instance, in our medical examples above, when Spengler and co-workers said, "In essence, the size of our cohort is not sufficient to detect accurately a low-dose radiation effect," they were saying that absence of a provable excess of leukemia in their study was within expectations.

The absence of a radiation effect in that study presented no mystery, no puzzle, and no challenge to the thesis that there is no safe dose or dose-rate. The Spengler Study is just another inconclusive study which is unable to address the threshold issue at all.

"A Myth with Every Shot" :

There will never be any shortage of inconclusive "no-effect-found" studies about ionizing radiation which people can cite. In fact, such studies could be designed in an infinite number if the sponsorship were to be sufficiently generous. I am reminded of a classic statement on the subject by F.A. Harper (Harpe57, p.537), a genuine free-market economist and expositor of liberty and harmony:

"As to the number of forms myths can take, consider the possible answers to 2 plus 2. The only non-mythical answer is 4. But there are infinite mythical answers ... So if [a person's] aim were perfect and he could shoot a myth with every shot, he could spend his entire lifetime shooting myths released by only one myth factory, without ever demolishing all this factory could produce."

There is no scientific obligation to shoot at myths, or to discuss the limits of EVERY inconclusive study. In Chapter 22, Part 5, readers will see the length sometimes required to discuss just ONE inconclusive study (Holm88) with appropriate thoroughness.

The samples discussed above are sufficient to illustrate the characteristics of studies which are

===

inconclusive with respect to the threshold issue, and to show why such studies are PROPERLY excluded from any genuine effort to settle the question of a safe dose or dose-rate.

3. Decisive Evidence on a Threshold : Types and Supply

"Proof" or "disproof" in the biomedical sciences is unlike possible proof and disproof in mathematics or logic, where some proofs may be claimed to be final. In the empirical sciences, proof is always a provisional matter, pending contrary evidence of an appropriate nature and amount.

We have repeatedly said in Chapter 18 that the evidence in Table 21-A amounts to disproof of any safe dose or dose-rate, by any reasonable standard. And if a series of decisive studies were to develop in which no excess cancer was observed, when it clearly should have been observed, we would certainly not reach the same conclusion as we do now. In other words, we are not trying to evade the meaning of such evidence, if it should develop. On the contrary. We would welcome it. We take no pleasure in reporting BAD news for human health.

But when the news is bad -- and Table 21-A shows that it is -- then human health is far better protected by facing reality than by ignoring it.

Thus we are critical of the 1988 UNSCEAR Report for appearing to ignore the implications of the studies in Table 21-A with regard to the threshold issue. Although all the studies except one were available, UNSCEAR-88 offers NO analysis of the rate of primary ionization tracks per nucleus associated with the doses in those studies. It offers NO hint that the positive cancer-excesses in those studies occurred from approximately the lowest conceivable doses and dose-rates in the cell-nuclei. It offers NO acknowledgment that these human studies can address the hypothesis of flawless repair and safe doses and dose-rates.

We wish that UNSCEAR-88 had addressed these matters, because current speculations about safe doses and dose-rates have profound implications for human health (Chapters 24 and 25).

The Decisive Nature of Table 21-A :

As we showed in Part 2 of this chapter, our Table 21-A properly excludes studies which are inconclusive.

Studies which are consistent with BOTH the existence and non-existence of a safe dose are irrelevant here.

By contrast, the nine studies which qualify for Table 21-A are highly relevant because they are NOT consistent with both positive and negative answers.

The results of these studies do NOT lie within threshold-expectations, because these are studies of human response to just about the Least Possible Disturbance from ionizing radiation. If a threshold is supposed to show up if the dose or dose-rate is just "low ENOUGH," how can one explain the observation that excess CANCER is what shows up in nine separate human studies, even when the average dose-rate is only a few primary ionization tracks per cell-nucleus? The combined weight of these nine studies is consistent with only ONE answer: There is no flawless repair and no safe dose or dose-rate with respect to radiogenic cancer.

So the crucial distinction between decisive evidence and inconclusive evidence is this: Decisive studies are consistent with only one answer to a question, and inconclusive studies are consistent with both positive and negative answers.

Reliance on Human Epidemiology :

Our disproof of the existence of any safe dose or dose-rate, with respect to human cancer-induction, relies exclusively on human epidemiological evidence, with the exception of cell-studies which we used for establishing the capacity for, and speed of, repair of radiation-induced lesions in DNA and chromosomes.

Our reliance on human epidemiological evidence is not a casual choice. It is by definite preference.

Everyone recognizes that evidence from other species can mislead us about humans, and that the same potential irrelevance surrounds evidence from in-vitro cell-studies. This is no denigration of those studies. It is just an acknowledgment that observations of real, whole humans are the only credible reality-check on ideas about how human beings "should" respond to low doses and irreducible dose-rates of ionizing radiation. The reality-check tells us how humans actually DO respond.

We readily acknowledge that single epidemiological studies can be flawed, just as laboratory experiments can be flawed, and mistaken conclusions can be drawn. For instance, an elevated cancer-rate can be falsely attributed to radiation, if the compared groups are not sufficiently comparable in their spontaneous

==

cancer-rates (the "Denver-Type" fallacy). In other words, a proper worry in epidemiology is that causation will be falsely inferred if some confounding variables -- which really explain the observations -- were not identified. In addition, it is inevitable that in any large body of studies, some statistical "flukes" will occur -- studies in which a highly significant result is nonetheless false. But experimental studies, with irradiated cells and irradiated animals of other species, ALSO suffer from occasional statistical "flukes," and they suffer enormously from confounding variables with respect to the response of real, whole humans.

Although we remain appropriately skeptical about single epidemiological studies, the nine epidemiological studies in Table 21-A reinforce and support each other, with features which make it reasonable to regard them as conclusive.

Basis for Confidence in the 9 Studies :

With respect to radiation as the cause of the excess cancer, readers will note that Table 21-A has five separate studies of excess breast-cancer in women. In addition to those five studies, excess breast-cancer is observed in the women of Hiroshima and Nagasaki, from their single acute exposure, in Swedish women irradiated for various benign breast lesions at the Radiumhemmet (Bara77) and in women irradiated for acute post-partum mastitis (Sho77; Sho86), both with some fractionation of dose, but not nearly so much fractionation as in the case of the fluoroscoped women. So, the epidemiologic studies available on radiation-induction of breast-cancer encompass virtually all the possible dose-rates and total doses. Moreover, the radiation sources include medical X-rays, A-bomb radiation, and gamma rays from radium-226 and daughters. In the aggregate, the case for causation is overwhelming.

In the studies -- singly -- of course there are bound to be some differences between the exposed and unexposed groups which will make the carcinogenic effect look bigger than it REALLY is in some studies, and smaller than it REALLY is in other studies. However, in studying the threshold issue, it is not necessary to know the EXACT magnitude of the effect. As long as the excess is real, the excess shows that repair-systems did NOT un-do all the carcinogenic damage flawlessly.

The breast-cancer studies are outstanding for their power. Four separate studies provide evidence of excess cancer after a large total dose was given in a series of very small doses, with the small doses well

enough separated in time that any repair which could operate has had an abundant opportunity to operate. These circumstances provide the best feature of high-dose studies -- namely large, clear results in terms of excess breast-cancers -- while still having the necessary features of low-dose studies with respect to the repair (threshold) issue. Thus analysts are not confronted by the usual problem at low doses: Small numbers of radiation-induced cancers against a background of large numbers of spontaneous cancers -- the low signal-to-noise ratio.

With the recent addition of breast-cancer evidence from the Israeli Scalp-Irradiation Study -- evidence gained from a single low total dose -- we have broadened the range of coverage to include females in the 5-15 year age-group at the time of their irradiation.

Three of the nine studies in our disproof of any safe dose or dose-rate are studies of in-utero irradiation at exceedingly low total doses of radiation, with a large effect in terms of excess cancers produced. Having three studies which mutually reinforce each other strengthens confidence in the meaning of each, and disposes of "third factor" ideas beyond a reasonable doubt.

It is possible that an important feature of the in-utero studies is that -- because they deal with children -- the studies are spared from many of the confounding variables which characterize radiation-studies of older groups. The focus on childhood cancers and leukemias means that the chance for non-radiation sources of cancer-induction to muddy the studies is reduced, because the studies can already become definitive in a single decade between exposure and cancer occurrence. Moreover, the greater radiation-sensitivity of the young makes for a larger excess than would be the case for older groups. Both features would tend to promote a favorable signal-to-noise ratio.

Lastly, in the Israeli Study, we now have two separate types of cancer induced -- thyroid and breast -- in a single large group of individuals, so that consistency of results is available to be checked. At this time, the consistency appears quite reasonable. The subjects should certainly be available for further follow-up, and therefore, the results, however they turn out, should not lack for adequate numbers of cases.

It is the combination of all these features which gives us full confidence that these nine studies are not aberrant or misleading. By any reasonable standard of evidence, their meaning is solid with respect to the threshold issue.

===

Epidemiology plus Track-Evaluation :

In recent years, it has been fashionable to suggest that epidemiologic investigations cannot usefully address the low-dose radiation question (e.g., Beir80, pp.22-23). The epidemiologic studies described here make it apparent that this is incorrect.

The effective use of case-control investigations, as in the in-utero studies, indicates that it is possible to overcome the difficulty of low cancer-rates. And the technique of "converting" high-dose studies to low-dose studies, as in the four breast-cancer investigations, permits having the large yield of cancers from a high-dose study while still providing full opportunity for any low-dose repair-mechanisms to prove their existence.

When the effort is made to evaluate the doses in such studies, in terms of tracks-per-nucleus, then it becomes evident that studies whose doses are not "next-to-zero" are nonetheless studies of truly minimal doses and dose-rates.

We suspect that, in terms of low-dose radiation questions, there must exist further opportunities of great value in still uninvestigated epidemiologic settings.

The "Not Proved in Peoria" Response :

The real-world, epidemiological evidence against any safe dose or dose-rate, summarized in Table 21-A, includes adults, children, high-energy gamma rays, diagnostic X-rays, acute single doses, and slow (chronic) occupational delivery. The average number of tracks per nucleus from each exposure was only 10-12 in the two studies with the HIGHEST track-rate. In five of the nine studies, the average track-rate was only 0.2937 up to 2.140. The observation of radiation-induced cancer in these studies is not compatible with the hypothesis that repair-systems un-do all carcinogenic damage, provided that the dose is sufficiently low and slow.

In the face of the evidence from Chapters 18 through 21, we anticipate that threshold proponents may demand that disproof of a threshold be made separately for each of over 100 sub-sets of cancer. Such a demand would be equivalent to saying, "So you've proven that the law of gravity is correct in Dallas, Texas, and in eight additional cities, but we don't accept that it is correct for Peoria, Illinois, until you prove it in Peoria specifically."

This position, which can be called "Not Proved in Peoria" or just "Peoria!" for short, has been the response to unwelcome evidence on a related issue (see Chapter 22). Therefore we anticipate it on the threshold issue, too.

We regard "Peoria!" as a scientifically inappropriate position, for the reasons below.

Scientists never have comprehensive data. We always are extending observations from a limited set of data and applying them to more general situations -- and the presumption of applicability is the reasonable presumption, in the absence of contrary evidence or logic. Indeed, when analysts refuse to do this and when they prefer sheer speculation to reasonable presumption grounded in evidence, then it may be a sign that objectivity has yielded to some sort of bias.

The radiation-inducibility of human cancer is now proven for most of the major sites of cancer-mortality, and also for many of the minor sites (Go85, pp.18-19). UNSCEAR is acknowledging it too: "It now appears that most (indeed, probably all) organs are vulnerable to radiation-induced cancer, given the right conditions of exposure" (Un88 p.460, para.394).

Here, then, we have a wide variety of cell-types which ALL display the SAME response to ionizing radiation, namely an excess of cancer above its spontaneous frequency. So the evidence demonstrates that, regardless of cell-type, there is a unity in the way human cells respond to ionizing radiation.

If this response were the only evidence at hand, and if there were no evidence available on the threshold-issue, it would be hard to find any scientist predicting, "When we get the evidence about the threshold-issue, it will turn out that some cell-types have a threshold and others do not." On the contrary. In view of the identical response of all cell-types to the agent (ionization tracks), the presumption would necessarily favor the SAME behavior by all cell-types on the threshold-issue. Most scientists understand the law of minimum hypotheses.

Additional Bases for Generalizing :

Now evidence on the threshold-issue DOES exist, and where it exists (childhood cancers, breast-cancer, thyroid-cancer), it shows that the threshold is provably absent. It would not be scientifically reasonable to presume that some cell-types have a threshold, when the threshold is provably absent where evidence DOES exist. The scientifically reasonable presumption clearly is that a threshold is absent in other cell-types also.

This presumption is further strengthened by related evidence, such as the evidence for a linear or supra-linear dose-response not only for breast-cancer and thyroid-cancer, but for all types of cancer in the aggregate (see Chapter 14), by strong evidence linking cancer with aberrations in DNA and chromosomal material, and by the evidence on the nature of radiation's interaction with cells regardless of their particular type (Chapter 19).

We do not overlook the fact that five of the nine decisive studies, in the disproof of any safe dose or dose-rate, are of breast-cancer. This fact increases the strength of the finding, because the evidence is arising from one of the two most serious and prominent cancers in women. Breast-cancer accounts for about 20 % of all their cancer mortality in the United States. Under the circumstances, it would be unthinkable to regard the disproof as limited to some RARE type of cancer. With respect to the no-threshold finding, it is fully reasonable to generalize from one of the most common cancer-sites to all cancer-sites.

=================

Table 21-A
Average Tracks per Nucleus, from Each Exposure in Nine Human Studies.

Number Assigned in the Text		Col.A Rads per Exposure	Col.B Tracks- per- Nucleus at 1 Rad	(Col.A times Col.B) Average Number of Tracks-per-Nucleus from Each Exposure	
1.	Nova Scotia Fluoroscopy	7.5	1.3378	10.0335	10 Rounded
2.	Israeli Scalp- Irradiation	7.5	1.3378	10.0335	10 Rounded
	(Authors' revised est.)	9.0	1.3378	12.0402	12 Rounded
3.	Massachusetts Fluoroscopy	4.6	1.3378	6.1539	6 Rounded
4.	Canadian Fluoroscopy (Excludes Nova Scotia)	4.6	1.3378	6.1539	6 Rounded
5.	Stewart In-Utero Series	0.5	1.3378	0.6689	< One 51 % with no track.
6.	MacMahon In-Utero Series	0.9	1.3378	1.2040	~ One
7.	British Luminizers	0.1	2.9370	0.2937	< One 75 % with no track.
8.	Harvey Twins In-Utero Series	1.0	1.3378	1.3378	~ One
9.	Israeli Breast-Cancer in Scalp-Irradiation Study	1.6	1.3378	2.140	~ 2

Entries in Column A come from the text of Chapter 21. Where more than one exposure
  occurred (Studies 1, 3, 4, 7), these entries are the average
  doses or delivery-rates at which higher total doses accumulated.
    See Chapter 18, Part 4 and Chapter 21, Part 1.
Entries in Column B come from Chapter 20, Table 20-K.
Entries on the righthand side are (Col.A times Col.B). For Studies 5 and 7, percents (of
  unhit nuclei) come from Tables 21-B and 21-C.

Table 21-B
Stewart In-Utero Study : Poisson-Predicted Distribution of Tracks per Nucleus.
Basis: The Poisson Equation (see Chapter 20, Part N).

For 30 KeV X-rays: The Stewart In-Utero Study
=================================
Mean number of TRACKS = 0.6689 TRACKS per cell-nucleus.
Question: How many nuclei will get 0,1,2,3,4,5,6,7,8 TRACKS?

```
  0.512272  PROBABILITY OF EXACTLY ZERO TRACKS PER CELL-NUCLEUS
  0.342659  PROBABILITY OF EXACTLY ONE TRACK PER CELL-NUCLEUS
  0.114602  PROBABILITY OF EXACTLY TWO TRACKS PER CELL-NUCLEUS
  0.025552  PROBABILITY OF EXACTLY THREE TRACKS PER CELL-NUCLEUS
  0.004273  PROBABILITY OF EXACTLY FOUR TRACKS PER CELL-NUCLEUS
  0.000572  PROBABILITY OF EXACTLY FIVE TRACKS PER CELL-NUCLEUS
  0.000064  PROBABILITY OF EXACTLY SIX TRACKS PER CELL-NUCLEUS
  0.000006  PROBABILITY OF EXACTLY SEVEN TRACKS PER CELL-NUCLEUS
 0.0000005  PROBABILITY OF EXACTLY EIGHT TRACKS PER CELL-NUCLEUS
  0.999999  SUM OF ALL THE ABOVE PROBABILITIES
```
===
0.145069 PROBABILITY OF TWO OR MORE TRACKS PER CELL-NUCLEUS
0.855 or 85.5 percent of nuclei receive either the Least Possible Disturbance (a single track) or no track at all, per exposure.

Table 21-C
British Luminizer Study : Poisson-Predicted Distribution of Tracks per Nucleus.
Basis: The Poisson Equation (see Chapter 20, Part N).

For Radium-226 and daughters: The British Luminizer Series.
=================================
Mean number of TRACKS = 0.2937 TRACKS per cell-nucleus.
Question: How many nuclei will get 0,1,2,3,4,5 TRACKS?

```
  0.745500  PROBABILITY OF EXACTLY ZERO TRACKS PER CELL-NUCLEUS
  0.218953  PROBABILITY OF EXACTLY ONE TRACK PER CELL-NUCLEUS
  0.032153  PROBABILITY OF EXACTLY TWO TRACKS PER CELL-NUCLEUS
  0.003148  PROBABILITY OF EXACTLY THREE TRACKS PER CELL-NUCLEUS
  0.000231  PROBABILITY OF EXACTLY FOUR TRACKS PER CELL-NUCLEUS
  0.000013  PROBABILITY OF EXACTLY FIVE TRACKS PER CELL-NUCLEUS
  0.999999  SUM OF ALL THE ABOVE PROBABILITIES
```
===
0.035546 PROBABILITY OF TWO OR MORE TRACKS PER CELL-NUCLEUS
Since the probability of more than five events (tracks) is so low, it is reasonable to refer to two-to-five events as "two or more".

0.9644 or 96.4 percent of nuclei receive either the Least Possible Disturbance (a single track) or no track at all, per exposure.

Additional tables in Chapter 20 provide additional Poisson distributions.

CHAPTER 22

The Popularity of Risk Reduction–Factors in the Radiation Community

This chapter is arranged in six parts:

1. Magnitude and Premise of Risk Reduction–Factors

The previous section of this book established that there is no safe dose or dose-rate of low-LET ionizing radiation, with respect to induction of human cancers.

This section takes up a separate issue: The general practice, by the radiation community, of REDUCING estimates of cancer-risk if the exposure is low or slow. This is the usual practice, whether or NOT any suggestion is made of a completely safe dose or dose-rate.

With the exceptions of breast-cancer and thyroid-cancer, the radiation community has been making its cancer risk-estimates for low-LET, low-dose exposures by asserting that the "effectiveness" or carcinogenic potency PER RAD is considerably less at low total doses than at high total doses, and also that the risk is considerably less if a dose is received slowly than if the same dose is received all at once.

In other words, the radiation community REDUCES estimates of risk-per-rad, observed in humans at acute high doses, by factors which are often called "dose effectiveness factors." There are two possible kinds of such factors: (1) one for the alleged reduction in cancer-risk per rad in going from a high total dose to a low total dose, all delivered acutely, and (2) one for going from a high dose-rate to a low dose-rate.

Definition and Magnitude of "DREFS" :

The NCRP (National Council on Radiation Protection) has, in essence, combined the two types as a single factor, referred to as the DREF, the dose-rate effectiveness factor. NCRP states that the DREF could also be called a "dose-magnitude effectiveness factor" (Ncrp80, p.9). A DREF is the ratio of two linear slopes: A steeper slope over a lower slope (Ncrp, p.176). The

significance of these slopes, demonstrated in the next chapter, need not be considered for now.

NCRP gives a range for its DREF factors as 2 to 10 for human carcinogenesis by low-LET radiation. Thus, if a human cancer-study provided cancer-risks per rad from observations at very high doses, these risk-rates would be DIVIDED by a factor of 2 to 10 to derive what NCRP considers appropriate estimates for cancer-risk per rad at low doses or low dose-rates.

Some users of DREFS refer to these very same factors as 0.5 to 0.1. They are simply MULTIPLYING the observed cancer-risks at high doses or high dose-rates by 0.5 to 0.1 instead of dividing by 2 to 10. The fractional formulation is in better accord with the formal meaning of "factor," which is defined by Webster's dictionary as "any of two or more quantities which form a product when multiplied together."

The Premise of DREFS :

The underlying premise of DREFS is that human dose-response for acute exposure is likely to have a concave-upward shape, except at extremely high doses. This premise is not only stated clearly in the NCRP report, but also in UNSCEAR 1977 and ICRP 1977 (see Part 3 of this chapter).

Of course, readers have seen for themselves in Chapters 13 and 14 that this premise is invalidated by the A-Bomb Study (1950-1982), whose dose-response has the opposite curve throughout the full dose-range. And readers are reminded that when RERF analysts, Shimizu and co-workers, examined all the A-bomb data 1956-1985, they too found the dose-response to be either linear or supra-linear (see Chapter 14, Part 2). Even if data in subsequent follow-ups were to produce a dose-response more linear than supra-linear, the underlying premise of a concave-upward shape would STILL be invalid.

==

Readers may wonder, "If the underlying premise of reduction-factors has already been invalidated, then why bother to discuss this topic at all?" Such a question assumes that human evidence will be ACCEPTED as the decisive reality-check on expectations concerning humans.

Our position is that it should be. Therefore, we are critical throughout this chapter whenever human epidemiological evidence of good quality is subordinated to non-human evidence.

Parts 2 and 3 of this chapter will show that "the general wisdom" of DREFS first emerged in the absence of good human epidemiological evidence, and also that, for many years already, good human evidence has been at variance with the underlying premise of DREFS.

Some readers will find it intrinsically interesting to see for themselves that, nonetheless, DREFS have been overwhelmingly popular and well embraced in the radiation community. This is demonstrated to mid-1989 by the statements provided in Part 3. Although we focus, in Part 2, on only three of the DREF documents, readers will find both earlier and later documents quoted in Part 3. (The quotations in this chapter may not be fully understood by readers who are unfamiliar with the linear-quadratic hypothesis of dose-response in this field. They may wish to study Chapter 23, Parts 1 and 2, BEFORE this chapter.)

In Chapter 23, we will show our own quantitative approach to risk-estimation for acute-low doses and for slow-low doses -- an approach which is CONSISTENT with the existing human evidence.

We call attention to our emphasis above on LOW doses: Acute-low and slow-low. As for HIGH total doses delivered slowly ("slow-high doses"), this topic is explored separately in Part 6 of Chapter 23.

2. A Historical Perspective

Although good human evidence on the shape of dose-response exists today, a couple of decades ago, the human evidence was very thin on this issue. Some animal experiments suggested that the dose-response relationships for tumorigenesis and certain other biological end-points were concave-upward, meaning that the cancer-risk per rad (cGy) could be higher at high doses than at low doses. If this were true for humans, then it would mean that extrapolation from high

doses to low doses in a linear fashion would overestimate the cancer-risk at low doses.

If one were to rely on some of the experimental animal data, and ASSUME the human dose-response relationship to be concave-upward, then reduction-factors would seem reasonable in trying to assess cancer-risks at low doses. And this was done. Over and over, one finds variants of the statement that "Radiobiological reasons exist for making this assumption in the absence of direct human data." (Allusions to radiobiology are allusions to evidence from other species and cell-studies, and to hypotheses derived therefrom.)

But by 1980, when NCRP produced its widely cited risk reduction-factors, human data were no longer absent.

1980 -- What the Record Shows :
=====================================

While the NCRP was preparing its 1980 report, its colleagues in the radiation community were concurrently preparing the BEIR-3 Report, with heavy reliance on the A-Bomb Study 1950-1974 (TR-1-77; Bee77; Bee78). For the reasons described in our Chapter 4, this is the key study. With respect to the A-Bomb Study, NCRP and BEIR-3 made five important admissions.

(1) Hiroshima -- Cancer Data :

As early as 1973, Baum (Baum73) noted that there was evidence in some of the Hiroshima-Nagasaki data for a DECREASING slope for cancer-risk per cSv with increasing dose -- just the opposite of what would be expected from some of the animal data. The radiation community suggested that the decreasing slope could be ascribed to cell sterilization (or killing) at very high doses.

In 1980, NCRP conceded that the effect was not limited to very HIGH doses: "Such an effect may be seen at relatively low doses in the Hiroshima data" (Ncrp80, p.160). In other words, the A-Bomb Study was warning that, in the human, the curve for cancer-risk versus dose might be supra-linear throughout the dose-range -- the opposite of the concave-upward expectation.

Besides the concave-DOWNWARD, supra-linear curvature in the Hiroshima dose-response (just mentioned), what were NCRP analysts able to see in 1980 ?

(2) Breast-Cancer Incidence :

In Ncrp80 (p.144, text and Table 10.3), the NCRP authors also acknowledged that breast-cancer incidence in the A-bomb survivors showed a supra-linear dose-response (a highly significant negative Q-coefficient in an L-Q model).

As we shall see below, BEIR-3 analysts were also unable to find any support in the A-bomb evidence for the concave-upward hypothesis.

(3) Nagasaki -- Cancer Incidence :

When the Nagasaki data for cancer-incidence were examined alone, the dose-response for all cancers combined (leukemia omitted) also warned against the use of risk reduction-factors for acute doses: "In the Nagasaki Tumor Registry data, the relationship between the radiation dose and the total incidence of all major cancers except leukemia is highly significant, and the observed dose-response relationship appears linear, with no suggestion of upward curvature" (Beir80, p.181).

(4) Both Cities -- Cancer-Deaths :

When all cancers (leukemia omitted) in Hiroshima and Nagasaki combined were analysed by BEIR-3, using the LQ-L model (the solitary L for the linear neutron-component), the dose-response was also found to be LINEAR. The Q-term was zero, as shown in Beir80, p.186, Table V-9, "Regression Analyses for LSS Mortality Data, 1955-1974 (excluding Leukemia)."

In the fine print, one discovers that BEIR-3 constrained the equation so that the quadratic term could NOT turn out negative. The Q term was "constrained to be nonnegative" (Beir80, p.186). We have noted elsewhere in this book that a negative Q-term means that a linear-quadratic model has a supra-linear (concave-downward) shape. Thus, when the BEIR-3 Committee constrained its equation to produce a nonnegative Q-term, the Committee had decided that a supra-linear dose-response must be ruled out. With the constraint upon it, the quadratic term turned out as zero -- the lowest value it could be, without being negative.

(5) Leukemia Registry Data :

With respect to dose-response for human leukemia in the A-bomb survivors, Beir80 gave enormous weight (as we shall see, in Part 3) to its concave-upward appearance in Nagasaki in the LSS sample. Because leukemia is only a single cancer among many, the data

were exceedingly thin -- especially when Nagasaki was examined alone. There were a total of 46 cases in all Dose-Groups combined.

RERF analysts (Bee78, p.198) had explicitly warned that, "In the face of the paucity of cases (or deaths) in the Nagasaki LSS sample in the low dose range, and the suggestion that the dose-response pattern for the entire Registry may be different, it would seem best not to invest too heavily in the nonlinear appearance of the LSS data."

By contrast, the Leukemia REGISTRIES for survivors in both cities contained far more data (Beir80, p.341). For Nagasaki, the Registry increased the cases from 46 (in the LSS sample) to 231, and for Hiroshima, from 120 (in the LSS sample) to 323 cases. BEIR-3 itself showed that the Registry data for leukemia were NOT concave-upward in either Hiroshima or Nagasaki (Beir80, p.343 Figure A-5).

Beside the A-Bomb Study :

The point is that, when the 1980 NCRP and BEIR-3 reports were issued, direct human data were certainly no longer lacking on the shape of dose-response for malignancies, and none of the data -- except the inappropriate leukemia sample -- supported the predicted concave-upward shape.

Indeed, NCRP itself described several minor human studies, at low doses, in which dose-response appeared concave-DOWNWARD (Ncrp80, pp.160-166). By the term "minor studies," we simply mean studies which inherently lack the scientific power of the A-Bomb Study (see Chapter 4). No disparagement of the work is implied.

And with respect to induction of human breast-cancer by low-LET radiation, there was already a succession of studies additional to the A-Bomb Study. Such studies pointed to a human dose-response which is linear, not concave-upward (Boi77, Boi79, Land80, My69, Sho77. It is proper to describe Land80 as an available analysis, because Land was a member of the BEIR-3 Committee -- see Chapter 37).

Breast-cancer is one of the two most prominent cancers in women (in the USA), and accounts for about twenty percent of all their cancer-mortality, as already noted in Chapter 21, Part 3. There is every reason to generalize from the breast-cancer data to dose-response for less important cancer-sites, in the absence of any contrary human evidence or contrary logic.

==

1980 -- The Evidence Was Seen :
==

Whether one considers only the A-Bomb Study, or additional studies too, the message from the direct human data was that risk reduction-factors were a mistake which would produce underestimates of cancer-risk at low acute doses. The direct human data were overwhelmingly suggesting linearity or supra-linearity by 1980. And I was not alone in seeing it (Go81). The record above shows that the NCRP and BEIR-3 radiation committees were seeing it too.

1980 -- Statement by NCRP :

Nonetheless, NCRP's 1980 report based DREFS on animal experiments rather than the available human epidemiology. NCRP explicitly admitted that its method could provide "no rigorously-defensible approach to deriving satisfactory DREFS for the human being" (Ncrp80, p.2):

"Because of the complexity and wide spectrum of the tumorigenic responses to radiation in the experimental animal, however, there appears to be no rigorously-defensible approach to deriving satisfactory DREFS for the human being, for either single tumor types or for all tumors collectively. Thus, the NCRP is reluctant at this time to go beyond providing a range of factors within which a single factor for the total yield of tumors in man after exposure of the whole body would probably lie. The DREF range is 2 to 10, when the actual absorbed dose is 20 rads or less, or the dose rate is 5 rads per year or less."

The tone of that statement suggests, to me, that NCRP was not eager to defend its DREFS. And if a lack of enthusiasm was present in NCRP's opening statement, it would have been appropriate, in my opinion. For in 1980 (Go81), I was examining the very same 1950-1974 evidence from the A-Bomb Study which NCRP had examined, and the evidence was indeed badly at variance with NCRP's underlying premise for DREFS -- namely, the premise of a concave-upward dose-response in the human.

1980 -- Statement by BEIR :

As for BEIR-3, the Committee split in bitter dispute over the shape of dose versus cancer-response in the human, with Harald Rossi arguing against any linear term at all, and for dominance of a quadratic term (Beir80, pp.254-260), and with the chairman, Edward Radford, arguing for a linear model (Beir80, pp.227-253).

In the end, the 1979 Draft Report was replaced by a compromise (Beir80, p.190), in which the Committee designated the linear-quadratic model (with a positive Q-term) as its preferred basis for making risk-estimates. (Details are in Part 3 of this chapter.) In other words, the human evidence was disregarded. According to Edward Webster, BEIR-3 member:

"A linear-quadratic dose/effect relationship, defensible in the light of current radiobiologic findings, has been adopted by most of the Committee members as a reasonable basis for prediction of risks of radiation-induced cancer" (Beir80, p.261).

1981 and 1983 -- Reduction-Factors Challenged :
==

Why Do Experts Disagree ?

By 1981, I reported that examination of the Hiroshima-Nagasaki evidence seriously pointed to a supra-linear relationship, between cancer-risk and dose of low-LET radiation, throughout the dose-range (Go81). This was the shape which the BEIR-3 Committee had ruled out, by actively constraining its equation (see above).

The finding in Go81 of supra-linearity, in agreement with Baum's earlier finding, had the additional weight of much more follow-up data since Baum's report. Furthermore, there was no basis for ascribing the supra-linearity to the presumed neutron-exposure at Hiroshima (see Chapter 8, Part 5).

People in and outside this field often ask, "Why do you experts disagree?" But it is not at all clear that we actually disagree about what the EVIDENCE is saying. If the BEIR-3 Committee had not artificially constrained its regression analysis (Table V-9), it probably would have found exactly what I reported from the same data in 1981 (Go81): A supra-linear, concave-DOWNWARD dose-response for radiation carcinogenesis in the human.

Of course, BOTH supra-linearity and linearity are incompatible with the use of risk reduction-factors for acute-low and slow-low doses. So the independent analysis in Go81 was a clear challenge to DREFS.

RERF Analysts Challenge DREFS :

In 1983, Wakabayashi and co-workers at RERF attempted to address the dose-response relationship in A-bomb survivors, by using cancer-incidence data for

Nagasaki. This choice was made because neutrons had never been considered prominent in the Nagasaki dose. These workers tried to compare a full quadratic model (Q), a linear-quadratic model (LQ), and a pure linear model (L) for the study of all cancers combined (omitting leukemia) in the Nagasaki cancer-incidence data. We quote the findings made by these workers directly (Waka83, pp.128-129). When they refer to "all cancers except leukemia," they do not mean that leukemia is different; they mean that leukemia is not part of the analysis:

"The Q model does not fit the incidence data on all cancers except leukemia, whereas the L and L-Q models fit equally well. The linear term is significant in the L-Q model, whereas the quadratic term is not. Thus the linear model appears to be the better for all cancers except leukemia. A similar tendency was observed for several specific sites of cancer, i.e. cancers of the lung, breast, thyroid, and stomach; the Q model either does not fit (for breast cancer) or fits more poorly than the L or L-Q model, and the quadratic term in the L-Q model does not differ from zero (the calculated value is negative). These findings, when compared with the analysis of the fit of these models to cancer-mortality in 1950-1978, where the neutron component was also considered, are seen to to be very similar.

"Thus it seems reasonable to use the linear model in risk estimation in the present analysis, though we cannot statistically distinguish one model from another among these three alternatives EXCEPT FOR CANCERS OTHER THAN LEUKEMIA AND FOR BREAST CANCER [emphasis added]. In the dissenting section in the BEIR III report, Rossi stated that the dose-response for mortality from all cancers in Nagasaki (1950-1974) fits a quadratic model best. The present analysis does not support this. Rather, the data suggest a linear model (see Radford's comments in the same dissenting section) or at least a linear-quadratic model, which the BEIR III Committee used as the basis of risk estimation." (Parentheses are in the original.)

Another Clear Warning :   So in 1983 -- only three years after the NCRP and BEIR-3 reports of 1980 -- Wakabayashi and co-workers were clearly alerting the radiation community (again) that for all cancers combined, and for breast-cancer specifically, the linear model fit best -- which meant that reduction-factors rested on a fantasy, with respect to the human evidence.

And in pointing out that the quadratic term in the L-Q model was negative (though not provably significantly so), they were alerting the radiation community (again) that supra-linearity might be the case.

1985 -- Refusal To Abandon DREFS :

In 1985, the radiation community produced two new reports on radiation risks: Nrc85 and Nih85. Both reports endorsed the use of DREFS in extrapolating from high acute to low acute doses, even though the real-world human evidence was at variance with the presumption on which the DREFS were based.

Exemptions from DREF-treatment have been made, however, one cancer-site at a time. If human evidence is conclusively against a concave-upward dose-response for a PARTICULAR kind of cancer, then DREFS are no longer used by the radiation community for that one site. Cancers of the breast and thyroid are examples of such exceptions.

For instance, the report of the NIH Working Group conceded that, for these two cancers, the linear model fit the data best, but its authors still were clinging to the concave-upward or linear-quadratic fit for all other cancers, with associated DREFS (Nih85, p.iv, p.55). In the quotation below, PC refers to Probability of Causation.

"In general, the Working Group has sought to use the dose-effect model for each cancer which is most consistent with both the human epidemiological data and the radiobiological data. For leukemia, the data are consistent with a so-called linear-quadratic model; hence this model is the basis for the PC tables calculated for leukemia. This model uses two constants and, in general predicts that small doses of radiation have a lesser effect per rad than do higher doses. There are radiobiological reasons for assuming that a linear-quadratic model is generally applicable to other cancers, which are discussed both in the BEIR III report and in Chapter III of the present report. Accordingly, we have used this approach for all cancers except those of the thyroid and breast. For carcinoma of the breast and thyroid, the data appear to be best described by a simple linear relationship in which the carcinogenic effect of radiation is directly proportional to dose; again the tables are based on this interpretation" (Nih85, p.iv).

An Eight-Point Commentary :

I consider the statements above to be faulted on several grounds:

(1) Human Evidence Disregarded :
Notwithstanding its claim of considering human epidemiological evidence as well as radiobiological data, the NIH report appears simply to disregard the findings

which show the LINEAR fit to be best for all human cancers combined, in both Beir80 (p.186, Table V-9) and in Waka83. The report also disregards my own 1981 analysis, which was highly suggestive of a SUPRA-linear fit for all human cancers combined, in the A-bomb survivor experience (Go81).

(2) Site-Specific Approach :

It is scientifically far better to use the findings based on all cancers combined, than to subdivide the observations by single sites of cancer. The NIH report invites error by examining each cancer-site separately. This approach CREATES the small-numbers problem, except for a very few common cancers. For all the other cancer-sites, when analysts attempt to analyse the sites one at a time, and the numbers pertaining to each are inadequate for reliable analysis, then spurious results are easily obtained.

(3) Leukemia Dose-Response :

The NIH Report rejected the data in the much larger Hiroshima and Nagasaki Leukemia Registries. As noted earlier in Part 2, those data do not fit the linear-quadratic, concave-upward model best; they fit the linear, or even the supra-linear model best. (See "1980 -- What the Record Shows" above; also Go81). It is interesting to note that, in the A-Bomb Study, the radiation community mounted a massive effort to revise the dose-estimates (DS86), but the community has made no meaningful effort to resolve the relatively minor problems which inhibit full use of the data-rich Leukemia Registries for both cities.

(4) Reasonable Presumption Rejected :

When all cancers combined (leukemia omitted) show a dose-response which is NOT concave-upward (Beir80, Go81, Waka83), and when two common types of cancer (breast and thyroid), analyzed separately, show a dose-response which is NOT concave-upward (Nih85), then the reasonable presumption is that the other cancers would NOT show a concave-upward dose-response either, if there were enough evidence to be reliable. However, in opting for the site-by-site approach, the NIH Working Group was rejecting the reasonable presumption.

(5) A Question of Consistency :

Substituting for the reasonable presumption, the NIH Working Group accepted "...radiobiological reasons for assuming that the linear-quadratic model is generally applicable to other cancers..." (Nih85, p.iv). Facing a choice between generalizing from strong, real-world evidence directly from the human, versus generalizing from other species and from their preferred radiobiological hypothesis, the NIH Working Group chose the latter -- and used risk reduction-factors.

The NIH Working Group appeared to require NO suitable human epidemiological evidence in order to embrace a concept (the concave-upward dose-response) which reduced risk-estimates, but appeared to require a MOUNTAIN of human epidemiological evidence -- extending to each cancer-site separately -- before embracing a concept (the linear dose-response) which would mean higher risk-estimates.

(6) "Not in Peoria!" :

Refusal by the NIH Working Group, to apply the findings from all cancer-sites combined to the individual cancer-sites, or from cancers of the breast and thyroid to other sites, amounted to the "Not in Peoria" response to evidence -- a response which we explained and criticized earlier (Chapter 21, Part 3). The Peoria approach, with special DREF-exemptions for cancers of the breast and thyroid, is found in additional reports from the radiation community (see Part 3).

No rational explanation has been offered in such reports for assuming that the shape of dose-response in one cancer would differ from the shape in another cancer -- an assumption which seems particularly irrational when, within the existing evidence, the shape is the SAME for thyroid-cancer, breast-cancer, and for all cancer-sites combined.

(7) No Demand from Radiobiology :

As we will show in Chapter 23, there was no reason for the NIH Working Group to have assumed that "radiobiological reasons" demand or even suggest the necessity of a concave-upward dose-response in the human.

For decades, it had been understood that a linear-quadratic equation can be modified away from a concave-upward shape by an exponential modifier, and that this should be done, if the modifier provides a better fit to actual observations than the equation without such a modifier. Indeed, the 1980 NCRP report itself is on record as recognizing this fact (Ncrp80, p.19, Figure 3.5).

However, it appears that the various radiation committees did not feel obliged to use the actual human observations. In the next chapter, we shall demonstrate how the linear-quadratic model, even with positive coefficients, can produce a curve which is concave-DOWNWARD (supra-linear) -- in accord with the the actual observations.

(8) Rejection of Human Evidence :

The NIH Working Group appears to have rejected the strong human evidence which was at variance with risk reduction-factors.

I do not object because the NIH Working Group appears to have paid no attention to my own work -- I object because it appears to have paid little attention to ANYONE'S work if that work was in conflict with DREFS.

3. The Exact Statements Which Convert Myth into Consensus

We call the supposed propriety of using DREFs a "myth" because the practice is in conflict with good human evidence. How a myth can become a general consensus may be illuminated by the chronological assembly of exact statements here about the expected concave-upward ("linear-quadratic") dose-response in humans and the consequent use of reduction-factors in risk-estimation. Our phrase above, "general consensus," is adapted from entry #9 below.

As far as we know, this assembly of exact statements has not been available before.
        1. UNSCEAR 1977
        2. ICRP 1977
        3. BEIR-3 1980
        4. NCRP 1980 (discussed above)
        5. NIH 1985 (discussed above)
        6. NRC 1985 and 1989
        7. Evans et al in 1986
        8. UNSCEAR 1986
        9. DOE 1987 and 1988
        10. Pierce 1987
        11. Preston and Pierce in 1987, 1988
        12. UNSCEAR 1988

Readers will see that some of these reports attempt to justify the use of risk reduction-factors, by prediction from non-human data and radiobiology, and that the rest simply quote the others as justification.

Although DREFS have spread throughout the literature and will be found at every turn, their basis is the same presumption stated by UNSCEAR and ICRP in 1977 -- a presumption which was invalidated in the same year by the reality-check of direct human data from the 1950-1974 A-Bomb Study (TR-1-77; Bee77).

1. The UNSCEAR Report of 1977 :

==

The United Nations Scientific Committee on the Effects of Atomic Radiation is UNSCEAR. Its individual analysts are acknowledged in our Chapter 37. These analysts addressed the topic of risk reduction-factors in Un77, Annex G, p.366, para.34-36 as follows.

(Para. 34): "Indeed, it has been suggested on theoretical grounds and microdosimetric grounds, that the tumour-inducing effect of radiation is likely to be represented substantially by the sum of a linear term in dose corresponding to the consequences of single events due to ionization tracks passing through sensitive cell structures, and of a quadratic term in (dose)^2 corresponding to damage due to two events. It must be emphasized therefore that the frequency of tumours induced per unit absorbed dose at a given dose level applies strictly to that dose level, and that the likely frequency per rad at low dose levels of a few rad or less, which are of most concern in radiation protection, cannot be assumed to be equal to the frequency observed per unit absorbed dose at higher levels."

A little further on, making use of the linear-quadratic relationship with 'a' being the coefficient of the linear term in dose and 'b' being the coefficient of the quadratic term in dose, UNSCEAR made some projections of what might be the "risk-reduction" at low doses. The authors then said the following:

"Data on the genetic effects of low-LET radiation in the mouse and on the induction of chromosome aberrations in several mammalian species including man which have been analysed in this way suggest values of b/a in the range of 0.01-0.03, and it has been suggested that similar values may apply for carcinogenesis. If this is so, it would indicate that estimates of carcinogenic effects per rad derived at doses of 100 rad of low-LET radiation could only overestimate the frequency of effects per rad at low dose by a factor of between 2 and 4."

A Strong Recommendation :

Later in its 1977 report, UNSCEAR strongly recommended that risk reduction-factors be used. Referring to its own central value of 1.0 per 10,000 per rad for the Cancer-Yield (including leukemia), the authors said (Un77, p.414, para.318):

"It is to be expected that low LET radiation is likely to be less carcinogenic per unit absorbed dose at doses of a few rads than at levels of one or a few hundred rads. For dose levels at which a leukemia induction rate of $(15-25)\ 10^{-6}\ rad^{-1}$ may apply (see 1196), a ratio of 4-6 between the frequency of other induced fatal malignancies and that for leukemia would imply a total for all fatal induced malignancies, including leukemia, of $(5-7)$ times $(15-25)\ 10^{-6}\ rad^{-1}$, suggesting a value of about 100 10^-6 rad^-1 at such dose levels. It must be emphasized again, however, that such a value is derived from mortalities induced at doses in excess of 100 rad. The value appropriate to the much lower dose levels involved in occupational exposure, and even more so in environmental exposures to radiation, may well be substantially less."

Basis -- An Assumption :

UNSCEAR's statements above ("... suggested on theoretical grounds...", "If this is so ...") made it very clear indeed that its suggestion of risk reduction-factors was based on its ASSUMPTION for humans of a linear-quadratic dose-response (with a positive coefficient for the quadratic term) -- in other words, the assumption of a concave-UPWARD dose-response. It is self-evident that the UNSCEAR risk reduction-factors of 2 to 4 (for going from high acute to low acute doses) would not apply at all, if the concave-upward dose-response relationship simply did not exist.

Subsequent information, published in 1977 and thereafter, has shown that the human dose-response is either concave-DOWNWARD or possibly linear, not concave-upward (see Part 2 of this chapter). The very basis of that early UNSCEAR suggestion of 2 to 4 as reduction-factors -- which was once reasonable enough as a hypothesis -- has been totally undermined by this later information.

Readers will see below what UNSCEAR had to say on the topic in its 1986 report.

2.   The ICRP Report of 1977 :
=======================================

In January, 1977, the International Commission on Radiological Protection (ICRP) adopted "Recommendations" which were published that year as ICRP Publication 26, in ANNALS OF THE ICRP (Icrp77). The publication identifies the editor and scientific secretary to have been Dr. F.D. Sowby, and the chairman to have been Dr. C.G. Stewart, Atomic Energy of Canada Ltd.

Paragraph 27 (p.6): "For radiation protection purposes it is necessary to make certain simplifying assumptions. One such basic assumption underlying the Commission's recommendations is that, regarding stochastic effects, there is, within the range of exposure conditions usually encountered in radiation work, a linear relationship without threshold between dose and probability of effect."

Paragraph 28 (pp.6-7): "The added risk from a given dose increment will depend on the slope of the dose-response relationship. If the dose-response relationship for stochastic processes is in fact highly sigmoid, the risk from low doses could be overestimated by making linear extrapolation from data obtained at high doses. There are radiobiological grounds for assuming that the dose-response curve for low-LET radiation will generally increase in slope with increasing dose and dose rate, over the absorbed dose range up to a few gray. For many effects studied experimentally, the response in this range can be represented by an expression of the form: $E = aD + bD^2$, where E denotes the effect, D the dose and 'a' and 'b' are constants. [ICRP footnote: "At high doses this expression would have to be modified to take account of the decreased tumour risk caused by cell sterilization."] The quadratic term (bD^2) in this expression predominates at high absorbed doses (generally above one gray) and high absorbed-dose rates (of the order of one gray per min); however, the linear term (aD) and the slope that it represents come to predominate as the dose and dose rate are reduced. Although a relationship of this form has been documented for a variety of effects, the relative values of the parameters 'a' and 'b' vary from one observation to another. The extent to which the relationship may differ for other situations remains to be determined. For human populations in particular, knowledge of dose-response relationships is too limited to enable confident prediction of the shapes and slopes of the curves at low doses and low dose rates. Nevertheless, in a few instances risk estimates can be based on results of irradiation of human populations involving single absorbed doses, of the order of 0.5 Gy or less, or to such doses repeated at intervals of a few days or more. In such cases it can be reasonably assumed that the frequency per unit absorbed dose of particular harmful effects resulting from such exposures is not likely to overestimate greatly the frequency of such effects in the dose range of concern in radiation protection, even though the latter may be received at much lower dose rates."

Paragraph 29 (p.7): "In many instances, however, risk estimates depend on data derived from irradiation involving higher doses delivered at high dose rates. In these cases, it is likely that the frequency of effects per unit dose will be lower following exposure to low doses or to doses delivered at low dose rates, and it may be appropriate, therefore, to reduce these estimates by a factor to allow for the probable difference in risk. The risk factors discussed later have therefore been chosen as far as possible to apply in practice for the purposes of radiation protection."

No Supporting Data Cited :

It is to be noted that ICRP Report 26 cites no evidence, no studies, and no sources whatsoever for any of its conclusions, and the report lacks even a list of references. One can assume, however, that Paragraph 28 includes early reports from the fluoroscopy studies cited in Chapter 21 of this book, when that paragraph refers to risk-estimates based on "single absorbed doses, of the order of 0.5 Gy or less, or to such doses repeated at intervals of a few days or more."

The ICRP's 1977 position on reduction-factors was interpreted as follows by Dr. Roger J. Berry, an ICRP member in 1987 (Berry87, p.122):

"The Commission also decided that for sparsely-ionizing radiations such as x- or gamma-rays the necessary interpolation between effects observed at high doses and those predicted at low doses ... should have some allowance for non-linearity of dose-response, with the vast majority of biological evidence to date suggesting that the dose-response would be concave-upwards."

Important Points Overlooked :

There are some important points made in the original ICRP statements, which are not widely appreciated.

(A) The ICRP stated very clearly in its Paragraph 28 that when the original estimates of risk are based upon observations at a total dose of 0.5 Gy (50 rads), or at higher doses which were fractionated into a series of individual exposures below 50 rads, it is reasonable to assume that NO risk reduction-factors are appropriate for the purpose of estimating "the frequency of such effects [risks] in the dose-range of concern in radiation protection."

(B) The ICRP was very clear in its Paragraph 28 in stating its uncertainty concerning the dose-response relationship in humans at low doses and dose-rates. What ICRP said was that, IF a concave-upward dose-response existed and IF risk-estimates were based on high doses delivered acutely, then risk reduction-factors would be indicated in order to derive risk-estimates for low-dose exposure.

One cannot disagree with this "if-then" position. But in 1977, apparently the ICRP was still unaware that the dose-response relationship in the 1950-74 A-Bomb Study was NOT concave-upward, but was linear or even concave-DOWNWARD. The ICRP's own words make it clear that, if ICRP had known the human dose-response relationship was going to be linear or

concave-downward throughout the dose-range, when enough data were in, ICRP would not have suggested any risk-reduction factors at all, for extrapolations from high acute to low acute doses.

3. The BEIR-3 Report of 1980 :

In 1972, the BEIR-1 Committee had adopted the linear model of dose-response for all cancers (Beir72). Its individual analysts are acknowledged in our Chapter 37.

By contrast, the BEIR-3 Committee was bitterly split over its position on dose-response, as already noted in Part 2 of this chapter. A compromise subcommittee was established (see Chapter 37), and in the end, the linear-quadratic, concave-UPWARD dose-response was declared as the model "which most members of the Committee prefer" for cancer-risk estimation (Beir80, p.190) -- (breast excepted, p.275, and thyroid excepted, p.301).

Where did the 1980 BEIR-3 Committee obtain this concave-upward curve, and a suitable equation, when its own analysis of the A-bomb survivors showed no positive Q-term at all in the linear-quadratic fit (see Part 2 of this chapter) ? BEIR-3 replaced the linear dose-response which it found for ALL cancers (Beir80, p.186, Table V-9), by adapting the LEUKEMIA curve -- which showed the preferred shape (see Part 2). This substitution is unmistakable in Beir80, pages 186-187, 250.

The record shows that the BEIR-3 Committee was fully acquainted with the evidence showing that dose-response for leukemia was also LINEAR (not concave-upward) when the Leukemia Registries were used instead of the tiny LSS sample (Beir80, p.341, p.343 - Figure A-5). Yet BEIR-3 chose to base its preferred risk-estimates for ALL cancers on the curve provided by the flimsy data for LEUKEMIA in the Nagasaki LSS sample.

The record shows also that in trying to fit the data for all cancers combined to the linear-quadratic model, the BEIR-3 Committee placed an "active constraint" upon the LQ equation so that the quadratic term could NOT be negative (Beir80, p.186). Constrained in this way, the Q-term then turned out as zero -- the lowest possible value without being negative (negative meaning supra-linearity).

Thus BEIR-3 was left with only a LINEAR term, and this too was incompatible with reduction-factors for

==

estimating risk at acute-low or at slow-low doses. However, BEIR-3's linear finding received little attention after the report endorsed the "preferred" concave-UPWARD model.

4. The NCRP Report of 1980 :
5. The NIH Report of 1985 :

====================================

These reports were discussed in Part 2 of this chapter. Both of them made the assumption of a concave-UPWARD dose-response, and so both of them supported the use of risk reduction-factors for extrapolating from high acute doses to low doses.

6. The NRC Report of 1985, and 1989 Up-Date :

====================================

In 1985, the (U.S.) Nuclear Regulatory Commission published its NUREG/CR-4214 report on health effects from a nuclear power accident (Nrc85). In May 1989, the NRC issued a revised version of the same report (Nrc89). In both versions, the section on radiation-induced cancer was written by Ethel Gilbert, an analyst at Battelle Pacific Northwest Laboratories.

This report addressed the issue of risk reduction-factors, but introduced nothing at all in the way of information concerning the issue. Instead, without any critical analysis, the NRC Report simply applied the mid-value of the range proposed by NCRP in 1980. We quote a passage which is identical in both the 1985 and 1989 versions:

"For most cancer-types, the central estimates are obtained by modifying the linear risk estimates ... by the factor 0.30 + 0.47D (where D is the dose in Gy), resulting in a linear-quadratic function of dose. The intent of using this factor is to account for the reduction in effects likely to result from the low doses and dose rates expected to be experienced by much of the exposed population in a nuclear power plant accident. The factor 0.3 is obtained as the midpoint of the range 0.1 to 0.5 suggested by NCRP (1980) ... " (Nrc85, p.II-99; Nrc89, p.II-125).

Appeal to Authority :

The range suggested by NCRP was indeed 0.1 to 0.5 (or 2 to 10). By citing Ncrp80, the NRC Report was using the "appeal to authority" device, as if Ncrp80 had presented a convincing scientific basis for the factors. The NRC Report does not warn its readers that the NCRP itself had warned that the reduction-factors (A)

were not based on human evidence, and (B) were NOT "rigorously defensible" as satisfactory for humans (Ncrp80, p.2).

The NRC Report simply copied NCRP in its use of a linear-quadratic relationship (except for breast and thyroid cancer). NRC provided no evidence for a linear-quadratic relationship, and it demonstrated no awareness of the considerable evidence already available that the human dose-response for all cancers combined was NOT concave-upward. By adopting the linear-quadratic relationship (with an inferred positive coefficient for the quadratic term), NRC was necessarily assuming a concave-upward dose-response.

The NRC Report, adopting the "Not in Peoria" approach like the NIH 1985 report, did concede the linear relationship for cancers of the breast and thyroid. Referring to DREFS, the NRC Report said: "Exceptions to the use of these reduction factors in obtaining central estimates are breast and thyroid cancer. For breast cancer, the non-age-specific linear estimate is used without modification of the central estimate" (Nrc85, p.II-99). In the 1989 version, the first sentence has been modified: "Exceptions to the use of these reduction factors in obtaining central estimates are breast cancer, thyroid cancer, and cancers resulting from in utero exposure" (Nrc89, p.II-125).

7. Evans and Co-Workers, 1986, New England Journal of Medicine :

====================================

John S. Evans, of the Harvard School of Public Health, was one of the three principal authors of the 1985 Nuclear Regulatory Report (Nrc85), and he is also one of three co-authors of the article in the NEW ENGLAND JOURNAL OF MEDICINE (Sept. 25, 1986), "The Influence of Diagnostic Radiography on the Incidence of Breast Cancer and Leukemia" (Evans86). Not surprisingly, the statements in the NEJM article pertaining to risk reduction-factors are just like the statements in Nrc85 and in Ncrp80. We quote from Evans86 (p.811). The parenthesis was in the original:

"Common approaches for extrapolating results to low doses involve one of two assumptions. In some types of cancer, low doses of radiation may be as effective (per unit of dosage) as high doses in inducing tumors. In others, low doses are perhaps only 1/10 to 1/2 as effective."

Thus, in two sentences, risk-reduction factors and the Peoria approach to dose-response have been conveyed to the medical community.

===

Building the Consensus :

A few paragraphs later, the authors speak specifically of breast cancer: "The equation describing the 'central estimate' relies on the relative risk projection method and includes only a linear term because there is little evidence to suggest that the risk is reduced at lower doses" (and they cite Boice79; Waka83; Kato82; Sho77). In other words, like Nrc85, Evans86 accepts the possibility that there is no reduction factor for breast-cancer.

For leukemia, however, Evans86 "assumes that a low dose of radiation is 30 percent as effective (per unit dosage) as a high dose in inducing leukemia" (parenthesis in the original), and the authors cite Gilbert (Nrc85) for support.

In summary, the assumptions of Ncrp80 and Nrc85 with regard to risk-reduction factors have been transmitted to the medical community. Nowhere in Evans86 is there acknowledgment that the human evidence for all cancers combined is totally at variance with the statement that, for some cancers, "... low doses are perhaps only 1/10 to 1/2 as effective ..." as high doses.

8. UNSCEAR Report of 1986 :

===

UNSCEAR-86, in its summary on radiation carcinogenesis, states (Un86, p.243, para.483): "Recent experimental findings on radiation-induced tumours in experimental animals have not substantially changed the main conclusions reached in annex I of the 1977 UNSCEAR report. Most data support the notion that dose-response relationships for x and gamma rays tend to be curvilinear and concave upward at low doses. Under these conditions, tumour induction is dose-rate dependent, in that a reduction of the dose rate, or fractionation, reduces the tumour yield. A linear extrapolation of the risk from doses delivered at high rates to zero dose would thus, as a rule, over-estimate the real risk at low doses and dose rates."

And (p.243, para.485): "Having reviewed existing data on dose-response relationships for radiation-induced tumours in man, UNSCEAR considers that this whole matter must be treated with caution because at the present time observations are fragmentary ... For sparsely-ionizing radiation, in some cases (lung, thyroid, breast), the data available are consistent with linear or linear-quadratic models ..." Bone sarcoma is the only solid cancer for which UNSCEAR-86 asserts that the linear model would "definitely" overestimate the risk in humans (p.243, para.486).

UNSCEAR takes a site-specific "Peoria" approach to analysis, one organ at a time. Since of course there is not a human database for each separate cancer with the size and statistical power which comes from all cancers COMBINED in the A-Bomb Study, the site-specific approach means that UNSCEAR is likely to say, indefinitely and perhaps forever, that human evidence is lacking at low doses. However, this lack is quasi-artificial -- a result of insisting that each organ be considered in isolation. In 1986, all cancers COMBINED in the A-Bomb Study (1950-1982) were clearly showing (A) radiation-induced excess at a LOW dose, and (B) a dose-response curve which was NOT concave-upward.

Instead of generalizing from the all-site human data, UNSCEAR-86 prefers to generalize from the non-human ("experimental") data. Referring to "other organs" besides breast, thyroid, lung, bone, Un86 states (p.244, para.490):

"For radiation-induced cancers of other organs, only experimental data are available. For sparsely-ionizing radiations upward concave curvilinear dose-response relationships with pronounced dose-rate and fractionation effects are usually found. If similar curves should apply to cancers in man, a linear extrapolation of risk coefficients (obtained at the intermediate dose region after acute irradiation) to the low dose and low dose rates, would very likely over-estimate the real risk, possibly by a factor up to 5."

Thus, UNSCEAR-86 becomes a recent source cited by others (for instance, by Preston and Pierce in TR-9-87 or Pr87b, p.34,35,36) as possibly justifying use of risk reduction-factors. The reduction-factors of 1.5 to 3.0 cited by Preston and Pierce come from Un86, p.191, para.153, as quoted below. The parentheses are in the original. "10 mGy" is the same as 1.0 rad.

"The linear-quadratic model may be characterized by the quotient of the induction constants ($a1/a2$), which varies with the radiation quality and the specific biological effect. For high-LET particles, this quotient is so high that the contribution of the dose-squared term may normally be neglected. The model then becomes linear. For low-LET radiation (considering chromosomal exchanges, mutations, and induction of some malignancies) the $a1/a2$ quotient is between 0.5 and 1.5 Gy. The over-estimation of the probability of effects at about 10 mGy from single-dose data at 1-2 Gy (acutely delivered) by linear (as opposed to linear-quadratic) extrapolation would vary from 1.5 to 3.0 for an assumed reasonable set of parameters."

Readers may note that Un86 uses a1 and a2 as the coefficients for the linear and quadratic terms, respectively, whereas other sources (including Un77) often use a and b for these coefficients. Also, readers may be perplexed that Un86 gives the ratio (a1/a2) in units of grays. This is done because the dose-units of a1 (the linear coefficient) are Gy^-1, the units of a2 (the quadratic coefficient) are Gy^-2. Therefore, on division we have Gy^-1 / Gy^-2, which is 1 / Gy^-1. Since this is the same as Gy, the ratio can be expressed in grays. This is awkward, so we use an alternative in Chapter 23, Part 2.

UNSCEAR is suggesting that, for "some malignancies," the dose at which the linear contribution to cancer-induction equals that for the quadratic contribution lies between 50 and 150 rads (0.5 and 1.5 Gy). We shall be returning in Chapter 23 to this issue of potential doses at which the linear and quadratic contributions to cancer may be equal, and to the issue of how such information is appropriately used.

9. The DOE Report of June 1987 and December 1988 :

In June 1987, the (U.S.) Department of Energy (DOE) published its estimates of the health consequences from the explosion of the Chernobyl nuclear power plant in a report DOE/ER-0332 (Doe87). On the issue of risk reduction-factors, Doe87 says the following (Section 7.2.1, pages 7.3 and 7.4). Parentheses are in the original:

"In the majority of epidemiologic studies, the excess cancer-risk coefficients depend on data derived from irradiation involving high doses delivered at high dose rates. The frequency of effects per unit dose is lower for exposures to low doses delivered at low dose rates. The UNSCEAR (1977) considered it appropriate to reduce these risk coefficients (and hence, risk estimates) by a factor on the order of 2.5 to 3 to adjust for the probable reduction in risk. Interpolation of risk coefficients from the high dose level at which effects in humans are observed down to zero has been done on a linear basis to assess an upper estimate of risk ..."

"In its 1980 report, the BEIR Committee (NAS/NRC 1980) considered the effect of dose-rate on dose-response relationships. For high-LET radiation, some evidence shows that protraction of dose over time, i.e., delivery of the same dose at lower rates, increases the cancer risk per unit of dose. For low-LET radiation, as encountered from the Chernobyl releases, human data on chronic exposure at low dose rates is limited; however, experimental data in animals strongly indicate

that a given dose of low-LET radiation would produce fewer effects at low dose rates than at high dose rates. A reduction factor of two to three has been considered in the 1980 BEIR Report, based on both human and animal data. However, evidence from all these studies indicates that, for a single exposure to low absorbed dose, e.g., between 0 and 0.2 Gy (0 and 20 rad), of low-LET radiation delivered at any dose rate, and from any total dose delivered at a dose rate of 0.05 Gy/yr (5 rad/yr) or less, dose-effect reduction factors are likely to be between two and ten (NCRP 1980)."

"General Consensus" Declared :

All that the DOE Report contributes on the issue of risk reduction-factors is to copy UNSCEAR 1977, BEIR-3 1980, and NCRP 1980.

In December 1988, when Doe87 was carried in abbreviated form by the journal SCIENCE, the presumption of a linear-quadratic (concave-upward) dose-response was presented as if it were scientifically solid:

"For latent health effects such as fatal cancers and genetic disorders, the scientific community has reached general consensus on a model derived from a linear-quadratic dose-risk relation ..." (Ansp88, p.1515).

10. Pierce, at OECD Meeting in Paris, October 1987 :

Donald Pierce, RERF analyst and co-author of TR-9-87 and TR-12-87, gave a paper in Paris in which he was discussing risk-estimates based on the recent follow-ups of the A-bomb survivors. In that paper, Pierce had the following to say about extrapolation to low doses (Pier87):

"A final element in risk estimation involves extrapolation to low doses. There is a substantial body of radiobiological theory which bears on this, and yet there remains great uncertainty. The primary reason for raising this here is to insure that the above discussion is not misinterpreted as pertaining directly to low-dose risks. The BEIR-III LQ-L model, which provided more or less the central value in their 'envelope' of low-dose extrapolations, had the effect of dividing their linear low-dose extrapolations by 2.25. A recent UNSCEAR Report (1986), containing very useful discussion of many aspects of radiogenic risk estimation, suggests using a range of 1.5 to 3.0 in place of this factor. Work in progress at RERF suggests that within the context of LQ-L models the upper part of the range of 1.5 to 3.0

===

suggested in UNSCEAR-86 is quite inconsistent with the RERF data. This should not be taken too strongly however, since it depends entirely on the LQ-L assumption and since there is a great deal of other scientific information to be taken into account."

Dr. Pierce does not comment on the fragmentary basis for the UNSCEAR 1986 factors, but he does point out in a somewhat obscure manner that the upper range of those projections is "quite inconsistent" with the RERF data.

High-Dose Data Need Increase-Factors :

It is hard to see why he is discussing LQ-L models at all, in view of the curve he presents in a figure in his paper -- a curve which is far more consistent with supra-linearity of dose-response. Indeed, in TR-9-87 (pp.29-32), Pierce acknowledges that the A-Bomb Study shows a non-linear dose-response which is concave-downward (supra-linear) at high doses. Thus, if high-dose data were used to make estimates at low doses, risk INCREASE-factors, not risk REDUCTION-factors, would be needed.

11. Preston and Pierce in RERF Report TR-9-87 :

=====================================

Preston and Pierce, co-authors of TR-9-87 (Pr87b), briefly mention DREFS or risk reduction factors as point (ii) in presenting their own estimates of Lifetime Fatal Cancer-Yields at low doses:

"To make such estimates requires a number of assumptions, the most critical of which involve: (i) extrapolation of the nonleukemia risks beyond the current follow-up, especially for those individuals who were young when exposed; and (ii) the method used for extrapolation to relatively small doses from the range of 1-2 Sv" (Pr87b, p.34).

In Table 13-A of this book, entries C3, C4, and C5 clearly show that there are direct observations in the A-bomb survivors at 14.6, 40.6, and 74.2 cSv (Dose-Groups 3, 4, and 5, in the DS86 dosimetry). It is utterly perplexing why RERF analysts are still discussing extrapolations downward from doses like 100-200 cSv. Not only are such extrapolations unnecessary, but the high-dose observations suffer from the small-numbers problem and are inherently LESS reliable than the lower-dose observations. Indeed, we combined Dose-Groups 6, 7, and 8 for that reason.

Preston and Pierce continue (in the same paragraph): "Regarding point (ii), it is suggested in a recent UNSCEAR report (Annex B, paragraph 153) that linear extrapolation in this setting will overestimate low-dose risks by a factor of 1.5 to 3.0. This is a major source of uncertainty which must remain in the following calculations" (Pr87b, p.34. Parentheses are in the original).

The last statement suggests that the authors had some reservations about the goodness of the UNSCEAR estimate of risk reduction-factors, and if so, such reservations would be in line with Pierce's statement quoted above (Pier87) that there was real inconsistency of Un86's factor of 3 with the RERF data.

The inconsistency is glaring. Readers are referred back to Chapter 14, Part 2, where we quoted from TR-12-87 (Shi87, p.28-30). The authors of that report -- and both Preston and Pierce are co-authors -- find that dose-response in the DS86 sub-cohort is linear or supra-linear -- not concave-upward.

Power of Persistence :

Nonetheless, in their tabulation of Lifetime Fatal Cancer-Yields, Preston and Pierce displayed their linear estimates and then showed reduction by factors of 1.5 and 3.0. Their tabulation is reproduced below (from Pr87b, p.35):

Lifetime Fatal Cancer-Yields from TR-9-87, p.35.

RBE	Linear Esti- mate	Range suggested by use of UNSCEAR factors for low-dose extrapolation
5	16.7	5.6 - 11.1
10	16.2	5.4 - 10.8
20	15.2	5.1 - 10.1

The tabulation above demonstrates the power of risk reduction-factors to persist in the radiation community and in the literature (A) despite the absence of any need for extrapolation from high to low doses -- since direct human observations exist at low doses, and (B) despite the presence of human evidence which invalidates the key premise on which the factors rest -- namely, a concave-upward dose-response.

When TR-9-87 appeared in its abbreviated form in the journal RADIATION RESEARCH (Pr88), the use of reduction-factors upon linear values was demonstrated again -- apparently for the purpose of facilitating comparisons with BEIR-3 and UNSCEAR.

(We use the linear risk-value from Pr88 in our

Chapter 24, Part 7. It is much lower than the linear value for RBE 10 shown above. We have made no error. Readers were warned in our Chapter 4 that the full RERF report and the abbreviated version are not the same on this key matter.)

12. UNSCEAR Report of 1988 :

Early in its 1988 report, UNSCEAR announces that some HUMAN evidence has developed to support the use of risk reduction-factors for slow delivery of low-LET radiation (Un88, p.34, para.208):

"The Committee concluded in 1986 that for some tumours, i.e., carcinomas of the female breast and perhaps of the thyroid a linear relationship at low and intermediate doses of low-LET radiations gave a good fit; for others a linear fit could not be rejected statistically but other models, e.g., linear quadratic and quadratic approximated the data equally well. These observations are still assumed to be basically correct, however, evidence presented recently to the Committee suggests that fractionated doses at very low doses per fraction may be less effective in inducing breast cancer than deduced previously from the linear relationship and apparent lack of dose-fractionation effects. [We are splitting the Un88 paragraph here.]

"Recent epidemiological studies on patients administered 131-iodine-iodides for diagnostic purposes suggest that low-LET radiation at low dose rates is also significantly less effective than intermediate and high doses delivered at high dose rates. This means probably that the dose-response relationship for induction of cancer of the thyroid gland is also non-linear (upward concave) as was suspected in the UNSCEAR 1986 Report" (Un88, p.34, para.208).

The breast-cancer study to which Un88 is referring is the Canadian Fluoroscopy Study as reported by Howe in 1984. The radio-iodine studies to which Un88 is referring are the studies in Sweden by Holm and co-workers (Holm80, Holm88).

UNSCEAR-88 presents the Holm studies as human evidence supportive for a risk reduction-factor of at least 3 and possibly even 4 for slow delivery (Un88, p.491, para.604).

And UNSCEAR-88 presents the Howe report as human evidence supportive for a risk reduction-factor of at least 3 for low dose or low dose-rate (Un88, p.492, para.605).

Then UNSCEAR-88 concludes its summary on

"Risks at Low Doses and Low Dose Rates" as follows (p.492, para.607):

"From examination of both experimental and human data the Committee concludes that the carcinogenic effects of low-LET radiation are generally smaller at low doses and at low dose rates compared with those at high doses and dose rates. The reduction factors will vary with dose and dose rate and with organ system but will generally fall within the range 2 to 10."

Readers will recognize, of course, the familiar "two to ten" range first suggested by NCRP in 1980. It was based almost exclusively on non-human data. When UNSCEAR-88 now adds the allusion to human evidence, Un88 is relying very heavily on the "recent" Howe and Holm studies.

Because the issue of risk reduction-factors is of such importance, we will examine the Howe Study (and its 1989 up-date) in Part 4 of this chapter, and then the 1988 Holm Study in Part 5 of this chapter.

4. Unwarranted Conclusions from the Canadian Fluoroscopy Study

As we explained in Chapter 21, Part 1, the Canadian Fluoroscopy Study consists of two distinct series: The Nova Scotia women (number 1 in Chapter 21) versus the other-Canadian women (number 4 in Chapter 21). The Nova Scotia series is distinct in at least two ways. First, the total breast-dose accumulated was much higher, and second, the per-rad risk appears higher than in the other-Canadian series.

UNSCEAR-88, as noted in our Part 3 above, is suggesting that the lower per-rad risk in the other-Canadian series (Howe84) is supportive evidence for a dose-RATE effect.

In at least three separate places, Un88 cites the conclusion by Howe 1984 that the dose-response in the Canadian Fluoroscopy Study is either linear-quadratic or quadratic -- in other words, concave-upward (Un88, p.439, para.241; p.455, para.361; p.456, para.367).

The next year, November 1989, an up-date of the Canadian Fluoroscopy Study was published (Miller 1989) on which Howe was a co-author. In the up-date, the authors now disagree with the statement which is so important to UNSCEAR-88. In Mi89, the authors state (Mi89, p.1287):

"... the evidence from Table 2 indicates that the most

appropriate form of dose-response relation is a simple linear one, with different slopes for Nova Scotia and the other provinces ... For these models there was no evidence of any upward curvature in the dose-response relation (i.e., the addition of a quadratic term did not significantly improve the fit ...).

We are not in any position to make an independent evaluation of the dose-response relationship in the Canadian Study. We would need raw data before their reduction, and these data are not published.

What needs emphasis is that UNSCEAR's statement is now in conflict with the more RECENT statement by the study's own authors.

UNSCEAR-88, in the search for human evidence to support its recommendation of risk reduction-factors for slowly delivered doses, suggests that the lower per-rad risk in the other-Canadian series compared with the Nova Scotia series is due to a 20-fold lower dose-rate per exposure for the other-Canadian series:

"In Nova Scotia, the patients were examined in the anterior-posterior position (facing the x-ray tube) whereas in the other provinces the patients were mainly examined in the reverse position, resulting in doses per fraction about 20 times smaller" (Un88, p.456, para.367).

Miller, Howe and co-workers make a similar comment in their discussion-section (Mi89, p.1288): "The only substantial difference in the dose-estimation procedures for Nova Scotia and the other provinces was in the proportion of women who faced the x-ray source. This difference is well established, and even varying the proportions substantially does not eliminate the difference in the slopes. One possible biologic reason for this difference is a dose-rate effect. Although the mean numbers of fluoroscopic exposures were similar, the rate per unit dose was more than an order of magnitude greater in Nova Scotia than in the other provinces."

Unwarranted Conclusions :

Both Un88 and Mi89 are mistaken in their conclusions that a dose-rate difference up to 20-fold EXISTS between the Nova Scotia series and the other-Canadian series. In reality, the biologically relevant rate at which total doses were accumulated in the two series was not even two-fold apart.

Readers are referred back to Chapter 21, Part 1, Study 3 (Massachusetts Fluoroscopy). There, we showed that the average delivery-rate of the rads in that study -- which is the same as the other-Canadian series, Study 4 -- is about 4.6 rads at one time. The average delivery-rate of the rads in the Nova Scotia series is about 7.5 rads at one time. The ratio of delivery-rates is (7.5 / 4.6), or 1.63 -- far below a factor of 20. This finding is due to the fact that only a very small fraction (about 13 %) of the total rads received in the other-Canadian series was received at the low dose-rate of 0.261 rad per exam.

Table 21-A provides a convenient way to compare all three fluoroscopy studies, not only in delivery-rate of the rads at one time, but in the tracks-per-nucleus at one time. In the Nova Scotia series, the tracks-per-nucleus are 10.0335 compared with 6.1539 in the other-Canadian series.

In other words, there is no meaningful difference in dose-rate between the studies.

Moreover, at such low doses and track-rates, the quadratic term (for inter-track carcinogenesis) is just negligible -- as is generally acknowledged -- and as is illustrated in our Chapter 23, Part 7. Thus, there is not even a basis in principle for invoking a dose-rate effect to explain the different slopes or per-rad risks in the Nova Scotia versus other-Canadian series.

In any case, we have shown that no appreciable difference in dose-rate EXISTS between the two series. Thus, the Canadian Fluoroscopy Study provides no human evidence supportive of a dose-rate effect.

5. Unwarranted Conclusions from the Holm Radio-Iodine Study

We are going to give some close attention here to a particular study of patients who received diagnostic radio-iodine, because the study has been recently featured by the 1988 UNSCEAR Committee as important human evidence supportive of a dose-rate effect (Un88, p.34, para.208, and p.459, para.389, and p.491, para.602, 604).

The study is "Thyroid Cancer after Diagnostic Doses of Iodine-131: A Retrospective Cohort Study," by Holm and eleven co-workers, published in the (U.S.) JOURNAL OF THE NATIONAL CANCER INSTITUTE, September 21, 1988 (Holm88). A preliminary report on a small fraction of the study-sample was published in 1980 (Holm80a, Holm80b).

The 1988 report states in its abstract, "Overall, these data provide little proof that I-131 is carcinogenic in humans and support the notion that the carcinogenic potential of internal I-131 beta particles might be as low as four times less than external x rays or gamma rays" (Holm88, p.1132). The same report states in its closing discussion, "... I-131 did not increase thyroid cancer risk in this cohort ..." (Holm88, p.1137).

This is the message which is used by others as human evidence supporting a safe-dose or at least a greatly reduced risk if exposure is gradual rather than acute. (A single dose of Iodine-131 decays gradually, and does not deliver its total dose to the thyroid all at one instant.)

As noted above, the 1988 UNSCEAR Committee features the Holm Study as important human evidence supporting the Committee's decision to recommend large risk-reduction factors, for radiation doses which are slowly delivered. Individual authors of the 1988 UNSCEAR Report are acknowledged in our Chapter 37. Lars-Erik Holm is among them.

Edward Webster, also a member of the 1988 UNSCEAR Committee (and a key member of the BEIR-3 Committee), features the 1980 Holm Study in the course of claiming that the cancer-consequences from Chernobyl will probably be small (see our Chapter 24, Part 9). Webster says (Webs87, p.424): "The effect of protraction [slow delivery of dose] may be the reason why iodine-131 has been judged to be three times less effective as a carcinogen per unit dose than x-rays delivered at high dose rates (Ncrp85, Table 11.3). This conservative judgment was largely based on the investigation by Holm et al (Holm80a) which found no excess thyroid cancer in 10,000 patients who had received gland doses between 58 rem (adults) and 159 rems (persons aged less than 20) after an 18-year follow-up."

Rosalyn Yalow, a co-author of the 1985 NIH Report on radiation risk (Nih85), also features Holm80a and Holm88 in a 1989 discussion of "radiation phobia" (Ya89, p.160): "Let us consider first what we know about the importance of dose-rate effects in radiation-induced malignancy for any given cumulative dose ... The relevant human evidence depends in part on the use of iodine-131 for diagnosis of thyroid disease and for the treatment of hyperthyroidism. Although only a small fraction of the more than one million patients who had I-131 uptake studies 20 or more years ago and received 50-100 rem thyroidal doses have [sic] been studied, no increase in thyroid cancer has been observed in this group (Holm80a; Holm88). Only 5 % of the more than 35,000 patients evaluated were less than

20 at the time of examination. These authors concluded (Holm80a) that the carcinogenic potential of I-131 would be fourfold less than would result from equivalent externally administered x- or gamma-ray exposure."

Reality -- An Epidemic of Thyroid Cancer :

In great contrast to the above statements -- which claim that no excess thyroid-cancer occurred in the Holm Study and therefore the slow delivery of dose from iodine-131 must account for this unexpected result -- it turns out (1) that a huge excess of thyroid-cancer occurred in the Holm Study, and (2) that the results of the study have not been clearly revealed.

Because the huge excess is revealed only indirectly in the 1988 Holm Study (half of one sentence, on page 1134 of Holm88), we had to go through a series of calculations to evaluate it. Before going through the steps with the reader, we must first describe the nature of the study.

Nature of the Holm Study :
==

The study-population consists of 38,653 patients (79 % females) who "were examined with diagnostic doses of iodine-131" between 1951 and 1969. These patients were "recruited from seven oncologic centers in Sweden ..." Twenty-nine percent were examined in the period 1951-1959, and 71 % in the period 1960-1969.

Age at the time of first I-131 examination ranged from one to 74 years, with a mean age of 44 years for the females and 46 years for the males. Only five percent of the total cohort was below age 20 at the time of examination.

Reason for performing the exam was obtained from the patients' medical records:
    31 % -- suspicion of thyroid tumor.
    42 % -- suspicion of hyperthyroidism.
    16 % -- suspicion of hypothyroidism.
    11 % -- other or unknown reasons.

One can certainly NOT assume that this is a study-population which will be just like the general population in risk of thyroid-cancer, except for its radiation-dose from I-131.

Far from it. People with histories of thyroid abnormalities such as enlarged (hyperplastic) thyroid, goiter, or history of thyroid nodules, go on to show a rate of thyroid-cancer enormously higher than patients without such conditions (Pre87, Table 2; McTier84, p.581; Ron87, p.4). By contrast, the evidence on

===

hyperthyroidism as a risk-factor is inconclusive. McTier84 and Ron87 report finding no basis for calling it a risk-factor. With regard to hypothyroidism, McTier84 shows suggestive evidence in a case-control study that people with hypothyroidism may have a LOWER risk of thyroid-cancer than people without hypothyroidism (Relative Risk = 0.40 in Table 6, McTier84), but she concludes: "In this study, a history of hypothyroidism was not associated with an altered risk of developing thyroid cancer" (McTier84, p.580).

In the Holm Study, mean radiation dose to the thyroid from the I-131 was estimated to be about 0.5 Gy or 50 rads (Holm88, p.1136). We independently checked this estimate of mean dose, by starting with microcuries of administered iodine-131, the mean weight of the gland, and the 24-hour uptake. We arrived at an estimate of 52 rads, in very good agreement with the estimate in Holm88. Holm and co-workers note that the distribution of doses was not random among the patients: "... patients who were examined for a suspected thyroid tumor received higher I-131 activities per examination than did others" (Holm88, p.1135). We shall return to this later.

"The follow-up period lasted from the time of the first I-131 examination until the date of diagnosis of thyroid cancer, the date of emigration or death, or December 31, 1984" (Holm88, p.1134). The mean follow-up was 20 years (p.1134).

"The cohort was matched against the nationwide Swedish Cancer Register (SCR) to identify malignant thyroid tumors occurring between 1958 and 1984. The SCR was started in 1958 and receives notifications on diagnosed cancers from pathologists/cytologists and clinicians ... The completeness of registration of thyroid cancers is higher than 97 % ..." (Holm88, p.1134).

Holm and co-workers assume that about 33 % of all the patients "had some sort of thyroid treatment at some time after the I-131 examination" (Holm88, p.1137). They specifically include thyroid surgery and thyroid hormone medication among the likely treatments.

Unabridged Results :

=======================================

"Within 5 years of follow-up, each of 136 patients had a thyroid cancer diagnosed, and an additional 3,443 patients died" (Holm88, p.1134). This is the only mention in the entire report of what happened during the first five years after the exposure.

Beyond 5 years, 50 (total) additional

thyroid-cancers were observed by December 31, 1984 (Holm88, p.1134, and Tables 4, 5, 7). Of these 50 additional cases, 34 occurred in the patients whose initial exam was due to suspicion of thyroid cancer. The Holm Study provides no way of knowing what fraction of the 136 early cancers came from this initially suspect group.

The figures above mean that at least 186 thyroid-cancers (136 + 50) were found in this study-population. We say "at least" for a reason. The number was assuredly greater than 186.

We must add some cases for the following reason. Holm and co-workers state (Holm88, p.1134) that "Thyroid cancers occurring between 1951 and 1957 could not be identified because of the lack of nationwide incidence data." And from the previous page, we know that 29 % of the 38,653 patients were examined in the 1951-1959 period. This means that all thyroid-cancers occurring in this segment (11,209 patients) before 1958 were missed. It also means that there were fewer than 38,653 patients in the base-population which gave rise to the 136 cases which were NOT missed during the first five years of the follow-up. We surely will not overestimate total cases if we add only 20 cases to the 136 observed within the first five years of follow-up.

Thus, a very reasonable approximation is that the number of post-irradiation thyroid cancers observed in 38,653 patients was: 136 + 20 + 50 = 206 cases, during a mean follow-up time (starting with the initial iodine-131 exam) of 20 years.

Was this an excess?

Observation of a Huge Excess :

Holm and co-workers say, "The expected numbers of malignant thyroid tumors were calculated by direct standardization; adjustment was made for age- (in 5-yr groups), sex-, and calendar year-specific cancer incidence rates for the whole country obtained from the SCR [Swedish Cancer Register] between 1958 and 1984" (Holm88, p.1134).

On this basis, they provide 39.4 as the expected number of thyroid cancers during the follow-up BEYOND the first five years. This expectation applies to the 35,074 persons still in the study as the sixth year begins (of the 38,653 initial patients, 3,443 have died, and 136 with identified thyroid-cancers have been dropped from follow-up). However, Holm and co-workers do not tell what the expected number was DURING the first five years of follow-up. Therefore, on this crucial issue, we will have to make an estimate on

===

our own. It is surprising that the peer-reviewers of this article did not insist on it.

As an approximation, we will assume that the expected incidence rate (39.4 cases per 35,074 persons) in the sixth through 20th year of follow-up will also apply to the first through fifth follow-up years. In the U.S., the incidence of thyroid cancer in women is flat from forty years of age onward through 80 years of age (Beir80, p.167), and we will use this for Sweden too.

A rate of (39.4 cancers per 35,074 persons during 15 years) is an average of (2.63 cases per 35,074 persons each year). Adjusting the cancers for the larger population during the first five years, we have (2.63 cancers) x (38,653 / 35,074), or (2.9 cancers per 38,653 persons each year). Finally, multiplying by 5 years, we have an expectation during the first 5 years of about 14.5 cancers. We can call it 14.

But the OBSERVATION during the first 5 years was about 156 cases. The ratio of observed over expected is (156 / 14), which means a rate some 11-fold above normal.

When we compare the O / E ratio (observed over expected) for the entire 20 years, we have:

Observed = 156 + 50 = 206 cancers.
Expected = 14 + 39.4 = 53.4 cancers.
Ratio of observed over expected = 3.86.

In other words, there is a huge excess of thyroid cancer in the patients who received the diagnostic radio-iodine. Readers of the Holm Study learn nothing about this.

What Became of the Excess ?

The Holm Study was undertaken by oncology centers to FIND OUT if their diagnostic use of radio-iodine is causing excess thyroid-cancer, and if it is, to estimate the magnitude of the elevated risk.

However, no effort was made to establish the expected rate from a control group having comparable thyroid conditions except for the exposure to Iodine-131. Instead, a predictably inappropriate control group -- the general population -- was used. By comparison with this inappropriate control group, a huge excess of thyroid-cancer was observed in the radio-iodine patients (an excess which the Holm Study does not evaluate or discuss at all).

This finding is handled in the Holm Study not by throwing out the 31 % of the sample suspected at the outset of thyroid tumor, and not by trying to establish a true expected rate for the remaining 69 % of the study population. The excess is not even mentioned. Instead:

"In the calculations of person-years at risk, the first 5 years after the initial I-131 administration were excluded for each patient. This was done to reduce the possibility of cancer being present but not diagnosed at the time of the examination and not detected clinically until some years later. All thyroid cancers occurring during the first 5 years after the initial iodine-131 examination were also excluded from the analyses for the same reason" (Holm88, p.1134).

This approach reduced 206 cancers to 50. Since Holm and co-workers used an expectation of 39.4, they report (50 / 39.4), or 1.27 as the Standardized Incidence Ratio (SIR), with a 95 % confidence interval of 0.94 to 1.67. In other words, with the 5-year exclusion, the excess is not provably different from zero.

With the 5-year exclusion, the following details are reported:

In the patients younger than 20 years old during the exam, 2 thyroid cancers were observed. The SIR was 2.02, with a confidence interval of 0.24 to 7.22. In the patients who received radio-iodine BECAUSE of suspicion of a thyroid tumor, the SIR was 2.77, with a 95 % confidence interval of 1.92 to 3.87. In the initially NON-suspect patients, the SIR was 0.62 (0.35 to 1.00).

The Holm Study also explores the effect of throwing away the first TEN years of results. This reduces the 206 cancers to 27, and the overall SIR to 0.93. Of the 27 remaining cases, 19 are in the group examined because of suspicion of thyroid tumor, and their SIR is 2.17.

A Fatally Flawed Study :
===

The Control Group :
The Holm Study relies on a control-group which may supply utterly inappropriate expected values, both for the initially suspect group and for the initially non-suspect group of thyroid patients. If the expected values are inappropriate, this would make all the risk ratios (Standard Incidence Ratios) and all the conclusions therefrom misleading, at best.

It seems self-evident that no one can possibly know, from the Holm Study, how much of the observed excess cancer in the initially suspect group is due to the radio-iodine and how much is due to the patients'

===

pre-radio-iodine condition. To say that NONE of the excess is due to the radiation would require some evidence. To say that ALL of the excess is due to radiation would certainly be foolish, too, in view of the higher risk of thyroid-cancer among patients suspected of thyroid-cancer.

Nor does the Holm Study provide a basis for confidence that the general population is an appropriate control group for the initially NON-suspect group. On the contrary. The finding by Holm88 (p.1135) that the risk-ratio is only 0.62, after the 5-year exclusion, strongly suggests that the "natural" risk (meaning, without radio-iodine experience) of thyroid-cancer in this special population of people with thyroid disorders, may be a lot LOWER than the natural risk in the general population.

Treatments Post-Radio-Iodine :
Moreover, no one can evaluate the impact, on the study's outcome, of post-radio-iodine treatments (including thyroid removal and thyroid hormones) received by an estimated one-third of the 35,000 patients in the study-population. UNSCEAR 1986, referring to the smaller Holm Study of 1980, rejects such post-radio-iodine treatments as a likely contributor to the study's presumed deficit of cancers (Un86, p.229, para.397). In 1988, Holm and co-workers dismiss this problem with a single sentence: "The absence of any increased thyroid cancer risk was considered not to be ascribable to the thyroid treatment" (Holm88, p.1137). Their allusion to the absence of excess risk is, of course, to an absence AFTER the first five years of results have been thrown away. Then the risk ratio becomes 1.27, which is not provably different from 1.00 under the circumstances.

Diseases in the Studied Organ :
It is interesting that the 1986 UNSCEAR Report, in listing several reasons for the claimed shortage of excess cancers in the overall preliminary (1980) results, points out that "... the subjects are a selected unhealthy population, with a high percentage of thyroid involvement, to whom specific rates of thyroid cancer induction, valid in the general population, may not apply" (Un86, p.229, para.397).

Such insights about the fatal flaws of the Holm Study seem to be discarded, however, in the 1988 UNSCEAR Report (Un88). Un88 relies heavily on the Holm Study on the key issue of risk reduction-factors.

Unknown Latency Period :
Another confounding variable in the Holm Study, not mentioned by UNSCEAR, is the real possibility that thyroid diseases themselves alter the latency period for radiation-induced cancer. For instance, one or another condition might induce promotional agents not present in healthy thyroid cells, and the peak incidence of radiation-induced cancer might occur 3, 5, or 8 years post-irradiation. Such early peaking is well-observed for radiation-induced leukemia, about 7.5 years after exposure.

Pre-Judgments versus Inquiry :
Throwing out the observed excess, in 5-year or 10-year stages, is no solution whatsoever to these very serious confounding variables. Throwing away any part of such a follow-up reflects an unwarranted pre-judgment, not a scientific inquiry, in our opinion.

We remind readers that the Holm Study is examining a study-population which -- during the first five years of follow-up -- showed an 11-fold excess of the exact variable (thyroid-cancer) which the investigators were hoping to study (see "Unabridged Results," above).

As an independent analyst, I cannot just pretend to myself that this is a NORMAL population showing normal behavior during a latency period, and that if I throw away these startling results, I can tell myself that I have a normal population entering the sixth year of a radiation follow-up study. It would really require some supernatural omniscience on my part to decide that truth would be best served by not mentioning the 11-fold excess and by throwing away the first five years of results.

Nonetheless, I am unaware that any other analysts, peer-reviewers, or radiation committees have (1) asked for an explanation of the 3.9-fold higher rate of thyroid-cancer in the exposed group (unabridged results), or (2) challenged use of the general population as a control group for this very abnormal study-population, or (3) challenged the failure even to divulge just how very abnormal the study-population is -- e.g., an 11-fold excess rate of thyroid-cancer during the first five years of follow-up, or (4) challenged the throwing out of the first five years of the results. What I think I see, so far, is an uncritical rush to EMBRACE this fatally flawed study with its welcome (welcome to me, also) but unwarranted conclusions.

Consistency in Standards ?

===

Radio-iodine studies have also tested consistency regarding reliance on human versus non-human evidence. This chapter has shown, with regard to risk reduction-factors (DREFS), how much of the radiation community greatly prefers to generalize from the non-human evidence than to generalize from the human evidence.

However, in 1982, Lee and co-workers published a rat-study in which they found NO lesser carcinogenicity of slow doses from iodine-131 compared with acute doses from 250 kVp X-rays, and the study extended down to thyroid doses of 80 rads (Lee82). Clearly, this finding is not as welcome as lesser carcinogenicity from iodine-131 would be.

The Lee Study was challenged as follows by Holm88 (p.1135):

"Iodine-131 has frequently been used to induce tumors in experimental animals, although its effectiveness relative to external photon exposures has been studied only to a limited extent. Earlier studies with high doses to the thyroid gland suggested that iodine-131 was one-tenth to one-fourth as effective as x rays in producing thyroid tumors. Lee et al. observed that with lower doses the difference in effectiveness between the two types of radiation was less pronounced and perhaps even the same at doses less than 3-4 Gy. [We are splitting the Holm88 paragraph here.]

"Like many other experiments on animals, their results are limited by the fact that iodine-131 is an efficient cancer inducer in certain animal species and strains only, such as the CBA mice and the Long-Evans rats. Lee et al. used female Long-Evans rats in their study, and the results may well have differed had they used male rats or a mixture of the two sexes. Regardless, there is a great deal of uncertainty in extrapolation from animal data to human populations. Epidemiologic data are therefore the preferred source of information for obtaining risk estimates in humans" (Holm88, p.1135).

We agree. But we would say "appropriate epidemiologic data."

Earlier, in 1985, NCRP commented on Lee82 in a different manner (Ncrp85, p.33): "For the production of thyroid carcinomas, the two radiation types appeared to be of equal effectiveness at all three doses although the results did not preclude a relative effectiveness of iodine-131 of as little as one-third compared to external radiation."

If one is going to discuss the confidence-limits on a best estimate, it is certainly not an appropriate practice to mention only the LOWER limit. Yet NCRP does not mention that the Lee82 findings are also consistent with a HIGHER risk from the slow exposure than from the acute exposure. There appears to be asymmetry in the

NCRP approach to the Lee82 Study.

UNSCEAR-86 shows the two dose-response curves from Lee82 practically superimposed on each other (and both looking supra-linear, not concave-upward), and comments (Un86, p.208, para.254): "Thus, there was no difference in the effectiveness of the two radiations over the observed range of doses, but a lower effectiveness of iodine-131 per unit dose (up to a factor of about 3) could not be excluded on statistical grounds (Ncrp85)." Thus, UNSCEAR-86 passes along the NCRP comment without any criticism of its asymmetry.

To help restore symmetry, we repeat: The best estimate from Lee82 does not support DREFS and is also consistent with HIGHER risk at slow-low doses.

Looking at the Initially Non-Suspect Group :
===

An obvious question with respect to the Holm Study is: What would this study have shown if the "initially suspect" 31 % of the study-population had never been included?

A Substantial Excess of Thyroid-Cancer :

Because Holm88 does not report what fraction of the early, discarded cancers occurred in the initially suspect group, and what fraction occurred in the intially NON-suspect group, the question cannot be answered with certainty. Indeed, the data do not exist at all for 1951-1957.

We can explore an answer by making an approximation. Of the total 50 cancers observed after the 5-year exclusion, 16 cancers occurred in the initially non-suspect group. The fraction was (16 / 50), or 0.32. And with the 10-year exclusion, no meaningful change occurred: The fraction was 8 cancers out of 27 total cancers, or 0.30. We shall use the approximation that the fraction which occurred DURING the 5-year exclusion was the same as the fraction which occurred afterwards: 0.32.

Since we estimated (see "Unabridged Results") that at least 156 thyroid-cancers occurred in the total study-sample during the first five years of follow-up, we would approximate that (0.32) x (156 cancers), or 50 cancers came from the initially non-suspect group. Beyond five years, another 16 thyroid-cancers occurred in this group, so the estimated total of observed thyroid-cancers would be 66.

What is the expectation, WITHOUT radio-iodine, if

===

the rate in this diseased group is comparable with the rate in the general population? We are using the same big "if" used (without discussion) by the Holm Study.

We showed above ("Unabridged Results") that the expectation in the full cohort during the first five years of follow-up was 14 cases. Since the initially non-suspect group represents 69 % of the total study-population, its expection is (0.69) x (14 cancers) = 9.66 cancers during the first five years of follow-up. For the follow-up beyond five years, its expection is (0.69) x (39.4 cancers) = 27.19 cancers during the rest of the follow-up. Total expectation, if radio-iodine had no effect, would be (9.66 + 27.19) = 36.85 cancers. And if the "natural" rate of thyroid-cancer in this special group is LOWER than in the general population, the expectation would also be LOWER than 36.85 cancers.

So this approach suggests that the relative risk, of observed cancers over expected cancers, might be (66 / 36.85) = 1.79 if the first five years of follow-up were included. This is about three-fold higher than the value of 0.62, reported in the Holm Study with the five-year exclusion for the initially non-suspect group. And if the appropriate EXPECTED value is even lower than 36.85, then the risk ratio would be HIGHER than 1.79.

We cannot know. We are only pointing out a good basis for thinking that the missing data on the first five years of follow-up might transform a "no provable excess" report into a highly significant excess. And this excess might even be wholly due to the radio-iodine administered. Only a pre-judgment would allow a claim that it was NOT.

Presence of a Dose-Response Trend :

One issue which the Holm Study may be capable of addressing is the issue of dose-response. On this issue, it does not matter whether the risk ratios are correct or INcorrect (correct meaning that they compare rates in two groups which are alike in risk, except for their radiation dose). What matters is how the risk ratios CHANGE (if they do) with rising dose.

Within the results which Holm and co-workers do report, there is a basis for thinking that there is a strong dose-response trend in the initially NON-suspect group.

Holm and co-workers, in their Table 5, divided the entire sample of 35,000 patients into three dose-levels as follows:

Microcuries of I-131	Observed Cancers	Risk Ratio: SIR (Obs / Expected)
<30	14	0.96
30-74	19	1.15
>74	17	2.04
All	50	1.27

Their Table 6 shows the comparable entries for just the patients who were examined for a suspected tumor:

Microcuries of I-131	Observed Cancers	Risk Ratio: SIR (Obs / Expected)
<30	12	3.69
30-74	11	2.06
>74	11	2.96
All	34	2.77

In Table 5, the total group (35,000) shows evidence of a dose-response trend, toward an increasing incidence of thyroid-cancer with increasing dose of radio-iodine. Holm and co-workers say (p.1135), "The thyroid cancer risk increased with increasing administered I-131 activity (Table 5)." In Table 6, by contrast, the initially suspect group by itself shows no evidence of a trend: "There was no relation between SIR and administered activity of I-131 (Table 6)."

This means that the study's inclusion of the initially suspect group is tending to dilute and to conceal a positive dose-response trend in the initially NON-suspect patients. Their dose-response trend must be even stronger than indicated in Table 5 -- where it is clear DESPITE dilution by the initially suspect patients. Rising incidence with rising dose is powerful supportive evidence for causality, of course. It is regrettable that Holm and co-workers chose NOT to evaluate the dose-response trend for the initially NON-suspect patients by themselves, in the same way that these authors evaluated the initially suspect patients by themselves.

No Evidence of a Dose-RATE Effect :

We shall continue our exploration of the Holm Study as if patients who were initially suspected of a thyroid tumor had never been included, and as if only the 69 % who had thyroid disorders (but were initially NOT suspected of a tumor) were in it.

Now we shall ask if there is any indication of a dose-RATE effect (for instance, reduced risk from slow exposure compared with acute exposure) in this group, when we make no pre-judgments -- which means that we look at the entire follow-up.

Readers who proceed step-by-step, through the two analyses which follow, will see for themselves that there is no evidence at all for a dose-rate effect from slow versus acute exposure.

Search for a Dose-Rate Effect :
===

In our work above ("A Substantial Excess"), we estimated 66 observed thyroid-cancers versus 36.9 expected. The difference, or radiogenic excess, is 29.1 thyroid-cancers.

Is this a smaller excess than we would expect, if we use expectations based on observations from ACUTE exposure?

We are going to answer this first in the way which we think is the scientifically best way, and then in the way used by Holm88.

Avoiding the Site-Specific Pitfall :

One of the most questionable practices in this field is the excessive subdivision of data, including undue reliance on site-specific risk-coefficients. (See our Index entries "Scientifically questionable practices" and "Site-specific analysis.")

Even a casual inspection of Studies 1 through 9, in Chapter 21, Part 1, demonstrates the delusion of thinking that reliable risk coefficients (K-values) can be directly determined for SPECIFIC sites of cancer.

Let us consider a K-value of 0.02, which is equivalent to a 2 % increase in spontaneous risk per rad. If K = 0.02, a dose of 50 rads causes a 100 % increment above the spontaneous expectation. The dose which adds as much cancer as the spontaneous rate is commonly called the doubling dose, so when K = 0.02, the doubling dose is 50 rads. In short, a dose which doubles the spontaneous rate is ONE doubling dose, and a dose which triples the spontaneous rate represents TWO doubling doses.

Now, we can inspect the breast-cancer doubling doses in Chapter 21, Part 1. The doubling dose in Study 3 (Massachusetts Fluoroscopy) was 150 rads, and the doubling dose in Study 7 (the British Luminizers) was about 80 rads -- even though the medical X-rays have a higher Relative Biological Effectiveness than the gamma rays from radium-226. So there is perhaps a 4-fold difference. (We cannot agree with any analyst who casually says that breast-cancer risk looks similar from one site-specific analysis to the next.)

A large range for the doubling dose occurs also in the in-utero studies of Chapter 21, Part 1. Even if we narrow the range by saying that in Study 5 (the Stewart Studies), a half rad causes a 50 % increment instead of a 94 % increment in childhood cancer, this choice would make the doubling dose 1 rad. By contrast, in Study 6 (the MacMahon Study), 0.9 rad provoked a 40 % increment, so (0.9 rad x 2.5) or 2.25 rads would provoke a 100 % increment -- a doubling. Thus there is more than a 2-fold difference in the magnitude of doubling dose derived from these studies of a single cancer-class (childhood cancer).

It is perfectly valid to use such studies to test the hypothesis of flawless repair. As long as a significant excess of radiogenic cancer occurs, the excess is evidence that repair was NOT flawless. The exact risk coefficient or doubling dose is irrelevant for such a test.

But it is a very DIFFERENT matter indeed when analysts attempt to use studies of specific kinds of cancers (such as childhood cancers, breast-cancers, thyroid-cancers) to test for an effect of slow versus acute exposure upon the magnitude of risk, when the magnitude of the ACUTE effect is so poorly known for single sites and classes of cancer. Such attempts just invite large errors, in my opinion.

I do not think site-specific studies are suitable for a dose-rate analysis, but if such analysis is done nonetheless, then I think there will be less likelihood of large errors, if analysts use the very reasonable approximation that all types of cancer have about the SAME fractional increase in their spontaneous rate per rad, if all other variables are held constant. Until and unless APPROPRIATE evidence develops which shows otherwise, I would regard myself as skating on scientifically "thin ice" NOT to make this approximation. (Go81, Chap.10; Go85, pp.19-20.)

All-Cancer K-Value from Our Table 15-L :

If we use the approximation that the thyroid gland is no more and no less radio-sensitive than other organs, we must use the all-cancer K-value from our Table 15-L in order to calculate the radiogenic expectation from 50 thyroid-rads in the Holm Study (initially non-suspect group).

Since 79 % of the Holm-Study patients were women,

==

with a mean age of 44 years, and since the dose-rate per day was far below 50 rads, and since the DS86 dosimetry is only supplemental in the A-Bomb Study, we shall use the low-dose K-value of 0.00615 from the T65DR dosimetry.

The average energy of beta particles from iodine-131 is about 189 KeV (Strom58). This may mean a somewhat higher RBE than A-bomb radiation, but we shall not raise the K-value directly. Instead, we shall use just the female K-value (which is higher than the male K-value), and we shall use 50 rads as the thyroid dose, even though Holm88 states that the initially non-suspect group received a LOWER average dose. (Holm88 does not say how MUCH lower.)

Results by Our Method :

The estimate is easy to make:

Expected number of cancers without I-131 = 36.9 .
Thyroid-dose = 50 rads.
K = 0.00615 per rad from acute exposure.
Estimated radiation-induced cancers =
   (36.9) x (50) x (0.00615) = 11.35 cases.
Radiation-induced plus spontaneous cancers =
   11.35 + 36.9 = 48.25 cases.

So do these calculations from the Holm Study suggest that the radiation-risk from radio-iodine would be 3-fold lower than the risk from ACUTE thyroid exposure?

Not at all. The estimated OBSERVED cases in this sample are 66 cancers, based on reasonable approximations (see "A Substantial Excess" above). This is a HIGHER number than 48.25 cases expected on the basis of acute exposure.

The number 66 is consistent even with a 3-fold HIGHER K-value from the radio-iodine than from the A-bomb radiation. With a 3-fold higher K-value, the radiation-induced cases would grow to (3 x 11.35) or 34.05 cases. So 34.05 radiation-induced cases plus 36.9 spontaneous cases would mean an observation of 70.95 cases -- STILL in good agreement with an estimated observation of 66 cases.

Readers who have followed this, step-by-step, can judge for themselves whether our approximations are reasonable or not.

We are certainly not claiming that this comparison, using the all-cancer K-value from the A-Bomb Study, means that slow dose-rate from iodine-131 is three-fold MORE carcinogenic than acute dose-rate.

We have tried to make it clear that we think the Holm Study is completely inappropriate for addressing the issue at all.

But, because of the weight given to the Holm Study by UNSCEAR 1988 and others, we have been obliged to point out that the Holm Study is consistent with exactly the OPPOSITE conclusions from the ones ascribed to it.

Analysis by the Holm Model :

We are not quite finished, because we promised that we would search for a dose-rate effect by using the Holm model too, although we think it is not a good model for such a purpose.

By "Holm model," we mean the use of a site-specific K-value, rather than an all-cancer K-value, to compute the radiogenic expectation of thyroid-cancer in this study. Holm and co-workers say (p.1136) that they used the site-specific K-value for thyroid from the 1985 NIH Report. The NIH Report (Nih85) in turn used thyroid incidence data from the A-Bomb Survivors, Hiroshima plus Nagasaki, 1958-1979 (Nih85, p.255). This would have meant no correction for the very large overestimate of neutron-dose at Hiroshima.

Perhaps because of the neutron-error for Hiroshima, the 1988 UNSCEAR Report (Un88, p.434, para.209) explicitly recommends the thyroid-cancer incidence data from Nagasaki alone as "the best," for which Un88 cites Wakabayashi and co-workers (Waka83). Nagasaki data never had a neutron problem. On the other hand, subdivision of the cities reduces the cases and thus increases uncertainty in the estimates. In any case, we should find out if, and how much, the site-specific K-value differs in Nih85 versus Waka83.

Checking the Site-Specific K-Value :

K-Value Based on Wakabayashi :

The Wakabayashi et al analysis divides the Nagasaki A-bomb survivors into two classes: Unexposed survivors and survivors receiving 100 kerma rads and more. On this basis, these analysts report on the relative risk (100+ rads versus zero rads) as follows in their Appendix Table 2:

RR = 1.70 for all cancers (leukemia omitted).
   Excess RR = 0.70 .
RR = 3.23 for thyroid cancers.
   Excess RR = 2.23 .

The ratio of excess relative risk (2.23 / 0.70 = 3.186) is for the same KERMA dose, but not for the same

ABSORBED dose in the organs from which the cancers arose. Site-specific analysis requires site-specific body transmission-factors (Chapter 8, Part 2). The body transmission-factor for thyroid is estimated at 0.7 in TR-12-87 (Shi87, p.43), which is higher than the factor for colon (see our Table 9-A).

We can proceed by establishing the KERMA dose to which the excess relative risks apply. Using our Table 9-B, we calculated the weighted mean dose received by the Waka83 exposed class (Dose-Groups 5,6,7,8) as 243.7997 kerma rads.

So, for all cancers, excess RR = (0.7 per 243.7997 kerma rads) = 0.002871 excess per kerma rad (or a K-value of 0.002871 per kerma rad).

But for equal KERMA rads, thyroid is 3.186 times more sensitive than all organs combined (if you take site-specific analysis seriously). So the K-value for thyroid is (3.186 x 0.002871), or 0.009147 per kerma rad.

But the thyroid's ABSORBED dose was lower than its kerma dose, so the K-value will be higher than 0.009147. It needs adjustment for the site-specific transmission-factor of 0.7 . So we divide (0.009147 / 0.7), and we obtain a site-specific K-value for the thyroid of 0.013067 per absorbed rad. This is the same as an excess relative risk of 0.013067 per thyroid-rad.

The value of 0.013067 arises from a population with an average age at the time of bombing of about 27. The value might be adjusted DOWNWARD to apply to the older study-population in Holm88, but we will simply compare it, as it is, to the site-specific K-value from Nih85.

K-Value from Nih85 :

In the 1985 NIH Report, Table X-12 (p.261) provides the following values for "Relative Excess by Exposure Age and Sex" per thyroid-rad:

Female, Exposure Age 44 = 0.0176 .
Male, Exposure Age 46 = 0.00935 .

The Holm Study (Table 1) has a female to male ratio of 3.8. If we say m = the male fraction, then 3.8m is the female fraction, and 4.8m = 1. Therefore m = 0.2083. And (1-m) or 0.7917 is the female fraction. So the weighted K-value for the overall Holm Study would be (0.0176 x 0.7917) + (0.00935 x 0.2083) = 0.01588 .

Results by the Holm Model :

We shall use BOTH site-specific K-values to compute the radiogenic expectation in the initially non-suspect group. The radiogenic expectation is (the spontaneous expectation of 36.9 cancers) x (site-specific K-value per rad) x (50 rads -- which is an exaggeration for this group).

With the K-value of 0.013067, based on Waka83, the radiogenic expectation = (36.9) x (0.013067) x (50) = 24.1 radiation-induced cancers. The spontaneous expectation (36.9 cancers) plus the radiogenic cancers (24.1) = 61.01 cases. And the estimated OBSERVED number was 66 cancers. So there is no indication of any risk-reduction from the slow delivery from iodine compared with acute delivery from A-bomb radiation here.

With the K-value of 0.01588, based on Nih85, the radiogenic expectation = (36.9) x (0.01588) x (50) = 29.3 radiation-induced cancers. The spontaneous expectation (36.9 cancers) plus the radiogenic cancers (29.3) = 66.2 cases. And the estimated OBSERVED number was 66 cancers. So there is no indication of any risk-reduction from the slow delivery from iodine compared with acute delivery from A-bomb radiation here.

For those who would say, "We want to look only at the period beyond 5 years," we say the following:

One must avoid distorting the outcome by pre-judgments which are totally unwarranted. Just what does anyone know about WHEN radiation-induced cancers will occur following radio-iodine in a group of manifestly abnormal people with diseased thyroids? If you see a large excess of thyroid cancers in the initially non-suspect group during the early follow-up, it needs explaining. There would be no basis whatsoever for simply CLAIMING that an early excess (if any occurred here) could not have been caused by the radiation.

Summary on Unwarranted Conclusions from the Holm Study :
=======================================

We wish to emphasize a point. Our exploration of what the Holm Study might have shown, if the 31 % of initially suspect patients had never been included, is NOT a statement by us that we think the initially non-suspect group is an appropriate group to compare with the general population. Far from it, as we already indicated above (see "A Fatally Flawed Study"). The general population appears to be an unsuitable control-group for BOTH the initially suspect and initially non-suspect study-samples.

We have shown our reasons for saying that (A) the Holm Study in its present state is consistent with OPPOSITE conclusions about dose-rate, and (B) no one should regard the Holm Study in its present state as meaningful about anything concerned with DREFS.

In other words, we disagree with its acceptance by the 1988 UNSCEAR Committee as a piece of notable human evidence in support of a dose-rate effect and risk-reduction factors.

Perhaps the Holm Study illustrates the fact that the peer-review system can perform unevenly. For instance, reviewers can be ultra-careful about the choice of control-groups for the in-utero studies (see Chapter 21, Part 1), and yet overlook glaring problems with the control group in a study like the Holm Study.

6. The Bottom Line

1. For over a decade, the radiation community has been using risk reduction-factors to make its estimates of cancer-risk at acute-low doses and at slow-low doses. These reduction-factors are based on the premise that dose versus cancer-response is concave-upward -- in other words, on the premise that the risk per rad (cGy) is smaller when dose is either acute-low or slow-low than when dose is high. This premise was explicitly stated in 1977 by both UNSCEAR and ICRP (see Part 3, above), and has been echoed again and again by other radiation committees. Of course, if dose-response is either linear or supra-linear, it would be a mistake to use risk reduction-factors, because they would produce underestimates of risk at both acute-low doses and at slow-low doses. The inappropriate use of reduction-factors with respect to Chernobyl-induced cancers is illustrated in Chapter 24, Part 7.

2. Since 1977 (TR-1-77, or Bee77), human epidemiological evidence has repeatedly shown that the premise of risk reduction-factors (the premise of a concave-upward dose-response in humans for radiation carcinogenesis) is fundamentally flawed. And the record shows that the radiation committees knew it by 1980 (see Part 2, above).

3. Nonetheless, from 1977 through mid-1989, almost all of the radiation community has subordinated the human evidence AGAINST using risk reduction-factors, in favor of using such factors on the basis of NON-human evidence and cell studies -- "radiobiology." I do not disparage radiobiological evidence, and we should learn all that we can from such work. But in science, when predictions from radiobiology are invalidated by the reality-check of direct human evidence, the direct evidence must prevail. This chapter shows that, for years, it has not.

Perhaps it will. In 1988, Warren Sinclair, president of the NCRP, conceded that in the A-Bomb Study 1950-1982, "... it appears that the dose-effect response is fitted about as well by a linear as by a linear-quadratic equation, and this may also influence risk estimates ..." (Sin88, p.154). And in 1988, Albrecht Kellerer (see Chapter 37) offered his opinion -- after studying the A-bomb survivors through 1985 -- that "Today, the use of a reduction factor in extrapolation from high doses to low doses which are relevant for radiation protection purposes, is less easily defensible ... Although even the extreme hypothesis remains unfalsifiable, that at the lowest doses there is no excess cancer incidence, a prudent extrapolation can nevertheless make use of a linear extrapolation and can drop the assumption of a reduction factor" (Kelle88, p.51; translated from the German by Dr. Rudi Nussbaum).

Such statements are hedged. Moreover, they are competing with vigorous pressure in the opposite direction from some other members of the radiation community, who are pressing for the ULTIMATE reduction-factor -- namely, for treating low doses as safe, and excluding them completely from risk-estimates (see Chapters 24 and 25).

4. The use of risk reduction-factors has meant that, for years, most radiation reports have been presenting linear estimates as the "upper limit" on risk, despite human evidence showing that linear estimates represent either the best values or a LOWER-limit of risk.

5. There is no longer any need to extrapolate from acute high-doses above 100 rads (100 cSv), in order to make risk-estimates at acute-low or at slow-low doses. The A-Bomb Study has already provided direct evidence at low doses for all cancers combined (see Chapter 13), and it will continue to do so, provided its legitimacy as a credible, prospective study is maintained (as proposed in Chapter 6).

==================

22 empty, after 22-25
===

Proper Risk-Estimates for "Low and Slow" Exposures :
No Conflict Between Human Epidemiology
and the Linear-Quadratic Hypothesis from Radiobiology

This chapter is arranged in seven parts:

1. Introduction

If a cherished hypothesis comes into apparent conflict with valid human epidemiological evidence -- and note the term, "valid" -- then we clearly do NOT throw away valid evidence and insist on the hypothesis. The proper approach is to find out how and why such a hypothesis is inadequate to explain the valid epidemiological evidence.

Risk-Estimates for Low Acute Doses :

As shown in the previous chapter, those who support the existence of risk reduction-factors for acute low-dose exposures -- in the presence of human evidence against such factors -- commonly invoke "radiobiological considerations" as the justification.

Radiobiological considerations include the hypothesis that both intra-track and inter-track events can result in fully competent carcinogenic lesions, and that in a linear-quadratic (LQ) equation, the linear term represents intra-track carcinogenesis and the quadratic term represents inter-track carcinogenesis (see Chapter 19, Part 4). Thus, the sign should be positive for both the linear (L) and quadratic (Q) terms, and dose-response should be concave-UPWARD.

Even if one accepts this hypothesis, the hypothesis can be readily reconciled with the real-world observation that, for carcinogenesis in the A-Bomb Study, human dose-response is supra-linear and concave-DOWNWARD throughout the dose-range.

The reconciliation is achieved by modifying the LQ equation with an exponential modifier which represents a cell-INACTIVATION function operating throughout the entire dose-range. By inactivation, we do NOT necessarily mean cell-killing, as we will explain in Part 4.

Recognition that the concave-upward shape, of an unmodified LQ equation, can be changed by an exponential modifier is nothing new. It has been recognized for decades. In fact, the format which we shall use in this chapter was displayed by NCRP in 1980 (Ncrp80, p.19) and by UNSCEAR-86 (p.188).

NCRP and all of the radiation committees recognized that an unmodified LQ equation was inherently false for human dose-response, when they all acknowledged that the curve flattens out "at high doses."   Ncrp80 (p.160) even conceded that the supra-linear curvature was seen "at relatively low doses in the Hiroshima data." Various reports and analysts have explored use of "cell-killing" terms to modify their LQ equations -- but only to change their curvature at very HIGH doses.

Since we all agree that the unmodified LQ equation does not match human dose-response, the task which remains is to modify an LQ equation so that it has what the human evidence requires: A supra-linear or a linear dose-response THROUGHOUT the dose-range. If this can be done -- with both the L and Q terms positive -- of course it means that "radiobiological reasons" do

NOT always predict a concave-upward dose-response at all.

It can be done, as this chapter demonstrates to any doubters.

Risk-Estimates for Slow Exposures :

Then, in Parts 6 and 7, we shall turn to the possible implications for dose-RATE.

It is possible (though not certain) that a HIGH acute dose is more carcinogenic than the same dose delivered slowly. We shall explore a range of possible values.

However, there is no reason at LOW total doses to expect more than trivial protection (reduction in risk) from slow delivery. ICRP itself acknowledged this, as noted in our Chapter 22, Part 3. In Part 7 of the present chapter, we have evaluated the maximum amount of protection which might occur if 5 rads, for instance, were given slowly instead of acutely. The amount would be very small indeed.

Therefore, the low-dose Cancer-Yields in Section 4 of this book are definitely valid for SLOW delivery as well as for acute delivery.

2. The Unmodified LQ Model, As Used by Radiation Committees

For the unmodified LQ model, depicted in Figures 23-B and 23-C, we use the following notation:

```
A cancers = intra-track cancers.
B cancers = inter-track cancers.
(A+B) cancers = total excess cancers.
    D^1 = dose in cSv to the first power.
    D^2 = dose in cSv squared.
(a cancers per cSv) = coefficient of the L term.
(b cancers per cSv^2) = coefficient of the Q term.

    The units cancel out when we write:
    -------------------------------------
● -- EQUATION (1) :
    A cancers = (a cancers cSv^-1) x (D^1 cSv^1)
            A = aD^1

● -- EQUATION (2) :
    B cancers = (b cancers cSv^-2) x (D^2 cSv^2)
            B = bD^2

● -- EQUATION (3) :  A+B = aD^1 + bD^2
```

In the radiation literature, one sees suggestions that

the linear and quadratic terms may make equal contributions to total excess cancer (radiation-induced cancer) at doses between 50 and 150 rads (cGy). These are purely speculative limits. We shall explore limits of 50 and 400 cSv.

A = B at 50 cSv :

If A = B at 50 cSv, we would write from Equations (1) and (2):

```
(a cancers cSv^-1) x (50 cSv) =
                (b cancers cSv^-2) x (2500 cSv^2)

    50a = 2500b
     a = 50b.
```

This is a ratio (a/b = 50), and we can set the value of b equal to 1.0 for the sake of clarity in producing Table 23-B.

Table 23-B shows the values of A, B, and (A+B) when b = 1.0, if A = B at 50 cSv. Because we have shown (above) that a = 50b in these circumstances, we can substitute (50b) for (a) in the equation A = aD^1. Thus the entries for Column A in Table 23-B are calculated from the equation A = (50b)(D^1).

In the row for 50 cSv, readers will find equal cancer-contributions from the intra-track and inter-track terms: 2,500 from each.

From Table 23-B, Columns A, B, and (A+B) are depicted by Figure 23-B, BB, BBB. This is a single figure in which 23-B examines the plots out to 400 cSv, 23-BB examines them out to 200 cSv, and 23-BBB examines them out to 100 cSv. In Figure 23-BBB, it is clear that A = B at 50 cSv. This is visible also in Figure 23-BB.

A = B at 400 cSv :

If A = B at 400 cSv, we would write a = 400b. Table 23-C shows the values of A, B, and (A+B) when b = 1.0, if A = B at 400 cSv. In the row for 400 cSv, readers will find equal cancer-contributions from A and from B: 160,000 from each.

From Table 23-C, Columns A, B, and (A+B) are depicted by Figure 23-C, CC, and CCC. Figure 23-C examines the plots out to 400 cSv, 23-CC examines them out to 200 cSv, and 23-CCC examines them out to 100 cSv. In Figure 23-C, it is clear that A = B at 400 cSv.

The Mistaken Risk-Reduction Factors for Acute Exposures :

==========================

It is self-evident from Figures 23-B and 23-C that the unmodified LQ model produces a concave-UPWARD curvature for total excess cancers -- Plot (A+B). This matches the presumption discussed in Chapter 22. Indeed, Figure 23-BB closely resembles the model displayed by Ncrp80 (p.16, Figure 3.4). Comparison of Figures 23-B and 23-C also shows that the concave-upward curvature is much greater if A = B at 50 cSv than if A = B at 400 cSv.

We shall calculate risk reduction-factors for both limits, for acute exposures, as if dose-response were actually concave-upward. Let us assume that we have observation of risk-rates only at 160 cSv of acute exposure and at zero dose (in other words, two datapoints), and we decide to estimate the risk from acute exposure at very low doses, by making a linear interpolation between 160 cSv and zero dose.

On Figures 23-BB and 23-CC, we have drawn a dashed straight line from Plot A+B at 160 cSv (the high-dose observation) to the origin. This dashed line lies above the A+B curve at low doses, and so linear interpolation would OVERestimate risk at low doses -- if dose-response were truly concave-upward.

When the dose is very low, readers can see for themselves that Plot B (the quadratic term) generates about zero excess cancer. At low doses, essentially all the excess cancers are coming from intra-track carcinogenesis (Plot A). This is not in dispute. Indeed, the Figures show that Plot A+B and Plot A are just about on top of each other, and their slopes are about the same in the low dose-range.

DREFS -- The Ratio of Slopes :

Under these circumstances of interpolation, it would be appropriate for everyone to estimate risk reduction-factors by dividing one slope by another: The slope of Plot A+B shown as the dashed line between zero and 160 cSv, by the slope of Plot A -- because the slope of Plot A approximates the actual slope of Plot A+B at low doses. As stated in Chapter 22, Part 1, a DREF is the ratio of the steeper slope over the lower slope (Ncrp80, p.176). Since slope in these circumstances means excess cancers per cSv, the centi-sieverts cancel out in such a division, and the ratio of excess cancers remains.

If A = B at 50 cSv, the slope of the dashed line is 33600 / 160, or 210. The value 33600 need not be read

off Figure 23-B; it comes from Table 23-B, the A+B column at 160 cSv. The slope of Plot A is 8000 / 160, or 50. The ratio of the slopes is 210 / 50, or 4.2. Therefore, if the plots shown in Figure 23-B were actually observed plots matching real-world data, linear interpolation from 160 cSv would overestimate risk at low doses by 4.2-fold. Under these circumstances, a risk reduction-factor of 4.2 would be appropriate.

If A = B at 400 cSv, the slope of the dashed line in Figure 23-CC is 89600 (from Table 23-C) divided by 160, or 560. The slope of Plot A is 64000 / 160, or 400. The risk reduction-factor under such circumstances would be 560 / 400, or 1.4-fold, to make interpolations from 160 cSv.

Visual comparison of Figure 23-BB with 23-CC shows why the presumption of A = B at 50 cSv "requires" a much larger risk reduction-factor than the presumption that A = B at 400 cSv, if linear interpolation is used. In Figure 23-BB, the linear term (Plot A) accounts for only a small share of Plot A+B. In Figure 23-CC, the linear term (Plot A) is not very distant from Plot A+B, and so linear interpolation from Plot A+B at 160 cSv "requires" less of a correction.

Nature of the Mistake :

We put "requires" in quotes because no risk reduction-factors are required for acute exposures at all, for two reasons: (1) dose-response in the human is NOT concave-upward, and (2) direct human observations at low doses leave no need to use high-dose data, in order to estimate low-dose risks.

The LQ Model -- Positive vs. Negative Q-Coefficient :

=============================

The underlying assumption of this model is that combined action of intra-track carcinogenesis and inter-track carcinogenesis gives rise to the total radiation-induced cancers (A+B). Therefore, both the linear and quadratic terms are presumed to be positive. It follows that at every dose, the points along Plot A+B are necessarily the sum of the corresponding points along Plot A and Plot B. If inter-track carcinogenesis is occurring at all, Plot A+B must always lie above Plot A. Moreover, the shape of Plot B guarantees that the shape of A+B is concave-upward.

However, when analysts try to fit the LQ model to a supra-linear set of datapoints, regression analysis produces a best-fit equation in which the quadratic term is NEGATIVE (see Chapters 14 and 22). This means that the points along the combined linear and quadratic plot are the A values MINUS the corresponding B values. The result is necessarily a supra-linear, concave-DOWNWARD plot, as illustrated by Figure 23-H.

The findings that (1) the Q-term is negative and (2) the dose-response is concave-downward, do not require any presumption, however, that intra-track lesions are carcinogenic and inter-track lesions are protective. Such a hypothesis would be utterly implausible, as shown in Chapter 19, Part 4.

The concave-downward dose-response, which is observed in the evidence, is perfectly consistent with POSITIVE signs for both the linear and quadratic terms -- as we shall show in Part 4 of this chapter.

3. Modified LQ Model, As Described by Radiation Committees

No one disputes that the concave-upward shape of an LQ model can be altered by adding an exponential modifier. Indeed, we will use the type of modifier suggested by Ncrp80 (p.19, Figure 3.5):

● -- EQUATION (4) :
$$I = [aD^1 + bD^2] \times [exp-(m'D^1 + m''D^2)]$$

where I = incidence of effect being studied (total excess cancers).

Equation (4) is clearly the unmodified Equation (3), except for the righthand term between brackets. The quantity between the righthand pair of brackets is the "exponential modifier" by which the quantity between the lefthand pair of brackets is multiplied. Some readers will want to review the meaning of "exp." See Chapter 19, Part 2, Poisson Equation, and the note below Table 23-A in this chapter. (We shall defer examination of Table 23-A, for its other purposes, until later.)

In Equation (4), the cSv-unit cancels out in the modifier, because the units of the m' and m'' coefficients are cSv^{-1} and cSv^{-2}, respectively.

Contribution of the NCRP :

Discussions of radiation carcinogenesis commonly refer to the necessity of modifying the LQ model, by some additional term, in order to fit the "leveling off" and "flattening" and "falling" of the incidence curve with rising dose. Almost invariably, these phenomena are described as occurring at HIGH doses. For instance, Ncrp80 (p.17) states:

"The phenomenon of the dose-response curve leveling off and then falling at high doses ... is seen frequently in radiobiology and specifically in curves for mutagenesis and carcinogenesis. Its cause, although incompletely understood, is frequently ascribed to cell killing. Since it is still seen in cell transformation experiments in tissue culture in which the results are normalized to surviving cells ... it could be due at least in part to intracellular processes that prevent the presumed 'induction' phenomenon from becoming manifest."

The NCRP statement above is very useful, and it is clear that NCRP does not consider cell-killing as necessarily the only explanation for the "leveling off" effect. We would agree on that point.

But we fault the NCRP statement for its general suggestion that the "leveling off" effect is necessarily a HIGH-dose effect. The understanding of why radiobiology and epidemiology are NOT in conflict depends upon not pre-judging how intense the "leveling off" effect is and at what dose it becomes appreciable.

The NCRP formulation using an exponential term, in order to take account of the "leveling off" effect, is quite reasonable. But after introducing the expression [exp-(m'Dose^1 + m''Dose^2)], it is totally unreasonable to pre-judge what the appropriate values for m' and m'' are going to be. (It might be noted that Ncrp80 uses the gamma and delta symbols instead of m' and m''.)

The values of the m' and m'' coefficients in the exponential term must be determined by curve-fitting with real data, not by some pre-judgment which can totally distort the reality of epidemiological evidence.

Pre-Judgment in NIH Report:

Other discussions in the literature, of the linear and quadratic terms, also tend to suggest that the "leveling off" effect can occur ONLY at very high doses -- a suggestion which I am sure has added wholly unnecessary confusion to the scene.

For example, in the 1985 NIH Report, the authors refer to how various "official bodies" (their term) have handled risk-reduction factors, and in this discussion, they say (Nih85, p.26):

"The BEIR III Committee did not incorporate the competing effect of cell inactivation, mainly at high dose levels, into its risk calculations, although it did consider the problem theoretically ..." The NIH Report also states, in discussing the Japanese A-bomb survivors (p.26-27):

"Doses high enough to reduce the carcinogenic response appreciably through the competing effect of cell inactivation might well be in the lethal range for man when delivered to his whole body."

The NIH Report clearly takes an extremely prejudicial position on how very high the doses might have to be, before cell inactivation could influence the dose-response for cancer. The NIH committee has decided, contrary to the evidence available in 1985 from the A-Bomb Study, that whole-body doses might have to be high enough to be lethal to man.

Implications of Breast-Cancer Data :

Moreover, it would appear that the NIH committee did not consider the implications of its own acceptance of the conclusion that the dose-response for human breast-cancer is linear over the entire dose-range (Chapter 22, Part 2).

The acceptance of linearity at all doses implies either (1) inter-track carcinogenesis is negligible over the entire dose-range, or (2) the "leveling off" effect from cell inactivation is appreciable enough at low doses to off-set the concave-UPWARD curve of Plot B. Indeed, where whole-body exposure occurred (the A-bomb survivors), the "leveling off" effect was appreciable enough to make the dose-response for breast-cancer concave-DOWNWARD rather than linear (Ncrp80, p.144; Go81, Chaps. 10,11).

"Radiobiologic Findings" :

It is my opinion that pre-judgments or "blind-spots" about the interaction of the linear term, quadratic term, and the cell-INACTIVATION term, have led to much nonsense about radiobiology being in conflict with human epidemiological evidence, and to suggestions that we must accept dose-response curves "based on radiobiology" even though the proposed curves are totally at variance with real human epidemiological data of good quality.

For instance, "radiobiologic findings" were named as the basis when BEIR-3 endorsed UPWARD curvature (Beir80, p.261), and substituted a leukemia curve for the all-cancer curve; see our Chapter 22, Part 3. This substitution was noted by RERF analysts in explaining why their own risk-estimates are higher than BEIR-3's:

[Some of the disparity] " ... may be ascribed to the fact that in BEIR III, the curvature in dose response for leukemia was used for all cancers except leukemia instead of the actual curvature which probably is much

closer to linearity, and this may cause much smaller estimates to be produced than if the actual dose-response curve were to be applied" (Shi88, p.51).

4. A Modified LQ Model, Fitting Supra-Linear, Linear, Sigmoid, and Other Dose-Responses

Unlike the radiation committees cited in Part 3, we shall NOT assume that the cell-inactivation term -- which is the exponential modifier in Equation (4) -- applies only at some arbitrarily high radiation dose. Instead, we shall investigate how this term can be used to fit actual human epidemiological data having supra-linear and linear dose-responses.

Moreover, we shall not pre-judge how prominent the linear term (A, or intra-track carcinogenesis) is in comparison with the quadratic term (B, or inter-track carcinogenesis). We shall explore two limits: A = B at 50 cSv, and A = B at 400 cSv.

When A = B at 50 cSv, the unmodified LQ dose-response has a markedly concave-upward curvature (Figure 23-B), but even such curvature becomes concave-DOWNWARD with the appropriate cell-inactivation function -- as we shall show.

Cell-Inactivation, and Table 23-A :
=====================================

To explain the observed "leveling off" of radiation carcinogenesis with rising dose, some analysts refer to the need for a "cell-killing" term. We do not regard cell-killing as the only possible explanation. Some other analysts make the presumption that "cell sterilization" occurs with rising dose, and that inability of cells to reproduce accounts for the observation. Also, it is possible that what accounts for the observation is redundancy of carcinogenic lesions, with rising dose, or dose-dependent changes in the biochemical milieu.

In the absence of evidence on the cause or causes of supra-linear and linear dose-responses, we prefer to use the term "cell-inactivation."

"Cell-inactivation" is a term compatible with all possibilities. It implies that, as dose rises, (1) a decreasing fraction of irradiated cells remains capable of providing the precursors of a clinical cancer, and (2) an increasing fraction of irradiated cells becomes "inactivated" with respect to developing into clinical cancers, even though radiation may have produced carcinogenic alteration in such cells.

It must be emphasized that there are no rules and no radiobiological principles which prevent variation of the cell-inactivation term, from one species to another. We shall return to this issue early in Part 5.

Table 23-A evaluates the cell inactivation term for various pairs of m' and m'' values in Equation (4) -- which is the modified LQ model. For convenience, it is provided again below.

● -- EQUATION (4) : Incidence = [aD^1 + bD^2] x [exp-(m'D^1 + m''D^2)]

In Table 23-A, one finds that the "active" fraction is 100 % at zero dose, and falls with rising dose. Figure 23-A shows that the fractions fall in a non-linear manner.

A = B at 400 cSv. Modified LQ Model Yields Supra-Linearity :
==================================

In Part 2, we showed how Table 23-C yields Figure 23-C -- a concave-upward dose-response with no "leveling off" or flattening at high doses. We plotted only the A, B, and A+B columns.

Now we return to Table 23-C, where A = B at 400 cSv, and we call attention to Column C. Column C shows dose-response (A+B) as modified by the cell-inactivation term when m' = 0.005 and m'' = -0.000004. In other words, Column C is the evaluation of Equation (4) when those are the values of m' and m''.

For instance, if we use 100 cSv as an example, the entry in Col. C is 50,000 excess cancers (from Column A+B, unmodified, at 100 cSv) times 0.63128 (the value of the cell inactivation term, from Table 23-A, Column D, at 100 cSv), or 31,564 excess cancers. The cell-inactivation term operates upon the intra-track and inter-track terms alike. One arrives at the same entry by modifying the A and B entries at 100 cSv separately: (40,000 x 0.63128) + (10,000 x 0.63128) = 31,564.

In Figure 23-D, we have plotted Column C as Plot M (for Modified). Otherwise, Figure 23-D is exactly the same as Figure 23-C.

It is self-evident, in Figure 23-D, DD, and DDD that Plot M has a supra-linear, concave-downward shape throughout the dose-range.

Figure 23-D and the A-Bomb Study :

Plot M of Figure 23-D, DD, DDD is in harmony with the human dose-response observed in the A-bomb survivors.

Examination of Figure 23-DDD shows that Plot M starts diverging from the unmodified LQ dose-response (which is Plot A+B) at very low doses. In other words, the cell-inactivation term is already operating below 30 cSv to produce a supra-linear bend which is appreciable and detectable. This is in accord with the curvature noted in Chapter 14 for the A-bomb survivors.

On the other hand, no one should expect PERFECT matching between Figure 23-D, DD, DDD and the dose-response depicted in Chapter 14. Figure 23-D is constrained only by its equation, whereas Figures 14-E and 14-F are constrained not only by different equations, but also by real-world datapoints. The plots in Chapter 14 are empirical best-fits to actual data, and thus do not pre-judge the interplay of factors such as possible population heterogeneity, possible lethargy of repair-systems at very low doses, possible effects of biochemical milieu, possible redundancy of injury, or other factors which may affect the steepness of slope in the very low dose-region.

A Spurious Conflict :

If we return to Figure 23-D, DD, DDD, the key point is that a modified LQ model resolves any alleged conflict between the real-world observation -- that supra-linearity (starting at very low doses) occurs throughout the entire dose-range of the A-Bomb Study -- and "radiobiology."

We cannot explain why the assumption is made, by so many, that the modifying term in an LQ model cannot operate below very high doses. There seems to be no logical or scientific basis for such an assumption. When we permit the modifying term in Equation (4) to have effect at quite low doses, we are not assaulting the LQ model. More importantly, we can attain a curve which is compatible with human epidemiology, instead of substituting a curve which assaults such evidence.

The Graphic Meaning of "Supra-Linear" and "Sub-Linear" :
==================================

Examination of Figure 23-DD shows clearly that Plot M has a concave-downward bend. If a straight line were to connect any two points along Plot M, the curve of Plot M would lie ABOVE the straight line. That is why it is correct to characterize a shape like Plot M as SUPRA-linear.

===

If confusion is to be avoided, the standard for describing the shape of a curve must be the curve itself, and not some other curve which may happen to be present in the same figure. Thus, the fact that Plot M lies beneath the linear Plot A does NOT make it appropriate to call it "sub-linear" -- a term encountered in the NRC's 1985 report (Gilb85, p.II-102). If Plot A were not in our figure at all, it would be impossible to guess the meaning of "sub-linear." By contrast, the term supra-linear is unambiguous with respect to shape.

As noted repeatedly in this book, another term commonly used for the supra-linear shape is "concave-downward." Far less common is the term "upward convex" -- a term encountered in Sho86 (p.693).

A = B at 400 cSv. Modified LQ Model Yields Linearity :

====================================

Next we will show that, with certain other values of m' and m" in the cell-inactivation term, the LQ model is also fully consistent with observing a LINEAR dose-response in human epidemiological studies.

We turn attention to Table 23-C again, where the linear and quadratic terms contribute equally to radiation-induced cancer at 400 cSv.

Column D modifies the LQ equation by using the following values in the cell-inactivation term: m' = 0.0025, and m" = -0.0000025. The details are in Note 2 of that table.

Column D is shown as Plot M (for Modified) in Figure 23-E. Except for Plot M, Figure 23-E is exactly the same as Figure 23-D.

It is self-evident, in Figure 23-E, that Plot M (the boxy symbol) looks linear from the origin out to about 250 cSv. Comparison of the entries in Table 23-C, Column A versus Column D, shows just how close the match is between the linear component (A) and the modified sum of A+B (Column D), out to 200 cSv. Indeed, Plot M is so very close to Plot A that one cannot distinguish the two plots from each other in Figure 23-EE, or EEE. In Figure 23-E, Plots A and M separate enough that, by about 250 cSv, we can discern that there are actually TWO plots, superimposed on each other, over most of the dose-range.

Thus, with a shift in the values of m' and m" in the cell-inactivation term, we can convert the concave-downward curve in Figure 23-D to a virtually perfect linear dose-response in Figure 23-E -- while the linear and quadratic terms are preserved intact.

Indeed, Figure 23-E shows that the effect of the exponential modifier (the cell-inactivation term), acting upon BOTH the linear and quadratic terms, can produce a "pseudo-linear" result -- as if no quadratic term existed at all.

Linearity and Supra-Linearity -- Different Faces of the Same Coin ?

====================================

We pointed out at the end of Part 2 that, if there is a positive linear term and a positive quadratic term in radiation carcinogenesis, then, without modification, the sum of these two types of terms must necessarily give a concave-upward dose- response.

It follows that observation of a linear dose-response means that a cell-inactivation term (or some equivalent) must be operating to convert the concave-upward dose-response to linearity. In other words, observed linearity is a step on the way from concave-upward curvature to supra-linearity with just the intensity of the modification separating linearity from supra-linearity. Ncrp80 (p.18) also points out that linearity can be derived in this way, and that several workers have made this suggestion in the past.

Nonetheless, the insight has been ignored for almost a decade, while "radiobiology" was mistakenly invoked to support a concave-upward dose-response and the popular risk reduction-factors -- in the face of contrary human evidence.

Figures 23-D and 23-E reconcile radiobiology with reality. They are based on assuming a positive linear term, a positive quadratic term, and an exponential modifying term.

Next, we will show that the reconciliation is feasible also at the other limit -- when A = B at 50 cSv.

A = B at 50 cSv. Modified LQ Model Yields Supra-Linearity

====================================

We now return to Table 23-B, where the linear term (A) and the quadratic term (B) are equally prominent at 50 cSv. The unmodified concave-upward shape of A+B was depicted in Figure 23-B.

We shall modify Column A+B of Table 23-B twice, as we did in Table 23-C. However, this time we shall illustrate conversion of Col. A+B into a sigmoid dose-response and then into a supra-linear dose-response.

Conversion to Sigmoid Shape :

Column C from Table 23-B has been depicted as Plot M in Figure 23-F, FF, FFF. Otherwise, Figure 23-F and Figure 23-B are the same.

Figure 23-FF and FFF show that Plot M is concave-upward below 100 cSv. Since dose-response in the A-Bomb Study is NOT concave-upward in this dose-range, it is clear that the values of m' and m" tested by Column C are at variance with reality.

Nonetheless, Figure 23-F is provided here in order to help demonstrate that the method itself is not ruling out the sigmoid shape. We rule out the sigmoid shape on the basis of the human epidemiological evidence. The method itself is capable of fitting just about any dose-response one has ever seen. We shall return to this point.

Conversion to Supra-Linearity :

In order to convert Figure 23-F to supra-linearity, we need only to change the values of m' and m". This has been done in Table 23-B, Column D.

Column D from Table 23-B has been depicted as Plot M in Figure 23-G, GG, GGG. Except for Plot M, Figure 23-G and Figure 23-F are the same.

In Figure 23-GGG, the particular pair of values for m' and m" in Column D happens to make Plot M very nearly linear between 0 and 50 cSv. Beyond 50 cSv, Plot M becomes supra-linear.

It is evident, from Figure 23-GG, that Plot M (which is A+B modified) diverges from the unmodified Plot A+B at very low doses. Indeed, Figure 23-GGG shows that, by the time dose rises to 50 cSv, the cell-inactivation term has cut the excess cancer depicted by Plot M in about half, compared with the unmodified Plot A+B.

A = B at 100 cSv.
Additional Conversions of the LQ Model :
=================================

Readers need not depend on our assertion that the modified LQ model is capable of fitting a vast variety of observed dose-responses.

For instance, Figure 23-I (Eye) shows how merely changing the values of m' and m" converts the

unmodified concave-upward model (where m' = 0, and m" = 0 also) into the other five shapes shown on that page. Using Tables 23-A and 23-B as examples, readers could generate the input and output for all six of those curves by using A = B at 100 cSv and by using the values of m' and m" shown in each figure.

A very important point is that shapes in Figure 23-Eye have actually been reported in the literature for certain dose-responses.

The shape shown by Figure 23-Eye-5, for instance, closely resembles the shape of dose-response shown in Ncrp80 Figure 4.12 for specific-locus mutation frequencies versus X-ray dose in mouse spermatogonia. It also resembles, in shape (not in scale), the dose-response shown in Ncrp80 Figure 9.1 for the incidence of myeloid leukemia in male RF mice versus dose, over a wide range of X-ray or gamma-ray doses.

Figure 23-Eye-6 -- with its initial rise followed by a flattening which is then followed by a secondary rise -- has the same pattern as a number of cell-transformation studies, such as those done by Hall and Miller with C3H10T1/2 mouse cells (Ha81). A similar shape was reported by Preston and Brewen in studies of translocations in mouse spermatogonial cells (Pres73).

A Warning about Other Species and about Cell-Studies :
=====================================

In the previous chapter, we showed that, (through mid-1989) the radiation committees have over-ruled direct human epidemiological evidence on the shape of dose-response for solid cancers, in favor of generalizations from NON-human evidence and from cell studies. (Breast-cancer is the significant exception to this practice.)

The errors which may be inadvertently introduced, by extrapolating from one species to another, are well known. What may be less fully appreciated by some readers are the serious confounding variables even within a single species. So we will provide an illustration, described by Little (Li81), in which an experimental dose-response was converted from concave-upward to linear, by changing the chemical milieu of the irradiated cells.

Little described experiments (Terz76; Kenn78) using mouse 10T1/2 cells to study cell transformation (from normal to cancerous). When the mouse cells were irradiated with various doses of X-rays, a clearly concave-upward dose-response was observed.

However, when the irradiated cells were exposed to the promoting agent commonly known as TPA (12-O-tetradecanoyl-phorbol-13-acetate) during the post-irradiation expression-period, two changes were observed. First, an enormous increase in transformation-yield per surviving cell occurred at all radiation doses. And second, the shape of dose-response changed from concave-upward to perfectly LINEAR.

Such cell-transformation data confirm that the biochemical milieu in which cell cultures are grown can profoundly influence the shape of the dose-response which investigators will observe. This is well known now, and probably explains much of the apparent inconsistency of results reported from experimental work, even within a single species.

In short, biochemical milieu makes a huge difference in dose-response, and if the biochemical milieu of human cells in a laboratory is unnatural -- and it is -- there is no guarantee that cells in intact human beings will have the same dose-response which they have in someone's laboratory.

Without denigrating the valuable experimental work done in laboratories, we simply remind readers that the only reliable data on human dose-response for radiation carcinogenesis are necessarily the human epidemiological data themselves.

5. Proper Risk-Estimates for Low Acute Exposures

We have worked our way back, now, to the title of this chapter.

We have demonstrated that there is no conflict between human epidemiology (which shows a supra-linear or linear dose-response, but not a concave-upward one) and the hypothesis from radiobiology that intra-track carcinogenesis can be expressed by a positive linear term, and inter-track carcinogenesis by a positive quadratic term.

The absence of conflict follows from the fact that the linear-quadratic hypothesis does NOT necessarily predict a concave-upward dose-response. It can predict ANY of the shapes (and more) which are depicted in Figure 23-Eye. It can certainly predict a supra-linear or linear dose-response, as we have shown -- provided that analysts exclude artificial

constraints, such as the presumption that the cell-inactivation term can operate only at very high doses.

Curve-Fitting to the Real Evidence :

There is a great deal of experimental evidence (from other species and cell studies), as well as the direct human evidence itself, which confirms that the LQ model needs an exponential modifier -- as shown in Equation (4) -- in order to fit actual observations.

It is crucial that the values and signs (positive, negative) for m' and m'' in the exponential modifier be chosen in order to fit the observations. It is the antithesis of objectivity for anyone to pre-judge these values, and then to discard reality-based observations if they do not fit the resulting curve.

Moreover, Figures 23-D through 23-Eye show that the LQ hypothesis would not be violated if it should turn out that dose-response for radiation carcinogenesis is concave-downward for some species (e.g., the human) and concave-upward or some other shape for other species. Such variation would be perfectly consistent with species-specific variation in values of m' and m''.

It is difficult to understand why this point has not been emphasized by the radiation committees for the past ten years. Instead, they have repeatedly suggested that analysts must choose between "radiobiology" and human epidemiological evidence, as if a conflict existed. We have shown that radiobiology and epidemiology can be in complete harmony with each other regarding the LQ hypothesis.

Risk Increase-Factors Needed :

We and the radiation committees (see for instance Un88, p.415, para.62) are in agreement that the best human epidemiological evidence on the shape of dose-response comes from the A-Bomb Study, for the reasons described in our Chapter 4. And within the A-Bomb Study, analysis for all cancers combined is, of course, far more reliable than single-site analysis.

For three consecutive follow-ups (1950-74, 1950-78, 1950-82), the A-Bomb Study has shown that the dose-response for acute exposure is not concave-upward. Within the data, dose-response for all cancers combined is supra-linear throughout the dose-range. (Beyond 1982, the data are not yet available for anyone to do a "constant-cohort, dual-dosimetry" analysis.)

The absence of a concave-upward dose-response means that risk reduction-factors are completely inappropriate for making risk-estimates at low acute exposures. Supra-linearity means that risk INCREASE-factors would be needed, if one insisted on estimating low-dose risks from high-dose data.

Illustrative Risk Increase-Factors :

Like risk reduction-factors, risk increase-factors derive from the ratio of the steeper linear slope over the lower linear slope (see Part 2).

Supra-Linearity, with A = B at 400 cSv :
Suppose Figure 23-D described reality, but one had datapoints only at 160 cSv and at zero dose. A linear interpolation, between 160 cSv on Plot M and the origin, would have the slope of 44,600.9 (from Table 23-C, Column C at 160 cSv) over 160 cSv, or 278.8 cancers per cSv. At low doses, the actual slope of Plot M, however, is almost identical with the unmodified slope of Plot A.

This can be verified by comparing low-dose entries in Column A with the corresponding entries in Column C of Table 23-C. The congruence at very low doses is expected, since the unmodified Column B makes only a small contribution to cancers, and the value of the cell-inactivation term is close to 1.0 at low doses (see Table 23-A).

Thus one can use the slope of the unmodified Plot A to approximate the slope of Plot M at low doses. The slope is 64,000 / 160, or 400. The appropriate risk INCREASE-factor, under these particular circumstances and values of m' and m", would be 400 / 278.8, or 1.43.

Supra-Linearity, with A = B at 50 cSv :
Under these circumstances and with the values of m' and m" used in Table 23-B, the linear slope of Plot M between 160 cSv and the origin would be 4361.97 (from Table 23-B, Column D) over 160, or 27.26. The slope of the unmodified Plot A would be 8000 / 160, or 50. The risk INCREASE-factor would be 50 / 27.26, or 1.83.

No Need to Use "Factors", Up or Down :

Section 4 of this book clearly shows that direct observations exist along the dose-response curve right down to 10-15 cSv (rems) of acute internal organ-dose. There is simply no need for anyone to use "factors" (up, or down) to estimate low-dose cancer-risk from high-dose data.

If "factors" are invoked anyway, we have shown that risk INCREASE-factors are needed for low acute exposures -- not risk REDUCTION-factors.

6. Risk-Estimates for Slow Delivery of High Doses

The observation of a supra-linear dose-response from acute exposure rules out risk reduction-factors for low acute exposures, but supra-linearity does NOT automatically rule out the possibility that a high dose is less carcinogenic if it is delivered slowly, than if it is delivered all at once. The various possibilities receive some quantitative examination in Part 6, here, for slow delivery of a high dose. Slow delivery of LOW doses is examined separately, in Part 7.

Lack of Conclusive Evidence for Moderate and High Doses :
=================================

I am not convinced that existing human epidemiological data are capable of reliably quantifying a dose-rate effect -- if one exists at all. It will not be an easy question to settle. If different human studies involve exposure to different distributions of gamma or X-ray energies, and if there is no reliable way to evaluate a valid RBE between such radiations, then a uncertainty factor of about 2 could be introduced on this basis alone. Moreover, dosimetry would have to be excellent.

The breast-cancer fluoroscopy studies cited in Chapter 21 are very reliable for testing whether or not all cancer-response was eliminated by flawless repair, but that is a totally different matter from asking those studies to tell us the exact magnitude of cancer-risk per rem -- well enough to discern a possible effect from dose-rate.

As for experimental data on a dose-rate effect, they are far from conclusive. Some results clearly challenge the conventional assumption that dose-fractionation or very slow delivery reduces the carcinogenic risk, compared with the risk from acute delivery of the same dose. For illustrative purposes, we will mention one such report on cell transformation following irradiation, by Hall and Miller (Ha81). They describe the complicated responses which have been observed with fractionation of X-ray dose (emphasis in the original):

"Experiments with fractionated doses of X-rays indicate that dividing the dose into two equal fractions separated by 5 hr results in a decrease of transformation incidence compared with a single exposure of the same total dose for doses above 1.5 Gy, but that at lower dose levels splitting the dose ENHANCES transformation incidence. In a further series of experiments, it has been shown that the transformation incidence resulting from a dose of 1 Gy delivered in two, three, or four equal fractions spread over 5 hr increases progressively with the number of fractions compared with the same total dose delivered in a single exposure. The same is true for continuous low-dose-rate irradiation, where 1 Gy delivered over 6 hr resulted in more transformations than an acute exposure of the same dose. Thus it has been clearly demonstrated with this IN VITRO system that the temporal distribution of dose, in particular its protraction over a period of time, significantly enhances transformation incidence at relatively low doses" (Ha81, p.208).

In my opinion, the combination of experimental work, human epidemiology, and hypothetical considerations, does not yet tell us whether dose-rate has any effect on human cancer-risk, when the total dose delivered is moderate or high.

As we shall see in Part 7, however, when the total dose is low, no basis exists for postulating a reduced cancer-risk from slow delivery.

Some General Considerations :

The presumption of the LQ model is that the Q term represents inter-track carcinogenesis. When we compare Column B (the Q term) with Column A+B in Tables 23-B and 23-C, we see that -- at low doses -- inter-track carcinogenesis contributes very little to total excess cancer. The linear term (single tracks, acting independently) accounts for virtually all of the radiation-induced cancer from low acute doses.

Therefore, if a high total dose like 100 cSv is delivered as a series of low doses -- say, one cSv per exposure -- it is widely presumed that the cancer-risk per cSv is reduced, because the inter-track contribution is virtually eliminated (see, for instance, Ncrp80, p.15).

As we illustrate how this presumption operates, it will become evident that a great deal depends upon the relative prominence of the linear and the quadratic terms in the LQ equation. We will evaluate slow versus fast delivery of 100 cSv, for the case where A = B at 400 cSv and, separately, where A = B at 50 cSv.

We will illustrate a range of risk reduction-factors, first by using the common -- but mistaken -- presumption that human dose-response is concave-

upward, and then by using the real-world observation that it is NOT.

With a Concave-UPWARD Dose-Response and 100 cSv Total Dose :

If A = B at 400 cSv and b = 1.0, then Table 23-C, Column A+B, shows that excess cancers = 50,000 at 100 cSv of acute dose. The inter-track term (Column B) is contributing substantially -- 10,000 out of 50,000. But the same table shows that cancer-risk from one cSv of dose is 401, to which the linear term contributes 400 cancers and the inter-track term contributes only 1.0.

We can neglect the inter-track term and can say that the risk, from 100 doses of one cSv each, would be (100 x 400 cancers), or 40,000 cancers -- instead of 50,000. Therefore, the risk from slow delivery would be (40,000 / 50,000), or 80 % of the risk from the same dose acutely delivered.

If A = B at 50 cSv and b = 1.0, then Table 23-B, Column A+B, shows that excess cancers = 15,000 at 100 cSv of acute dose. The inter-track term (Column B) is contributing very substantially -- 10,000 out of 15,000. But the same table shows that cancer-risk from one cSv of dose is 51, to which the linear term contributes 50 cancers and the inter- track term contributes only 1.0.

Again we can neglect the inter-track term and can say that the risk, from 100 doses of one cSv each, would be (100 x 50 cancers), or 5,000 cancers -- instead of 15,000. Therefore, the risk from slow delivery would be (5,000 / 15,000), or 33.3 % of the risk from the same dose acutely delivered.

With a Concave-DOWNWARD Dose-Response and 100 cSv Total Dose :

If one accepts the linear-quadratic hypothesis, it follows that when dose-response is concave-downward, one is dealing with Equation (4) -- the modified LQ equation with the cell-inactivation term. At low doses, the quadratic term virtually disappears and only the linear term operates -- and so the cell inactivation term operates essentially on the linear term alone.

But we must ask, "Which cell-inactivation term?" It seems clear that the appropriate choice of cell-inactivation term is dependent upon the rate of delivery of the radiation. Therefore, if 100 cSv is delivered acutely, then the cell-inactivation term, for any particular choice of m' and m", will be found on the line for 100 cSv in Table 23-A. However, if 100 cSv is delivered in the form of 100 doses, each of one cSv, then the cell-inactivation term, for those same values of m' and m", will be found on the line for 1 cSv in Table 23-A.

The consequences of these presumptions will be demonstrated with specific examples.

If A = B at 400 cSv :

Excess cancers will be calculated for acute delivery of 100 cSv, and for 100 cSv delivered in 100 separate doses, each of 1 cSv. The entries from Table 23-C, Column C, will be used. The cell inactivation values will be obtained from Table 23-A, Column D. Those values for the active fraction of cells remaining are:

```
For dose =    1 cSv: Active fraction = 0.99502
For dose = 100 cSv: Active fraction = 0.63128

For acute delivery of 100 cSv:
A + B = 50,000 (from Table 23-C)
Excess cancers = (50,000)(0.63128)
               = 31564
This value is in Column C of Table 23-C.
```

The calculation for "slow" delivery -- one hundred separate doses of 1 cSv -- requires more detail, now provided.

The first dose of 1 cSv has an associated active fraction of 0.99502 . Each subsequent dose also has an associated active fraction of 0.99502 BUT these subsequent doses are operating on cells which already have had their active fraction reduced by the operation of prior 1 cSv doses. Thus, the total active fraction for the FIRST 1 cSv dose-increment is 0.99502. The total active fraction for the SECOND 1 cSv dose is (0.99502) x (0.99502), or 0.990064. The total active fraction for the THIRD 1 cSv dose is (0.990064) x (0.99502), or 0.985134 .

This procedure is repeated 100 total times, and provides the active fraction left for carcinogenesis from each of the 100 separate 1 cSv doses. The 100th active fraction has the value (0.99502)^100, or 0.606989. The AVERAGE active fraction, for these 100 doses of 1 cSv each, is 0.785248.

Since each 1 cSv dose provides 401 excess cancers, and since the average active fraction is 0.785248, it follows that the total excess cancers from 100 doses will be (100) x (401 cancers) x (0.785248), or 31,488 excess cancers.

The result is extremely close to the 31,564 excess cancers produced by a single dose of 100 cSv. The single dose is associated with a lower modifier (0.63128), operating on a larger number of cancers (50,000). The serial doses are associated with a higher average modifier (0.785248), operating on a lower number of cancers (100 x 401, or 40,100).

No Reduced Cancer-Risk :

The conclusion is that there is NO protection (no reduced cancer-risk) from slow delivery of 100 cSv IN THIS CASE. We stress "IN THIS CASE" because this result is obtained for the case where A = B at 400 cSv, and for a particular set of m' and m" values, chosen to illustrate a concave-downward dose-response.

Intuitively, we are not surprised at the result. When the linear term is so much more important than the quadratic term -- that is, where B does not reach a contribution equal to that of A until a dose of 400 cSv -- the lessening of the quadratic response with dose-delivery in small increments is far smaller than it would be in the case where A = B at some much lower value, e.g. 50 cSv. Indeed, we shall now explore that case.

If A = B at 50 cSv :

Excess cancers will be calculated for acute delivery of 100 cSv, and for 100 cSv delivered in 100 separate doses, each of 1 cSv. The entries from Table 23-B, Column D, will be used. The cell inactivation values will be obtained from Table 23-A, Column H. Those values for the active fraction of cells remaining are:

```
For dose =    1 cSv: Active fraction = 0.98513
For dose = 100 cSv: Active fraction = 0.25666

For acute delivery of 100 cSv:
A + B = 15,000 (from Table 23-B)
Excess cancers = (15,000)(0.25666)
               = 3849.9
This value is in Column D of Table 23-B.
```

For the "slow" delivery -- 100 separate doses of 1 cSv each -- we must go through the same type of iterative procedure as was done for the case of A = B at 400 cSv.

The active fraction for the FIRST 1 cSv dose-increment is 0.98513. The total active fraction for the SECOND 1 cSv dose is (0.98513) x (0.98513), or 0.970481 . The total active fraction for the THIRD 1 cSv dose is (0.970481) x (0.98513), or 0.956049 .

This procedure is repeated 100 total times, and provides the active fraction left for carcinogenesis from each of the 100 separate 1 cSv doses. The 100th active fraction has the value (0.98513)^100, or 0.223539 . The AVERAGE active fraction, for these 100 doses of 1 cSv each, is 0.514401 .

Since each 1 cSv dose provides 51 excess cancers, and since the average active fraction is 0.514401, it follows that the total excess cancers from 100 doses will be (100) x (51 cancers) x (0.514401), or 2623.445 excess cancers.

Yes, Reduced Cancer-Risk :

By contrast, the expectation from acute delivery of 100 cSv, for this case, is 3849.9 excess cancers (above).

Therefore, under these circumstances and assumptions, we would invoke a risk-reduction factor of (2623.445 / 3849.9), or 0.68, for slow delivery of 100 cSv.

Summary on Slow Delivery of 100 cSv :

We have shown in Part 6 that estimates of risk reduction-factors, for slow delivery of 100 cSv compared with acute delivery, are affected not only by the shape of the ACUTE dose-response, but also by the dose at which the linear and quadratic terms (A,B) are presumed to be equal.

It may not be appropriate to invoke any risk reduction-factors at all, for slow delivery. Above, under the concave-downward dose-response, we provided one illustration where the presumption of risk reduction-factors would not be warranted under the linear-quadratic model, and one illustration where it would be warranted.

Pending more evidence on this issue, we regard it as premature for anyone to count on a much lower cancer-risk from 100 cSv slowly delivered than from 100 cSv acutely delivered. As we said at the outset of Part 6, we do not believe the issue can yet be settled, for moderate and high total doses, on an objective scientific basis.

7. Risk-Estimates for Slow Delivery of Low Doses

We have already shown, in Section 5 of this book, that there is no dose or dose-rate which is SAFE, with respect to induction of fatal human cancer.

However, Section 5 did not examine the possibility that low doses received slowly might be LESS carcinogenic than the same low doses received acutely. Now, in Part 7, we shall show why risk reduction-factors are NOT appropriate for slow delivery of low total doses.

Doses in the Range of Millirems :

It is unnecessary to look at this issue below 100 millirems. Readers who refer back to Chapter 20 (especially Part 3 and Table 20-M) will see that, at the level of the cell-nucleus, a few hundred millirems can be regarded as the slowest conceivable dose-rate.

Since in the very low dose-range, we are dealing with essentially a single track through a nucleus, there is no difference in dose-rate between a few hundred millirems delivered all at once, and the same total dose spread out over years. In both cases, the dose-rate is virtually instantaneous delivery of the entire dose to those cell-nuclei which receive any dose at all.

It follows that in the entire dose-range between zero dose and a few hundred millirems, the issue is already settled about possible risk-reduction from slow delivery: There is NO reduction of risk to be considered because there is no reduction in dose-rate.

Next, we shall consider a somewhat higher dose.

Slow Delivery of 5 cSv :

Using the approach demonstrated in Part 6, we will examine the possible risk-reduction if a total dose of 5 cSv is delivered in five fractions of one cSv each.

If A = B at 400 cSv :

Excess cancers will be calculated for acute delivery of 5 cSv, and for 5 cSv delivered in 5 separate doses, each of 1 cSv. The entries from Table 23-C, Column C, will be used. These are entries for a dose-response which is concave-DOWNWARD between zero and 5 cSv. The cell-inactivation values will be obtained from Table 23-A, Column D. Those values for the active fraction of cells remaining are:

```
For dose =    1 cSv: Active fraction = 0.99502
For dose =    5 cSv: Active fraction = 0.97541

For acute delivery of 5 cSv:
```

A + B = 2,025 (from Table 23-C)
Excess cancers = (2,025)(0.97541)
              = 1975.20
This value is in Column C of Table 23-C.

For the "slow" delivery -- 5 separate doses of 1 cSv each -- we must do what we did in Part 6.

The first dose of 1 cSv has an associated active fraction of 0.99502 . Each subsequent dose also has an associated active fraction of 0.99502 BUT these subsequent doses are operating on cells which already have had their active fraction reduced by the operation of prior 1 cSv doses. Thus, the total active fraction for the FIRST 1 cSv dose-increment is 0.99502. The total active fraction for the SECOND 1 cSv dose is (0.99502) x (0.99502), or 0.990064.

Since there are only 5 doses of 1 cSv involved, we can show the full set of active fractions, and the excess cancers calculated for each 1 cSv dose. Each modifier operates on an A+B value of 401 cancers per cSv. Therefore, in each line below, Excess Cancers = 401 x 1 x Active Fraction:

Dose-Increment	Active Fraction	Excess Cancers
First	0.995020	399.0030
Second	0.990064	397.0157
Third	0.985134	395.0387
Fourth	0.980228	393.0714
Fifth	0.975346	391.1137
Total Excess Cancers		1975.243

We could have made the same calculation here as we did for the case of 100 separate 1 cSv doses: The average active fraction = 0.985158
Excess cancers = 5 x 401 x 0.985158
              =   1975.242

For A = B at 400 cSv, the fast delivery and the slow delivery of 5 cSv yield identical results.

We shall now examine this same comparison, of slow versus fast delivery of 5 cSv, for the case where the quadratic component is more prominent.

If A = B at 50 cSv :

Excess cancers will be calculated for acute delivery of 5 cSv, and for 5 cSv delivered in 5 separate doses, each of 1 cSv. The entries from Table 23-B, Column D, will be used. These are entries for a dose-response which is slightly concave-UPWARD between zero and 5 cSv. The cell inactivation values will be obtained from Table 23-A, Column H. Those values for active fraction of cells remaining are:

For dose =   1 cSv: Active fraction = 0.98513
For dose =   5 cSv: Active fraction = 0.92807

For acute delivery of 5 cSv:
A + B = 275 (from Table 23-B)
Excess cancers = (275)(0.92807)
              = 255.219
This value is in Column C of Table 23-C.

For the "slow" delivery -- 5 separate doses of 1 cSv each -- we can show the full set of active fractions, and the excess cancers calculated for each 1 cSv dose. Each modifier operates on an A+B value of 51 cancers per cSv. Therefore, in each line below, Excess Cancers = 51 x 1 x Active Fraction:

Dose-Increment	Active Fraction	Excess Cancers
First	0.985130	50.24163
Second	0.970481	49.49454
Third	0.956050	48.75855
Fourth	0.941833	48.03351
Fifth	0.927828	47.31926
Total Excess Cancers		243.8475

We could have made the same calculation here as we did for the case of 100 separate 1 cSv doses: The average active fraction = 0.956264
Excess cancers = 5 x 51 x 0.956264
              243.847

By contrast, the expectation from acute delivery of 5 cSv, for this case, is 255.219 excess cancers (above).

Therefore, under these circumstances and assumptions, we would expect cancer-risk from slow delivery to be (243.8474 / 255.219), or 95.5 % of the risk from acute delivery of the same dose -- a negligible difference by most standards.

Summary on 5 cSv :

So at one extreme, where A = B at 400 cSv, the LQ model suggests no risk-reduction factor at all, and at the other extreme, where A = B at 50 cSv, the LQ model suggests a risk reduction-factor of approximately 0.95 .

Slow Delivery of 1.0 cSv :

Lastly, we will temporarily ignore our own remarks, "Doses in the Range of Millirems," in order to push this other approach below 1.0 cSv.

We will compare 1 cSv of acute delivery with ten doses of 0.1 cSv each, for the case where A = B at 50 cSv. Since Table 23-A, Column H, and Table 23-B do not include values for 0.1 cSv, we provide them below:

```
Active fraction    = 0.998501
(A+B) = (5 + 0.01) = 5.01 cancers
```

```
        In each line below, excess cancers = 5.01 x
Active Fraction.
Dose            Active              Excess
Increment       Fraction            Cancers
First           0.99850             5.00249
Second          0.99700             4.99499
Third           0.99551             4.98750
Fourth          0.99402             4.98003
Fifth           0.99253             4.97256
Sixth           0.99104             4.96511
Seventh         0.98955             4.95767
Eighth          0.98807             4.95023
Ninth           0.98659             4.94281
Tenth           0.98511             4.93540

Total Excess Cancers                49.68880
```

```
The average active fraction =  0.991792
So we can check the calculation as follows:
Excess cancers =  10 x 5.01 x 0.991792
               =        49.68880
```

For comparison, the expectation from acute delivery of 1 cSv, for this case, is 50.2414 excess cancers (from Table 23-B, Column D).

Therefore, under these circumstances and assumptions, we would expect cancer-risk from slow delivery of 1 cSv to be (49.6888 / 50.2414), or 98.9 % of the risk from acute delivery of the same total dose.

In other words, this final fractionation hardly alters the expected risk at all. Thus this analysis is in good accord with the conclusion from track-analysis concerning the meaning of dose-rate at very low tissue-doses (Chapter 20, Part 3).

Slow Exposure --
Validity of Our Cancer-Yields :

Earlier in this book, we have stated that our low-dose Cancer-Yields are applicable to both acute-low and slow-low exposure. Those Cancer-Yields are based on the best-fit curve for acute exposure at 5 cSv (rems) of internal organ-dose. The analyses above indicate that this conclusion -- applicability to both acute-low and slow-low exposure -- is well supported by considerations related to the linear-quadratic model of dose-response.

Indeed, the expectation that there is no meaningful difference between acute and "slow" delivery of radiation dose, in the dose-region of zero to 5 cSv, is consistent with the near convergence in Table 23-B of the unmodified linear term alone (Column A) with the modified linear-quadratic term (Column D), and with the same near convergence in Table 23-C of Column A with Column C, in this dose-region.

It is not possible to state, within the evidence available currently, whether the human data are more consistent with A = B at 400 cSv, or with A = B at 50 cSv. In either case, the analyses above, in Part 7, indicate that no meaningful error at all will be introduced by use of our low-dose Cancer-Yields both for acute and for "slow" delivery of radiation dose.

A Warning about Risk UNDERestimates :

By contrast, meaningful underestimates of aggregate cancer-risk could develop if low doses, slowly received, were simply ignored -- as currently discussed under "de minimis" and "below regulatory concern" notions (see Chapter 24, Parts 9 and 10).

As shown by Sections 5 and 6 of this book, we cannot find any scientific justification within the evidence for excluding such exposure from risk-estimates or from associated protective measures. We have shown that the per-rad risk from acute-low and slow-low exposure is just as great or even greater than the per-rad risk from acute-moderate or acute-high exposure.

Table 23-A

Evaluation of Cell–Inactivation Function in Equation (4), for Various Pairs of m' and m″ Values.

Equation (4): Incidence = [aDose^1 + bDose^2] x [exp–(m'Dose^1 + m″Dose^2)]. See text, Part 3.

Dose^1 cSv	Dose^2 cSv^2	m'--> / m″-->	0.005 0.000008 Col. A	0.005 0.000004 Col. B	0.005 0 Col. C	0.005 -0.000004 Col. D	0.005 -0.000006 Col. E	0.00001 0.000005 Col. F	0.0025 -0.0000025 Col. G	0.015 -0.000014 Col. H
0	0		1	1	1	1	1	1	1	1
1	1		0.99500	0.99501	0.99501	0.99502	0.99502	0.99999	0.99751	0.98513
5	25		0.97511	0.97521	0.97531	0.97541	0.97546	0.99983	0.98764	0.92807
10	100		0.95047	0.95085	0.95123	0.95161	0.95180	0.99940	0.97555	0.86191
20	400		0.90195	0.90339	0.90484	0.90629	0.90701	0.99780	0.95218	0.74498
30	900		0.85453	0.85761	0.86071	0.86381	0.86537	0.99521	0.92983	0.64571
40	1600		0.80832	0.81351	0.81873	0.82399	0.82663	0.99164	0.90846	0.56124
50	2500		0.76338	0.77105	0.77880	0.78663	0.79057	0.98708	0.88803	0.48919
60	3600		0.71979	0.73023	0.74082	0.75156	0.75699	0.98157	0.86849	0.42759
70	4900		0.67760	0.69101	0.70469	0.71864	0.72571	0.97511	0.84980	0.37479
80	6400		0.63686	0.65338	0.67032	0.68770	0.69656	0.96773	0.83194	0.32943
90	8100		0.59762	0.61730	0.63763	0.65863	0.66938	0.95945	0.81485	0.29037
100	10000		0.55990	0.58275	0.60653	0.63128	0.64404	0.95028	0.79852	0.25666
110	12100		0.52372	0.54969	0.57695	0.60556	0.62039	0.94026	0.78290	0.22750
120	14400		0.48909	0.51809	0.54881	0.58135	0.59834	0.92941	0.76797	0.20222
130	16900		0.45603	0.48792	0.52205	0.55856	0.57776	0.91778	0.75371	0.18025
140	19600		0.42452	0.45914	0.49659	0.53708	0.55856	0.90538	0.74008	0.16112
150	22500		0.39455	0.43171	0.47237	0.51685	0.54064	0.89226	0.72706	0.14442
160	25600		0.36612	0.40560	0.44933	0.49778	0.52393	0.87845	0.71462	0.12982
170	28900		0.33919	0.38075	0.42741	0.47979	0.50834	0.86398	0.70275	0.11702
180	32400		0.31374	0.35715	0.40657	0.46283	0.49381	0.84891	0.69143	0.10578
190	36100		0.28973	0.33474	0.38674	0.44682	0.48027	0.83327	0.68062	0.09589
200	40000		0.26714	0.31349	0.36788	0.43171	0.46767	0.81709	0.67032	0.08716
210	44100		0.24591	0.29335	0.34994	0.41745	0.45594	0.80043	0.66051	0.07945
220	48400		0.22600	0.27428	0.33287	0.40398	0.44504	0.78333	0.65116	0.07263
230	52900		0.20738	0.25625	0.31664	0.39125	0.43492	0.76583	0.64227	0.06658
240	57600		0.18999	0.23921	0.30119	0.37923	0.42554	0.74796	0.63381	0.06120
250	62500		0.17377	0.22313	0.28650	0.36788	0.41686	0.72979	0.62578	0.05642
260	67600		0.15869	0.20796	0.27253	0.35715	0.40885	0.71134	0.61816	0.05215
270	72900		0.14468	0.19367	0.25924	0.34701	0.40148	0.69267	0.61094	0.04834
280	78400		0.13170	0.18022	0.24660	0.33743	0.39471	0.67381	0.60411	0.04494
290	84100		0.11970	0.16756	0.23457	0.32837	0.38852	0.65482	0.59765	0.04189
300	90000		0.10861	0.15567	0.22313	0.31982	0.38289	0.63572	0.59156	0.03916
310	96100		0.09839	0.14451	0.21225	0.31174	0.37780	0.61656	0.58582	0.03671
320	102400		0.08899	0.13404	0.20190	0.30410	0.37322	0.59738	0.58042	0.03451
330	108900		0.08036	0.12423	0.19205	0.29689	0.36913	0.57822	0.57537	0.03254
340	115600		0.07245	0.11505	0.18268	0.29008	0.36553	0.55912	0.57064	0.03076
350	122500		0.06522	0.10646	0.17377	0.28365	0.36240	0.54010	0.56623	0.02916
360	129600		0.05861	0.09843	0.16530	0.27759	0.35973	0.52121	0.56214	0.02772
370	136900		0.05259	0.09094	0.15724	0.27188	0.35751	0.50248	0.55836	0.02643
380	144400		0.04711	0.08394	0.14957	0.26649	0.35572	0.48394	0.55488	0.02526
390	152100		0.04214	0.07743	0.14227	0.26143	0.35437	0.46561	0.55170	0.02422
400	160000		0.03763	0.07136	0.13534	0.25666	0.35345	0.44754	0.54881	0.02328
			See Table 23–B, Column C		See Table 23–C, Column C				See Table 23–C, Column D	See Table 23–B, Column D

Each entry evaluates e (e = 2.71828) raised to the power: –(m'D^1 + m″D^2).
For Lotus 123 spreadsheets, each entry has the form: @EXP(–((m'D^1)+(m″D^2))).

Entries are the active fraction remaining (see text, Part 4). When dose = 0, the active fraction is 100%. It falls with rising dose, in a non–linear fashion. Figure 23–A depicts Columns A through F.

Table 23-B

Contributions from Intra-Track Cancers (A) and Inter-Track Cancers (B) to the Total Excess Cancers (A+B), When A = B at 50 cSv (rems).

This table provides the input depicted in Figures 23-B, 23-F, and 23-G.

Dose^1 in cSv	Dose^2 in cSv^2	Intra-Track Cancers = (50b)(D^1)	Inter-Track Cancers = (b)(D^2)	Combined Excess Cancers	m'--> 0.005 m"--> 0.000004	0.015 -0.000014
					[(A+B) x Exponential Term]	
		A	B	A+B Concave-Up Fig.23-B	Col. C Sigmoid Fig.23-F	Col. D Supra-Linear Fig.23-G
0	0	0	0	0	0.00	0.000
1	1	50	1	51	50.75	50.241
5	25	250	25	275	268.18	255.219
10	100	500	100	600	570.51	517.148
20	400	1000	400	1400	1264.75	1042.970
30	900	1500	900	2400	2058.28	1549.711
40	1600	2000	1600	3600	2928.63	2020.477
50	2500	2500	2500	5000	3855.26	2445.961
60	3600	3000	3600	6600	4819.50	2822.067
70	4900	3500	4900	8400	5804.49	3148.203
80	6400	4000	6400	10400	6795.13	3426.043
90	8100	4500	8100	12600	7777.98	3658.659
100	10000	5000	10000	15000	8741.22	3849.912
110	12100	5500	12100	17600	9674.55	4004.020
120	14400	6000	14400	20400	10569.10	4125.284
130	16900	6500	16900	23400	11417.37	4217.894
140	19600	7000	19600	26600	12213.13	4285.817
150	22500	7500	22500	30000	12951.32	4332.728
160	25600	8000	25600	33600	13627.99	4361.980
170	28900	8500	28900	37400	14240.22	4376.594
180	32400	9000	32400	41400	14786.00	4379.265
190	36100	9500	36100	45600	15264.16	4372.381
200	40000	10000	40000	50000	15674.31	4358.043
210	44100	10500	44100	54600	16016.73	4338.089
220	48400	11000	48400	59400	16292.33	4314.124
230	52900	11500	52900	64400	16502.53	4287.542
240	57600	12000	57600	69600	16649.24	4259.554
250	62500	12500	62500	75000	16734.76	4231.210
260	67600	13000	67600	80600	16761.74	4203.421
270	72900	13500	72900	86400	16733.08	4176.977
280	78400	14000	78400	92400	16651.94	4152.568
290	84100	14500	84100	98600	16521.64	4130.801
300	90000	15000	90000	105000	16345.63	4112.209
310	96100	15500	96100	111600	16127.42	4097.271
320	102400	16000	102400	118400	15870.61	4086.418
330	108900	16500	108900	125400	15578.76	4080.047
340	115600	17000	115600	132600	15255.45	4078.532
350	122500	17500	122500	140000	14904.19	4082.226
360	129600	18000	129600	147600	14528.41	4091.477
370	136900	18500	136900	155400	14131.44	4106.629
380	144400	19000	144400	163400	13716.52	4128.034
390	152100	19500	152100	171600	13286.74	4156.055
400	160000	20000	160000	180000	12845.03	4191.073

1. When A (intra-track cancers) = B (inter-track cancers) at 50 cSv, then a = 50b (see text, Part 2). 50b is substituted for a, in the equation of Col.A. In Col.B, the absolute value of the quadratic dose-coefficient (b) has been set equal to 1.0, to make the relationship between A and B very clear.

---

2. Column C is depicted as Plot M in Figure 23-F, FF, FFF. The exponential modifier for Col.C was evaluated in Table 23-A, Col.B. Thus, when we use 210 cSv as an example, the entry in Col.C above is 54,600 (from the A+B column at 210 cSv) times 0.29335 from Table 23-A, Col.B., at 210 cSv.

---

3. Column D is depicted as Plot M in Figure 23-G, GG, GGG. The exponential modifier for Col.D was evaluated in Table 23-A, Col.H. Thus, when we use 80 cSv as an example, the entry in Col.D above is 10,400 (from the A+B column at 80 cSv) times 0.32943 from Table 23-A, Col.H, at 80 cSv.

Table 23-C

Contributions from Intra-Track Cancers (A) and Inter-Track Cancers (B) to the Total Excess Cancers (A+B), When A = B at 400 cSv (rems).

This table provides the input depicted in Figures 23-C, 23-D, and 23-E.

Dose^1 in cSv	Dose^2 in cSv^2	Intra-Track Cancers = (400b)(D^1)	Inter-Track Cancers = (b)(D^2)	Combined Excess Cancers	m'--> 0.005 m"--> -0.000004	0.0025 -0.0000025
					[(A+B) x Exponential Term]	
		A	B	A+B Concave-Up Fig.23-C	Col. C Supra-Linear Fig.23-D	Col. D Linear Fig.23-E
0	0	0	0	0	0.00	0.000
1	1	400	1	401	399.00	400.000
5	25	2000	25	2025	1975.20	1999.970
10	100	4000	100	4100	3901.60	3999.770
20	400	8000	400	8400	7612.81	7998.321
30	900	12000	900	12900	11143.18	11994.849
40	1600	16000	1600	17600	14502.18	15988.967
50	2500	20000	2500	22500	17699.13	19980.670
60	3600	24000	3600	27600	20743.14	23970.305
70	4900	28000	4900	32900	23643.13	27958.539
80	6400	32000	6400	38400	26407.75	31946.335
90	8100	36000	8100	44100	29045.39	35934.929
100	10000	40000	10000	50000	31564.18	39925.811
110	12100	44000	12100	56100	33971.97	43920.703
120	14400	48000	14400	62400	36276.32	47921.549
130	16900	52000	16900	68900	38484.52	51930.494
140	19600	56000	19600	75600	40603.58	55949.880
150	22500	60000	22500	82500	42640.24	59982.227
160	25600	64000	25600	89600	44600.96	64030.230
170	28900	68000	28900	96900	46491.97	68096.752
180	32400	72000	32400	104400	48319.23	72184.813
190	36100	76000	36100	112100	50088.49	76297.588
200	40000	80000	40000	120000	51805.26	80438.406
210	44100	84000	44100	128100	53474.84	84610.740
220	48400	88000	48400	136400	55102.32	88818.214
230	52900	92000	52900	144900	56692.61	93064.598
240	57600	96000	57600	153600	58250.45	97353.805
250	62500	100000	62500	162500	59780.41	101689.902
260	67600	104000	67600	171600	61286.90	106077.100
270	72900	108000	72900	180900	62774.21	110519.767
280	78400	112000	78400	190400	64246.49	115022.426
290	84100	116000	84100	200100	65707.77	119589.763
300	90000	120000	90000	210000	67161.99	124226.627
310	96100	124000	96100	220100	68613.00	128938.041
320	102400	128000	102400	230400	70064.55	133729.209
330	108900	132000	108900	240900	71520.34	138605.520
340	115600	136000	115600	251600	72984.02	143572.556
350	122500	140000	122500	262500	74459.18	148636.107
360	129600	144000	129600	273600	75949.39	153802.173
370	136900	148000	136900	284900	77458.18	159076.981
380	144400	152000	144400	296400	78989.10	164466.992
390	152100	156000	152100	308100	80545.67	169978.916
400	160000	160000	160000	320000	82131.45	175619.724

1. When A (intra-track cancers) = B (inter-track cancers) at 400 cSv, then a = 400b (see text, Part 2). 400b is substituted for a, in the equation of Col.A. In Col.B, the absolute value of the quadratic dose-coefficient (b) has been set equal to 1.0, to make the relationship between A and B very clear.

----

2. Column C is depicted as Plot M in Figure 23-D, DD, DDD. The exponential modifier for Col.C was evaluated in Table 23-A, Col.D. Thus, when we use 50 cSv as an example, the entry in Col.C above is 22,500 (from the A+B column at 50 cSv) times 0.78663 from Table 23-A, Col.D, at 50 cSv.

----

3. Column D is depicted as Plot M in Figure 23-E, EE, EEE. The exponential modifier for Col.D was evaluated in Table 23-A, Col.G. Thus, when we use 160 cSv as an example, the entry in Col.D above is 89,600 (from the A+B column at 160 cSv) times 0.71462 from Table 23-A, Col.G, at 160 cSv.

Figure 23–A

Cell–Inactivation Functions. Depiction of Columns A through F of Table 23–A.

The cell-inactivation function is the term between the righthand pair of brackets in the modified linear-quadratic Equation (4): Excess Cancers = [aD^1 + bD^2] x [exp-(m'D^1 + m"D^2)] . The functions depicted here were evaluated in Table 23-A. Thus "Col.A", "Col.B", etc. in this figure refer to Column A and Column B in that table.

In this figure, all six curves have a value of 1.0 or 100 % at zero dose, and the fraction falls below 1.0 in a non-linear fashion as dose increases. The fractions at 400 cSv of dose in the figure correspond with the bottom entries in Columns A through F of Table 23-A.

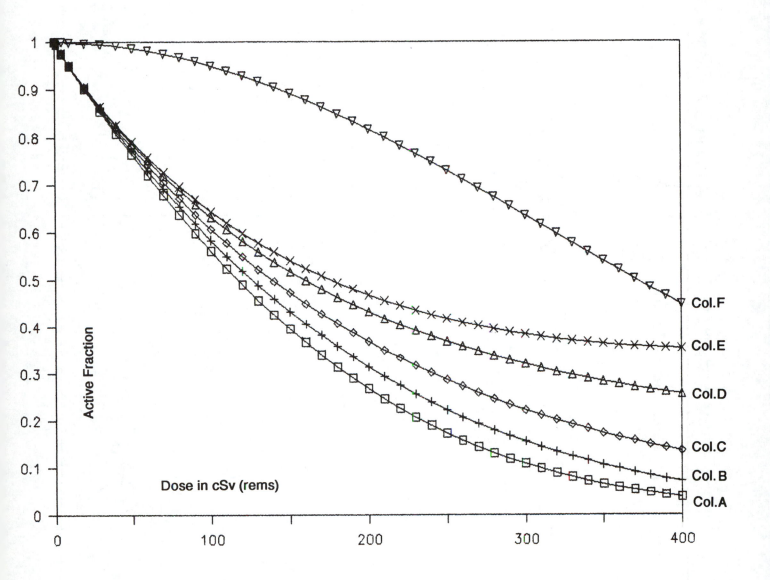

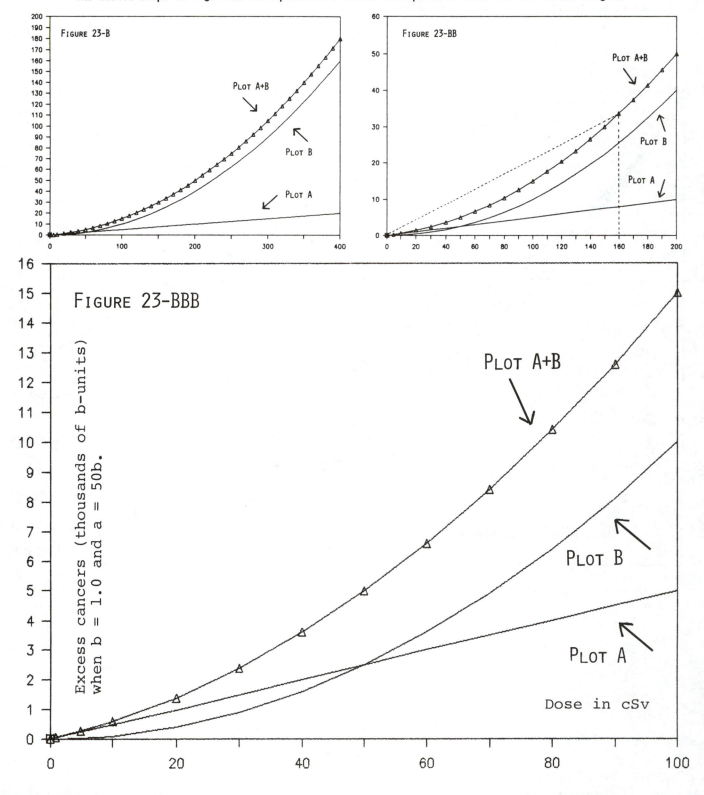

Figure 23-B

Unmodified LQ Model of Dose-Response. Contributions from Intra-Track Cancers (A) and from Inter-Track Cancers (B) to the Total Excess Cancers (A+B), When A = B at 50 cSv.
Total Excess = aD^1 + bD^2 (see text, Part 2), and a = 50b.

Input for these figures comes from Table 23-B :
Column A = Plot A, Column B = Plot B, and Column A+B = Plot A+B.
Depicted: Dose-range out to 400 cSv, out to 200 cSv, and out to 100 cSv.
The dashed slope in Figure 23-BB represents a linear extrapolation from 160 cSv to the origin.

Figure 23-C

Unmodified LQ Model of Dose–Response. Contributions from Intra–Track Cancers (A) and from Inter–Track Cancers (B) to the Total Excess Cancers (A+B), When A = B at 400 cSv.
Total Excess = aD^1 + bD^2 (see text, Part 2), and a = 400b.

```
Input for these figures comes from Table 23-C :
Column A = Plot A, Column B = Plot B, and Column A+B = Plot A+B.
Depicted: Dose-range out to 400 cSv, out to 200 cSv, and out to 100 cSv.
The dashed slope in Figure 23-CC represents a linear extrapolation from 160 cSv to the origin.
```

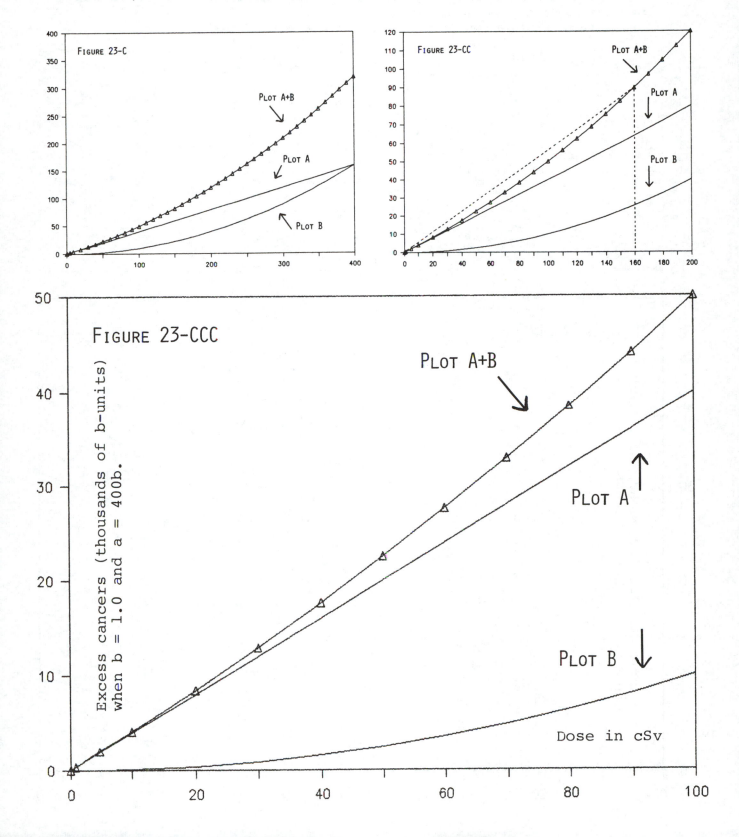

Figure 23-D

Example of a Linear-Quadratic Model with a Supra-Linear Dose-Response at Low Doses. A = B at 400 cSv.

● -- Input comes from Table 23-C. Col.A = Plot A. Col.B = Plot B. Col.A+B = Plot A+B. Col.C = Plot M.
● -- Col.C (Plot M) is the original equation (Plot A+B), after modification by a cell inactivation term.
● -- Comparison of Plot A+B, with Plot M, shows that a cell inactivation term can convert the shape of a linear-quadratic equation from concave-UPWARD to concave-DOWNWARD (supra-linear). Figure 23-DDD shows that Plot A+B and Plot M diverge at very low doses.
● -- Except for the addition of Plot M, Figure 23-D is the same as Figure 23-C.

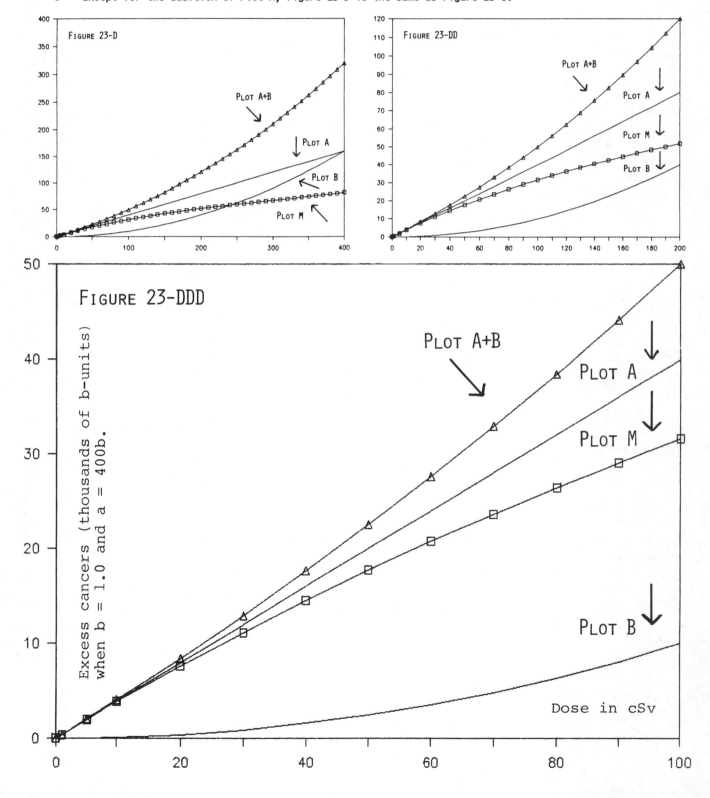

Figure 23-E

Example of a Linear–Quadratic Model with a Linear Dose–Response. A = B at 400 cSv.

● -- Input comes from Table 23-C. Col.A = Plot A. Col.B = Plot B. Col.A+B = Plot A+B. Col.D = Plot M.

● -- Col.D (Plot M) is the original equation (Plot A+B), after modification by a cell inactivation term.

● -- Comparison of Plot A+B, with Plot M, shows that a cell inactivation term can convert the shape of a linear-quadratic equation from concave-UPWARD to LINEAR. Between zero and 200 cSv of dose, Plot A (the linear term) and Plot M are virtually on top of each other. Compare entries in Table 23-C.

● -- Except for the altered nature of Plot M, Figure 23-E is the same as Figure 23-D.

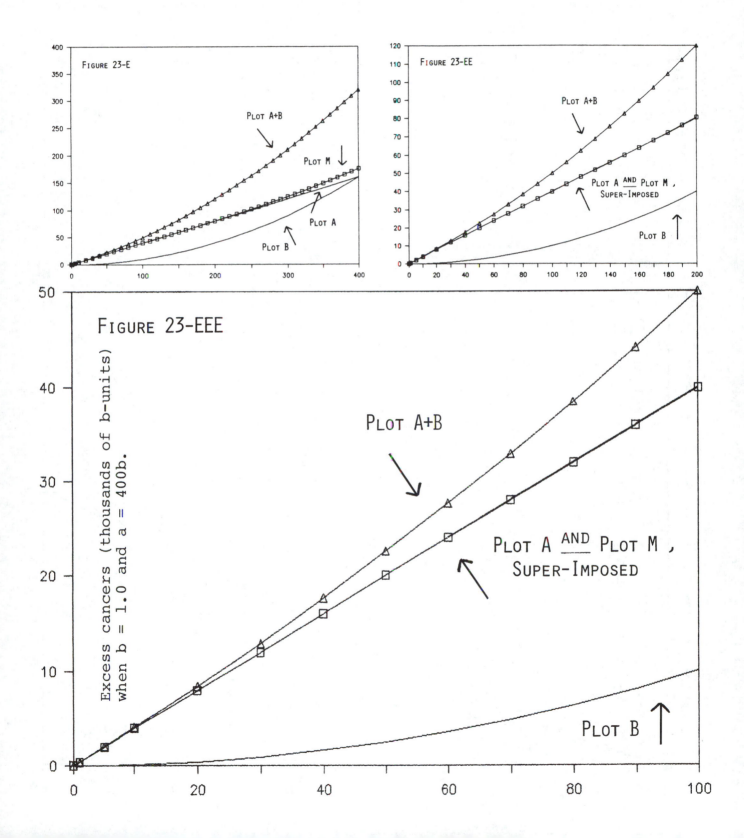

Figure 23-F

Example of a Linear–Quadratic Model with a Sigmoid Dose–Response. A = B at 50 cSv.

- -- Input comes from Table 23-B. Col.A = Plot A. Col.B = Plot B. Col.A+B = Plot A+B. Col.C = Plot M.
- -- Col.C (Plot M) is the original equation (Plot A+B), after modification by a cell inactivation term.
- -- Comparison of Plot A+B, with Plot M, shows that a cell inactivation term can convert the shape of a linear-quadratic equation from concave-UPWARD to SIGMOID. Between zero and 130 cSv of dose, Plot M is concave-upward, and beyond 130 cSv, Plot M is concave-downward.
- -- Except for the addition of Plot M (and some vertical scaling), Figure 23-F is the same as Figure 23-B.

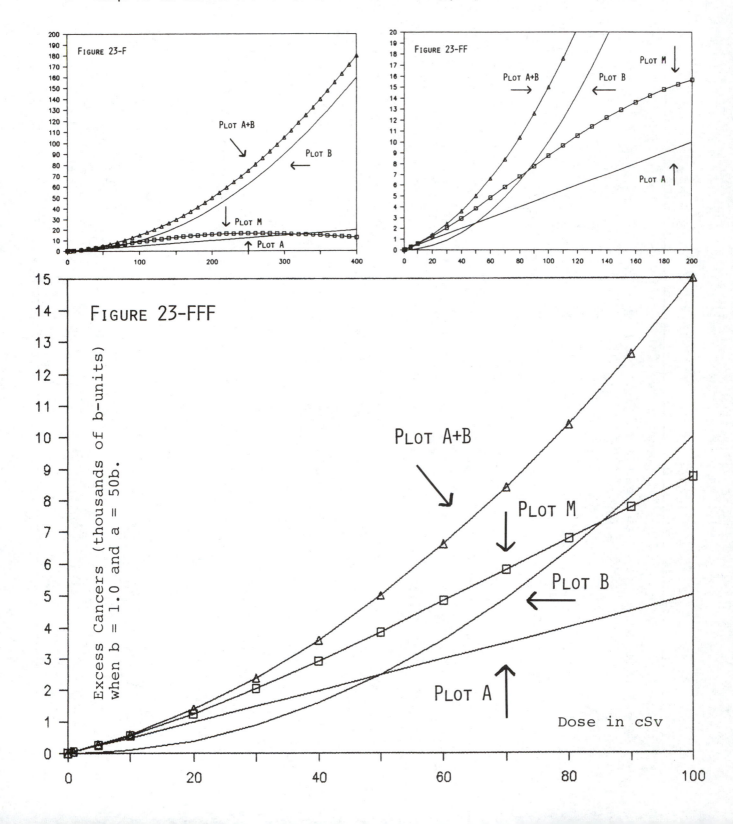

Figure 23–G

Example of a Linear–Quadratic Model with a Supra–Linear Dose–Response at Low Doses. A = B at 50 cSv.

● -- Input comes from Table 23-B. Col.A = Plot A. Col.B = Plot B. Col.A+B = Plot A+B. Col.D = Plot M.

● -- Col.D (Plot M) is the original equation (Plot A+B), after modification by a cell inactivation term.

● -- Comparison of Plot A+B, with Plot M, shows that a cell inactivation term can convert the shape of a linear-quadratic equation from concave-UPWARD to concave-DOWNWARD. Between zero and 20 cSv of dose, Plot M is very nearly linear, and beyond 20 cSv, Plot M is concave-downward.

● -- Except for the altered nature of Plot M, Figure 23-G is the same as Figure 23-F.

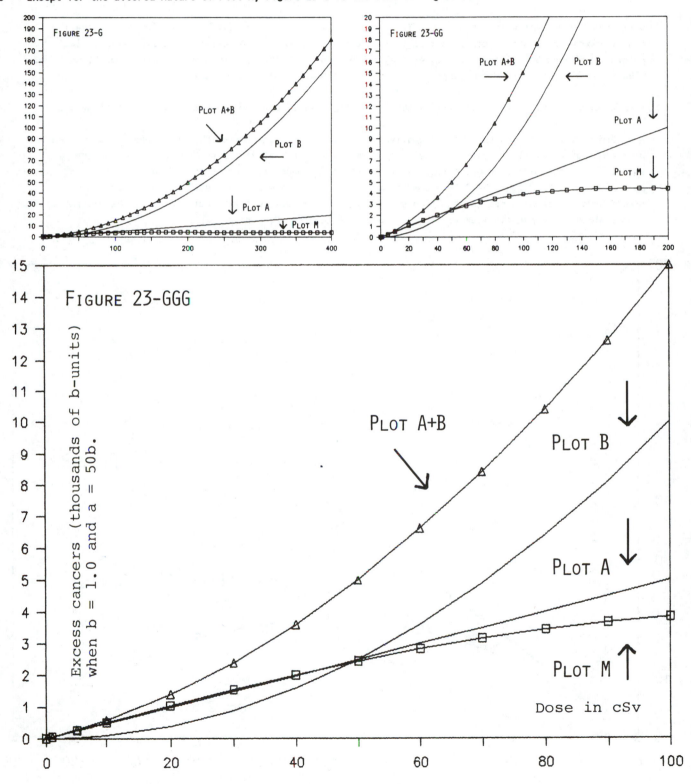

Figure 23–H

Example of a Negative Quadratic Term, in the LQ Model, Producing a Supra–Linear Curve. A = B at 200 cSv.
See text, Part 2, "LQ Model: Positive vs. Negative Q–Coefficient."

● -- Input for Figure 23-H is like the input for Figure 23-B and 23-C, except that here, A = B at 200 cSv.

● -- When both the linear and quadratic terms are POSITIVE, the plot of an unmodified linear-quadratic equation is necessarily concave-upward, because it is the sum of the points along Plot A (always a straight line) and along Plot B (always a concave-upward curve).

● -- When the quadratic term has a NEGATIVE sign, the plot of an unmodified LQ equation is necessarily concave-downward (supra-linear), because it is the points along Plot A (always a straight line) MINUS the points along Plot B. In the example below, A = B at 200 cSv. Thus at 200 cSv, Plot (A minus B) would be (200 minus 200), or zero excess cancers -- if the Q-term (Plot B) were negative.

● -- A curve is supra-linear if it lies ABOVE a straight line, drawn between any two points along itself.

● -- Ordinarily, the sign (positive, negative) of the Q-term is determined by the evidence, not by the preference of a set of analysts. The sign (positive, or negative) "falls out" of a regression analysis, in which analysts permit actual datapoints to "say" which shape fits them best and which sign is appropriate. [EXCEPTION: The BEIR-3 Committee -- in its analysis of dose-response for cancer in the A-Bomb Study -- constrained the equation so that the Q-term could NOT turn out negative: The Q-term was "constrained to be nonnegative" (Beir80, p.186). See Chapter 22, Part 2.]

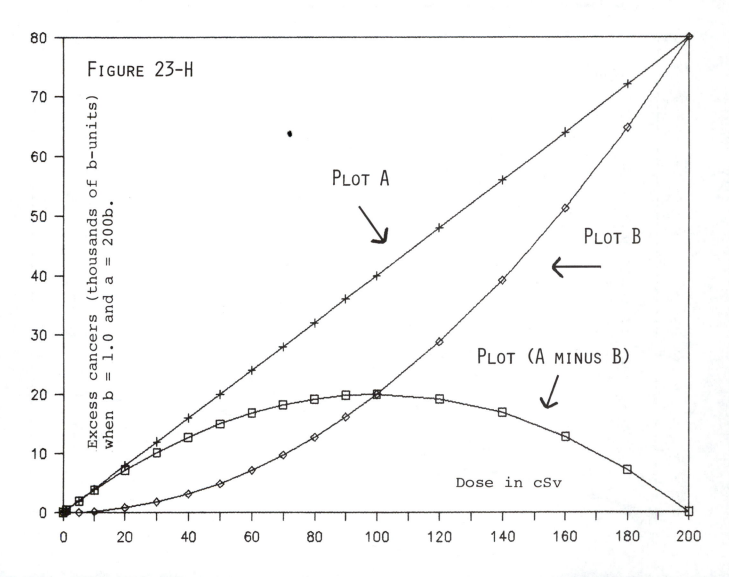

FIGURE 23-H

PLOT A

PLOT B

PLOT (A MINUS B)

Excess cancers (thousands of b-units) when b = 1.0 and a = 200b.

Dose in cSv

Figure 23-Eye

Variety of Dose-Responses Fit by a Single Linear-Quadratic Equation, with Changes in Its Modifier.
See text, Part 4, "Additional Conversions of the LQ Model."

● -- The equation for all six figures here is Equation (4) from Part 3 of the text:
   Excess Cancer = [aD^1 + bD^2] x [exp-(m'D^1 + m"D^2)] .
● -- For all six figures on this page, A = B at 100 cSv. Thus in all the figures alike, a = 100b, as
shown in the text, Part 2. The X-axis is Dose in cSv, and the Y-axis is Excess Cancers (in thousands)
when b = 1.0.
● -- The ONLY input which changes from one figure to the next is the value of m' and m". Those values are
indicated within each figure.
● -- Figure 23-Eye-1 represents the unmodified LQ equation, because m' and m" both are zero.

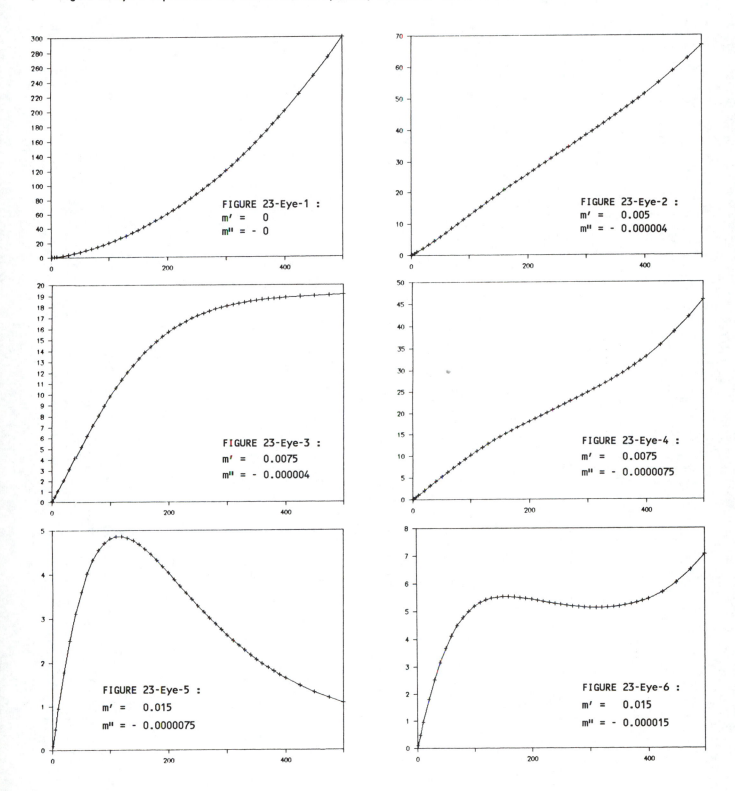

FIGURE 23-Eye-1 :
   m' =   0
   m" = - 0

FIGURE 23-Eye-2 :
   m' =   0.005
   m" = - 0.000004

FIGURE 23-Eye-3 :
   m' =   0.0075
   m" = - 0.000004

FIGURE 23-Eye-4 :
   m' =   0.0075
   m" = - 0.0000075

FIGURE 23-Eye-5 :
   m' =   0.015
   m" = - 0.0000075

FIGURE 23-Eye-6 :
   m' =   0.015
   m" = - 0.000015

23-empty, after figures.
===

| Chernobyl : |
| A Crossroad in the Radiation Health Sciences |

This chapter is arranged in 10 parts:

Then tables.

Introduction :

=======================================

This chapter will compare our independent analysis of Chernobyl's cancer consequences, with three estimates from influential segments of the radiation community. We will account for the huge disparity in such estimates. In addition, we shall provide some new estimates which use the Cancer-Yields developed in this book, as well as the Cancer-Yields published in 1987 and 1988 by RERF analysts.

In the process, we will suggest how the response by segments of the radiation community to the Chernobyl accident could have serious implications -- extending to nuclear issues far beyond this single accident, and beyond ionizing radiation to other health issues and to the practice of science itself.

1. Chernobyl's Cancer Consequences -- Integrity of the Data

On September 9, 1986, I presented my analysis of (A) the doses committed for people globally from the Chernobyl accident, and (B) the estimated cancer consequences from the doses -- namely, a half-million radiation-induced cancer fatalities. The Chernobyl analysis was part of a longer paper (mentioned already in Chapter 18, Part 1) which I presented at the Symposium on Low-Level Radiation at the 192nd National Meeting of the American Chemical Society -- the ACS.

The analysis was one of the very earliest detailed estimates of the cancer consequences of the Chernobyl accident, and was widely reported by the Associated Press, United Press International, and Reuters. The paper itself (Go86) has been widely distributed in the USA and abroad by the Committee for Nuclear Responsibility, inside and outside the radiation community.

As a permanent record, the entire sections dealing with the Chernobyl accident are reprinted in precisely the form in which they originally apppeared, as Chapter 36 of this book.

Original versus Revised Dose-Data :

There is a very special reason for reprinting the 1986 Chernobyl analysis in its exact form as originally presented. The doses recorded in the 1986 paper are those reported, within the first four months of the accident, by sources such as the World Health Organization, the U.S. Environmental Protection Agency, several separate country reports, and originally by the Soviet Union itself (citations are in Chapter 36). There may be good reasons to have more confidence in these original reports than in the many revisionist efforts.

The Chernobyl accident dismayed the promoters of nuclear power in virtually every country on the globe. After the accident, there has been a continuous effort, by governmental and private arms of the nuclear enterprise, to put the best face on the consequences of the accident. One way to "improve" the consequences of the accident would be, of course, to reduce estimates of the public's radiation exposure from it. For this reason, there is a realistic basis for skepticism concerning "revised" dose-estimates -- revisions which may continue to appear for years to come.

In short, it is impossible to know which "revisions" of dose are truly valid, and which are simply window-dressing on behalf of the nuclear enterprise.

As we shall see in Part 6, the Soviet Union has revised the Soviet doses downward, which may or may not be correct. Analysts for the U.S. Department of Energy accept and use the downward revisions with apparent contentment (Doe88, p.1515-1517).

Elsewhere, however, items like the following news reports make it exceedingly difficult to have confidence in Soviet candor about Chernobyl. The numbers are clearly at the mercy of politics.

On March 6, 1989, the WALL STREET JOURNAL (Wsj89, p.A-1) reported from Ukraine that "Records of radiation levels [from the accident] have been deemed so secret that top Soviet scientific researchers, let alone local residents, can't get access to them" -- a statement supported by considerable detail in the full article.

On April 27, 1989, the NEW YORK TIMES (Nyt89b) reported from Moscow that -- according to IZVESTIA -- the Soviet Minister of Energy, Anatoly Mayorets, had signed an order strictly curbing press coverage of nuclear power accidents. According to IZVESTIA, the new directive designated as classified nearly all reports on nuclear and conventional power accidents, breakdowns, or contaminations of any severity. The order prohibits disclosure of such information in "non-classified documents and in telegraphic communications, as well as in material intended for publication in the open press or for export abroad."

And the Health-Data?

On July 30, August 9, and August 15, 1989, the ASSOCIATED PRESS (As89) filed reports from Moscow on the dispute between the government and scientists in Byelorussia. Because of continuing exposure from the Chernobyl fallout, scientists were saying that an additional 106,000 people currently need evacuation from Byelorussian villages, whereas the government there was saying only 11,000 new evacuations would be needed. The Associated Press cited the official Tass news agency as the source for all its reports.

On November 13, 1989, TIME magazine devoted a full page to a report entitled, "The Chernobyl Cover-Up -- Are Soviet Officials Still Concealing the Truth about the Disaster?" (Time89, p.73). Among other things, TIME notes that leukemia and other radiation-related disorders "have allegedly been misreported as more innocent sounding conditions."

Sadly, all the reports above constitute a reminder that studies of delayed health effects (including leukemia and other malignancies) among Chernobyl-exposed Soviet populations could become grossly distorted by government interference at many levels.

We commonly hear statements from the radiation community that observation of the Chernobyl survivors will provide valuable additional evidence on the magnitude of the cancer effect. (See for instance, Webs87, p.424; Doe88, p.1517; Ya89, p.160). We ask: What reason is there for scientists anywhere to trust the INPUT to studies of the Chernobyl survivors?

One Aspect of the "Crossroad" :
=======================================

There are several aspects to the "crossroad" mentioned in this chapter's title. One aspect is the choice between credulous acceptance -- versus diligent exclusion -- of data from any nation with a world-class record of distorting truth in the service of state policy, and punishing those who object.

Both the USSR and the People's Republic of China are such countries. Nonetheless, certain data coming out of both countries are immediately embraced by parts of the radiation community.

Suppose the data are "doctored" at some step in the system? Is human health everywhere to be placed at the mercy of possibly spurious data which can never be verified? I can think of no protection other than making a presumption of "guilt" instead of "innocence" until such countries gradually EARN the trust of the world. Meanwhile, the unfairness to individual, innocent Soviet and Chinese analysts (who can receive false data without knowing it) is undeniably another injustice in a long series of injustices suffered due to such regimes.

A Distasteful Subject
=======================================

Readers may find the subjects of deceit and bias in research distasteful. So do I.

==

But they are not imaginary problems anywhere. In this country, too -- where temptation ought to be less -- standards in health research have been sinking so fast that, according to an estimate from the U.S. Public Health Service (PHS), about one out of every 200 principal investigators is involved in some type of scientific misconduct.

The PHS estimate above is incorporated into a report on the problem of misconduct in research, issued by the Academic Senate of the University of California to the entire faculty in November 1989 (Uni89, p.2). The same report also notes:

"A curious fact about known instances of research fraud is that most of them have taken place in the health sciences" (Uni89, p.4).

Indeed, in 1986, the American Medical Association decided to sponsor a "Congress on Peer Review in Biomedical Publication." According to Drummond Rennie, M.D., Deputy Editor,West of the JOURNAL OF THE AMERICAN MEDICAL ASSOCIATION (JAMA), and Elizabeth Knoll, Ph.D., Assistant to JAMA's Editor, one of the reasons for the meeting was to look into the responsibilities of institutional authorities and editors in preventing publication of work involving "fraud and slippery dealing in research" (Renn88). Additional problems with peer review are well described in Renn86. The conference took place in May 1989 (Nyt89c).

In 1988, the Association of American Universities felt the need to release a report entitled "Framework for Institutional Policies and Procedures to Deal with Fraud in Research," and in August 1989, the U.S. Public Health Service (PHS) began requiring all institutions which receive PHS grants to develop a process for investigating allegations of scientific misconduct and fraudulent research.

The "Downstream" Victims :

The report of the Academic Senate of the University of California includes an immensely important warning, expressed by Karl Hittleman, Associate Vice Chancellor for Academic Affairs at the University of California San Francisco -- the medical center. Commenting on scientific misconduct-rates like one per 200, Hittleman said (Uni89, p2):

"It is the view of Congress, and should be the view of the scientific community, that no amount of fraud is acceptable, because of the corrosive effects on science and the bad effects on public trust."

Then the report paraphrased additional comments from Hittleman as follows: "Regarding science itself, he says, there is a 'multiplier' effect to fraud: Any instance of it can destroy the worth of related 'downstream' research. Worse, fraud can have potentially disastrous effects on those touched by research -- on patients involved in medical clinical trials, for example."

How Much Would It Matter?

======================================

How much would "slippery dealing" (Rennie's phrase, Renn88) and spurious data matter in the low-dose radiation health sciences? How many people downstream would be touched?

In medicine, almost every patient would be affected because of diagnostic uses of X-rays and radionuclides. In addition, millions of workers in this country receive occupational exposure to ionizing radiation.

But the human species as a WHOLE has by far the biggest stake in an honest evaluation of the risks from ionizing radiation.

Billions of people (many not yet born) will receive exposure from the Chernobyl accident, and people everywhere could pay the price if underestimated risk were to become accepted in this field. Everyone would face nuclear pollution not just from accidents, but also by INTENTION (see Part 10).

Examination of the Chernobyl accident by this chapter will illustrate how very small dose-increases for millions and billions of people produce huge collective dose commitments. This is not even in dispute, as this chapter shows. The CONSEQUENCES are. The human race cannot afford serious underestimates of risk in this field. Readers will understand why, after they have compared various sets of numbers provided in this chapter.

2.   The Two Keys to Estimating Cancer Consequences from Chernobyl

This chapter will compare several estimates of Chernobyl's cancer consequences, by myself and by others.

No matter who is estimating those consequences, only two kinds of values are needed in order to make an estimate.

The first value is an estimate of the all-time collective dose commitment caused by the accident. This value is in the "person-rad" unit (or some variant, such as person-gray). It is calculated by multiplying (the average whole-body dose in rads in each affected country) x (the country's population), and then summing all these person-rad values to obtain the collective dose commitment in all countries combined.

The second value is the conversion-factor from dose to cancer-fatalities. Most analysts make the conversion by using a Lifetime Fatal Cancer-Yield for whole-body exposure of a mixed-age population -- though they may call it "risk factor" or other names. This value is in the units "cancers per 10,000 persons, per rad (or cGy)," or cancers x 10^-4 persons^-1 rad^-1. Or more clearly: (cancers / 10,000 person-rads).

Thus in the appropriate equation for radiation-induced cancer-deaths, both the persons and the rads cancel out, as shown in the following illustration -- which uses a dose-commitment of 127.4 million person-rads and the Cancer-Yield of 37.313 fatal cancers per 10,000 person-rads (from Go81).

Sample Calculation :

```
Radiation-induced cancer-deaths =
   (dose commitment) x (Lifetime Fatal Cancer-Yield).

Cancers = (127,400,000 person-rads)
            x (37.313 cancers / 10,000 person-rads).

Cancers = 475,368 cancers.
```

One purpose of this chapter is to show whether the grave disparity, in estimates of Chernobyl's cancer consequences, arises primarily from differences in dose-estimates, or whether it arises primarily from differences in Cancer-Yields.

Percent Increase per Rad, and Cancer-Yield :

Analysts (including myself) sometimes express the radiation-induced cancer-risk in terms of "percent increase per rad" in the spontaneous cancer death-rate. In Chapter 16, Part 2, we illustrated the conversion from Lifetime Fatal Cancer-Yield to "percent increase per rad." Now we will illustrate the reverse. It requires the estimated fraction of all deaths which are cancer-deaths in the population under discussion.

Suppose that approximately 17 % of all deaths in a population are from cancer. Then the lifetime spontaneous cancer death-rate per 10,000 persons =

1,700. For many purposes, one can omit adjustment for cancer-deaths which occurred in a mixed-age population before the radiation exposure. If the percent increase per rad is, say, 2.0 percent, then (1,700 cancer-deaths x 0.02), or 34 cancer-deaths is the Lifetime Fatal Cancer-Yield -- namely, the number of radiation-induced fatal cancers which occur among 10,000 persons over their remaining lifspan after an average whole-body internal organ-dose of one rad (or rem).

3. Bottom Line from Our September 1986 Estimate of Chernobyl's Cancer Consequences

Collective Dose Commitment :

In Section 7 of our 1986 estimate -- which is now Chapter 36 -- we developed and demonstrated three different methods to estimate the average per capita dose commitment from the dominant source of exposure (the radio-cesiums), according to the particular kind of measurements which a country was supplying during the weeks right after the accident.

In Chapter 36, the Technical Appendix 2 describes the types of measurements, country by country.

In that paper, Table 6 (now on page 36-19) provides our estimate of average dose commitment in millirads per capita, country by country, along with each country's population. The countries which are omitted had made no report available for inspection, and it was not possible to estimate doses by interpolation from neighboring countries.

Readers who multiply a country's population by its average per capita dose, and then sum all the person-millirad values, will find that our estimate of 475,500 fatal cancers (plus 19,500 leukemias) is based on a collective dose commitment of 127.4 billion person-millirads -- or 127.4 million person-rads. The geographical distribution of our dose estimate is:

```
EUROPEAN USSR:          56.9 million person-rad.
NON-USSR EUROPE:        65.6 million person-rad.
OTHER, AS INDICATED:    4.9 million person-rad.
```

As we shall see when we come to dose-estimates by others, it is important to note that our dose commitments are all-time commitments (also called "infinite time" commitments). Although cesium-134 decays with a radioactive half-life of only 2.3 years (page 36-5), cesium-137 has a radioactive half-life of 30.2 years. When 151 years (five half-lives) have passed since the accident, one part in 32 of the cesium-137 released by the accident will still exist. (See page 36-29 for the estimated time-distribution of the combined dose from both cesiums.)

Cancer-Yield Conversion Factor :

Our 1986 analysis uses the Lifetime Fatal Cancer-Yield of 37.313 fatal cancers per 10,000 person-rads, which is the estimate developed in Go81 from the worldwide epidemiological evidence.

This value appears on page 36-4 in another form -- namely a Whole-Body Cancer Dose of 268 person-rads per fatal radiation-induced cancer. The conversion from Cancer Dose to Cancer Yield is straight-forward:

```
Number of cancers from 10,000 person-rads
    = (1 cancer / 268 person-rads)
          x (10,000 person-rads) = 37.313 cancers.


  The Cancer-Yield of 37.313 excludes leukemia.


Number of leukemia cases from 10,000 person-rads
    = (1 leukemia / 6,500 person-rads)
          x (10,000 persons-rads) = 1.54 case.
```

It might be noted that this value of 1.54 (from Go85) is in good agreement with RERF's linear value of 1.2 (Pr88, p.460). There is no science-based reason for applying any reduction-factor for low and slow exposure, because the leukemia dose-response is NOT concave-upward when the full database is used (see Chapter 22, Part 2).

Estimate of Chernobyl-Induced Cancers :

As already shown in Part 2 of this chapter, the estimate of fatal radiation-induced cancers is the product of the dose commitment times the Cancer-Yield. So:

```
(127.4 x 10^6 person-rads)
      x (37.313 cancers / 10,000 person-rads)
   = 475,368 cancers, fatal.
```

In Table 6 of Chapter 36, this was rounded off to 475,500 fatal cancers. In addition, approximately one non-fatal cancer is expected for each fatal cancer produced. The geographical distribution of the Chernobyl-induced cancers in Go86, Table 6 (Chapter 36, page 36-19) is:

```
EUROPEAN USSR:     212,150 fatal + 212,150 non-fatal.
NON-USSR EUROPE:   244,786 fatal + 244,786 non-fatal.
OTHER:              18,512 fatal +  18,512 non-fatal.
```

The combined and rounded number, 951,000 radiation-induced cancers, does not include additional cancers expected from the unestimated doses delivered by radionuclides less prominent than the radio-cesiums, nor does it include thyroid and other cancers induced by the sizable radio-iodine doses which were received. All such cancers are additional to the 951,000 cases. The leukemias are also additional:

```
Number of leukemias from 127.4 million person-rads
    = (1 leukemia / 6,500 person-rads)
          x (127.4 million persons-rads) = 19,600.
This was rounded down to 19,500 cases.
```

So the bottom line from the 1986 estimate is 970,500 malignancies, from the radio-cesium dose.

4. Bottom Line from the 1987 Estimate Issued by the Nuclear Regulatory Comm'n.

The report named below, and dated January 1987, was issued by the U.S. Nuclear Regulatory Commission or NRC (our reference Nrc87):

REPORT ON THE ACCIDENT AT THE CHERNOBYL NUCLEAR POWER STATION. NUREG-1250.

According to the report's title page, it was prepared by:
Department of Energy
Electric Power Research Institute
Environmental Protection Agency
Federal Emergency Management Agency
Institute of Nuclear Power Operations
Nuclear Regulatory Commission

The report's Chapter 8, "Health and Environmental Consequences," was prepared by J. Puskin, C. Nelson, D. Janes, and S. Myers of the Environmental Protection Agency.

Collective Dose Commitment :

The dose commitments in this report appear to be primarily 50-year "lifetime" estimates (Nrc87, p.8-10, 8-13), and are characterized by the authors as tentative:

```
EUROPEAN USSR:  50 million person-rem (at p.8-10).
NON-USSR EUROPE:  20 million person-rem (at p.8-14).
```

How did Nrc87 arrive at these dose estimates? For the European USSR, whose exposed population is estimated at 75 million people in the report, the authors accepted the estimates provided by the Soviets

(Ussr86), except that they reduced the Soviet estimate of dose via ingestion (Nrc87, p.8-10). As for dose in Non-USSR Europe, the authors say that any estimate "must be regarded as highly tentative" and perhaps good "within about a factor of 2" (Nrc87, p.8-13). They make their estimate by excluding Spain, Portugal, England, Ireland, Denmark, and most of France, and then estimating that the remaining population of about 350 million received an average individual dose of about 60 millirems "spread over a period of years" (Nrc87, p.8-14).

Cancer-Yield Conversion Factor :

The authors used a Cancer-Yield of 2 fatal cancers per 10,000 person-rads.

They state: "For illustrative purposes in this chapter, the staff used a risk factor of 2×10^{-4} fatal cancers per rad of (low-LET) radiation to the whole body, corresponding approximately to the linear-quadratic, relative risk model described in the National Academy of Sciences 'BEIR III' report (NAS, 1980). With minor modifications, this model has recently been adopted by two panels of experts as providing a reasonable central estimate of the risk from low-level radiation" (Nrc87, p.8-6). The two panels of experts cited are our references Nrc85 and Nih85.

Elsewhere (Nrc87, p.8-10), the authors also state that one should expect one non-fatal cancer for each fatal cancer induced by radiation.

Estimate of Chernobyl-Induced Cancers :

This is the product of the dose commitment times the Cancer-Yield. So:

```
(70 x 10^6 person-rads)
        x (2 cancers / 10,000 person-rads)
    = 14,000 cancers, fatal. Plus 14,000 non-fatal.
```

The geographical distribution in the estimate is (Nrc87, pages 8-10, 8-14):

```
EUROPEAN USSR:    10,000 fatal + 10,000 non-fatal.
NON-USSR EUROPE:   4,000 fatal +  4,000 non-fatal.
```

5. Bottom Line from the 1987 Estimate Issued by the Department of Energy

The report named below, and dated June 1987, was issued by the U.S. Department of Energy or DOE (our reference Doe87):

HEALTH AND ENVIRONMENTAL CONSEQUENCES OF THE CHERNOBYL NUCLEAR POWER ACCIDENT. DOE/ER-0332.

Report to the U.S. Department of Energy
    Office of Energy Research
    Office of Health & Environmental Research
From the
    Interlaboratory Task Group on Health and
    Environmental Aspects of the Soviet Nuclear
    Accident.
Prepared by
    The Committee on the Assessment of Health
    Consequences in Exposed Populations.

Authors:

Marvin Goldman (Chairman), University of
    California, Davis.
Robert J. Catlin, Electric Power Research Inst.
Lynn Anspaugh, Livermore National Laboratory.

Co-Authors:

Richard G. Cuddihy, Lovelace Inhalation Toxicology
    Research Institute.
William E. Davis, Pacific Northwest Laboratory.
Jacob I. Fabrikant, Lawrence Berkeley Laboratory.
Andrew P. Hull, Brookhaven National Laboratory.
Rolf Lange, Livermore National Laboratory.
David Robertson, Pacific Northwest Laboratory.
Robert Schlenker, Argonne National Laboratory.
Edward Warman, Stone & Webster Engineering.

Collective Dose Commitment :

Although the authors of Doe87 demonstrate the difference between 50-year and infinite-time dose commitments (for instance, at their pages 5.33 and 5.35), they choose to use the lower dose commitment in making their cancer estimates. We will evaluate the impact of this preference. Their Table 5.16 provides the "50-year collective dose commitments" which they use. The same estimates are called "lifetime collective doses" in their Table J.4.

```
EUROPEAN USSR:    47 million person-rad.
ASIAN USSR:       11 million person-rad.
NON-USSR EUROPE:  58 million person-rad.
NON-USSR ASIA:     2.7  million person-rad.
UNITED STATES:     0.11 million person-rad.
CANADA:            0.0094 million person-rad.

SUM:             118.82 million person-rad.
```
Doe87 rounds this off to 120 million person-rad.

===

How did Doe87 arrive at these dose estimates, from what it calls (at p.vii) the Chernobyl reactor's "violent disassembly"?

As shown in Doe87 Table 7.1, the 50-year dose commitment for the European USSR is the Soviet's own estimate, including the May 1987 report by the Soviet Ministry of Health (Ussr87a). Doe87 supplies its own estimate for Asian USSR, and calls it "a very rough estimate" (Doe87, p.5.60). For non-USSR Europe, the estimates in Doe87 are derived from analytical methods and data quite similar to our own in Chapter 36 -- except for Doe87's effort to stop exposure at 50 years.

Beyond the fiftieth year, some twenty percent of the all-time dose commitment is yet to come -- an estimate from our Chapter 36, page 29, with which DOE agrees (Doe88, p.1514). Therefore, Doe87's all-time collective dose commitment would be

```
(118.82 million person-rad)
            = (0.8) x (All-Time Dose Commitment).
148.6 million person-rad = All-Time Dose Commitment.
```

Cancer-Yield Conversion Factor:

Doe87 is explicit at page 7.6 about using the risk model suggested by the Nuclear Regulatory Commission in its NUREG/CR-4214 Report (our Reference Nrc85). On page J.3, the authors describe the Nrc85 model as a "composite" absolute-relative risk model with linear and linear-quadratic dose-responses, which work out to a "risk coefficient (fatal cancers / rad) of 2.3×10^{-4}," for "long-term" carcinogenesis.

In other words, Doe87 uses a Lifetime Fatal Cancer-Yield of 2.3 fatal cancers per 10,000 person-rads.

Estimate of Chernobyl-Induced Cancers :

This is the product of the dose commitment times the Cancer-Yield. So:

```
(120 million person-rads)
        x (2.3 cancers / 10,000 person-rads)
    = 27,600 cancers, fatal.  Doe87 rounds off to
      28,000.
```

In the key table, Table 7.11 (Doe87, Chapter 7, page 7.22), the authors do not mention any non-fatal cancers. The geographical distribution of the 28,000 "estimated possible radiation-induced fatal cancers" in that table is:

```
EUROPEAN USSR:     11,410 fatal cancers.
ASIAN USSR:         2,500 fatal cancers
NON-USSR EUROPE:   13,000 fatal cancers.
NON-USSR ASIA:        620 fatal cancers.
USA + CANADA:          27 fatal cancers.
```

6. Bottom Line from the 1988 Up–Date of DOE's 1987 Estimate

The article named below was published by the journal SCIENCE in its Volume 242 (December 16, 1988), pages 1513-1519:

"The Global Impact of the Chernobyl Reactor Accident," by Lynn R. Anspaugh, Robert J. Catlin, and Marvin Goldman. This is our reference Ansp88.

However, since this article is basically an abbreviation of Doe87, we shall refer to it as Doe88 in this chapter. The article itself states the following in its Note 2, in which their reference (3) is DOE/ER-0332 or Doe87:

"This article is based on work published by the authors and others for the Department of Energy (3); this reference can be consulted for methodological details not reported here. The present article contains several updates to (3); a major one is a revision of the collective dose commitment reported for the Soviet Union."

Collective Dose Commitment :

The "collective 50-year total-body dose" given in Table 3 of this article is 93 million person-rad (we converted person-Gy to person-rad). The geographical distribution is given below. As indicated above (and noted already in Part 1 of this chapter), these authors accept the Soviets' downward estimate of the dose commitment in European USSR. Anspaugh et al cite Ussr87b and Ussr88 in this article. The figure in Doe87 was 47 million person-rad; it goes down to 32 million person-rad in Doe88.

```
EUROPEAN USSR:     32 million person-rad.
ASIAN USSR:        0.69 million person-rad.
NON-USSR EUROPE:   58 million person-rad.
NON-USSR ASIA:     2.71 million person-rad.
UNITED STATES:     0.11 million person-rad.
CANADA:            0.0094 million person-rad.

SUM:               93.52 million person-rad.
```

Anspaugh and co-workers attempt to justify using a 50-year dose commitment as follows (Doe88, p.1514):

===

"We used a time period of 50 years, a standard interval over which to calculate the doses for lifetime cancer risks. Exposures over the first-year period and over infinite time were also derived. As an approximation, the first-year exposure is 10 % of the 50-year exposure, and the 50-year exposure is more than 75 % of the exposure over infinite time."

As noted in Part 5 above, it is about 80 % .

This practice of throwing away the dose commitment beyond fifty years is simply an arbitrary way of reducing the cancer expectation. Anspaugh et al refer to this as "standard," but one wonders whose standard this might be, and why it is used.

If we were dealing with one set of persons and there were no "new entries" to the exposed population, it might be a more reasonable practice, since even the youngest persons in 1986 would not be very radio-sensitive after age 50. But this is clearly NOT the situation.

In this situation, we are dealing with mixed-age populations from which some are departing by death, and into which others are entering by birth, every year following the accident. New young people are always being added to the group exposed by the Chernobyl accident, in great contrast to the A-bomb study, where no new persons are added to the exposed group over time.

When about 20 % of the radio-cesium dose will occur beyond the year 2036, it is a mistake to treat that dose as if it did not exist. Therefore, we shall convert Doe88's 50-year total-body dose commitment into an all-time dose commitment:

```
(93 million person-rad)
        = (0.8) x (All-Time Dose Commitment).
116 million person-rad = All-Time Dose Commitment.
```

Cancer-Yield Conversion Factor :

Although Anspaugh and co-workers are content to incorporate, into their up-date, new information provided in 1987 and 1988 by Soviet officials about the dose, they are silent about the new estimates of cancer-risk provided in 1987 and 1988 by two sets of RERF analysts. Both RERF reports (Pr87b and Shi88) cast very serious doubt upon the Cancer-Yield used in Doe87. Both reports mean that the value used in Doe87 needs to be a great deal HIGHER. We shall return to this in Part 7.

While Doe87 was explicit about using a Cancer-Yield from NUREG/CR-4214 of 2.3 fatal cancers x 10^{-4} person-rad, Doe88 is never explicit. Although Doe88 lists "radiogenic risk factors" and "reduction factors" from NUREG/CR-4214 (Nrc85), Doe88 never states that the model works out to a Cancer-Yield of 2.3 cancers. The statement is absent for good reason.

The operative Cancer-Yield used by Anspaugh and co-workers in Doe88 turns out to be LOWER than 2.3 cancers per 10,000 person-rads. It is 1.87, as we shall show in a moment. The change is just there, and it represents a decrement of about 20 percent in the estimate of Chernobyl-induced cancers.

Estimate of Chernobyl-Induced Cancers :

This number is given as 17,400 fatal cancers in Tables 3 and 5 of Doe88.

Since the same tables confirm that this number arises from a dose commitment of 93 million person-rad, the rate is 17,400 fatal cancers per 93,000,000 person-rad, or 0.000187 fatal cancer per person-rad. Multiplying by 10,000 to obtain the rate per 10,000 person-rad, we find that the operative Cancer-Yield in Doe88 is 1.87 fatal cancer per 10,000 person-rad.

The distribution of the 17,400 Chernobyl-induced fatal cancers is stated in Doe88, Table 5:

```
USSR:                 6,500 fatal cancers.
NON-USSR EUROPE:     10,400 fatal cancers.
NON-USSR ASIA:          500 fatal cancers.
USA + CANADA:            20 fatal cancers
```

7. Reason for the Great Disparity

Part 7 focuses on two tables. Table 24-A facilitates comparison of our 1986 estimate with the three estimates already discussed, and thereby makes the source of the disparities self-evident. Table 24-B compares our 1986 estimate with additional estimates based on (A) the new data in this book, and (B) the recent findings by RERF analysts.

Obviously, we regard the range of estimates in Table 24-B as the scientifically reasonable range. However, this book does not ask readers to accept our OPINION. Previous sections of this book have presented the scientific input which caused us to develop this opinion. And those chapters did not evade the inherent uncertainties.

Now it is up to the readers to make their own judgments about which range of estimates is the more likely to be correct, on a strictly scientific basis.

The Message of Table 24-A :

People unfamiliar with this field, and unfamiliar with the details of the various reports, have expressed surprise to me that the consequences of the Chernobyl accident can be so differently estimated. And surprise is natural. A range of 14,000 to 475,500 is startling.

Because the low estimates were published subsequent to my own estimate, it is widely assumed that the radiation dose must have truly been far smaller than initially estimated, and that this is the reason for the markedly lower estimates by the radiation community.

Nothing could be farther from the truth. Table 24-A makes it almost self-evident that the massive difference in cancer estimates has practically nothing to do with the issue of estimated dose commitment from the Chernobyl accident. Indeed, the Gofman and DOE estimates of collective dose in Column B are remarkably close. The NRC estimate of dose deserves no attention at all, in view of its superficial nature (see Part 4). Even Doe87 (at page J.6) heavily criticizes the dose estimate in Nrc87. As for Gofman-DOE differences in dose estimates for some specific countries, these differences are of no consequence here, because the bottom lines in Column D come from the aggregate dose estimates.

No Mystery :

There is no mystery about what causes the difference in the estimates of Chernobyl-induced cancers. The disparity arises overwhelmingly from Column C -- the Cancer-Yield, or conversion factor from dose to cancers.

The radiation community uses some Cancer-Yields even lower than the range of 1.87 to 2.3 shown in Table 24-A. For instance, Doe87 (at page 7.17) reports that UNSCEAR's 1977 value of 1.0 was used by the U.K. Central Electricity Generating Board to evaluate Chernobyl-induced cancers.

And Doe87 itself claims (mistakenly) that 1.0 is approximately the "lifetime fatal cancer risk" produced by the A-Bomb Study in the T65DR dosimetry (Doe87, p.7.4). For low-dose exposure, the Doe87 authors are wrong about this by at least l3-fold, as proven in our Chapters 13 and 14.

The value of 1.0 as a Lifetime Fatal Cancer-Yield was promoted also by the 1986 president of the American Nuclear Society (see Chapter 34, Bertram Wolfe), and 1.0 is called the "official" estimate by BEIR-3 member Edward Webster -- who seems to regard 1.0 as too high (Webs87).

After Chernobyl, we heard the value of 1.0 used too many times to count.

The NRC and DOE, however, must have been obliged to make use of the higher estimate issued earlier by the NRC itself, in NUREG/CR-4214 (Nrc85), some aspects of which are discussed in Chapter 22, Part 3. The Nrc87, Doe87, and Doe88 reports all claim that they base the values of 1.87 to 2.3 in Column C upon Nrc85.

Correcting One of the Errors:

In Chapter 22, Part 3, readers have seen for themselves ONE of the obvious errors in this Fatal Lifetime Cancer-Yield from Nrc85. Except for breast-cancer and thyroid cancer (which is rarely fatal), the Nrc85 risk-value rests on replacement of the real-world human epidemiological evidence by the preferred radiobiological hypothesis that dose-response is concave-upward. The A-Bomb Study has been invalidating this hypothesis for many years, and Chapter 22 shows that the radiation committees were aware of this in 1980 already.

Nonetheless, the Nrc85 risk-model rejects both the supra-linear and linear dose-responses, and erroneously incorporates DREFS for low and slow exposure. This is no small matter, as we shall see.

As shown by Doe88 (Table 2, p.1515), this Nrc85 model incorporates a DREF of 0.3 for low and slow exposure -- which characterizes almost the entire dose commitment from Chernobyl. This means Doe87 and Doe88 are using a cancer risk-estimate 0.3 times the LINEAR estimate. In other words, just correcting for this one error would make the Cancer-Yields about 3-fold higher. So 2.3 would become 6.9, and 1.87 would become 5.6 fatal cancers per 10,000 person-rad.

Result -- 84,000 Fatal Cancers :

The corresponding linear estimates of Chernobyl-induced fatal cancers would also rise by a factor of about three. For instance, the estimate of 28,000 would become about 84,000 Chernobyl-induced fatal cancers.

As we said, this is no small matter. Nor is it any small matter to reject real-world human evidence on dose-response shape, in favor of a preferred but hypothetical shape.

As our "Crossroad" title suggests, Chernobyl demands evaluation in various circles of the radiation health sciences. If the evaluations use unrealistically low Cancer-Yields like 1.0 or 2.0 -- completely at variance with the existing human evidence -- it is no surprise to me if the nuclear enterprise has credibility problems (see Part 8, "Chickens Come Home to Roost").

The Message of Table 24-B :
====================================

Other analytical efforts at this time are showing conversion values (of dose to cancers) of 11, 12, 16, 25, 31, 37 per 10,000 person-rad. Table 24-B presents all of them, not just the highest or the lowest.

The message from Table 24-B is that, when estimates of Cancer-Yield are scientifically reasonable, they place estimates of Chernobyl-induced fatal cancers in the range between 140,000 and 475,000, plus an equal number of non-fatal cancers.

The two RERF entries in Table 24-B need some discussion here.

First, their inclusion should not be interpreted as approval of the non-constant-cohort, non-dual-dosimetry approach currently used by RERF. The RERF entries are characterized as "realistic" in Table 24-B because they are tied to real-world epidemiological observations -- unlike the NRC and BEIR-3 models which are tied to a preferred but invalidated presumption that human dose-response would be concave-upward (see Chapter 22).

Second, as far as we know, RERF analysts have made no public estimates of Chernobyl's cancer consequences. However, we (and others) are entitled to use RERF's Cancer-Yields in order to estimate those consequences, just as everyone else has been using Cancer-Yields from NRC, BEIR, UNSCEAR, and ICRP for the same purpose.

Readers are reminded, of course, that RERF Cancer-Yields from the A-Bomb Study are not directly comparable with our own. We enumerated several of the reasons in Chapter 14, Part 2.

Our own Cancer-Yields from the A-Bomb Study are explicitly based on low-dose exposure. In Table 14-C,

the estimates are based on linear interpolation between 11 cSv and less than one cSv (rem). (In the supplemental DS86 analysis, 11 cSv becomes 15 cSv.) Our other Cancer-Yields from the A-Bomb Study are based on the best-fit curve (supra-linear), with linear interpolation between 5 cSv and zero dose.

Now let us consider the two RERF estimates in Table 24-B.

Shimizu + Kato + Schull (Shi88) :

In TR-5-88, page 53, Table 19, Shimizu, Kato, and Schull explicitly confine their estimates of Lifetime Fatal Cancer-Yield to acute exposure of 10 rems (cSv). We have already commented on this in Chapter 14, Part 5, "Venturing below 10 Rems." If they cannot use their curve BELOW ten rems, we wonder why they can use it anywhere at all. In the region ABOVE ten rems, the small-numbers problem makes it increasingly unreliable.

The only science-based reason we can imagine, for not interpolating along their curve below ten rems, would be positive, credible evidence that the dose-response changes in this little dose-segment, or that there is a threshold dose below which no carcinogenesis occurs. Shimizu, Kato, and Schull neither provide such evidence nor suggest that they believe any exists.

We have already stated (Chapter 14, Part 5) that, in the absence of contrary evidence or logic, we consider it highly reasonable and perhaps obligatory for analysts to presume that the dose-response which derives from the dose-range as a whole ALSO characterizes the little segment between 10 rems and zero dose.

Moreover, in Chapters 18 through 23, we showed by any reasonable standard of proof that there is no safe dose or dose-rate, and no basis for invoking DREFS for low and slow exposures.

Therefore, it is perfectly appropriate to use the Cancer-Yield from Shi88 to estimate Chernobyl-induced cancers in Table 24-B.

However, there is not just ONE Cancer-Yield listed in Shi88, Table 19. Cancer-Yields are given separately for males and females. For each sex, these analysts present values from their best-fit linear analysis, with all eight Dose-Groups included and also with the high-dose groups thrown out. And then they do it all again, for their best-fit linear-quadratic analysis, with all the Dose-Groups included and with the high-dose groups thrown out.

===

All their values are derived from the DS86 sub-cohort, 1956-1985, with an RBE of 10 for neutrons.

The abundance of Cancer-Yields in Shi88 is not surprising, in view of the authors' finding (Shi88, pp.50-51) that their data fit linearity and supra-linearity equally well -- when they include all the evidence, as we do. In other words, the quadratic term was NEGATIVE in their LQ analysis when they used ALL the evidence. In order to obtain a POSITIVE quadratic term in their LQ analysis, they threw away the high Dose-Groups. We have already criticized this practice in Chapter 14, Part 2.

The value of 12.4 for Cancer-Yield which appears in Table 24-B is the average of males and females from the LQ analysis, all Dose-Groups included.

Preston + Pierce (Pr88) :

Unlike Shimizu, Kato, and Schull above, Preston and Pierce do not confine their estimated Cancer-Yields to an acute dose of 10 rems. In Pr88, at page 458, it is described as a linear value per 10,000 persons per 10 mSv (one rem).

As Preston and Pierce did in the unabbreviated version of TR-9-87, they show the effect of using the reduction-factors (DREFS) suggested by others, but Preston and Pierce avoid any direct endorsement of their use.

It would be perplexing if they did endorse DREFS, because the presumption of DREFS is the concave-upward dose-response, and these authors do NOT find dose-response to be concave-upward. Both Preston and Pierce are co-authors of Shi87 (TR-12-87). This RERF Technical Report finds that linearity and supra-linearity (the LQ model with a NEGATIVE Q-term) fit the data equally well (Shi87, pp.28-29). The authors comment:

"For those sites other than leukemia and colon, the fitted curve associated with the LQ model is invariably concave downwards, not upwards ..." (Shi87, p.29), and "... since the curvature is invariably downwards when a curvilinear model gives an acceptable fit, this would imply a higher risk at low doses than that which obtains under a linear model" (Shi87, p.30).

It is clearly appropriate to use the Preston and Pierce Cancer-Yield in our Table 24-B, without a reduction-factor, to estimate Chernobyl-induced fatal cancers.

The value of 11 for Cancer-Yield which appears in our Column C is their linear result for the DS86 sub-cohort, 1950-1985, with Dose-Group 8 omitted and with an RBE of 10 assumed for neutrons. It is found in Pr88 at page 458.

8. Some Important Comments from the NRC and DOE Reports

It is self-evident that private and governmental segments of the nuclear enterprise, worldwide, have an interest in helping the public to perceive the Chernobyl accident as a non-disaster -- as the accident which killed 31 people from acute radiation sickness. (Robert Alexander of the NRC is particularly candid about the importance of shaping perception, as we will see in Part 9 of this chapter.)

In Part 8, below, we will illustrate some of the help offered by the Nrc87, Doe87, and Doe88 reports with respect to perception.

How is perception of the Chernobyl accident related to a "crossroad in radiation health sciences" ? The answer will become clear in Parts 9 and 10, and most of our own comments are deferred until then. Right here, we will only point out that public perception of the Chernobyl accident might be quite different if the geographical distribution of the radio-cesium fallout had been more concentrated.

Distribution of the fallout was a matter of chance. For instance, if the rain and wind conditions had been different during the accident, the same amount of fallout might have been concentrated upon a much smaller area -- with high per capita dose commitments. Indeed, if the plume had carried the radio-cesiums right to the city of Kiev, evacuation of the whole metropolitan area might have meant visible misery for a couple of million radiation refugees.

Instead, the fallout was spread all over Europe (European USSR and non-USSR Europe), so per capita dose commitments are low. It is the collective dose commitment which is huge. The resulting radiation-induced malignancies will occur gradually and undetectably, over many decades. They will not be distinguishable from the very large number of spontaneous cancers occurring for other reasons among 500,000,000 Europeans.

This one aspect of the accident-induced cancer-deaths is emphasized very favorably by parts of the radiation community, as we shall show.

Comments by the Authors of Nrc87 :

=====================================

ABOUT EUROPEAN USSR -- The authors of Nrc87, Chapter 8, call 10,000 fatal cancers plus 10,000 non-fatal cancers "quite substantial" as potential health effects from an accident (Nrc87, p.8-10):

"The estimated effect of the Chernobyl accident on the exposed population of 75 million is, from the standpoint of potential health effects induced, quite substantial. Even if the Soviet report overestimates the dose via the food pathway by an order of magnitude, one estimates a total collective dose of about 5×10^7 person-rem. Assuming a risk factor of 2×10^{-4}/rem, about 10,000 fatal cancers (plus a comparable number of nonfatal cancers) would be projected over the next 70 years."

ABOUT NON-USSR EUROPE -- The authors of Nrc87, Chapter 8, suggest a perspective on the accident which will be frequently echoed in other reports from the radiation community. They compare the accident-induced dose with the unavoidable natural dose, and the accident-induced death-rate with the entire cancer death-rate from other causes (Nrc87, p.8-14):

"Thus, as a tentative approximation, the average individual in Europe (outside the Soviet Union and the other countries named above) will receive a 60-mrem dose from the accident, this dose being spread over a period of years. For comparison, this individual will receive about 100 mrem EACH YEAR [their emphasis] from background radiation. Using this estimated average dose and a total population of about 350 million people in that part of Europe being considered, a collective dose of 2×10^7 person-rem is calculated. Based again on a risk factor of 2×10^{-4}/rem, about 4000 excess cancer deaths outside the Soviet Union may be calculated to result from the accident. These deaths would be completely masked by the 70 million or so cancer deaths predicted in the population over the next 70 years."

Comments by the Authors of Doe87 :

=====================================

Return of the Threshold :

In their Chapter 7 (at page 7.5), the authors state that there may be a safe dose or dose-rate: "A variety of models and assumptions can be employed in predicting possible latent health effects in exposed populations. For example, when radiation doses are only a few percent of natural background radiation, such doses might be considered negligible in producing detectable adverse health effects. For example, annual doses of 10 micro-sieverts (1 mrem), or a lifetime dose of about 500 micro-sieverts (50 mrem), would likely produce no additional risk; thus, a major portion of the Northern Hemisphere might produce no additional radiological risk from the Chernobyl fallout. As noted in NCRP Report No. 64 (1980), there are no direct data that confirm that a few random ionizations in tissue cause fatal cancers. Moreover, the BEIR Committee noted that for low dose and dose rates, the likelihood of zero deleterious health effects is not precluded."

Notwithstanding 1980 statements by NCRP and the BEIR-3 Committee, direct human data DO exist which confirm that random ionizations from SINGLE TRACKS, acting independently, have caused fatal cancers. Readers have seen the evidence themselves in Section 5 of this book. Most of that evidence circulated widely (as Go86) within the radiation community. The authors of Doe87 do not refute the evidence against any safe dose or dose-rate. They just ignore it.

Moreover, it is utterly misleading for the Doe87 authors to use the phrase "a few random ionizations." As readers know from Chapter 19, Part 1, the smallest possible unit of ionizing radiation is a single primary electron track. Even for the low-energy X-rays (30 KeV), one track from one photo-electron will produce about (30,000 eV x one ionization per 30 eV), or about ONE THOUSAND ionizations concentrated along its track. And not only does single-track carcinogenesis occur -- but it might even turn out to be overwhelmingly dominant in radiation carcinogenesis compared with inter-track action. No one presently knows.

"Zero-Risk Model" :

The Doe87 authors announce, somewhat urgently, that their report definitely includes the threshold model in its analyses, whereas Nrc87 -- which is NUREG-1250 -- did not. We quote (Doe87, p.J.8):

"While NUREG-1250 does not recognize the zero risk model for low-dose, low-LET exposure, the data do not rule out the possibility that the cancer increase will be zero. The DOE Report, however, contains this provision, and all cancer mortality projections are expressed as a range, starting at zero. The zero risk projection alternative is set forth both in the risk projection models given in NUREG/CR-4214 (NRC 1985) and used in the preparation of the DOE report, as well as in the BEIR report (NAS/NRC 1980)."

And the "threshold" or zero-risk model is displayed or mentioned everywhere throughout Doe87. We will

==

demonstrate with two examples.

The first is from the key table, Doe87 Table 7.11, p.7.22, where the authors flag their column of 28,000 "Estimated Possible Radiation-Induced Fatal Cancers" with the following note: "The possibility of zero health effects at very low doses and dose rates cannot be excluded." The same note appears in several tables.

The second is from Doe87 Table J.5 at p.J.7:

Location	Excess Radiogenic Cancer Mortality
EUROPEAN USSR	0 to 11,000
ASIAN USSR	0 to 2,500
NON-USSR EUROPE	0 to 13,000
NON-USSR ASIA	0 to 600
NORTHERN HEMISPHERE	0 to 28,000

Setting the lower end of the range at zero is a statement that a threshold may exist, with no cancer-risk at all at doses below that threshold.

The statement in digits and words, that Chernobyl may cause NO cancer-deaths, is made so many times in Doe87 that we lost count. It is mentioned four times even in the "Executive Summary."

Comparison with Entire Cancer Problem :

Also more times than we can count, Doe87 makes the comparison between the 28,000 "estimated possible radiation-induced fatal cancers" and the entire number of cancers which will occur anyway. It starts in the Executive Summary.

The table on page xii tabulates spontaneous and radiation-induced fatal cancers side by side. Among 3.5 billion people in the Northern Hemisphere, Doe87 expects about 600,000,000 "natural" fatal cancers (about one death in six), and lists 28,000 Chernobyl-induced fatal cancers -- annotated with the speculation that the possibility of zero cancers "cannot be excluded."

On the next page, the text makes the comparison in words: "Estimates of excess cancer cases, which may be as low as zero for the majority of exposed populations, are so small that they are negligible compared to the higher cancer mortality from natural or spontaneous causes in those populations" (Doe87, p.xiii). The 28,000 possible Chernobyl-induced deaths are described as a possible 0.004 percent increase in cancer-mortality (p.xiii, p.7.22). The percent is (28,000 / 600,000,000) x (100), of course.

Comparison with Natural Dose :

Another recurring theme, in the authors' own comments, is the comparison of per capita dose commitments from Chernobyl with the dose commitment received by humans from natural background sources. One example suffices. Discussing 50-year dose-commitments in Non-USSR Europe, Doe87 says (p.5.62):

"... the calculated average dose commitment to the population of any listed country is less than 5 mGy (500 mrad). Thus, although the calculated total collective dose commitment is large, the average individual dose commitments for even the European countries are equivalent to that received from background radiation in a few years."

Comments by the Authors of Doe88 :
====================================

At the Beginning :

The abstract of the SCIENCE version is very brief, and features this statement: "The best estimates for the lifetime expectation of fatal radiogenic cancer would increase the risk from 0 to 0.02 % in Europe and 0 to 0.003 % in the Northern Hemisphere" (Doe88, p.1513).

Immediately following the abstract are three introductory paragraphs in which Anspaugh, Catlin and Goldman describe the Chernobyl accident as "the largest reported accidental release of radioactive material." They wish to put this into perspective:

"The purpose of this article is to present a global perspective of the significance of the release." They add, "The dominant concern for the world's citizenry after the Chernobyl accident has been future risks to health. This concern continued even after it was clear that the individual risks outside the Soviet Union would be quite small," at which point they cite their own DOE 1987 report.

"Chickens Come Home to Roost" :

Why did the public continue to be concerned in spite of the reassuring report from DOE in 1987?

In the Preface of the 1987 report, Goldman, Catlin, and Anspaugh describe themselves and the co-authors as dedicated scientists: "A dedicated group of scientists from 11 research institutions [mostly DOE-funded laboratories] have contributed to making this report possible ... Many of the models and values chosen for parameters used in this report stem from

===

research that has been sponsored by the U.S. Department of Energy. The spectrum of such radiological health and environmental research over the past 4 decades includes... pioneering advances in risk assessment" (Doe87, p.vi). And Doe87 was the mother of Doe88.

These authors seem unaware that DOE reports have no credibility at all with much of the public, in view of DOE's inherent conflict of interest coupled with its record of covering-up the careless radioactive contamination around many of its own facilities and its record of other problems.

Indeed, soon after Doe88 -- and following pressure from citizen lawsuits, FBI investigations, and the prospect of criminal prosecution of some DOE employees -- Energy Secretary James Watkins would admit in June 1989:

"... the chickens have finally come home to roost, and years of inattention to changing standards and demands regarding the environment, safety and health are vividly exposed to public examination, almost daily. I am certainly not proud or pleased with what I have seen over my first few months in office" (Wat89a).

And even more recently, Watkins is still expressing dismay over DOE performance. Referring in December 1989 to DOE's plans for waste burial in Nevada and New Mexico, he said that "the whole set of schedules was not scientifically sound, not fiscally sound, not technically sound... They were incomplete, misleading, and not properly done" (Wat89b).

On the problem of candor, Watkins said that DOE will soon issue rules to protect lower-level employees who make allegations about safety, competence or the honesty of their superiors. "We've been totally unresponsive to whistle-blowers," Watkins said (Wat89b).

In the Middle :

In Doe88, between its beginning and its end, the authors assert ten times in six pages that there may be zero Chernobyl-induced cancers. As justification, they say only, "We have taken the bottom of the range [of cancers] to be zero, which is consistent with the NUREG report" (Doe88, p.1515.)

There is a lack of symmetry here. If Anspaugh, Catlin and Goldman wish to stress NUREG's absolutely lowest risk at every opportunity, they are scientifically obliged to give equal emphasis to NUREG's so-called "upper bound estimate" (from the linear model). They

quantify it only once in their summary (p.1518), as quoted below, and they do not show that NUREG's "upper-bound" risk-factor would increase the Doe88 estimate of 17,400 Chernobyl-induced cancers by about 3-fold, to at least 50,000 fatal cancers.

In Their Summary :

Anspaugh, Catlin, and Goldman provide a summary of the "global perspective" as follows:

"Outside of the immediate Chernobyl region, the magnitude of radiation doses to individuals is quite small, leading to extremely low incremental probabilities of any person developing a fatal radiogenic cancer over a lifetime ... Probably no adverse health effects will be manifest by epidemiological analysis in the remainder of the Soviet population [outside the immediate Chernobyl region] or the rest of the world. Projections of excess cancer risk for the Northern Hemisphere range from an incremental increase of 0 % to 0.003 %. An upper bound estimate would range from 0 % to about 0.01 %, still undetectable ... The social consequences are more difficult to quantify, but public concerns, whether justified or not, have increased, necessitating attention by medical, public health, and other authorities" (Doe88, p.1518).

Their perspective has the familiar format -- many more people will NOT be killed than WILL be killed. Perhaps a global perspective is adaptable for Bhopal, famine, World War Two, or even homicide.

If a "global perspective" is considered today, why not an inter-stellar perspective tomorrow? With a bit more advance in the space program, we will find out how many other places support life, and then someone can estimate the INTER-STELLAR impact of nuclear accidents which occur on Earth ... and the inter-stellar impact will surely be much smaller than the global impact.

9. The Threshold and Dose-Exclusion : Ultra-Low Cancer Estimates

It is undeniable that the Chernobyl accident has made the concept of a safe dose or dose-rate more attractive than ever. It is understood that 17,400 to 475,000 cancer-deaths from a single accident do not provide a fertile ground for the nuclear enterprise, which funds (via its governmental and private arms) most radiation research worldwide. A perception of ZERO cancer-deaths would be much more favorable.

Can this need for a threshold be met on a scientific basis? Having presented our DISPROOF of any threshold, we answer "No," of course. But elswehere, as we have already shown, one may face temptation to presume a threshold, without having any appropriate basis in science and without even dealing with the conclusive evidence AGAINST it. Under such a presumption, the Chernobyl problem could be "solved" by throwing away about 95 percent of the collective dose commitment, because it would lie BELOW the presumed threshold. Handling scientific issues in such a manner would be truly a "crossroad in the radiation health sciences."

Some ultra-low Chernobyl estimates follow.

An Article
in the Official Journal of
the Society of Nuclear Medicine
==================================

The first article we will examine is by a member of all the key BEIR-3 Committees (see Chapter 37): Edward W. Webster, Ph.D., Department of Radiological Sciences, Massachusetts General Hospital.

The article is entitled "Chernobyl Predictions and the Chinese Contribution," in the April 1987 issue of THE JOURNAL OF NUCLEAR MEDICINE (Webs87). It is based on a paper given on November 6, 1986.

Webster begins by calling Chernobyl-induced cancers "obviously speculative" and offering a perspective of his own: "As of this writing, the only certain effect has been the 31 early deaths, and therefore to-date the casualties are much smaller than the hundreds who died in each of the several recent crashes of jumbo jet aircraft, and the thousands who died in the chemical disaster at Bhopal, India" (Webs87, p.423).

He goes on to point out, correctly, that the issue of predicted cancers will interest nuclear medicine physicians since individual doses from the accident are typically "well below those administered in diagnostic nuclear medicine" (Webs87, p.423).

Also correctly, Webster states: "The predictions cover a wide range, heavily dependent on the assumptions made concerning the relation of cancer to low-level radiation exposure, and somewhat less dependent on dose assessments. At the high end of the range are those of John Gofman, PhD, MD," and he cites my estimate given at the American Chemical Society meeting (Go86).

Webster continues : "Dr. Gofman's prediction is unique insofar as it employs his own estimate of lifetime cancer risk per rem, whereas most other predictions utilize the risk estimates adopted by the International Commission on Radiological Protection (ICRP), the United Nations Scientific Committee on the Effects of Atomic Radiation (UNSCEAR), and other international bodies."

By definition, independence from the official line is the ESSENCE of an independent analysis -- although independence alone does not make the analysis CORRECT, as we pointed out in Chapter 2.

In the same chapter, we also pointed out a set of circumstances (chiefly funding) which can produce an ARTIFICIAL consensus of experts. It is interesting to contrast the views of Dixy Lee Ray, a former head of the U.S. Atomic Energy Commission (AEC), with the predicament of James Watkins, current head of AEC's replacement, DOE. Moghissi and Ray (Mog89) have been insisting that consensus in science means everything, whereas Watkins is finding that experts can be persuaded to reach a consensus on managing radioactive waste which is "not scientifically sound ... misleading, and not properly done" (see Part 8).

Webster's First Recommendation :

Webster continues, still correctly (Webs87), p.423: "The Gofman risk estimate... is about 40 times higher than the above 'official' estimate of 100 [cancer-deaths] per million person-rems" -- which is a Cancer-Yield of 1.0. Webster appears to prefer the 1977 UNSCEAR value to the higher BEIR-3 value of about 2.0.

Webster makes two recommendations for resolving the disparity between my estimates and 'official' estimates, and for estimating Chernobyl-induced cancers.

First, he suggests that the world will find out the "correct" value for Cancer-Yield from an epidemiologic follow-up of 24,000 highly exposed persons near the Chernobyl explosion (Webs87, p.424).

By contrast, we strongly caution against any policy which would make the radiation health sciences and human health itself dependent, in any measure at all, upon Soviet data on a radiation issue. Readers are referred back to Part 1 of this chapter.

===

Webster's Second Recommendation :

Webster also recommends that meanwhile, the radiation community should give great weight to a recent "Denver-Type" study (our term, not his) from the People's Republic of China, in order to resolve the disparity in Cancer-Yields: "The Gofman estimate appears particularly improbable in the light of the Chinese study" (Webs87, p.425).

The study to which he refers is by Zufan and Luxin (Zu86) entitled "An Epidemiological Investigation of Mutational Diseases in the High Background Radiation Area of Yangjiang, China," in the JOURNAL OF RADIATION RESEARCH (JAPAN). Zufan and Luxin thank RERF in Hiroshima for editorial assistance. Luxin is a Chinese delegate on UNSCEAR-88.

The study (Zu86) finds the cancer-rate in the high background area to be lower than the cancer-rate in the low background area. The paper is one of several earlier and later Chinese reports on their high background area (see also Chapter 35, Part 7).

This type of study is inherently unable to resolve anything about the low-dose and threshold issues, as explained in Chapter 21, Part 2. The BEIR-3 Committee made much the same point with respect to some earlier "Denver-Type" studies (Beir80, pp.469-471). Therefore we are critical of reliance on this study and of its representation to the physicians as a key study.

The Need for Proper "Blinding" :

Moreover, another aspect of the paper by Zufan and Luxin deserves attention. The study may have an open doorway for bias to confound its results. The authors state the following (Zu86, p.143):

"Cancer mortality in the high background radiation area and the control area has been investigated for more than 14 years. The early data (1970-1978) were obtained by means of a retrospective survey. In 1979, a cancer registry system was established for the study areas whereby local physicians, with the help of many hospitals and administrative organizations, report all incident cancer cases and cancer deaths to the registry. Diagnoses are confirmed by an expert group who meet to evaluate cases once or twice a year."

In other words, this is not even a Denver-Type study based on Vital Statistics compiled by persons with no knowledge of the study. In the Zufan study, the statistics are first collected with a well-known purpose, and then re-evaluated by an "expert group" with full knowledge of the purpose.

The opportunities for bias to enter are self-evident. The paper mentions not even one precaution against such bias. If input to the study's database were to include some over-diagnosis of cancer in the low background area, or some under-diagnosis in the high background area, the study's output -- its "answer" -- could be easily pre-determined at the outset.

We are disappointed that peer-reviewers did not insist that the "blinding" problem be shown as solved, or be acknowledged if NOT solved.

Embracing Data from China :

Ideally, a scientific report deserves to stand or fall on its own merits, and not because of its source. We made that point emphatically at the end of Chapter 2.

But also one is obliged to be realistic about the misuse of science in the service of policy. (See also warnings by Dr. Sheldon Wolff on this same subject, in Chapter 35, Part 4).

As stated with regret in part 1 of this chapter, I warn against acceptance of uncheckable data or findings coming out of any country whose authorities have recently or currently demonstrated no regard for truth when it undermines policy.

In China, the policy has been to undertake nuclear power generation. By 1982, plans were underway to build such plants just north of Hong Kong (Nyt82). And the policy has been pursued against popular protest -- a million signatures in Hong Kong against it, according to the WALL STREET JOURNAL of April 13, 1987 (Wsj87). Under the circumstances, it is common sense to say that the government would welcome reports suggesting that a little radiation is harmless or possibly even good for people.

It is realistic to worry that radiation analysts in the People's Republic of China -- especially in the absence of a free press there -- may expect to pay a heavier price than radiation analysts elsewhere, if they were ever to question whether data sponsored by the state (on background doses, cancer mortality-rates, or anything else) were rearranged, falsified, selectively abbreviated, or just plain fabricated. Individual analysts, fully innocent themselves, could be deceived under such regimes without even knowing it for certain.

100 Chernobyl–Induced Cancers :

Notwithstanding all these problems, Webster looks very favorably on what his title calls "the Chinese Contribution." His article ends as follows:

"The Chinese evidence at present suggests that the excess cancer mortality from the long–term exposure to low levels of external and internal radioactivity of many millions in Russia and Europe could be less than 100 and is almost certainly below a few thousand. The Chinese contribution to our knowledge of low–level radiation is still developing, and the present provocative findings may change or may reveal an explanation which will admit support for current risk estimates. Potentially, the impact of a larger statistical study with a zero or negative index of low–level radiation effect could be very far reaching."

Nowhere do the nuclear physicians receive warning about the inherent limits of Denver-Type studies, about the "blinding" issue in this study, and about the even bigger issue of caution toward unverifiable reports from certain nations.

These physicians may infer, mistakenly, that the "Chinese contribution" is valid evidence in favor of a safe dose -- an inference which could have unintended consequences for their patients and staffs. Webster himself must assume a safe dose when he suggests Chernobyl-induced cancers "below a few thousand" or even "less than 100." As for the conclusive evidence AGAINST any safe dose -- presented in Go86, which Webster cites -- Webster does not refute it or even mention it.

An Article in the Official Journal of the Health Physics Society

====================================

The second article we will examine is by Robert E. Alexander. He is the 1988-89 President of the Health Physics Society. Elsewhere, he identifies himself also as (A) a scientist with the U.S. Nuclear Regulatory Commission, and (B) a member of the Science Panel preparing a report for the Veterans Administration to "assist in the adjudication of claims of service-related radiogenic cancer" (Alex88a, p.145; Alex88b, p.592).

The article is entitled "A New Intellectual Atmosphere," in the June 1988 issue of HEALTH PHYSICS, which describes itself as "the radiation protection journal" on its cover. This article (Alex88b) is a guest editorial. Sections of this article also appear in a much shorter article entitled "Health Effects from Radiation," in the February 1988 issue of ENVIRONMENTAL SCIENCE & TECHNOLOGY (Alex88a).

Concern about "Decision Makers" :

Alexander is quite forthright about the importance to the nuclear enterprise of shaping the perception of Chernobyl's cancer consequences -- especially the perception of decision-makers:

"... predictions of delayed deaths from radiation-induced cancer seem to me to be the most significant reactor accident consequences in terms of impressions left with decision makers. I suspect it is these estimates that are more likely to prompt the word 'catastrophic' and to alarm decision makers" (Alex88b, p.589).

"... very small doses to very large numbers of people can yield very alarming results" (Alex88b, p.592), at which point he cites the Doe87 estimate of 28,000 Chernobyl-induced cancer-deaths.

Then he calls the Doe87 estimates for European USSR and for Non-USSR Europe "conjecture, i.e., inference from insufficient evidence and not useful for decision making" (p.592). On the next page and also in the shorter article he says:

"In my opinion there is a very limited place for conjecture and speculation in science. Even hypotheses must always be clearly identified as such, particularly when the results of hypothetical calculations can reach unsuspecting legislators and agency heads, influencing their decision-making process in a manner detrimental to the best interests of the nation" (Alex88a, p.145; with minor differences, Alex88b, p.593).

"There is a larger picture that should be considered. The catastrophe that I am worried about is that the energy needs of many people may be delayed by those who fear that the sky is falling" (Alex88b, p.593).

Speculations about a Threshold

Alexander recognizes, as everyone must, that acceptance of nuclear energy would be vastly easier if there were acceptance of a threshold.

In support of the threshold hypothesis, he cites (Alex88b, p.592) a number of Denver-Type studies and the A-Bomb Study 1950-1978. We have already explained why all of these studies are inherently incapable of answering the threshold question, however.

==

Alexander does not refute or even mention the conclusive and appropriate human evidence AGAINST any safe dose. Mostly, he relies upon quoting threshold allusions from Doe87 and from the 1980 BEIR-3 Report (provided, respectively, to readers by us in Part 8 of this chapter and in Chapter 34).

The threshold speculation is competing with good human evidence. When the speculation about upward curvature for human dose-response was competing with good human evidence, the speculation prevailed. If the threshold speculation prevails, then 95 percent of the dose commitment and consequences from Chernobyl can be thrown out.

Goldman, Catlin, and Anspaugh appear to have been the pioneers in this -- which is consistent with their description of DOE as the sponsor of "pioneering advances in risk assessment" (Doe87, p.vi). Although Doe87 made its range of Chernobyl-induced cancers "0 to 28,000," it also explored dose-levels at which a threshold would be important (Doe87, p.5.46):

"Another question of interest is how much the total collective dose might be reduced if the calculation were made with the exclusion of very small, but nonzero, individual total-body doses of, for example, less than 0.5 mGy (50 mrad)." The authors report that with this exclusion, "... the calculated total collective dose commitment would decrease by less than 6% ."

So it would seem that a speculative threshold at 50 millirads cannot solve the Chernobyl problem. In the next paragraph, the authors explore 500 millirads:

"To put these dose estimates into further perspective, it should be noted that if individual lifetime dose commitments below 5 mGy (500 mrad) are excluded, all but the more heavily affected portion of the USSR would be removed from the global collective dose summary" (Doe87, p.5.46).

Now this could be USEFUL threshold information.

410 Chernobyl-Induced Cancers :

And it is soon used. On page 7.8, Goldman, Catlin, and Anspaugh suggest that the population evacuated from the 30 kilometers around the former reactor will experience between zero and 410 cancer fatalities from their external exposure. (Doe87 used the Soviet estimate of 135,000 evacuated persons in this context; the Soviets reduced the number to 115,000 persons before Doe88.)

The number "410" is picked up by Alexander and featured in both his long and short articles (Alex88b, p.591 quoted below; abbreviated in Alex88a, p.145):

"Consider the example of the 28,000 cancer death estimate for Chernobyl. If individual doses below 0.1 Gy (10 rads), and dose rates below 0.01 Gy y^{-1} (1 rad y^{-1}) lifetime, are excluded from the calculation, only the evacuees are affected and the theoretical result is 410 cancer deaths. A difference of this magnitude is sufficient to alter conclusions." Indeed.

10.   Beyond Chernobyl :
The Much Bigger Agenda

Chernobyl is only "the tip of the iceberg" with respect to the concept of dose-exclusion. There is a bigger agenda under discussion, and Alexander's article serves as one illustration. Alexander makes it clear, by his own words below, that he disapproves in GENERAL of including individual doses below 10 rads and dose-rates below one rad per year in current risk-benefit considerations. Those levels are the ones below which the BEIR-3 Report declined to quantify risk coefficients (our Chapter 34), even though its own analysis of solid cancer in the A-Bomb Study produced a linear dose-response. Alexander writes:

"It is understandable that many health physicists are dismayed by the now common practice of including extremely low doses in collective dose calculations. When doses obtained in this manner are multiplied by risk coefficients, valid at best for doses and dose rates exceeding those specified by the BEIR-III Committee, the results can be alarming, misleading and they may have detrimental influence on decision makers" (Alex88b, p.591).

After telling readers that the Nuclear Regulatory Commission is proposing to establish a "de minimis" dose of one millirad for collective dose calculations, Alexander says that the Environmental Protection Agency is opposing the NRC proposal. He blames the behavior of EPA and "government officials" on their ignorance:

"It is inconceivable to me, to mention only three examples, that government officials actually aware of the assumptions made in connection with low-level radiation risk assessments would have (1) approved $2 billion for decommissioning of formerly used U.S. Atomic Energy Commission (AEC) facilities and other aspects of the DOE Remedial Action Program, (2) established NRC effluent-control design criteria of ...8 mrem y^{-1} for nuclear power plants or (3) taken the

U.S. Environmental Protection Agency (EPA) position that Environmental Impact Statements using non-zero lower limits of collective dose integration are not acceptable" (Alex88b, p.593).

"Reasonable people will not knowingly want to support proposals for large expenditures to protect against risks that have an entirely theoretical basis, that may not exist, and that can never be demonstrated" (Alex88b, p.594).

"The nation is expending enormous resources to protect the public against risks believed by an overwhelming, but silent, majority of the scientific community to be trivial or even non-existent" (Alex88b, p.594).

"Below Regulatory Concern" :

Silent? Regulatory bodies seldom respond to silence, and yet proposals are moving forward in the U.S. Nuclear Regulatory Commission to declare a large share of radioactive waste to be "below regulatory concern" and to treat it just like non-radioactive waste in local landfills, incinerators, sewage plants, and recycling circles.

So Sorry If We're Wrong ...

Some segments of the radiation community appear to believe passionately that no one should impede the nuclear enterprise on the basis of what they label as speculation and conjecture about injury from low doses and dose-rates. Instead, they ask the world to accept THEIR speculation and conjecture that low doses and dose-rates are safe -- a notion which would surely result in increased exposures.

But if the threshold speculation is wrong (as shown in this book), and nonetheless we contaminate the planet irreversibly with radioactive poisons, the results might be hundreds of millions of unnecessary cancers over time -- as well as a presently unquantifiable price in heritable genetic damage.

Price of Past Presumption :

Society has acted before, in previous decades, on the basis of rosy but mistaken presumptions promoted by parts of the radiation community.

In the absence of conclusive evidence, optimistic assumptions in this field have led to past "benefit-risk" judgments in which the benefit was sometimes real, but the cancer-risk from the associated doses was casually

dismissed. Today some of the practices in the list below continue, but usually at much lower doses than in the past. The following is merely a partial listing:

● - Use of luminous radium dials in wrist-watches and airplane instruments (chronic gamma irradiation of the cockpit crew).
● - The promotion of radon spas and radium-laced water as health-enhancers.
● - Use of fluoroscopy machines in shoe stores, with some unavoidable dose not only to the pelvis, but also to the face and neck of people looking down to enjoy the sight of their foot-bones.
● - Use of the fluoroscope by voice teachers to show the position of the diaphragm at the beginning, middle, and end of a singer's phrase.
● - Irradiation of infants in utero during maternal pelvimetry.
● - Routine irradiation of infants for a "disease" (thymic enlargement) which was later admitted never to have needed any treatment at all.
● - Routine irradiation of tuberculosis patients to monitor pneumothorax treatment.
● - Irradiation of women for post-partum mastitis.
● - Irradiation of people for ringworm of the scalp.
● - Cobalt treatment for blocked eustachian tubes.
● - Radium treatments for "sinus trouble."
● - Use of X-ray exams to monitor the advance or regression of curvature of the spine (scoliosis), mostly in young girls.
● - Fluoroscopic exams of babies as part of routine "check-ups."
● - Use of radioactive thorotrast as a routine contrast medium in diagnostic radiography.
● - The practice of giving full-spine X-rays, "GI series" and barium enemas as part of the routine "annual check-up" in the 1940s.
● - The smoking of cigarettes whose tobacco-smoke is contaminated by radioactive decay-products from uranium, present in the soil or in phosphate and raffinate fertilizers.
● - The use of young nurses and young mothers to hold small children during X-ray exam of the child.
● - Absence of lead-shielding between X-ray offices and adjacent offices and elevators.

Several of these past practices provided the early epidemiological proof that ionizing radiation can induce fatal human cancers.

One needs to wonder seriously how much of the current cancer-rate is due to past exposure to ionizing radiation from such practices. It could be a meaningful part of the so-called "spontaneous" rate.

"De Minimis" -- Beyond Chernobyl :

"De minimis non curat lex", or "the law does not concern itself with trifles," is referred to simply as "de minimis" in proposals NOT to count a certain amount of population exposure from ionizing radiation in risk-analysis -- and NOT to regulate certain amounts of radioactive pollution. Of course, the two issues are closely related to each other.

The most extreme position, probably supported by very few in the radiation community, favors the exclusion from risk-considerations of all individual doses when the individual's risk is small, regardless of the magnitude of the COLLECTIVE dose.

This is another way of saying that even 950,000 Chernobyl-induced cancers would not be worth attention, because -- although the collective dose and health-price might be huge -- each INDIVIDUAL's dose and risk would be very small. If this type of "de minimis" proposal ever prevails, the health consequences from Chernobyl-size accidents (or the equivalent from gradual PLANNED emissions) could be officially treated as negligible.

Less drastic "de minimis" proposals would give some consideration to the magnitude of the collective dose -- with some limit on the person-rads per source which would not "count." Of course, if sources were subdivided into regions, facilities, or ultimately into particular vents or pipes, the true collective dose "not counted" could become larger and larger.

"De minimis" proposals are a "hot" topic, and certainly NOT everyone in the radiation community supports the concept. Whatever decisions are made, it seems safe to predict that policies accepted in the radiation health sciences will influence policies set in other health sciences, too.

We will quote Bo Lindell of Sweden's National Institute of Radiation Protection. He is also a member emeritus of the ICRP's Main Commission, and is a Swedish delegate to UNSCEAR (see Chapter 37). In a thoughtful letter to HEALTH PHYSICS, he concludes (Linde89):

"... I suggest that the profession of radiation protection should adopt a cautious attitude rather than belligerently crying for a de minimis, a concept which I consider untenable on both logical and ethical grounds."

"De Minimis" -- Beyond Radiation :

Many people have observed that human nature incorporates some contradictory tendencies. It seems contradictory to me that, on the one hand, there is a readiness to inflict cancer-death on undetectable victims who will not be noticed, while there is a competing tendency which causes some people in Oakland, California, to risk their own lives on an unstable structure and work themselves to exhaustion following the October 1989 earthquake, just on the very slim chance that they might SAVE one life from under the collapsed freeway.

People of goodwill need to look closely at the aggregate consequences of individually small risks. If pollution sources of all types are regulated individually, and each is allowed under the "de minimis" concept to kill one person in 100,000 (a low individual risk), then only 10,000 sources could kill up to one tenth of the population. And no one would ever be able to prove it.

A Reality-Check on Confidence :

When various experts advocate that we neglect to "count" or evaluate exposure to some pollutant below an arbitrary dose or dose-rate, they generally claim that the low dose or dose-rate will be too trivial to matter: "A smaller hazard than getting out of bed." Thus such experts should not object to pre-testing their own proposals before scaling them up to everyone.

After all, if the proposed doses are such a trivial hazard that the experts say the general public should not object, then why should these same experts object to exposing their OWN children and grandchildren intentionally to all the proposed doses, for the next 10 to 20 years?

I wonder if such guardians of the public's health might think twice, before agreeing to a personal kind of pre-testing for their policies -- BEFORE they are applied to children everywhere.

Table 24–A
Comparison of Chernobyl–Induced Fatal Cancers, Estimated by Gofman, NRC, and DOE.

Col.A Source of Estimate:	Col.B Whole–Body Dose Commitment in Person–Rad	Col.C Fatal Cancer–Yield (Fatal Cancers per 10,000 Person–Rad)	Col.D Chernobyl–Induced Fatal Cancers (estimated)
Gofman Sept. 1986. Part 3 of this chapter.	127.4 million person–rad. *All-time commitment.*	37.313	475,500
NRC January 1987. Part 4 of this chapter.	70 million person–rad. *Fifty-year cut-off.*	2.0	14,000
DOE June 1987. Part 5 of this chapter.	120 million person–rad. *Fifty-year cut-off.*	2.3	28,000
	If Doe87 had used the corresponding all–time commitment: 150 million person–rad.	2.3	34,500
DOE December 1988 Part 6 of this chapter.	93 million person–rad. *Fifty-year cut-off.*	1.87	17,400
	If Doe88 had used the corresponding all–time commitment: 116 million person–rad.	1.87	21,700

There is no mystery about the disparities in Column D.

These differences cannot be blamed on the relatively small differences in estimated dose. Indeed, the Gofman and DOE estimates are remarkably close. Part 6 explains why DOE needs to use the all–time dose commitment –– not the 50–year cut–off.

The differences in the estimated Chernobyl–induced cancers lie overwhelmingly in an independent evaluation of Cancer–Yield (cancer–risk) versus the Cancer–Yields used by the radiation community.

Table 24-B
A Realistic Range for Chernobyl-Induced Fatal Cancers, Based on Gofman and RERF.

Every estimate here is based on a collective all-time dose commitment of 127.4 million person-rad. This value (from Go86) lies between the DOE all-time dose commitments of 116 and 150 million person-rad. See Table 24-A, Column B.

Col. A Source of the Estimate of Fatal Cancer-Yields	Col.B Lifetime Fatal Cancer-Yield T65DR Dosimetry	Col.C Lifetime Fatal Cancer-Yield DS86 Dosimetry	Col.D Chernobyl-Induced Cancer Fatalities T65DR	DS86
Gofman Cancer Difference Method. A-Bomb Study, 1950-1982. Low-Dose Exposed vs Ref. Grp. Table 14-C, Row 1.	16.2	12.23	206388	155810
Gofman Cancer Difference Method. A-Bomb Study, 1950-1982. Best Fit by Regression. Table 14-C, Row 2.	12.9	12.03	164346	153262
Gofman Cancer-Rate Ratio Method. A-Bomb K-values and A-Bomb Survivors. Table 16-B.	31.65	30.43	403221	387678
Gofman Cancer-Rate Ratio Method. A-Bomb K-values and U.S. Population. Table 16-C.	26.64	25.56	339394	325634
RERF: Shimizu and co-workers. Sub-cohort, A-Bomb Study, 1956-85. Table 19, page 53, Shi88. Details in our text, Part 7.	NOT DONE	12.4	NOT DONE	157976
RERF: Preston and Pierce. Sub-cohort, A-Bomb Study, 1950-85. Pr88, page 458. Details in our text, Part 7.	NOT DONE	11	NOT DONE	140140
Gofman: Worldwide Low-LET Human Evidence, with Variable Rel. Risk. A-Bomb Study, 1950-1974 included. Go81.	37.313	NOT DONE	475368	NOT DONE

The entries in Column D for the T65DR dosimetry are (127.4 million x Col.B) / (10,000).
The entries in Column D for the DS86 dosimetry are (127.4 million x Col.C) / (10,000).

The Cancer-Yields in Columns B and C are central estimates based on the best available real-world human evidence. By contrast, Cancer-Yields in the range of 1.0 to 2.3 used by the radiation community are grossly at variance with this evidence, as we demonstrated in this book by showing step-by-step what really does emerge from the evidence.

If DOE, for instance, would just use reality-based Cancer-Yields instead of Cancer-Yields based on preferred speculations, the disparity among estimates of Chernobyl-induced cancer-deaths would shrink to about three-fold, as shown in Column D above.

Each entry in Column D needs doubling, if one wishes to include non-fatal cancers. Table 24-B shows that scientifically reasonable estimates of Chernobyl-induced cancers range in the hundreds of thousands, not the tens of thousands.

CHAPTER 25

Closing Statement

This closing statement is arranged in five parts:

At the close of this book, we must return to the question posed by the book's title, and by Chapter 2: Do conclusions in this field come out differently from an independent analysis, than from analyses provided by the radiation community?

The answer is yes. This book has examined five main topics, listed above. (Hormetic speculations are in a class by themselves, and are examined in Chapter 35.) Except on the least important topic -- the cancer-risk from acute exposure at moderate and high dose-levels -- we differ seriously with most of the radiation community.

Moreover, we are severely critical of scientifically questionable practices and apparent inconsistencies which exist in some other analyses, and which we have identified in the preceding chapters.

In this closing chapter, we shall compare our own conclusions on each of the five main topics with those of most of the radiation community, and in particular, with those of the 1988 UNSCEAR and 1990 BEIR-5 Committees.

1. Method for Handling the Retroactive Alteration of Dose Estimates in the A-Bomb Study

Uncertainties remain in the field of radiation epidemiology, and the database which is most capable of resolving them in the future is the A-Bomb Study. Thus humankind as a whole has a stake in protecting this uniquely valuable study from practices which can destroy its credibility in the future.

We have shown in Chapter 5 that a process is now underway of substituting a retroactively altered database for the study's previous database. This is not planned as an ADDITION of new dose-estimates to the study. What is occurring is REPLACEMENT of the previous dose-estimates and even replacement of the ENTIRE STRUCTURE of the A-Bomb Study.

Everyone welcomes possible new insights about dosimetry in the A-Bomb Study, but there are right ways and wrong ways to add new information to an on-going prospective study. It is essential to show the scientific community that introduction of new information is not creating opportunities for intentional or unintentional bias to enter a revised study, for such opportunities by themselves are sufficient basis for the scientific community to reject a study as unreliable.

Introduction of the new DS86 dosimetry has placed the A-Bomb Study at a crossroad. In Chapter 5, we have shown -- using the very principles of epidemiological science -- that the A-Bomb Study's foundation as a legitimate prospective study will sink into quicksand, unless a way for handling the new dosimetry is developed which restores the study's continuity and maintains the continuity during the study's remaining decades of follow-up.

The farthest thing from the truth would be for anyone to say that we are objecting to possible new insights about dosimetry in the A-Bomb Study. (Indeed, the new DS86 dosimetry confirms the correctness of our own handling, almost ten years ago, of the mistaken neutron dose-estimates.) Far from objecting, we are just determined that improvements in dosimetry be handled in a way which will not ever impair the credibility of this never-to-be-repeated study.

● -- Part 1, Our Finding :

====================================

This book not only proposes, but also demonstrates, a practical "constant-cohort, dual-dosimetry" method for having the benefit of possible new insights about dosimetry, while maintaining the continuity and identity of the A-Bomb Study as a first-class prospective study with a permanent structure.

Our method (described in Chapter 6) keeps the cohorts of survivors together, exactly as they were before the new DS86 dosimetry. For each cohort, we just calculate a DS86 dose-estimate which is additional to the cohort's previous T65DR dose-estimate, and then we analyse cancer-hazard in BOTH the old and new dosimetries for the SAME sets of people.

In this way, scientists can have the potential benefits of the new DS86 dosimetry, but DS86 never REPLACES the previous dose-estimates and never disturbs the study's permanent prospective structure. The unaltered database would remain, forever, the stable and objective foundation ensuring the scientific credibility of the whole study. With our method, there would be no retroactive changes of input at all -- only some SUPPLEMENTAL information about doses. Therefore, the "constant-cohort, dual-dosimetry" approach protects the A-Bomb Study from rejection based on concern that the current version of the new dosimetry and its FUTURE revisions might be opportunities for bias to enter.

A Warning from "Lizzie Borden" :

A major purpose of this book is to help redirect the handling of the A-Bomb Study along sound epidemiological lines. We wish to emphasize the importance of this issue for science in general.

Poor choices regarding a world-famous database would not only set back THIS field for decades, but would influence work in other fields, too. If it were ever to become universal practice to alter a prospective study's original input after any of the outcome is known, never to reveal what the study would have shown with its unaltered input, and to commit mayhem on the study's original architecture and cohorts, then epidemiology as a credible science would be finished. Some worst-case scenarios were described in our Chapter 5, Part 2. Surely we are not alone in wanting to avert "Lizzie Borden Methods" of database management:

> "Lizzie Borden took an axe
> And gave her mother forty whacks.
> When she saw what she had done,
> She gave her father forty-one."   (Anonymous.)

Leading figures in the radiation community acknowledge that the retroactive alterations of the A-Bomb Study, now underway, are massive. We would

have thought that this obvious challenge to the most basic rules of prospective research would merit thoughtful discussion and remedial proposals by the radiation committees. Nothing of the sort has occurred.

● -- Part 1, Radiation Committees :
===

UNSCEAR 1988 :

There is no discussion of this issue, nothing to quote, except phrases which imply full approval of what is going on:

For instance, the DS86 dosimetry is described in the executive summary as "a revised dosimetric system for the survivors of Hiroshima and Nagasaki that allows a better analysis of this important epidemiological series" (Un88, p.32, Para.192).

Later, the word "replace" appears: "It is particularly propitious that risk assessments be made now, in light of the revised dosimetric evaluations of the Japanese survivors of the atomic bombings, the most important study population. This re-evaluation, completed in 1986 and known as the dosimetry system 1986 (DS86), replaces the previous estimates of 1965 (T65)" (Un88, p.407, Para.3).

BEIR-5 Committee :

Like the UNSCEAR Committee, the BEIR-5 Committee appears ready to REPLACE the T65DR dosimetry by the new DS86 dosimetry, and the report does not show results for the T65DR cohorts or dosimetry.

"The analyses of radiation effects among the Japanese A-bomb survivors in this report make use of new dose estimates developed in a five-year study by Japanese and American scientists. This binational study resulted in a new dosimetry system, designated DS86, which is documented in two recent Radiation Effects Research Foundation (RERF) reports ..." (Beir90, p.190).

"As the aim of this report is to provide risk estimates based on the best available data, the committee confined itself to analyses using just the DS86 data" (Beir90, p.198).

● -- Part 1, Discussion :
===

We note that both UNSCEAR-88 and BEIR-5 may leave the impression on their readers that retroactive

==

alterations are limited to new dose-estimates. Even if that were the situation, it would not justify sending the T65DR dose-estimates to oblivion. A "dual-dosimetry" analysis would be required in order to maintain the study's legitimate prospective status, with the new dose-estimates handled as a supplement -- not a REPLACEMENT.

And, unfortunately, the retroactive alterations now underway are certainly NOT limited to new dose-estimates. We have shown in detail (Chapter 5, and Tables 10-A,B, and Tables 26-N,O) that all the former cohorts are destroyed, and participants are shuffled into new groupings with new distribution of the previous cancer-deaths and new mean ages at the time of bombing and new male-female ratios. Without a "constant-cohort" approach, continuity is gone.

In effect, the prospective study was terminated with the 1982 follow-up, its database was marked for oblivion, and with 37 years of results in hand, a new database was created.

It is hard to imagine a MORE "questionable practice" in epidemiological research than this. Thus I find it amazing, particularly in a report which carries the imprint of the National Academy of Sciences, National Research Council, that this treatment of a database merits no discussion at all.

By contrast, we say that such handling will unnecessarily send the A-Bomb Study's scientific BELIEVABILITY into oblivion -- and we say "unnecessarily" because Chapters 10 through 17 of this book demonstrate a "constant-cohort, dual-dosimetry" approach to the current and future follow-ups which can easily maintain the study's status as an objective, first-rate prospective inquiry.

The "constant-cohort, dual-dosimetry" approach offers everything to gain and nothing to lose.

In Part 3 of this chapter, readers will see for themselves the urgency of a "constant-cohort, dual dosimetry" analysis. Without it, there is trouble even sooner than we expected.

2. Cancer-Risk at Moderate and High Dose-Levels, Acute Delivery Only

Since this is a book about radiation-induced cancer from LOW-dose exposure, only one of our tables includes any estimate of Lifetime Fatal Cancer-Yield from moderate or high dose-levels. But for the purpose

of comparing our work with the new estimates from the radiation committees, we will make the necessary estimates right here.

Readers will see for themselves that there is substantial agreement between the analysis in this book and the 1988 UNSCEAR and 1990 BEIR-5 Reports with respect to cancer-risk per rad from moderate and high doses acutely delivered -- now that those committees have greatly increased their past estimates. On the other hand, we can only compare apples with oranges, as readers will see below.

Preparation of Estimates :

First we can look at Table 13-A, where Row 10 shows that the average internal organ-dose for ALL the exposed A-bomb survivors combined (Reference Group excluded, of course) was 41.7 cSv in the T65DR dosimetry, and 47.4 cSv in the DS86 dosimetry.

Then we can look at Table 13-B, which includes Lifetime Fatal Cancer-Yields based on all the exposed Dose-Groups (3,4,5,6,7,8) combined. For the T65DR dosimetry, Column D shows the Cancer-Yield to be 7.37 radiation-induced cancers per 10,000 persons, per cSv (or, 7.37 cancers x 10^{-4} person^{-1} x rem^{-1}). For the DS86 dosimetry, Column J shows 6.50 as the Cancer-Yield.

We must make two adjustments, in order to make these values properly comparable with the UNSCEAR-88 and the BEIR-5 values.

First Adjustment :

The values in Table 13-B do not take account of the fact that cancers in future follow-ups will be arising in the A-Bomb Study from the most radio-sensitive age-groups. The values in Table 16-B do take this important fact into account. The impact can be measured by the ratio of LOW-dose Cancer-Yields from Table 16-B over the LOW-dose Cancer-Yields from Table 14-C.

```
Table 16-B, T65DR:          Yield = 31.65
Table 14-C, Col.C, Row 2:   Yield = 12.90
Ratio = 2.45


Table 16-B, DS86:           Yield = 30.43
Table 14-C, Col.E, Row 2:   Yield = 12.03
Ratio = 2.53
```

Therefore, to take account of the radio-sensitivity, we should raise the Cancer-Yields for the combined Dose-Groups by these ratios.

```
JAPANESE SURVIVORS,
acute gamma-ray doses of moderate level,
LIFETIME FATAL CANCER-YIELD (excl. leuk.) :


T65DR:  7.37 x 2.45 = 18.06
DS86:   6.50 x 2.53 = 16.44
```

This is all we need to make the comparison with the Cancer-Yield in UNSCEAR-88. For the comparison with BEIR-5, we need to adjust our Japanese value to a United States value.

Second Adjustment :

To adjust the two values above for a United States' population, we shall use the ratio of our Lifetime Fatal Cancer-Yields for a U.S. population in Table 16-C, over the Cancer-Yields for the A-Bomb Survivors in Table 16-B:

```
UNITED STATES POPULATION,
acute gamma-ray doses of moderate level,
LIFETIME FATAL CANCER-YIELD (excl. leuk.) :

T65DR:  (26.64 / 31.65) x (18.06) = 15.20
DS86:   (25.56 / 30.43) x (16.44) = 13.80
```

● -- Part 2, Our Finding :
===================================

We will assemble our findings from above.

```
LIFETIME FATAL CANCER-YIELD excluding leukemia.
Radiation-induced fatal cancers per 10,000 persons,
per rad, from a single, acute gamma-ray dose of
moderate level :

Japanese              United States

T65DR = 18.06         T65DR = 15.20
DS86 = 16.44          DS86 = 13.80
```

These Cancer-Yields should be doubled if exposure is from diagnostic X-rays.

● -- Part 2, Radiation Committees :
===================================

At the end of this section, we will assemble all the values for comparison.

UNSCEAR 1988 :

UNSCEAR-88 says: "The atomic bomb survivors have been used in this report as the main source of risk estimates, while the Committee notes that other sources of data such as the ankylosing spondylitis patients are in general terms consistent with these estimates, especially when the mode of delivery of the exposure is taken into account. The Committee has not itself made primary estimates of risk in the Japanese atomic bomb survivors, but has relied on risk estimates developed in recent publications ..." (Un88, p.490, para.594). Elsewhere, Un88 acknowledges Shi87 and Shi88 (TR-12-87 and TR-5-88) as the source of its risk-coefficients. Only the DS86 dosimetry, and only the abridged cohort of 75,991 survivors, were used.

Values in the UNSCEAR-88 tables do not include the correction-factor of 1.23 for underascertainment of cancer in the A-Bomb Study (see our Chapter 11). UNSCEAR warns its readers (Un88, p.485, para.557): "... the risk coefficients that are used have been obtained from published reports and do not take into account the underreporting of cancer deaths on death certificates. BEIR III, in its projections, increased these coefficients by 23 % to take account of underreporting. A comparable action here would increase the Committee's projections of excess lifetime mortality by 20-25 %."

In its Table 62 (at page 527), UNSCEAR-88 provides its estimate of Lifetime Fatal Cancer-Yield for a Japanese population of both sexes (50 % male, 50 % female) and all ages, exposed to 100 rads "of organ absorbed dose of low-LET radiation at high dose rate, using age-specific risk coefficients" (from the Japanese A-bomb survivors). Since UNSCEAR-88 states (p.479, para.510) that "linear risk estimates are a reasonable summary of the dose-response," the per-rad value from 100 rads in its Table 62 will be the same at a total acute dose of 42-47 rads -- the dose used in our own estimate above.

In Table 62's multiplicative model, the per-rad value for all malignancies (excluding leukemia) is 9.7 fatal cancers per 10,000 persons per rad. (The value for leukemia alone is 1.) The value of 9.7 needs multiplying by 1.23 for underascertainment.

Thus the UNSCEAR-88 value which compares with our "Japanese" value above is 11.93.

It should be noted that UNSCEAR's previous value -- which even INCLUDED leukemia -- was 1.0. The new estimate in UNSCEAR-88's Table 62 is more than 12-fold higher than its previous one.

BEIR-5 Committee :

Like UNSCEAR-88, the BEIR-5 Report relies heavily on the A-bomb survivors (abridged DS86 cohort) for arriving at its Cancer-Yields: "... the risk estimates that

===

are presented in this report are derived chiefly (or exclusively) from the Japanese experience" (Beir90, p.218). Indeed, the report acknowledges Dale Preston as its scientific advisor. And practices by RERF analysts which we criticized earlier in this book are carried on in the BEIR-5 Report too.

For instance, in addition to excessive subdivision of data, and replacement of the entire T65DR database, and exclusion of 15,000 of the study's 91,231 survivors, there are even exclusions of data from the abridged DS86 database and there are pre-judgments. A few illustrations are in order here.

Five Years of Follow-Up Discarded :

In BEIR-5, there is pre-judgment of a 10-year minimal latency period with the exception of leukemia and breast-cancer. Cancers occurring before 1956 are just not counted in BEIR-5's "preferred risk models" (page 168). The 1950-1955 follow-up has been discarded. This is an extremely questionable practice, as we noted earlier in the book. UNSCEAR-88 (p.524) also assumes a 10-year "minimum latency," for all malignancies except leukemia.

Discarding the 1950-1955 evidence becomes an even more questionable practice when BEIR-5 (p.274, Fig. 5-13) seems to be claiming a time-dependence for lung-cancer which would imply that the ten-year exclusion may result in MISSING much of the radiation-induced excess with respect to lung-cancer -- one of the most common of all cancers.

Two Dose-Groups Discarded :

In BEIR-5, there is also pre-judgment that dose-response cannot be supra-linear except at very high doses, where cell-KILLING is regarded by BEIR-5 as an acceptable explanation. This pre-judgment leads to additional throwing out of evidence : "The RERF data show a tendency toward decreased risk per Gy in the highest dose groups, which may reflect either cell-killing or overestimation of the doses in this group. The committee considered various ways of dealing with this problem, including adding terms to the dose-response part of the model and adjusting the highest doses downward. In the end, it was decided simply to exclude the two highest dose groups" (Beir90, p.199).

We note the subjective view of a supra-linear dose-response: It is called a "problem" to find that risk per rad INCREASES progressively as dose decreases toward lower levels. Supra-linearity was viewed as such a BAD problem by BEIR-5 that desperation measures were considered (described in BEIR's statement above) -- including even CHANGING the DS86 doses which had just been newly estimated by a group of presumably objective physicists after almost ten years of study (our Chapter 5). The attitude toward the findings, as they fall out of the data, was such that the only solution for BEIR-5, "in the end," was to get RID of part of the data.

One may ask what the BEIR-5 Committee would have done if these two Dose-Groups had contributed to a concave-UPWARD dose-response. Would the Committee have thrown them out?

We regard the exclusion of two Dose-Groups on the basis cited by BEIR-5 as scientifically unacceptable. If there were a solid basis for regarding the finding of supra-linearity as spurious, it would be scientifically objective to call it a problem. But there is no such basis. On the contrary. The finding has been turning up for a decade (our Chapter 22), and now is turning up in both the T65DR and DS86 dosimetries. BEIR-5's own Table 4D-2 (p.200) again confirms that dose-response is supra-linear for all non-leukemic cancers combined, throughout the dose-range shown there. We shall return to the shape of dose-response in Part 3.

Cancer-Deaths beyond Age 75 Discarded :

We will mention one MORE example of throwing out data. All cancers occurring after age 75 have been excluded from the BEIR-5 risk analysis. "Records of cancer mortality at attained ages greater than 75 years were omitted because of the lesser reliability of death certificate information in such cases, as outlined in Annex 4D" (Beir90, p.165). In Annex 4F (p.218), a statement suggests that the severity of this problem may be magnified by BEIR's own choice to do site-specific analysis. We cannot be sure: "... in that body of data [from RERF], the accuracy of diagnosis from death certificates declines rather sharply beyond age 75, to the point that little reliance can be placed on the data for specific sites. The Committee has refrained from basing analyses on data that it considers unreliable."

BEIR's exclusion of cancer-deaths after age 75 must already affect two of the five age-bands (see our Table 4-B): The age-band 35-49 years old at the time of the bombings, and the age-band 50-years and older (average = 58.5 years) ATB.

An Urgently Needed Remedy :

These three exclusions (follow-up years, Dose-Groups, cancers occurring beyond an attained age of 75) amount to major retroactive revisions in the study's database, all made with 35 years of follow-up results at hand. Each of the three exclusions has its own impact on risk-estimates and on the curvature of dose-response, but presently, only RERF and the radiation committees know what those impacts are.

The three changes are ADDITIONAL to the replacement of the T65DR database and cohorts by the DS86 database and cohorts, and these additional changes presently represent ANOTHER assault against the continuity of the A-bomb Study and its credibility as a legitimate prospective inquiry with a permanent structure.

The urgently needed remedy would be similar to the "constant-cohort, dual-dosimetry" approach. If ALL the data are made available by RERF, in a form which maintains analytical continuity with the 1950-1982 follow-up, then no one should object to SUPPLEMENTAL analytical work carefully showing the separate impact of each retroactive exclusion upon risk-estimates and upon curvature of the dose-response. Every type of analysis should be welcome PROVIDING nothing interferes with the continuity of the on-going study in its unaltered form.

Cancer-Yield -- BEIR-5 vs. BEIR-3 :

After making its chosen exclusions, BEIR-5 does provide Lifetime Fatal Cancer-Yields based on the abridged DS86 subcohort.

BEIR-5's "preferred model" for estimating Lifetime Fatal Cancer-Yield is based on subdivision of the solid cancers into four classes, with separate equations for each class (pp.168-170). For two of the four classes, namely respiratory and breast cancers, BEIR's equations forecast that the radiation effect will fall with various times after exposure. Of course, different equations are used for different ages at exposure. The BEIR-5 Committee acknowledges that its choices were influenced by its idea of how much the risk should vary between those young at exposure and old at exposure (Beir90, p.203):

"The committee considered a variety of models before selecting the preferred models described in Chapter 4 ... In general, the preferred models fit the data as well as the alternatives and have fewer terms. This was not the sole criterion for model selection. The committee paid particular attention to how risks were proportioned between various age groups."

BEIR-5 does not provide Lifetime Fatal Cancer-Yields explicitly for moderate or high doses. In its Table 4-2 (at page 172), BEIR-5 provides a value for a single, acute whole-body exposure of a mixed-age United States population to 10 rems. However, since BEIR-5 states emphatically that it finds the dose-response to be linear (for instance, p.5, p.200), the per-rem or per-rad value from 10 rems in its Table 4-2 is necessarily its per-rem value for moderate and high acute doses too.

In Table 4-2, the per-rem value, for a population of 50 % males and 50 % females, is 6.95 radiation-induced cancer-deaths (leukemia excluded) per 10,000 persons, per rad. (The value for leukemia alone is 0.95.) The value of 6.95 needs multiplying by 1.23 for underascertainment.

Thus the BEIR-5 value which compares with our "USA" value above is 8.55.

It should be noted that BEIR's previous value -- which excluded leukemia and bone cancer -- was 2.0 (Beir80, page 206, Table V-19). BEIR's new estimate is about 4-fold higher than its previous estimate.

● -- Part 2, Discussion :
=====================================

Now we will assemble all the values from above.

LIFETIME FATAL CANCER-YIELD excluding leukemia. Radiation-induced fatal cancers per 10,000 persons, per rad, from a single, acute gamma-ray dose of moderate level :

Japanese Pop'n	United States Pop'n
Gofman est.	Gofman est.
T65DR = 18.06	T65DR = 15.20
DS86 = 16.44	DS86 = 13.80
UNSCEAR-88 est.	BEIR-5 est.
DS86 = 11.93	DS86 = 8.55

All the Cancer-Yields above should be doubled if exposure is from diagnostic X-rays (see our Chapter 13, Part 4; also Beir90, p.218).

Readers can see for themselves that there is less than a factor of two separating our estimates and those of the radiation committees.

On the other hand, assessment of the agreement must remain approximate, due to the fact that we have necessarily compared apples with oranges. The radiation committees and we are no longer working with the same A-bomb database. We alone are providing estimates which use the unabridged, legitimate prospective database, with its constant cohorts and its objectivity ensured by continuity.

==

We are eager to acquire the necessary data -- with none pre-discarded -- to extend our "constant-cohort, dual-dosimetry" analysis (which presently covers 1950-1982) to include 1950-1985 and beyond.

3. Cancer-Risk at Low Doses, Acutely and Slowly Delivered

Where risk-estimates really matter -- for acute-LOW and for slow-LOW exposures, our independent analysis indicates that the radiation committees are underestimating cancer-risk by up to 30-fold.

In other words, although the radiation committees have made progress toward realism by greatly increasing their previous risk-estimates for acute moderate-to-high exposures, we think they still lack realism with respect to acute-low and slow-low exposures. These committees are continuing the practice, documented by our Chapter 22, of rejecting good human evidence pertaining to such estimates, and substituting a preferred hypothesis based on non-human evidence.

The preferred hypothesis is that human dose-response is concave-upward. However, our Figure 14-C clearly shows that upward curvature does NOT describe the human evidence.

If dose-response really were concave-upward, the cancer-risk PER RAD would progressively diminish as either dose or dose-rate decreased, due to the diminishing opportunity for inter-track carcinogenesis (Chapter 23).

However, the direct human evidence shows a dose-response relationship which is supra-linear (like Figure 14-A) and supports no expectation of reduced risk per rad from acute-low or slow-low exposures compared with acute-high. UNSCEAR-88 makes a claim that some human evidence supports a dose-rate effect, but we have shown the fallacy of the claim in Chapter 22, Parts 4 and 5.

It should be emphasized, also, that even if human dose-response were linear (Figure 14-B) instead of supra-linear, linearity would NOT support any expectation of reduced risk per rad from acute-low or slow-low exposures compared with acute-high.

"Q.E.D." Summary :

As we illustrated in Chapter 23, Parts 5 and 7, the following relationships occur between risk and dose.

In the absence of a concave-upward dose-response relationship, there is no REDUCTION in per-rad risk between an acute dose of 160 rads and an acute dose of one rad. Indeed, when dose-response is SUPRA-linear, we illustrated how the per-rad risk INCREASES at acute-low doses compared with 160 rads. Thus, one writes:

● -- EQUATION (1) for supra-linear & linear:

    Per-rad risk at acute-low => per-rad risk at
    acute-high.

Virtually no one denies that the contribution to cancer-risk from inter-track carcinogenesis (the quadratic term in a linear-quadratic dose-response equation) is extremely small at acute-low doses. Therefore, removal of opportunities for inter-track carcinogenesis by SLOW delivery of a low total dose has a negligible effect on per-rad risk. Thus one writes:

● -- EQUATION (2) for supra-linear & linear :

    Per-rad risk at slow-low = per-rad risk at
    acute-low.

    Then by substitution or direct logic, one writes:

● -- EQUATION (3) for supra-linear & linear :

    Per-rad risk at slow-low => per-rad risk at
    acute-high.

In short, in the absence of the concave-upward dose-response relationship, there is no basis whatsoever for expecting per-rad risk of radiation-induced cancer to be LOWER from acute-low or slow-low exposures than from acute-high.

However, we do not rule out the possibility (as indicated in Chapter 23, Part 6) that per-rad risk may be lower for slow-HIGH than for acute-HIGH. On the other hand, in Chapter 23 we showed that slow delivery of a high total dose may NOT reduce the per-rad risk at all. It may turn out in the human that inter-track carcinogenesis accounts for only a minor part of the radiation-risk, even at moderate to high acute doses. Pending more evidence on the issue, we regard it as premature for anyone to count on any reduction of risk if a moderate or high total dose is delivered slowly.

==

Conflict over the Shape :
=================================

As shown in Chapters 13 and 27, radiation-induced cancer is now provable in the A-bomb survivors from an internal organ-dose as low as 11 rems (15 rems in DS86). Radiation-induced cancer-risk between 11 rems and zero dose (or 15 rems and zero) is necessarily estimated by interpolation. Thus such estimates depend on the SHAPE of the dose-response curve along which analysts make their interpolation.

We will compare our finding about shape with the reports from the radiation committees.

Our Own Finding of Supra-Linearity :

In Chapters 14, 29, and 30, we showed that that dose-response is supra-linear, with the highest cancer-risk per rad in the lowest dose-range. And this finding is shown to be significant. The 1950-1982 evidence fits a supra-linear relationship significantly BETTER than it fits a linear relationship.

We ask no one to accept, on faith alone, our assertion that this is so. Our finding of supra-linearity has been reached openly, step-by-step, from the unabridged evidence. All the work is checkable and verifiable.

We have stated clearly, in Chapter 14, Part 4, that credible evidence might develop in the future to alter the current finding of supra-linearity. Only time, and objectively conducted studies, will tell. Meanwhile, we note that supra-linearity is the shape which has been showing up for three consecutive follow-ups of the A-bomb survivors (1950-1974, 1950-1978, 1950-1982).

Within the 1950-1982 evidence, the dose-response relationship turns out supra-linear no matter how we approach the data. It turns out supra-linear with the T65DR dose-estimates, and with the DS86 dose-estimates. It turns out supra-linear when we test cancer-deaths per 10,000 initial persons versus dose, and when we test cancer-deaths per 10,000 person-years versus dose. And it turns out supra-linear whether we combine males and females, or test them separately.

Very important is the finding that supra-linearity is the dose-response relationship THROUGHOUT the dose-range, not just at high doses (see Table 13-B).

A great deal has been written about the alleged necessity of basing low-dose risk-estimates on dose-response curves limited to high-dose observations. Now that radiation-induced cancer is provable in the A-bomb survivors at an internal organ-dose of only 11 rems (or 15 rems in DS86), interpolation of radiation-risk is required only in the short segment of the dose-range between zero rems and 11 (or 15) rems. Any suggestion that low-dose Cancer-Yields must be based on high-dose observations would be plainly inappropriate.

UNSCEAR 1988 on Shape :

UNSCEAR-88, introducing its section on radiation carcinogenesis, states (p.407, para.5): "A main concern that cannot be adequatetly resolved is how to relate the results obtained at high doses and dose rates to the low levels of exposure that may be expected in environmental and routine occupational settings."

The suggestion that estimates still depend on high-dose observations is made again soon thereafter: (Un88, p.416, para.68): "Estimates of low-dose risks based largely on high-dose data must depend heavily on the assumptions about the shape of the dose-response curve and are, of necessity, no better than the model is applicable. Current data suggest that resolution of these difficulties will not be easy, and it seems likely that there will be many site-specific differences."

Earlier in this book, we have criticized the practice of subdividing databases by specific organs, creating horrific small-numbers problems, and then taking the results seriously. It is in the nature of numbers that there will never be a database so large that it cannot be rendered inconclusive and unreliable by excessive subdivision. It should be evident that one can lose the prospect of ever obtaining answers to certain questions simply by excessive subdivision of the data.

What does UNSCEAR-88 say about the shape of dose-response in the A-Bomb Study? The report acknowledges that linearity provides a good fit, and not only for all cancers combined, but even for subdivisions -- which would seem to undermine the suggestion about "many site-specific differences" above. We quote (Un88, p.479, para.510):

"Over the range of doses from 0 to 6 Gy, there is no clearly significant evidence of non-linearity (although other forms of response fit the data), so from a purely statistical point of view linear risk estimates are a reasonable summary of the dose-response. Moreover, when linear, quadratic, and linear-quadratic models (with or without provision for cell-killing) are fitted to the data on all cancers except leukaemia and on those five sites where a clear dose-response curve had previously been obtained (i.e., leukaemia, and cancers of the stomach, colon, lung, and female breast), a simple linear model fits the data on leukaemia, cancers of the stomach, lung and female breast, and all cancers except leukaemia better than the quadratic model and as well as the linear-quadratic model, as judged by the deviance ... Inclusion of cell-killing does not significantly improve the fit, except in one instance where leukaemia mortality under either the linear or linear-quadratic model fits somewhat better with a cell-killing term. These findings hold true both for organ absorbed doses and shielded kerma."

Nonetheless, on the very next page, UNSCEAR-88 appears to retreat from the linear model and to endorse use of the model which yields lower risk-estimates (Un88, p.480, Para.519): "Most current studies use a linear model for breast and thyroid cancer and a linear-quadratic model for other sites; these are the best-available models only, for the data do not really permit the validation of a specific model with confidence."

We note a real conflict between the UNSCEAR assertion and our own findings. We find that the data permit us to rule OUT the concave-upward dose-response with a great deal of confidence, and even to establish that the linear response is significantly inferior to the supra-linear dose-response.

Can it be that failure of UNSCEAR and its sources to use a "constant-cohort, dual-dosimetry" approach causes them to miss the supra-linearity? And what is the effect of their throwing out the 1950-1955 evidence? We will return to this after reviewing what BEIR-5 says about shape.

BEIR-5 on Shape :

Referring to the A-Bomb Study, BEIR-5 says in its Executive Summary (p.5): "The dose-dependent excess of mortality from all cancer other than leukemia, shows no departure from linearity in the range below 4 sievert (Sv), whereas the mortality data for leukemia are compatible with a linear-quadratic dose response relationship."

BEIR-5 restates this finding several times within the report, and shows no quadratic term in its best-fit equations for its several subdivisions of solid cancers (pp.168-170). Except for leukemia, all the BEIR-5 Cancer-Yields are based on the linear dose-response (Beir90, p.6).

Above, in our Part 2, we already discussed how

BEIR-5 responded to its finding of supra-linearity: It threw out the high-dose groups. Our finding, however, is that supra-linearity is not limited to the high-dose groups. So we differ on shape with the BEIR Committee, too.

Can it be that failure of BEIR-5 to use a "constant-cohort, dual-dosimetry" approach causes it to miss the supra-linearity throughout the dose-range? And what is the effect upon shape of their throwing out the 1950-1955 evidence? And the effect upon shape of their throwing out cancers occurring after age 75?

First Crisis for the A-Bomb Study :

In first proposing that RERF support a "constant-cohort, dual-dosimetry" approach to the A-bomb database (Chapter 6), we predicted that problems of believability for new findings were certain to arise in the absence of such an approach.

We have shown above that the first crisis has arisen even earlier than we expected. A difference, or a change, in the shape of dose-response is a matter of the greatest seriousness. The entire A-Bomb Study's credibility can appropriately be called into question unless the reason for this difference can be fully traced and explained. And a comparison of apples with oranges permits no such explanation.

The simplistic suggestion can be made that all of the difference arises because three more years of follow-up (1983, 1984, 1985) have been provided for the abridged DS86 database used by the radiation committees (and by Muirhead; see Chapter 30) than for our "constant-cohort, dual-dosimetry" analysis for 1950-1982. It is possible that this is the explanation, and we wish to find out.

On matters of such importance, no one should have to speculate concerning what the truth is. If RERF provides the additional cancer-death data through 1985 for the T65DR cohorts used in this book, and reported on in RERF's TR-1-86 (91,231 persons), then we can calculate the up-dated dose-response for 1950-1985 in the T65DR and DS86 dosimetries, by our method of "constant-cohorts." If the results show that the last three years of follow-up have altered the shape of dose-response (after 12-years of a supra-linear shape), such a finding will be of profound importance.

But if the results show that dose-response remains supra-linear in both dosimetries with the "constant-cohort" method, despite the additional three years of follow-up, then a very serious problem exists. It would mean that the radiation committees' failure to find supra-linearity is caused by all the retroactive alterations, including deletion of 15,000 persons and shuffling of the remaining 75,000 into new cohorts.

A full explanation would be required of just how it could happen that a DS86 analysis by the "constant-cohort" method could possibly give a different answer from a DS86 analysis with the cohort-shuffling method currently in practice at RERF.

The credibility of the A-Bomb Study is going to hang in the balance until such questions are resolved. These questions and others which may arise in the future could all be resolved on a permanent basis if RERF itself would adopt a "constant-cohort, dual-dosimetry" approach along the lines we have proposed in Chapter 6.

● -- Part 3, Our Finding :
=================================

Next, we are going to compare our own risk-estimates for acute-low and slow-low exposures with those of UNSCEAR-88 and BEIR-5. As usual, we will assemble the final values from the three sources afterwards.

Our own low-dose Lifetime Fatal Cancer-Yields come from Table 16-B for the A-Bomb Survivors and from Table 16-C for the United States population. These tables, unlike the tables in Chapters 13 and 14, are based on age-specific risk-coefficients -- as are the UNSCEAR-88 and BEIR-5 Cancer-Yields.

Our age-specific risk-coefficients or K-values for low-dose exposure incorporate (A) our finding from Chapter 14 that dose-response is supra-linear, with the highest cancer-risk per rad in the lowest dose-range, and (B) an interpolation within the short segment of the dose-range lying between 15 rads and zero rads.

Thus Equation (2) from our "Q.E.D." section applies, and there is no reason whatsoever to reduce our low-dose Cancer-Yields for slow delivery. They are proper risk-estimates for both acute-low and slow-low exposures.

LIFETIME FATAL CANCER-YIELD (excl. leuk.) for the dose-range 0-5 rads, any dose-rate. Number of fatal radiation-induced cancers per 10,000 persons, per rad.

Data are in next column.

---------------   ------------------
Table 16-B,   Table 16-C,
A-bomb   United States'
survivors :   population :

T65DR = 31.65   T65DR = 26.64
DS86 = 30.43   DS86 = 25.56

Values need doubling for exposure by X-rays.

● -- Part 3, Radiation Committees :
=====================================

Both UNSCEAR-88 and BEIR-5, having conceded that the best available human evidence shows a LINEAR dose-response, nonetheless refuse to USE the information. If they were to use it, their risk-estimates for acute-low and slow-low exposures would be exactly the same per rad as their moderate-to-high acute risk-estimates per rad.

Instead, both committees recommend dividing their risk-estimates by numbers like 2 up to 10 -- which is equivalent to reducing them by factors of 0.5 to 0.1. UNSCEAR-88 makes this recommendation for both acute-low and slow-low estimates, whereas BEIR-5 recommends the reduction only for slow-low exposures.

UNSCEAR 1988, Low-Dose Cancer-Yield :

UNSCEAR-88, in its executive summary, states (Un88, p.39, para.249): "In this Report, the problems in deriving risk coefficients at low doses and for low dose rates remain. The Committee agreed that there was a need for a reduction factor to modify the risks shown in Table 9 and Table 10 for low doses and low dose rates. [UNSCEAR's Tables 9 and 10 apply to 100 rads of organ absorbed dose delivered at high dose rate.] The Committee considered that such a factor certainly varies very widely with individual tumour type and with dose rate range. However, an appropriate range to be applied to total risk for low dose and low dose rate should lie between 2 and 10. The Committee intends to study this matter in detail in the near future." This same statement is repeated, almost verbatim, at page 494, para.623. In "typical situations," the number which UNSCEAR-88 recommends is five (Un88, p.491,para.602).

We cannot find any effort by UNSCEAR-88 to reconcile its endorsement of either "five" or "two to ten" with its statement, cited above, that "there is no clearly significant evidence of non-linearity" in the A-Bomb Study, so that "linear risk estimates are a reasonable summary of the dose-response."

Readers of our Chapter 22 will recognize the familiar "two to ten" range, suggested in 1980 by NCRP and based not on the human evidence already available then, but rather on other animals. UNSCEAR-88 (p.491, para.602) explicitly cites Ncrp80.

    The UNSCEAR-88 multiplicative-model
Cancer-Yield for acute exposure to 100 rads is
11.93 (see Part 2 of this chapter), excluding
leukemia and based on a Japanese population. Thus,
for acute-low and slow-low exposure, UNSCEAR's
Cancer-Yields have the following range:

        (11.93) / (2) = 5.96
        (11.93) / (5) = 2.39
        (11.93) / (10) = 1.19

Values need doubling for exposure by X-rays.

BEIR-5, Low-Dose Cancer-Yield :

BEIR-5, referring to its Cancer-Yield for a single exposure to 10 rems, says in its Executive Summary (p.6): "For low LET radiation, accumulation of the same dose over weeks or months, however, is expected to reduce the lifetime risk appreciably, possibly by a factor of 2 or more."

In BEIR-5's Chapter 1 (p.22), the report acknowledges: "There are scant human data that allow an estimate of the dose-rate effectiveness factor (DREF)." The discussion procedes to confirm what we have explained in Chapters 22, 23, and earlier in this chapter -- that DREFS depend on dose-response having an upward-concave curvature. Then BEIR-5 mentions leukemia, the only malignancy where it is claiming a concave-upward dose-response. No comment is made that this one site-specific finding may be spurious, in view of BEIR's failure to find such curvature for any other subset of cancer with the same type of analysis. Instead, BEIR-5 reports (p.23) that the leukemia curvature indicates a DREF of 2.1.

After singling out leukemia from the human data, BEIR-5 completely retreats from human evidence -- evidence which shows that no reduction for slow dose-rate is appropriate. Instead, BEIR-5 focuses on laboratory animal studies. So its Table 1-4, "Summary of Dose-Rate Effectiveness Factors for Low-LET Radiation," consists of three types of entries: (1) DREF of 2.1 from human leukemia as analyzed by BEIR-5, (2) DREF of 2.0 to 2.5 from human leukemia as analyzed by BEIR-3 (a very questionable analysis; see our Chapter 22), and (3) the familiar DREF-range of 2-10

from laboratory animals. For the latter range, BEIR-5 lists "4" as the "single best estimate."

This evidence from other species is clearly the only basis for what BEIR-5 refers to as "the consensus" (Beir90, p28): "For low-LET radiations, the consensus is that decreasing the dose rate or dividing a given dose into a number of fractions spread over a period of time reduces the biological effectiveness." And indeed, as noted in Chapter 23 and above, we do not rule out the possibility that risk is reduced if a HIGH total dose is delivered slowly. But BEIR-5 is recommending "dreffing" (reducing) the Cancer-Yield which applies to an acute dose of only ten rems, if the ten rems are accumulated slowly. We have shown, and BEIR-5 will admit at a later page, that there is no basis in either the human evidence or in logic for any such reduction.

Substitution of Non-Human for Human Data :

BEIR-5 addresses its retreat to the animal evidence in the most superficial way, in our opinion: "The committee felt strongly that its risk assessments should be based on human data to the extent that they were available and that animal data should be used only to address questions for which human data were unavailable or inadequate. Questions in the latter category included the RBE of neutrons and gamma rays and the effect of dose rate" (Beir90, p.55).

We call this explanation "superficial" because it offers no reason for regarding the A-Bomb Study as "inadequate" -- the very same study on which BEIR-5 relies for its leukemia DREF and most everything else in its risk-analysis (see Part 1 of this chapter, above).

And the statement by BEIR-5 certainly does not explain how one could possibly trust other species MORE than the human species, for evaluating the human dose-response. Everyone recognizes that "... the transfer of inferences from animal studies to humans is perilous" (Ncrp85, p.1), and that "Extrapolation from animal data to humans remains a difficult process of uncertain validity" (Ncrp85, p.36).

One cannot justify the substitution of non-human data for human data just because we have MORE of the non-human data. A mountain of stable and elegant animal data is worse than none at all, if it is mistakenly assumed to be relevant where it is not, and if it is used to REPLACE the direct human evidence whose relevance is self-evident.

BEIR-5 offers no justification. The following quote shows that BEIR-5 makes a key recommendation which is ADMITTED to be in conflict with the human

==

evidence (Beir90, p.171):

"Since the risk models were derived primarily from data on acute exposures ... the application of these models to continuous low dose-rate exposures requires consideration of the dose rate effectiveness factor (DREF), as discussed in Chapter 1 [see quotations above]. For linear-quadratic models, there is an implicit dose-rate effect, since the quadratic contribution vanishes at low doses and, presumably, low dose-rates leaving only the linear term which is generally taken to reflect one-hit kinetics. The magnitude of this reduction is expressed by DREF values. For the leukemia data, a linear extrapolation indicates that the lifetime risks per unit bone marrow dose may be half as large for continuous low dose rate as for instantaneous high dose rate exposures. [We are splitting the BEIR-5 paragraph here.]

"For most other cancers in the LSS [A-Bomb Life Span Study], the quadratic contribution is nearly zero, and the estimated DREFS are near unity. Nevertheless, the committee judged that some account should be taken of dose rate effects and in Chapter 1 suggests a range of dose rate reduction factors that may be applicable."

The range suggested in BEIR's Chapter 1 (Table 1-4) is the familiar 1980 NCRP value of two to ten. At a later page (p.220), BEIR-5 mentions "2," whereas at page 6 it recommends "2 or more," and at page 23, it calls 2 to 4 the best estimates.

In the BEIR-5 statement above (p.171), which maintains the pattern documented in our Chapter 22, "nevertheless" introduces the key action. A scientific basis for this action escapes us.

The BEIR-5 Cancer-Yield for acute exposure to ten rads is 8.55 (see Part 2 of this chapter), excluding leukemia and based on a United States population. Thus, for slow-low exposure, BEIR-5's Cancer-Yields have the following range:

        (8.55) / (2) = 4.28
        (8.55) / (4) = 2.14
        (8.55) / (10) = 0.86

BEIR-5 is explicit in suggesting that all its values may need doubling for X-ray exposure (Beir90, p.26, p.218, p.220).

• -- Part 3, Discussion :

==

Now we will assemble all the values from above.

Gofman Estimate from A-Bomb Study:
LIFETIME FATAL CANCER-YIELD (excl. leuk.)
for the dose-range 0-5 rads, any dose-rate.
Number of fatal radiation-induced cancers
per 10,000 persons, per rad.
---------------   ------------------
Table 16-B,   Table 16-C,
A-bomb   United States'
survivors :   population :

T65DR = 31.65   T65DR = 26.64
DS86 = 30.43   DS86 = 25.56

Values need doubling for exposure by X-rays.

The UNSCEAR-88 multiplicative-model Cancer-Yield for acute exposure to 100 rads is 11.93 (see Part 2 of this chapter), excluding leukemia and based on a Japanese population. Thus, after "dreffing" for acute-low and slow-low exposure, UNSCEAR's Cancer-Yields have the following range:

        (11.93) / (2) = 5.96
        (11.93) / (5) = 2.39
        (11.93) / (10) = 1.19

Values need doubling for exposure by X-rays.

The BEIR-5 Cancer-Yield for acute exposure to 10 rads is 8.55 (see Part 2 of this chapter), excluding leukemia and based on a United States population. Thus, after "dreffing" for slow-low exposure, BEIR-5's Cancer-Yields have the following range:

        (8.55) / (2) = 4.28
        (8.55) / (4) = 2.14
        (8.55) / (10) = 0.86

BEIR-5 is explicit in suggesting that all its value may need doubling for X-ray exposure (Beir90, p.26, p.218, p.220).

Our analysis, above, indicates that the radiation committees are underestimating risk from slow-low exposure by up to 30-fold. It is easy to see how the close agreement in Part 2 converted into a big disparity. We began in Part 2 with a difference of about 1.5-fold. Our own estimate for LOW-dose exposure goes up by about a factor of two from its value at 45 rads, because of supra-linearity. So the disparity widens to 3-fold. And if the radiation committees cut their own estimates to one-tenth, in adjusting them from acute-moderate to slow-low exposure, then the disparity can widen to a factor as big as 30.

We have already discussed what is needed in order to resolve the difference over shape. As for our difference over "dreffing," there is no foreseeable reconciliation if one party is going to REPUDIATE good human evidence and replace it by non-human evidence which gives a reduced risk-estimate.

It seems to me that BEIR-5 is trying to sit on both ends of a teeter-totter at the same time. At the one end, BEIR-5 takes the position that human dose-response is LINEAR in the study on which it relies for most of its report. And at the other end of the see-saw, it repudiates its own statement of linearity by taking a dose rate reduction-factor.

BEIR-5 has produced neither evidence nor logic to support any speculation that the shape of human dose-response may suddenly change below ten rads. And BEIR-5 has correctly noted that if the shape WERE to change below 10 rads for reasons unknown, it could change in either the direction of increased risk or decreased risk per rad (Beir90, p.6, p.181). But the scientifically objective presumption, in the absence of contrary evidence or logic, is that the shape does NOT suddenly turn below 10 rads.

Thus we regard it not only as scientifically reasonable, but virtually obligatory, to USE the reasonable presumption. And as far as we can tell, BEIR-5 is willing to use the linear model to estimate risk at ACUTE doses below 10 rads, for it suggests the use of DREFS only in association with slow-low (not acute-low) exposures.

In the dose-range below ten rads, with respect to speculation about diminished risk if delivery is slow, we recommend close attention to track-analysis -- and particularly to "The Fallacy of Slow Delivery of Very Low Doses" in our Chapter 20.

For instance, our Table 20-M estimates that at a total tissue-dose from X-rays of one rad, cell-nuclei are experiencing only about one primary ionization track, on the average. Since, at the level of cell-nuclei, there is no conceivable dose-rate LOWER than one track at a time, it would approach absurdity to speculate that such a dose may be less hazardous if it is delivered slowly than if it is delivered all at once.

4. Disproof of Any Safe Dose or Dose-Rate

As demonstrated in our Chapters 24 and 34, influential segments of the radiation community have been speculating in favor of a "threshold" -- the notion that low doses and dose-rates may be completely safe ("without effect"). The U.S. Department of Energy calls this the "zero risk" model (Doe87, p.J.8). It received widespread attention when an abbreviated version of Doe87 was published by the journal SCIENCE (Ansp88).

Indeed, opportunities for disseminating such speculations have increased, because slow-low exposure of populations has been much in the news after the Chernobyl accident and after the series of recent revelations about radioactive pollution inside, outside, and beneath many Department of Energy facilities. The estimated cost to clean up DOE's contamination ranges from $63 billion (DOE estimate) to $175 billion (Government Accounting Office estimate), according to the press (Nyt88; Nyt89a).

The BEIR-3 Report of 1980 (see our Chapter 34) "chose not to include the class of functions with a threshold, i.e., functions in which the cancer risk is zero up to some positive value on the dose-scale" (Beir80, p.181).

At the same time, the BEIR-3 Committee encouraged threshold speculation (A) by stating "It is by no means clear whether dose rates of gamma or x radiation of about 100 mrads/yr are in any way detrimental to exposed people" (Beir80, p.139), and by stating that the BEIR-3 Committee itself felt "uncertainty as to whether a total dose of, say, 1 rad would have any effect at all" (Beir80, p.193), and (B) by stating that it was not possible to settle the question within the available evidence (Beir80, p.22).

We disagreed (Go81). And we disagree today even more emphatically.

● -- *Part 4, Our Finding :*
=====================================

In Chapters 18 through 21 of this book, plus supporting Chapters 32 and 33, we prove beyond reasonable doubt and by any reasonable standard that no safe dose or dose-rate exists for the human with respect to radiogenic cancer. Our disproof of a threshold is based on the human evidence (much of which existed in 1980, too).

Our finding means that when very large populations are exposed to very small increments of ionizing radiation, the cancer-fatalities can be enormous even though each individual's personal risk is low. Chapter 24 uses the small individual doses from the Chernobyl explosion as just an illustration. Chapter 3 (page 1) mentions another illustration -- our 1985 estimate of the cancer-deaths induced in the United States by unnecessarily high doses given during diagnostic X-ray exams.

Disproof of any safe dose or dose-rate means that such cancer-deaths are not "hypothetical" and not "imaginary." They are real.

Thus, there is no issue of greater importance to the public and to the radiation community, than the threshold issue.

● -- *Part 4, Radiation Committees :*
=====================================

UNSCEAR 1988 on Threshold :

On the threshold issue, the UNSCEAR-88 Report (p.411, para.26) refers its readers to its previous report of 1986, Annex B. And there one finds various statements like the ones quoted in our Chapter 34.

UNSCEAR-86, p.166, para.3: "Although the absence of the threshold is often assumed, this has not been proved for any form of radiation-induced malignancy and must be regarded as a working hypothesis ... Proving or disproving a threshold below the levels of direct observation may be impossible, due to statistical fluctuations of the spontaneous level and of the presumably induced response ..."

At a later page, UNSCEAR-86 makes a statement (about dose-response curvature) which suggests that UNSCEAR should approve of our own approach to the threshold question: "What may happen at the low doses, where direct information is lacking, may only be inferred from a combination of empirical data and theoretical assumptions, linked together into some

models of radiation action" (Un86, p.241, para.474).

Our disproof of any safe dose or dose-rate takes the the human epidemiological observations at low tissue-doses, and combines them with track-analysis (number of primary ionization tracks per cell-nucleus), to show that the empirical observations DO tell us what is happening at even lower tissue-doses.

BEIR-5 on Threshold :

The repair of carcinogenic lesions, inflicted by a single primary ionization track upon genetic molecules in a cell-nucleus, is a key issue in speculations about a safe dose or dose-rate of ionizing radiation.

The BEIR-5 Committee alludes to the issue very early in its report (Beir90, p.4):

"Of the various types of biomedical effects that may result from irradiation at low doses and low dose rates, alterations of genes and chromosomes remain the best documented. Recent studies of these alterations in cells of various types, including human lymphocytes, have extended our knowledge of the relevant mechanisms and dose-response relationships. In spite of evidence that the molecular lesions which give rise to somatic and genetic damage can be repaired to a considerable degree, the new data do not contradict the hypothesis, at least with respect to cancer induction and hereditary genetic effects, that the frequency of such effects increases with low-level radiation as a linear, nonthreshold function of the dose."

However, the statement which is likely to be quoted by several segments of the radiation community is the statement which the BEIR-5 Committee provides much later (p.181):

"... epidemiologic data cannot rigorously exclude the existence of a threshold in the millisievert dose range. Thus the possibility that there may be no risks from exposures comparable to external natural background radiation cannot be ruled out. At such low doses and dose rates, it must be acknowledged that the lower limit of the range of uncertainty in the risk estimates extends to zero."

We are disappointed that BEIR-5 would issue such a statement without first TESTING the epidemiologic evidence against a track-analysis of the type demonstrated in this book.

==

● ── Part 4, Discussion :

====================================

Readers of Chapters 24 and 34 will not be surprised if there is great resistance in parts of the radiation community to our disproof of any safe dose or dose-rate.

If it is claimed by anyone that the nine human epidemiological studies in our disproof do not constitute ENOUGH evidence, such a claim would establish quite a contrast of standards, for NO human evidence is demanded in order for the radiation committees to recommend REDUCING risk-estimates (by "dreffing," as discussed in Part 3). Indeed, the recommendation is made CONTRARY to good, human evidence.

For all the reasons stated in our Chapter 21, we think that we have disproven any safe dose or dose-rate, beyond reasonable doubt. But we do not expect readers to accept anyone's assertion on faith alone. The entire case has been laid out -- from the evidence, step-by-step, to the conclusion -- for readers to judge for themselves.

5. Some Practical Implications for Human Health

How seriously need we take ionizing radiation, as a human carcinogen?

There is just no doubt that ionizing radiation is a cause of some unrepaired injuries to our genetic material (DNA and chromosomes). There is a vast body of work connecting genetic anomalies with human cancer. Indeed, the Nobel Prize in Medicine has just been awarded for work showing that disruption of our genes can trigger cancer. And the human epidemiological reality-check leaves no doubt that exposure of people to ionizing radiation, even at the lowest possible doses and dose-rates, results in excess fatal cancer.

The Most Important Single Carcinogen ?

A prominent member of the radiation community, Rosalyn Yalow (see Chapter 34), has asserted that "... exposure to ionizing radiation is only weakly carcinogenic" (Ya88, p.11). Weak on the basis of whose estimate? The question really matters, when estimates differ by factors of 2, 5, 10, 15, 20, 25, or even 30.

And weak compared with what?

The separate contributions from OTHER carcinogens to the population's total cancer mortality are hardly quantified at all. My estimates of the risk-per-rad from ionizing radiation are consistent with some 15 to 25 percent of all human cancer being caused by ionizing radiation (see box). Radon injects considerable uncertainty into the range. Ionizing radiation may even turn out to be the MOST important single carcinogen to which large numbers of humans are actually exposed. No one can possibly be sure yet, in the absence of equally good epidemiological data on all the other human carcinogens and on the magnitude of human exposure to them.

"A Ball-Park Estimate" : For U.S. Population
Radiation's Contribution to the Cancer Problem

~2,200 persons out of 10,000 die of cancer. We will use 60-year accumulation of dose. Lifetime Fatal Cancer-Yield, rounded from Table 16-C, is ~ 26 cancer-deaths per 10,000 persons per rem. (Basis is A-bomb radiation.)
Annual dose estimates in Col.B below are taken unchanged from BEIR-5, Table 1-3.
For our estimate below, the medical dose-estimate should be cut in half because children receive little from this source, and should be doubled for the greater carcinogenicity of X-rays. Thus, we need no net change in this BEIR-5 value.
BEIR presents all doses in Whole-Body Effective Dose Equivalents in rems (cSv).

Col.A	Col.B	Col.C	Col. D	Col.E
Source	Dose(rems)	Dose(rems)	Lifetime Fatal	Fatal Cancers /
	(Annual)	(60 year,cumulative)	Cancer-Yield	10,000 persons
Radon	0.2	12.0	26	312
Other natural	0.094	5.64	26	147
Medical X-rays	0.039	2.34	26	61
All other	0.024	1.44	26	37
TOTAL EXPECTED CANCERS PRODUCED IN 10,000 PERSONS =				557
Radiation-induced share of cancer-mortality = (557/2200)(100%) = 25.3 % .				

Other Human Carcinogens :

Even if human carcinogens could be reliably ranked, we certainly do not wish to imply that only the Number One killer deserves to be taken seriously. Far from it.

And we are troubled by the implications of what we see, in the radiation field, for the possible chemical carcinogens. Is the position going to be taken that it is acceptable to release "low-levels" of possible chemical carcinogens into the common indoor and outdoor environment, unless the public can prove from direct human epidemiological evidence for each of them that there is no safe dose?

Certain unique features of ionizing radiation PERMIT us to know more about it than about other human carcinogens. For instance, in this field of research, we do not need to depend on possibly irrelevant, and therefore eternally inconclusive, evidence from non-human species or cell-studies. Without conducting immoral human experimentation, human data exist for ionizing radiation because it is widely used in medicine, diagnostically and therapeutically. In addition, as a result of the two atomic bombings in Japan, genuinely comparable groups of humans exist who were exposed to very different dose-levels. This situation is important in many ways (discovering the shape of dose-response, proving causality beyond a reasonable doubt, etc.), and yet the situation is unlikely to occur for many other carcinogens. And lastly, the unique physical properties of ionizing radiation make it possible to prove that there is NO safe dose or dose-rate, even in the absence of human studies conducted at the lowest conceivable doses.

A Giant Gamble with Human Health ?

When we think over the fierce resistance to giving up the threshold idea with respect to ionizing radiation, even when there is such compelling human evidence against any safe dose or dose-rate, we wonder what behavior will prevail with respect to all those chemical substances where compelling human epidemiological evidence is lacking.

In Chapter 24, with respect to ionizing radiation, we have mentioned that proposals are pending to omit very low-dose exposure entirely from evaluations of human health effects ("de minimis non curat lex," or "the law does not concern itself with trifles"), and to treat a large share of "low-level" radioactive wastes (possibly some consumer items too) as if they were not radioactive at all -- "below regulatory concern."

If such proposals prevail, it is self-evident that less of the past radioactive contamination will be cleaned up, that future nuclear pollution will increase, and that human exposures to ionizing radiation will rise.

The "Global Perspective" :

The UNSCEAR 1988 Committee has raised the issue of public perception of radiation risk -- a timely issue after the Chernobyl nuclear accident has called worldwide attention to such risk. UNSCEAR makes no estimate itself of the cancer-fatalities which will occur from the accident, but it comments (Un88, p.42, para.268):

" ... the way in which basic scientific facts are presented influences the impression they give. For example, thousands of cancer deaths from a single accident would undoubtedly be a high number of deaths. However, since such deaths could be expected to occur over a long period of time, the annual incidence will be low. This means a very small increase of the normal incidence of cancer, an increase which is not expected to be noticeable in health statistics. This shows that it is possible, by selecting the form of presentation, to convey different impressions."

Not surprisingly, parts of the radiation community have been extremely active in trying to shape public perception of the Chernobyl accident. In Chapter 24, we documented the repeated comparison of any estimate of people receiving a cancer-death from Chernobyl, with the far greater number of people who will die of cancer ANYWAY in the northern hemisphere during the next 50 to 100 years.

The authors of the Department of Energy's Chernobyl assessment call this the "global perspective" (Ansp88, p.1513). If there is another accident -- or equivalent nuclear pollution from intentional releases -- we expect to hear about the "inter-stellar perspective."

To illustrate the consequences of "giving" small per-capita doses to entire populations, we presented some realistic estimates of Chernobyl's all-time cancer-consequences.

The range in Table 24-B, based on Cancer-Yields from both Gofman and from RERF analysts, is from 140,000 to 475,000 fatal cancers (leukemia excluded). Because such estimates come from very low per-capita doses received by hundreds of millions of people, such estimates could just be erased from the slate of a benefit-risk analysis, if risk-evaluation were ever to exclude all slow-low exposures (as in "de minimis" proposals).

===

Just One Part in a Thousand ?

It may sound like a trifle to put only one part per thousand of a poison into the environment, but we will show what one part per thousand means with respect to radioactive cesium.

The cesium-137 produced each year by a 1000-megawatt (electrical) nuclear power plant amounts to nearly 4 million curies. Since its radioactive half-life is 30.2 years, very little of it decays during a year.

The Chernobyl reactor contained a two-year cesium-inventory of about 8 million curies. Recent estimates are that the Chernobyl reactor released about 2.5 million curies of cesium-137, which is equivalent to (2.5 / 4.0) or 62.5 % of a ONE-year inventory.

Now let us consider 100 large nuclear power plants each operating in the USA for a lifespan of about 25 years each. Call "A" the yearly cesium-137 production by one plant.

```
Then 100A = the yearly production by 100 plants.
Lifetime production = 25 yrs x 100A/year = 2,500A.
99.9 % containment = release of 1 part per 1,000.
With 99.9 % perfect containment, loss = 2.5A.
Chernobyl lost 0.625A.
The ratio of 2.5A and 0.625A is 4.0.
```

This ratio, 4, has an enormous meaning. It means that achieving 99.9 % PERFECT containment of the cesium-137 produced by 100 plants during 25 years of operation, through all steps of the cesium's handling up through final burial, would STILL result in cesium-137 contamination equivalent in curies to 4 Chernobyl accidents.

Worldwide, there are about 400 plants underway, so the same scenario (99.9 % perfection in containing cesium) would mean cesium-loss equivalent to 16 Chernobyl accidents per 25 years of operation. And this assault on human health could occur without blowing the roof off any single plant.

Best Estimates ... Semi-Prudence :

The stakes in the correct evaluation of cancer-risk from low-dose exposure extend far beyond one spectacular accident like Chernobyl. Not only do such evaluations affect hundreds of millions of medical and dental patients, and millions of occupationally exposed workers, but correct evaluation necessarily affects the decisions which will determine the ultimate and aggregate levels of radioactive pollution, everywhere, from current and contemplated nuclear activities worldwide.

It is possible that new evidence developing in the future will show that our estimates in this book, of cancer-risk from low-dose, low-LET ionizing radiation, are too high -- and it is equally possible that new evidence will show that our estimates are too low. In other words, there is as much chance that sampling variation and forecasting are producing UNDERestimates of hazard as OVERestimates.

Pending future evidence, it is scientifically appropriate to produce and disseminate the best risk-estimates which come from the available human epidemiological evidence of good quality.

But we will repeat a warning.

What is scientifically appropriate behavior is only SEMI-prudent with regard to public health protection. True prudence with respect to human health would require the operating assumption that current uncertainties in sampling and forecasting are causing us to UNDERestimate the real risk.

25-empty, after 25-17.

==

Master Table and Special RERF Data for the A–Bomb Study (1950–1982)

In the Master Table 26-A,B,C,D, all entries come from RERF diskette R10ALL.DAT (R-Ten-All), unless noted otherwise below. As pointed out in Chapter 7, the observed deaths in Columns M through R are the aggregate numbers counted during all the follow-ups between 1950-1982. These are the raw numbers (see Chapter 11).

Column A = City. H = Hiroshima. N = Nagasaki.
Column B = Sex. M = male. F = female.
Column C = Nominal Mean Age ATB, as provided on the diskette R10ALL.
Column D = True Mean Age ATB, from special Tables 26-E through 26-M.
Column E = Dose-Group. RERF sorted all participants into 8 dose-groups.
Column F = Nominal Mean Kerma Dose, T65DR dosimetry, from disk R10ALL.
Column G = True Mean T65DR Kerma Dose, from Tables 26-E through 26-M.
Column H = Mean Internal Organ-Dose, T65DR dosimetry with neutron RBE=2.
  These entries were obtained as demonstrated in Chapter 9.
Column I = True Mean DS86 Kerma Dose. These entries were obtained from
  Tables 26-N and 26-"O" as demonstrated in Chapter 10.
Column J = Mean Internal Organ-Dose, DS86 dosimetry with neutron RBE=20.
  These entries were obtained as demonstrated in Chapter 10.
Column K = Initial Persons who entered the study in 1950.
Column L = Person-Years of follow-up through 1982.
Column M = Number of Deaths from All Causes Combined, 1950-1982.
Column N = Number of Deaths from All Diseases Combined, 1950-1982.
Column O = Number of Deaths from Any Type of Neoplasm, 1950-1982.
Column P = Number of Deaths from Any Type of Malignancy, 1950-1982.
Column Q = Number of Deaths from Leukemia alone, 1950-1982.
Column R = Number of Cancer-Deaths Excluding Leukemia, 1950-1982.

The arrangement in Master Table 26-A,B,C,D is by age-band. In Tables 11-B and 11-D, the arrangement is by Dose-Group, and the two cities have been combined. Additional arrangements by age-band are provided in Chapters 15 and 17.

Special Tables 26-E through 26-"O" :
================================

These tables, already described in Chapter 7, are exactly as RERF provided them. Tables 26-E through 26-M provide the data on persons, true dose, and true age ATB which were missing from diskette R10ALL. Tables 26-N and 26-"O" provide data which were missing from Appendix Table 2 of TR-12-87, on the neutron and gamma components of DS86 doses; we use these data in Tables 10-A and 10-B.

Table 26-A
Basic Data for Hiroshima Males, A–Bomb Study 1950–1982

C	D	E	F	G	H	I	J	K	L	M	N	O	P	Q	R
			DISK	TRUE	RBE=2	TRUE	RBE=20								ALL
			T65DR	T65DR	T65DR	DS86	DS86								CANCER
DISK	TRUE	RERF	KERMA	KERMA	ORGAN	KERMA	ORGAN		PERSON	DEATHS	DEATHS	DEATHS	DEATHS	DEATH	DEATHS
AGE	AGE	DOSE-	DOSE	DOSE	DOSE	DOSE	DOSE	INITIAL	YEARS	ALL	ALL	ALL	ALL	LEUK	EXCEPT
ATB	ATB	GRP	(rads)	(rads)	(rems)	(rads)	(rems)	PERSONS	(PYR)	CAUSE	DISEASE	NEOPLAS	MALIG		LEUK
5	4.0	1	0	0.0	0.00	0.16	0.12	2586	81756	109	66	9	9	3	6
5	4.0	2	3.3	3.1	1.56	3.54	2.77	1446	45611	71	39	11	11	1	10
5	3.9	3	22.1	21.4	10.74	21.27	16.77	1024	32420	40	23	2	2	2	0
5	3.7	4	70.3	70.2	35.23	58.63	48.31	228	7153	9	2	0	0	0	0
5	4.5	5	139.0	139.1	69.85	104.81	88.89	100	3168	4	2	2	1	1	0
5	3.8	6	243.5	238.5	119.81	167.81	147.98	49	1468	8	7	4	4	0	4
5	3.6	7	346.4	340.2	171.00	234.75	212.54	22	657	3	1	1	1	1	0
5	3.9	8	524.4	519.1	260.98	379.43	359.76	29	843	4	4	4	4	3	1
15	14.2	1	0	0.0	0.00	0.16	0.12	2314	70732	263	179	41	41	4	37
15	14.1	2	3.3	4.1	2.06	4.68	3.66	1655	50865	181	140	40	37	2	35
15	14.3	3	22.1	22.2	11.14	22.07	17.40	730	22540	72	59	20	18	5	13
15	14.5	4	70.3	70.4	35.33	58.79	48.45	162	4993	17	11	5	5	1	4
15	15.2	5	139.0	137.0	68.80	103.22	87.54	147	4428	17	14	3	3	1	2
15	15.6	6	243.5	255.8	128.50	179.98	158.71	65	1974	7	5	2	2	0	2
15	15.8	7	346.4	353.9	177.89	244.21	221.10	38	1148	6	5	4	3	1	2
15	15.4	8	524.4	532.8	267.86	389.44	369.25	69	2007	17	14	4	4	1	3
27	28.2	1	0	0.0	0.00	0.16	0.12	1424	41170	393	359	111	106	7	99
27	27.8	2	3.3	3.4	1.71	3.88	3.04	939	27206	231	209	68	65	2	63
27	28.4	3	22.1	22.4	11.24	22.27	17.56	535	15235	153	134	43	42	2	40
27	27.8	4	70.3	68.0	34.13	56.79	46.80	130	3633	42	41	8	7	1	6
27	28.1	5	139.0	140.8	70.71	106.09	89.97	107	3083	28	26	10	10	2	8
27	27.9	6	243.5	242.8	121.97	170.84	150.65	50	1477	12	11	6	6	2	4
27	26.4	7	346.4	339.3	170.55	234.13	211.97	26	753	8	8	2	2	2	0
27	27.0	8	524.4	546.9	274.95	399.75	379.03	35	1062	8	8	2	2	0	2
42	42.5	1	0	0.0	0.00	0.16	0.12	2701	63531	1749	1640	469	447	10	437
42	42.6	2	3.3	3.5	1.76	4.00	3.13	1570	37481	1029	971	260	246	4	242
42	42.8	3	22.1	22.6	11.34	22.47	17.71	1067	25397	691	658	198	193	6	187
42	42.6	4	70.3	69.6	34.93	58.13	47.90	283	6586	186	180	57	56	2	54
42	42.4	5	139.0	135.3	67.94	101.94	86.45	238	5696	142	136	47	47	1	46
42	42.7	6	243.5	238.7	119.91	167.95	148.10	71	1618	50	50	17	17	3	14
42	42.7	7	346.4	340.7	171.26	235.10	212.85	35	663	28	28	4	4	0	4
42	42.8	8	524.4	528.3	265.60	386.15	366.13	61	1372	47	46	21	20	3	17
60	58.2	1	0	0.0	0.00	0.16	0.12	2230	29452	2171	2096	379	362	2	360
60	58.1	2	3.3	3.3	1.66	3.77	2.95	1329	17662	1281	1230	221	212	2	210
60	58.3	3	22.1	21.9	10.99	21.77	17.16	869	12097	835	819	139	134	4	130
60	57.2	4	70.3	71.1	35.69	59.38	48.93	223	3495	212	208	40	39	0	39
60	56.8	5	139.0	142.8	71.71	107.59	91.25	171	2149	168	160	31	29	0	29
60	55.9	6	243.5	245.3	123.22	172.60	152.20	47	723	45	43	13	13	1	12
60	57.8	7	346.4	354.3	178.09	244.48	221.34	23	335	23	23	2	2	0	2
60	57.7	8	524.4	529.5	266.21	387.03	366.97	43	526	43	42	5	5	2	3
								24871	634163	10403	9697	2305	2211	84	2127

A Column represented Hiroshima; B Column represented Males. Since all data in this Table are for Hiroshima Males, those two columns are eliminated here.

Table 26-B
Basic Data for Nagasaki Males, A–Bomb Study 1950–1982

C	D	E	F	G	H	I	J	K	L	M	N	O	P	Q	R
			DISK T65DR KERMA DOSE (rads)	TRUE T65DR KERMA DOSE (rads)	RBE=2 T65DR ORGAN DOSE (rems)	TRUE DS86 KERMA DOSE (rads)	RBE=20 DS86 ORGAN DOSE (rems)		PERSON YEARS (PYR)	DEATHS ALL CAUSE	DEATHS ALL DISEASE	DEATHS ALL NEOPLAS	DEATHS ALL MALIG	DEATH LEUK	ALL CANCER DEATHS EXCEPT LEUK
DISK AGE ATB	TRUE AGE ATB	RERF DOSE-GRP						INITIAL PERSONS							
5	4.4	1	0	0.0	0.00	0.00	0.00	1201	37729	69	41	6	5	1	4
5	4.4	2	2.6	2.7	1.35	0.71	0.52	1585	49944	81	50	8	6	1	5
5	4.5	3	21.2	20.0	10.00	8.85	6.58	523	16557	24	13	3	1	0	1
5	4.3	4	71.2	68.0	34.00	32.56	24.96	131	4094	7	6	0	0	0	0
5	4.8	5	146.9	147.3	73.66	70.80	54.70	89	2798	4	4	3	3	1	2
5	4.2	6	243.7	241.0	120.53	115.27	89.70	56	1667	9	6	5	4	3	1
5	4.1	7	343.7	340.4	170.25	174.40	136.48	21	677	0	0	0	0	0	0
5	4.1	8	529.2	505.2	252.70	329.89	261.44	35	1082	3	3	2	2	2	0
15	13.5	1	0	0.0	0.00	0.00	0.00	976	29456	129	84	16	12	0	12
15	13.7	2	2.6	2.6	1.30	0.68	0.50	1433	43720	175	132	33	31	2	29
15	13.7	3	21.2	22.1	11.05	9.78	7.27	382	11858	34	27	7	7	1	6
15	14.6	4	71.2	70.3	35.15	33.66	25.80	180	5548	21	18	5	5	0	5
15	15.2	5	146.9	147.5	73.76	70.90	54.77	224	6940	23	19	4	3	0	3
15	15.4	6	243.7	244.6	122.33	116.99	91.03	102	3155	11	11	5	5	0	5
15	14.9	7	343.7	330.7	165.40	169.43	132.59	32	962	4	4	2	2	0	2
15	14.5	8	529.2	527.0	263.60	344.12	272.72	57	1702	9	8	4	4	1	3
27	28.2	1	0	0.0	0.00	0.00	0.00	436	12574	119	111	37	34	0	34
27	27.9	2	2.6	2.4	1.20	0.63	0.46	494	13921	141	129	29	29	1	28
27	27.6	3	21.2	25.2	12.60	11.15	8.29	168	4956	46	44	14	14	0	14
27	26.7	4	71.2	74.5	37.25	35.67	27.34	107	3235	21	18	5	5	0	5
27	27.5	5	146.9	143.1	71.56	68.78	53.14	117	3224	44	40	18	15	1	14
27	28.9	6	243.7	248.5	124.28	118.86	92.49	72	1989	27	24	13	13	0	13
27	28.4	7	343.7	343.7	171.90	176.09	137.80	27	821	5	5	2	2	0	2
27	27.9	8	529.2	540.7	270.46	353.07	279.81	22	650	4	4	2	2	1	1
42	42.8	1	0	0.0	0.00	0.00	0.00	822	19314	546	529	137	134	5	129
42	42.8	2	2.6	2.5	1.25	0.65	0.48	906	20025	643	611	164	156	1	155
42	42.5	3	21.2	23.8	11.90	10.53	7.82	314	7056	207	191	57	54	1	53
42	42.3	4	71.2	74.0	37.00	35.43	27.16	155	3666	102	98	28	28	0	28
42	42.0	5	146.9	144.4	72.21	69.41	53.62	130	3110	91	88	26	26	0	26
42	42.0	6	243.7	242.0	121.03	115.75	90.07	62	1466	43	42	12	12	2	10
42	42.7	7	343.7	342.3	171.20	175.37	137.24	35	772	24	24	8	8	0	8
42	41.0	8	529.2	536.3	268.26	350.20	277.54	50	932	39	36	14	13	2	11
60	58.1	1	0	0.0	0.00	0.00	0.00	716	8717	698	678	92	88	1	87
60	58.1	2	2.6	2.5	1.25	0.65	0.48	822	10297	807	791	99	92	2	90
60	57.7	3	21.2	22.5	11.25	9.96	7.40	276	3527	271	266	27	26	1	25
60	57.0	4	71.2	71.2	35.60	34.09	26.13	85	1138	81	79	13	12	0	12
60	55.6	5	146.9	147.3	73.66	71.29	55.08	63	912	60	59	12	12	1	11
60	54.1	6	243.7	243.7	121.88	116.56	90.70	27	438	24	24	4	3	0	3
60	53.3	7	343.7	350.2	175.16	179.42	140.41	11	152	11	11	2	2	1	1
60	56.0	8	529.2	553.4	276.81	361.36	286.38	22	272	21	21	5	5	0	5
								12966	341049	4678	4349	923	875	32	843

A Column represented Nagasaki ; B Column represented Males. Since all data in this Table are for Nagasaki Males, those two columns are eliminated here.

Table 26-C
Basic Data for Hiroshima Females, A–Bomb Study 1950–1982

C	D	E	F	G	H	I	J	K	L	M	N	O	P	Q	R
			DISK T65DR KERMA DOSE (rads)	TRUE T65DR KERMA DOSE (rads)	RBE=2 T65DR ORGAN DOSE (rems)	TRUE DS86 KERMA DOSE (rads)	RBE=20 DS86 ORGAN DOSE (rems)								ALL CANCER DEATHS EXCEPT LEUK
DISK AGE ATB	TRUE AGE ATB	RERF DOSE-GRP						INITIAL PERSONS	PERSON YEARS (PYR)	DEATHS ALL CAUSE	DEATHS ALL DISEASE	DEATHS ALL NEOPLAS	DEATHS ALL MALIG	DEATH LEUK	
5	3.9	1	0	0.0	0.00	0.16	0.12	2621	83712	57	43	14	12	1	11
5	3.7	2	3.3	3.0	1.51	3.43	2.68	1519	48437	39	22	11	11	0	11
5	3.7	3	22.1	21.9	10.99	21.77	17.16	1014	32289	29	24	9	9	4	5
5	3.9	4	70.3	70.1	35.18	58.54	48.24	229	7300	6	6	3	3	1	2
5	4.3	5	139.0	136.7	68.65	103.00	87.35	128	3939	10	8	5	5	2	3
5	4.0	6	243.5	244.3	122.72	171.89	151.57	51	1620	3	2	2	2	1	1
5	3.2	7	346.4	346.7	174.27	239.24	216.60	22	710	0	0	0	0	0	0
5	4.1	8	524.4	521.4	262.13	381.11	361.35	29	917	1	1	1	1	0	1
15	15.2	1	0	0.0	0.00	0.16	0.12	3020	94015	202	167	51	49	4	45
15	15.2	2	3.3	3.3	1.66	3.77	2.95	1589	50120	84	74	21	18	0	18
15	15.2	3	22.1	21.4	10.74	21.27	16.77	1156	36046	81	67	19	18	2	16
15	15.3	4	70.3	72.3	36.29	60.38	49.76	291	9109	19	13	4	4	0	4
15	14.9	5	139.0	137.8	69.20	103.83	88.06	217	6721	21	17	9	9	3	6
15	15.3	6	243.5	248.1	124.63	174.57	153.94	84	2571	9	9	5	5	1	4
15	14.0	7	346.4	341.6	171.71	235.72	213.41	71	2164	10	9	6	6	0	6
15	16.0	8	524.4	531.7	267.31	388.64	368.49	63	1949	10	8	5	5	0	5
27	26.8	1	0	0.0	0.00	0.16	0.12	4011	122883	503	482	163	157	5	152
27	26.8	2	3.3	3.3	1.66	3.77	2.95	2329	71003	303	286	109	101	3	98
27	26.8	3	22.1	22.2	11.14	22.07	17.40	1657	50438	217	204	101	97	5	92
27	26.6	4	70.3	70.9	35.59	59.21	48.79	480	14596	74	70	27	23	2	21
27	26.3	5	139.0	142.5	71.56	107.37	91.06	253	7690	33	31	18	15	2	13
27	25.7	6	243.5	244.0	122.57	171.68	151.39	98	2859	26	25	19	19	2	17
27	26.3	7	346.4	347.4	174.62	239.72	217.03	59	1744	15	15	8	7	3	4
27	25.3	8	524.4	505.6	254.19	369.56	350.40	97	2802	24	23	13	13	2	11
42	41.7	1	0	0.0	0.00	0.16	0.12	4029	108973	1749	1687	430	409	12	397
42	41.5	2	3.3	3.2	1.61	3.66	2.86	2140	58273	911	874	257	244	3	241
42	41.6	3	22.1	22.4	11.24	22.27	17.56	1803	48549	802	772	223	214	3	211
42	41.7	4	70.3	69.2	34.73	57.79	47.62	462	12306	218	203	69	68	3	65
42	41.6	5	139.0	138.8	69.70	104.58	88.69	267	7168	124	120	42	38	1	37
42	41.3	6	243.5	239.4	120.26	168.45	148.54	100	2624	50	50	17	16	1	15
42	41.7	7	346.4	350.6	176.23	241.93	219.04	51	1293	25	25	12	12	3	9
42	42.3	8	524.4	517.0	259.92	377.89	358.30	62	1579	38	36	16	16	2	14
60	58.9	1	0	0.0	0.00	0.16	0.12	2633	42350	2458	2383	314	303	2	301
60	59.4	2	3.3	3.2	1.61	3.66	2.86	1415	22266	1310	1286	154	141	2	139
60	58.5	3	22.1	22.2	11.14	22.07	17.40	1054	17268	978	951	134	121	2	119
60	58.2	4	70.3	70.3	35.28	58.71	48.38	295	4507	276	265	39	36	2	34
60	57.8	5	139.0	138.7	69.65	104.50	88.62	112	1753	103	99	21	21	1	20
60	57.2	6	243.5	236.4	118.75	166.33	146.67	44	746	41	40	10	8	1	7
60	56.4	7	346.4	351.0	176.43	242.20	219.28	22	308	21	21	4	4	1	3
60	59.0	8	524.4	536.5	269.72	392.14	371.81	22	292	21	19	5	5	0	5
								35599	985888	10901	10437	2370	2245	82	2163

A Column represented Hiroshima; B Column represented Females. Since all data in this Table are for Hiroshima Females, those two columns are eliminated here.

Table 26-D
Basic Data for Nagasaki Females, A–Bomb Study 1950–1982

C DISK AGE ATB	D TRUE AGE ATB	E RERF DOSE-GRP	F DISK T65DR KERMA DOSE (rads)	G TRUE T65DR KERMA DOSE (rads)	H RBE=2 T65DR ORGAN DOSE (rems)	I TRUE DS86 KERMA DOSE (rads)	J RBE=20 DS86 ORGAN DOSE (rems)	K INITIAL PERSONS	L PERSON YEARS (PYR)	M DEATHS ALL CAUSE	N DEATHS ALL DISEASE	O DEATHS ALL NEOPLAS	P DEATHS ALL MALIG	Q DEATH LEUK	R ALL CANCER DEATHS EXCEPT LEUK
5	4.5	1	0	0.0	0.00	0.00	0.00	1221	38650	45	36	9	8	1	7
5	4.4	2	2.6	2.7	1.35	0.71	0.52	1574	50010	52	42	12	11	2	9
5	4.5	3	21.2	20.3	10.15	8.98	6.67	533	16868	23	18	4	4	0	4
5	4.6	4	71.2	67.6	33.80	32.37	24.81	143	4471	6	5	1	1	0	1
5	4.4	5	146.9	145.6	72.81	69.99	54.07	85	2724	1	1	0	0	0	0
5	4.2	6	243.7	243.1	121.58	116.27	90.70	48	1500	4	4	3	3	0	3
5	4.8	7	343.7	355.5	177.81	182.14	142.53	19	611	1	1	1	1	0	1
5	4.9	8	529.2	540.7	270.46	353.07	279.81	41	1146	6	4	2	2	2	0
15	14.3	1	0	0.0	0.00	0.00	0.00	1165	36281	78	66	22	21	0	21
15	14.4	2	2.6	2.7	1.35	0.71	0.52	1629	50683	112	94	37	33	1	32
15	14.1	3	21.2	21.3	10.65	9.42	7.00	507	15830	34	30	8	8	1	7
15	15.0	4	71.2	73.3	36.65	35.10	26.90	252	7970	11	10	3	3	0	3
15	15.3	5	146.9	149.0	74.51	71.62	55.33	339	10534	30	25	13	12	0	12
15	15.4	6	243.7	243.3	121.68	116.37	90.55	180	5534	19	18	7	6	2	4
15	15.2	7	343.7	346.1	173.10	177.32	138.76	47	1456	5	5	2	2	0	2
15	14.9	8	529.2	515.9	258.05	336.88	266.98	48	1493	4	4	2	2	1	1
27	26.4	1	0	0.0	0.00	0.00	0.00	1182	35768	167	164	64	62	1	61
27	26.5	2	2.6	2.6	1.30	0.68	0.50	1738	52269	260	247	91	87	2	85
27	26.9	3	21.2	21.0	10.50	9.29	6.90	532	15977	84	74	30	29	0	29
27	26.6	4	71.2	71.3	35.65	34.14	26.17	190	5681	35	34	15	15	0	15
27	24.8	5	146.9	148.0	74.01	71.14	54.96	183	5585	22	21	9	9	0	9
27	24.7	6	243.7	244.3	122.18	116.85	90.93	94	2839	15	14	5	5	0	5
27	24.6	7	343.7	339.5	169.30	173.94	136.12	44	1369	4	3	2	2	0	2
27	25.3	8	529.2	519.4	259.80	339.16	268.79	55	1558	11	10	3	2	0	2
42	41.7	1	0	0.0	0.00	0.00	0.00	1055	27943	492	478	113	106	2	104
42	42.0	2	2.6	2.6	1.30	0.68	0.50	1614	41847	798	766	191	187	4	183
42	41.6	3	21.2	20.1	10.05	8.89	6.61	488	12474	248	242	64	64	1	63
42	41.4	4	71.2	68.7	34.35	32.89	25.21	120	3229	58	55	12	11	0	11
42	42.6	5	146.9	141.7	70.86	68.11	52.62	99	2573	50	49	5	5	0	5
42	41.3	6	243.7	243.5	121.78	116.46	90.62	55	1472	26	26	6	5	0	5
42	40.4	7	343.7	356.6	178.36	182.70	142.97	23	616	12	11	3	3	0	3
42	41.4	8	529.2	531.9	266.06	347.32	275.25	35	948	16	15	4	4	0	4
60	59.3	1	0	0.0	0.00	0.00	0.00	830	11648	801	785	79	73	1	72
60	58.8	2	2.6	2.6	1.30	0.68	0.50	1129	16820	1054	1026	104	97	1	96
60	59.4	3	21.2	19.5	9.75	8.63	6.41	311	4385	301	296	41	40	0	40
60	59.6	4	71.2	71.2	35.60	34.09	26.13	79	1262	75	73	5	5	0	5
60	58.8	5	146.9	151.4	75.71	72.77	56.22	59	797	54	54	7	7	0	7
60	60.2	6	243.7	239.0	119.53	114.31	88.95	26	375	26	26	3	2	0	2
60	56.2	7	343.7	344.8	172.45	176.65	138.24	11	170	10	9	0	0	0	0
60	58.3	8	529.2	563.8	282.01	368.15	291.76	12	145	11	11	2	2	0	2
								17795	493510	5061	4852	984	939	22	917

A Column represented Nagasaki; B Column represented Females. Since all data in this Table are for Nagasaki Females, those two columns are eliminated here.

Tables 26–E through 26–M

RERF Data on Persons, T65DR Shielded Kerma Dose, and Age ATB, for the Full Cohort

RERF's eight, undivided dose-groups are presented in the top row as shielded kerma dose-ranges in rads (0, 1–9 rads, 10–49 rads, etc.).

RERF's five age-bands are presented in the left, vertical column as a range of Ages at Time of Bombing (e.g., 0–9 years ATB, 10–19 years ATB, etc.).

Persons ("cases") are participants originally enrolled in the Life Span Study in 1950.

These nine tables are the printouts as provided by RERF in August 1988.

Table 26–E

Both Cities, Both Sexes Combined

```
REPORT 10TH CROSS TABLE      BOTH CITIES

SEX : TOTAL
--------------------------------------------------------------------------------------------------
                                                           T65DR
AGE ATB
                   TOTAL      0      1-9    10-49   50-99  100-199  200-299  300-399   400+
--------------------------------------------------------------------------------------------------
TOTAL    CASE      91231    37173   28855   14943    4225    3128     1381      639      887
TOTAL    MEANDOSE   23.9      0.0     3.0    21.8    70.6   142.5    243.6    345.2    526.4
TOTAL    MEAN AGE   28.4     28.7    27.8    28.9    29.1    27.9     26.1     26.6     27.1


0-9      CASE      18402     7629    6124    3094     731     402      204       84      134
0-9      MEANDOSE   18.4      0.0     2.8    21.1    69.3   141.5    241.7    345.4    522.6
0-9      MEAN AGE    4.1      4.1     4.1     4.0     4.1     4.5      4.0      3.9      4.3


10-19    CASE      19224     7475    6306    2775     885     927      431      188      237
10-19    MEANDOSE   29.8      0.0     3.2    21.7    71.8   144.1    246.4    343.3    527.7
10-19    MEAN AGE   14.6     14.5    14.4    14.6    14.9    15.2     15.4     14.8     15.2


20-34    CASE      17691     7053    5500    2892     907     660      314      156      209
20-34    MEANDOSE   27.1      0.0     3.0    22.2    71.0   143.8    244.9    343.2    519.8
20-34    MEAN AGE   27.0     27.1    27.0    27.2    26.8    26.4     26.5     26.2     25.9


35-49    CASE      20903     8607    6230    3672    1020     734      288      144      208
35-49    MEANDOSE   24.1      0.0     3.0    22.3    70.0   139.1    240.6    347.1    527.5
35-49    MEAN AGE   42.0     42.0    42.1    42.0    42.0    42.1     41.8     42.0     42.0


50+      CASE      15011     6409    4695    2510     682     405      144       67       99
50+      MEANDOSE   19.1      0.0     2.9    21.8    70.8   143.6    241.1    351.0    540.5
50+      MEAN AGE   58.5     58.6    58.7    58.4    57.9    57.2     56.7     56.3     57.7
```

Table 26–F

Both Cities, Males Only

REPORT 10TH CROSS TABLE   BOTH CITIES

SEX : MALE

AGE ATB		TOTAL	0	1-9	10-49	50-99	100-199	200-299	300-399	400+
										T65DR
TOTAL	CASE	37837	15406	12179	5888	1684	1386	601	270	423
TOTAL	MEANDOSE	25.0	0.0	3.1	22.1	70.6	141.9	244.3	343.2	530.9
TOTAL	MEAN AGE	27.9	28.3	26.8	28.4	29.2	29.9	27.0	28.2	28.5
0-9	CASE	9125	3787	3031	1547	359	189	105	43	64
0-9	MEANDOSE	18.1	0.0	2.9	21.0	69.4	142.9	239.8	340.3	511.5
0-9	MEAN AGE	4.1	4.1	4.2	4.1	3.9	4.6	4.0	3.9	4.0
10-19	CASE	8566	3290	3088	1112	342	371	167	70	126
10-19	MEANDOSE	28.6	0.0	3.4	22.1	70.4	143.3	248.9	343.3	530.2
10-19	MEAN AGE	14.1	14.0	13.9	14.1	14.6	15.2	15.4	15.4	15.0
20-34	CASE	4689	1860	1433	703	237	224	122	53	57
20-34	MEANDOSE	31.6	0.0	3.0	23.1	70.9	142.0	246.2	341.6	544.5
20-34	MEAN AGE	28.0	28.2	27.8	28.2	27.3	27.8	28.5	27.4	27.3
35-49	CASE	8500	3523	2476	1381	438	368	133	70	111
35-49	MEANDOSE	27.8	0.0	3.2	22.9	71.2	138.5	240.2	341.5	531.9
35-49	MEAN AGE	42.6	42.6	42.6	42.7	42.5	42.3	42.4	42.7	42.0
50+	CASE	6957	2946	2151	1145	308	234	74	34	65
50+	MEANDOSE	21.9	0.0	3.0	22.1	71.1	144.0	244.7	353.0	537.6
50+	MEAN AGE	58.0	58.2	58.1	58.1	57.2	56.5	55.2	56.4	57.1

Table 26–G

Both Cities, Females Only

REPORT 10TH CROSS TABLE   BOTH CITIES

SEX : FEMALE

AGE ATB		TOTAL	0	1-9	10-49	50-99	100-199	200-299	300-399	400+
										T65DR
TOTAL	CASE	53394	21767	16676	9055	2541	1742	780	369	464
TOTAL	MEANDOSE	23.1	0.0	2.9	21.7	70.6	142.9	243.1	346.7	522.4
TOTAL	MEAN AGE	28.7	29.1	28.5	29.3	29.0	26.3	25.4	25.5	25.8
0-9	CASE	9277	3842	3093	1547	372	213	99	41	70
0-9	MEANDOSE	18.7	0.0	2.8	21.3	69.1	140.2	243.7	350.8	532.7
0-9	MEAN AGE	4.1	4.1	4.1	3.9	4.2	4.3	4.1	4.0	4.6
10-19	CASE	10658	4185	3218	1663	543	556	264	118	111
10-19	MEANDOSE	30.8	0.0	3.0	21.4	72.8	144.6	244.8	343.4	524.9
10-19	MEAN AGE	14.9	15.0	14.8	14.9	15.1	15.2	15.3	14.5	15.5
20-34	CASE	13002	5193	4067	2189	670	436	192	103	152
20-34	MEANDOSE	25.4	0.0	3.0	21.9	71.1	144.8	244.2	344.1	510.6
20-34	MEAN AGE	26.6	26.7	26.7	26.8	26.6	25.7	25.2	25.6	25.3
35-49	CASE	12403	5084	3754	2291	582	366	155	74	97
35-49	MEANDOSE	21.5	0.0	3.0	21.9	69.1	139.6	240.8	352.4	522.4
35-49	MEAN AGE	41.7	41.7	41.7	41.6	41.6	41.9	41.3	41.3	42.0
50+	CASE	8054	3463	2544	1365	374	171	70	33	34
50+	MEANDOSE	16.7	0.0	2.9	21.6	70.5	143.1	237.4	348.9	546.1
50+	MEAN AGE	58.9	59.0	59.1	58.7	58.5	58.1	58.3	56.3	58.8

Table 26-H

Hiroshima Only, Both Sexes Combined

REPORT 10TH CROSS TABLE   HIROSHIMA

SEX : TOTAL

AGE ATB		TOTAL	0	1-9	10-49	50-99	100-199	200-299	300-399	400+
TOTAL	CASE	60470	27569	15931	10909	2783	1740	659	369	510
TOTAL	MEANDOSE	21.3	0.0	3.3	22.1	70.3	139.0	243.5	346.4	524.4
TOTAL	MEAN AGE	29.6	29.5	29.2	30.1	31.0	30.7	28.7	27.6	28.8
0-9	CASE	11097	5207	2965	2038	457	228	100	44	58
0-9	MEANDOSE	16.8	0.0	3.0	21.7	70.1	137.7	241.5	343.5	520.3
0-9	MEAN AGE	3.9	4.0	3.9	3.8	3.8	4.4	3.9	3.4	4.0
10-19	CASE	11671	5334	3244	1886	453	364	149	109	132
10-19	MEANDOSE	24.1	0.0	3.7	21.7	71.7	137.5	251.5	345.9	532.3
10-19	MEAN AGE	14.8	14.8	14.6	14.9	15.0	15.0	15.4	14.6	15.7
20-34	CASE	12230	5435	3268	2192	610	360	148	85	132
20-34	MEANDOSE	23.5	0.0	3.3	22.2	70.3	142.0	243.6	345.0	516.5
20-34	MEAN AGE	27.1	27.2	27.1	27.2	26.9	26.9	26.4	26.3	25.8
35-49	CASE	14940	6730	3710	2870	745	505	171	86	123
35-49	MEANDOSE	22.3	0.0	3.4	22.5	69.4	137.2	239.1	346.6	522.6
35-49	MEAN AGE	42.0	42.0	41.9	42.0	42.1	42.0	41.9	42.1	42.5
50+	CASE	10532	4863	2744	1923	518	283	91	45	65
50+	MEANDOSE	19.0	0.0	3.2	22.1	70.6	141.2	241.0	352.7	531.8
50+	MEAN AGE	58.5	58.6	58.8	58.4	57.8	57.2	56.5	57.1	58.1

Table 26-Eye

Nagasaki Only, Both Sexes Combined

REPORT 10TH CROSS TABLE   NAGASAKI

SEX : TOTAL

AGE ATB		TOTAL	0	1-9	10-49	50-99	100-199	200-299	300-399	400+
TOTAL	CASE	30761	9604	12924	4034	1442	1388	722	270	377
TOTAL	MEANDOSE	29.1	0.0	2.6	21.2	71.2	146.9	243.7	343.7	529.2
TOTAL	MEAN AGE	26.0	26.5	26.1	25.8	25.4	24.4	23.6	25.4	24.7
0-9	CASE	7305	2422	3159	1056	274	174	104	40	76
0-9	MEANDOSE	20.9	0.0	2.7	20.2	67.8	146.5	242.0	347.6	524.4
0-9	MEAN AGE	4.4	4.5	4.4	4.5	4.5	4.6	4.2	4.5	4.5
10-19	CASE	7553	2141	3062	889	432	563	282	79	105
10-19	MEANDOSE	38.7	0.0	2.7	21.6	72.0	148.4	243.7	339.9	522.0
10-19	MEAN AGE	14.2	13.9	14.1	13.9	14.9	15.3	15.4	15.1	14.6
20-34	CASE	5461	1618	2232	700	297	300	166	71	77
20-34	MEANDOSE	35.2	0.0	2.6	22.0	72.5	146.1	246.1	341.1	525.5
20-34	MEAN AGE	26.8	26.9	26.8	27.0	26.6	25.9	26.5	26.0	26.0
35-49	CASE	5963	1877	2520	802	275	229	117	58	85
35-49	MEANDOSE	28.6	0.0	2.6	21.6	71.7	143.2	242.7	348.0	534.5
35-49	MEAN AGE	42.2	42.2	42.3	42.0	41.9	42.3	41.7	41.8	41.2
50+	CASE	4479	1546	1951	587	164	122	53	22	34
50+	MEANDOSE	19.3	0.0	2.6	20.9	71.2	149.3	241.4	347.5	557.1
50+	MEAN AGE	58.5	58.8	58.5	58.6	58.3	57.1	57.1	54.7	56.8

Table 26-J

Hiroshima Only, Males Only

REPORT 10TH CROSS TABLE   HIROSHIMA

SEX : MALE

AGE ATB		TOTAL	0	1-9	10-49	50-99	100-199	200-299	300-399	400+
							T65DR			
TOTAL	CASE	24871	11255	6939	4225	1026	763	282	144	237
TOTAL	MEANDOSE	21.7	0.0	3.5	22.1	70.0	138.6	244.4	346.0	531.4
TOTAL	MEAN AGE	29.3	29.1	28.7	29.8	30.8	33.4	29.3	29.1	30.4
0-9	CASE	5484	2586	1446	1024	228	100	49	22	29
0-9	MEANDOSE	16.5	0.0	3.1	21.4	70.2	139.1	238.5	340.2	519.1
0-9	MEAN AGE	4.0	4.0	4.0	3.9	3.7	4.5	3.8	3.6	3.9
10-19	CASE	5180	2314	1655	730	162	147	65	38	69
10-19	MEANDOSE	23.4	0.0	4.1	22.2	70.4	137.0	255.8	353.9	532.8
10-19	MEAN AGE	14.3	14.2	14.1	14.3	14.5	15.2	15.6	15.8	15.4
20-34	CASE	3246	1424	939	535	130	107	50	26	35
20-34	MEANDOSE	24.4	0.0	3.4	22.4	68.0	140.8	242.8	339.3	546.9
20-34	MEAN AGE	28.1	28.2	27.8	28.4	27.8	28.1	27.9	26.4	27.0
35-49	CASE	6026	2701	1570	1067	283	238	71	35	61
35-49	MEANDOSE	23.7	0.0	3.5	22.6	69.6	135.3	238.7	340.7	528.3
35-49	MEAN AGE	42.6	42.5	42.6	42.8	42.6	42.4	42.7	42.7	42.8
50+	CASE	4935	2230	1329	869	223	171	47	23	43
50+	MEANDOSE	21.5	0.0	3.3	21.9	71.1	142.8	245.3	354.3	529.5
50+	MEAN AGE	58.1	58.2	58.1	58.3	57.2	56.8	55.9	57.8	57.7

Table 26-K

Nagasaki Only, Males Only

REPORT 10TH CROSS TABLE   NAGASAKI

SEX : MALE

AGE ATB		TOTAL	0	1-9	10-49	50-99	100-199	200-299	300-399	400+
							T65DR			
TOTAL	CASE	12966	4151	5240	1663	658	623	319	126	186
TOTAL	MEANDOSE	31.5	0.0	2.6	22.2	71.5	146.0	244.3	340.0	530.2
TOTAL	MEAN AGE	25.1	25.9	24.2	24.9	26.5	25.7	24.9	27.1	26.2
0-9	CASE	3641	1201	1585	523	131	89	56	21	35
0-9	MEANDOSE	20.6	0.0	2.7	20.0	68.0	147.3	241.0	340.4	505.2
0-9	MEAN AGE	4.4	4.4	4.4	4.5	4.3	4.8	4.2	4.1	4.1
10-19	CASE	3386	976	1433	382	180	224	102	32	57
10-19	MEANDOSE	36.5	0.0	2.6	22.1	70.3	147.5	244.6	330.7	527.0
10-19	MEAN AGE	13.8	13.5	13.7	13.7	14.6	15.2	15.4	14.9	14.5
20-34	CASE	1443	436	494	168	107	117	72	27	22
20-34	MEANDOSE	48.0	0.0	2.4	25.2	74.5	143.1	248.5	343.7	540.7
20-34	MEAN AGE	27.9	28.2	27.9	27.6	26.7	27.5	28.9	28.4	27.9
35-49	CASE	2474	822	906	314	155	130	62	35	50
35-49	MEANDOSE	37.9	0.0	2.5	23.8	74.0	144.4	242.0	342.3	536.3
35-49	MEAN AGE	42.6	42.8	42.8	42.5	42.3	42.0	42.0	42.7	41.0
50+	CASE	2022	716	822	276	85	63	27	11	22
50+	MEANDOSE	22.9	0.0	2.5	22.5	71.2	147.3	243.7	350.2	553.4
50+	MEAN AGE	57.8	58.1	58.1	57.7	57.0	55.6	54.1	53.3	56.0

Table 26–L

Hiroshima Only, Females Only

REPORT 10TH CROSS TABLE   HIROSHIMA

SEX : FEMALE

AGE ATB		TOTAL	0	1-9	10-49	50-99	100-199	200-299	300-399	400+
						T65DR				
TOTAL	CASE	35599	16314	8992	6684	1757	977	377	225	273
TOTAL	MEANDOSE	21.0	0.0	3.2	22.1	70.5	139.3	242.9	346.6	518.4
TOTAL	MEAN AGE	29.8	29.8	29.5	30.3	31.1	28.7	28.3	26.6	27.5
0-9	CASE	5613	2621	1519	1014	229	128	51	22	29
0-9	MEANDOSE	17.0	0.0	3.0	21.9	70.1	136.7	244.3	346.7	521.4
0-9	MEAN AGE	3.8	3.9	3.7	3.7	3.9	4.3	4.0	3.2	4.1
10-19	CASE	6491	3020	1589	1156	291	217	84	71	63
10-19	MEANDOSE	24.6	0.0	3.3	21.4	72.3	137.8	248.1	341.6	531.7
10-19	MEAN AGE	15.2	15.2	15.2	15.2	15.3	14.9	15.3	14.0	16.0
20-34	CASE	8984	4011	2329	1657	480	253	98	59	97
20-34	MEANDOSE	23.1	0.0	3.3	22.2	70.9	142.5	244.0	347.4	505.6
20-34	MEAN AGE	26.8	26.8	26.8	26.8	26.6	26.3	25.7	26.3	25.3
35-49	CASE	8914	4029	2140	1803	462	267	100	51	62
35-49	MEANDOSE	21.3	0.0	3.2	22.4	69.2	138.8	239.4	350.6	517.0
35-49	MEAN AGE	41.6	41.7	41.5	41.6	41.7	41.6	41.3	41.7	42.3
50+	CASE	5597	2633	1415	1054	295	112	44	22	22
50+	MEANDOSE	16.8	0.0	3.2	22.2	70.3	138.7	236.4	351.0	536.5
50+	MEAN AGE	58.9	58.9	59.4	58.5	58.2	57.8	57.2	56.4	59.0

Table 26–M

Nagasaki Only, Females Only

REPORT 10TH CROSS TABLE   NAGASAKI

SEX : FEMALE

AGE ATB		TOTAL	0	1-9	10-49	50-99	100-199	200-299	300-399	400+
						T65DR				
TOTAL	CASE	17795	5453	7684	2371	784	765	403	144	191
TOTAL	MEANDOSE	27.3	0.0	2.6	20.5	70.9	147.6	243.2	346.9	528.2
TOTAL	MEAN AGE	26.6	26.9	27.4	26.4	24.4	23.3	22.7	23.8	23.3
0-9	CASE	3664	1221	1574	533	143	85	48	19	41
0-9	MEANDOSE	21.2	0.0	2.7	20.3	67.6	145.6	243.1	355.5	540.7
0-9	MEAN AGE	4.4	4.5	4.4	4.5	4.6	4.4	4.2	4.8	4.9
10-19	CASE	4167	1165	1629	507	252	339	180	47	48
10-19	MEANDOSE	40.5	0.0	2.7	21.3	73.3	149.0	243.3	346.1	515.9
10-19	MEAN AGE	14.5	14.3	14.4	14.1	15.0	15.3	15.4	15.2	14.9
20-34	CASE	4018	1182	1738	532	190	183	94	44	55
20-34	MEANDOSE	30.6	0.0	2.6	21.0	71.3	148.0	244.3	339.5	519.4
20-34	MEAN AGE	26.4	26.4	26.5	26.9	26.6	24.8	24.7	24.6	25.3
35-49	CASE	3489	1055	1614	488	120	99	55	23	35
35-49	MEANDOSE	21.9	0.0	2.6	20.1	68.7	141.7	243.5	356.6	531.9
35-49	MEAN AGE	41.8	41.7	42.0	41.6	41.4	42.6	41.3	40.4	41.4
50+	CASE	2457	830	1129	311	79	59	26	11	12
50+	MEANDOSE	16.4	0.0	2.6	19.5	71.2	151.4	239.0	344.8	563.8
50+	MEAN AGE	59.1	59.3	58.8	59.4	59.6	58.8	60.2	56.2	58.3

Doses are shielded kerma doses, given in cGys or rads. Except for dose–ranges in the column headed "T65DR", all doses refer to the DS86 dosimetry. To the left of RERF's table, we have added the dose–group legends which apply to the column marked "DS86, cGy".

If we consider Dose–Group 2–A, as an example, this table shows that RERF plans to compose the new 2–A cohort for Hiroshima as follows: 4,898 persons transferred from the Dose–Group 1 cohort of the T65DR database, plus 7,716 persons already in the Dose–Group 2–A cohort in the T65DR database, plus 130 persons transferred from the Dose–Group 2–B cohort of the T65DR database, plus one person transferred from the Dose–Group 3–A cohort of the T65DR database.

MEAN DOSE DS86

CITY : HIROSHIMA

Legend	DS86 (cGy)	T65DR	SUBJECT	TOTAL	NEUT	GAMMA
	TOTAL	TOTAL	51390	18.4	0.6	17.8
	TOTAL	0	25244	0.2	0.0	0.2
	TOTAL	1-5	8903	3.3	0.0	3.2
	TOTAL	6-9	1984	7.9	0.1	7.8
	TOTAL	10-19	4904	14.1	0.2	13.9
	TOTAL	20-49	4684	31.6	0.5	31.1
	TOTAL	50-99	2670	58.7	1.4	57.4
	TOTAL	100-199	1642	105.0	3.3	101.8
	TOTAL	200-299	595	172.3	6.8	165.5
	TOTAL	300-399	328	241.0	11.0	230.0
	TOTAL	400+	436	385.2	22.3	362.8
	0	TOTAL	20346	0.0	0.0	0.0
	0	0	20346	0.0	0.0	0.0
	0	1-5				
Dose–Group 1	0	6-9				
	0	10-19				
	0	20-49				
	0	50-99				
	0	100-199				
	0	200-299				
	0	300-399				
	0	400+				
	1-5	TOTAL	12745	2.0	0.0	2.0
	1-5	0	4898	0.8	0.0	0.8
	1-5	1-5	7716	2.7	0.0	2.7
	1-5	6-9	130	4.8	0.0	4.8
Dose–Group 2–A	1-5	10-19	1	5.1	0.1	5.0
	1-5	20-49				
	1-5	50-99				
	1-5	100-199				
	1-5	200-299				
	1-5	300-399				
	1-5	400+				
	6-9	TOTAL	3376	7.2	0.1	7.2
	6-9	0				
	6-9	1-5	1074	6.2	0.0	6.2
	6-9	6-9	1631	7.5	0.1	7.4
Dose–Group 2–B	6-9	10-19	671	8.3	0.1	8.2
	6-9	20-49				
	6-9	50-99				
	6-9	100-199				
	6-9	200-299				
	6-9	300-399				
	6-9	400+				
	10-19	TOTAL	4360	13.8	0.2	13.7
	10-19	0				
	10-19	1-5	113	11.0	0.1	10.9
	10-19	6-9	221	12.3	0.1	12.2
Dose–Group 3–A	10-19	10-19	3668	13.7	0.1	13.5
	10-19	20-49	358	17.5	0.3	17.2
	10-19	50-99				
	10-19	100-199				
	10-19	200-299				
	10-19	300-399				
	10-19	400+				

Continues ---->

Continuation of Table 26-N

Hiroshima: RERF'S Supplementary Data for TR-12-87, Appendix Table 2, for the LSS "Sub-Cohort"

CITY : HIROSHIMA

	DS86	T65DR	SUBJECT	TOTAL	NEUT	GAMMA
	20-49	TOTAL	5407	31.9	0.6	31.3
	20-49	0				
	20-49	1-5				
Dose-Group 3-B	20-49	6-9	2	19.7	0.2	19.5
	20-49	10-19	564	23.6	0.3	23.3
	20-49	20-49	4035	31.0	0.5	30.5
	20-49	50-99	806	42.3	1.0	41.4
	20-49	100-199				
	20-49	200-299				
	20-49	300-399				
	20-49	400+				
	50-99	TOTAL	2911	68.6	1.7	66.9
	50-99	0				
	50-99	1-5				
	50-99	6-9				
Dose-Group 4	50-99	10-19				
	50-99	20-49	291	57.9	1.1	56.8
	50-99	50-99	1806	64.5	1.5	63.0
	50-99	100-199	814	81.6	2.4	79.2
	50-99	200-299				
	50-99	300-399				
	50-99	400+				
	100-199	TOTAL	1422	138.9	4.9	134.0
	100-199	0				
	100-199	1-5				
	100-199	6-9				
Dose-Group 5	100-199	10-19				
	100-199	20-49				
	100-199	50-99	58	107.5	2.7	104.8
	100-199	100-199	819	127.1	4.0	123.1
	100-199	200-299	475	157.1	6.1	151.0
	100-199	300-399	63	176.9	8.1	168.7
	100-199	400+	7	191.4	8.7	182.6
	200-299	TOTAL	483	242.5	11.0	231.4
	200-299	0				
	200-299	1-5				
	200-299	6-9				
Dose-Group 6	200-299	10-19				
	200-299	20-49				
	200-299	50-99				
	200-299	100-199	9	206.8	7.7	199.1
	200-299	200-299	118	231.0	9.4	221.6
	200-299	300-399	214	239.4	10.8	228.6
	200-299	400+	142	258.9	13.0	245.9
	300-399	TOTAL	167	336.9	17.4	319.5
	300-399	0				
	300-399	1-5				
	300-399	6-9				
Dose-Group 7	300-399	10-19				
	300-399	20-49				
	300-399	50-99				
	300-399	100-199				
	300-399	200-299	2	304.9	14.2	290.7
	300-399	300-399	51	327.4	15.5	311.9
	300-399	400+	114	341.7	18.2	323.5
	400+	TOTAL	173	525.3	33.3	492.1
	400+	0				
	400+	1-5				
Dose-Group 8	400+	6-9				
	400+	10-19				
	400+	20-49				
	400+	50-99				
	400+	100-199				
	400+	200-299				
	400+	300-399				
	400+	400+	173	525.3	33.3	492.1

Table 26–"O"

Nagasaki: RERF'S Supplementary Data for TR–12–87, Appendix Table 2, for the LSS "Sub-Cohort"

Doses are shielded kerma doses, given in cGys or rads. Except for dose-ranges in the column headed "T65DR", all doses refer to the DS86 dosimetry. To the left of RERF's table, we have added the dose-group legends which apply to the column marked "DS86, cGy".

MEAN DOSE DS86

CITY : NAGASAKI

	DS86 (cGy)	T65DR	SUBJECT	TOTAL	NEUT	GAMMA
	TOTAL	TOTAL	24601	11.6	0.1	11.5
	TOTAL	0	9431	0.0	0.0	0.0
	TOTAL	1-5	8744	0.4	0.0	0.4
	TOTAL	6-9	1069	2.5	0.0	2.5
	TOTAL	10-19	1702	5.4	0.0	5.4
	TOTAL	20-49	1165	15.0	0.0	14.9
	TOTAL	50-99	953	33.5	0.2	33.3
	TOTAL	100-199	667	71.2	0.5	70.6
	TOTAL	200-299	426	116.7	1.1	115.6
	TOTAL	300-399	175	178.4	2.0	176.3
	TOTAL	400+	269	342.2	5.0	337.2
	0	TOTAL	13926	0.0	0.0	0.0
	0	0	9431	0.0	0.0	0.0
	0	1-5	4495	0.0	0.0	0.0
	0	6-9				
Dose-Group 1	0	10-19				
	0	20-49				
	0	50-99				
	0	100-199				
	0	200-299				
	0	300-399				
	0	400+				
	1-5	TOTAL	6447	1.8	0.0	1.8
	1-5	0				
	1-5	1-5	4249	0.9	0.0	0.9
	1-5	6-9	1069	2.5	0.0	2.5
Dose-Group 2-A	1-5	10-19	1124	4.3	0.0	4.3
	1-5	20-49	5	5.2	0.0	5.2
	1-5	50-99				
	1-5	100-199				
	1-5	200-299				
	1-5	300-399				
	1-5	400+				
	6-9	TOTAL	753	7.2	0.0	7.2
	6-9	0				
	6-9	1-5				
	6-9	6-9				
Dose-Group 2-B	6-9	10-19	506	6.8	0.0	6.8
	6-9	20-49	247	8.1	0.0	8.1
	6-9	50-99				
	6-9	100-199				
	6-9	200-299				
	6-9	300-399				
	6-9	400+				
	10-19	TOTAL	812	14.1	0.0	14.1
	10-19	0				
	10-19	1-5				
	10-19	6-9				
Dose-Group 3-A	10-19	10-19	72	11.1	0.0	11.1
	10-19	20-49	676	14.1	0.0	14.1
	10-19	50-99	64	17.5	0.1	17.4
	10-19	100-199				
	10-19	200-299				
	10-19	300-399				
	10-19	400+				

Continues ----->

Continuation of Table 26-O

Nagasaki: RERF'S Supplementary Data for TR-12-87, Appendix Table 2, for the LSS "Sub-Cohort"

CITY : NAGASAKI

	DS86	T65DR	SUBJECT	TOTAL	NEUT	GAMMA
	20-49	TOTAL	1151	31.6	0.2	31.4
	20-49	0				
	20-49	1-5				
	20-49	6-9				
Dose-Group 3-B	20-49	10-19				
	20-49	20-49	237	24.8	0.1	24.7
	20-49	50-99	805	32.1	0.2	32.0
	20-49	100-199	109	42.2	0.3	41.9
	20-49	200-299				
	20-49	300-399				
	20-49	400+				
	50-99	TOTAL	705	72.2	0.6	71.7
	50-99	0				
	50-99	1-5				
	50-99	6-9				
	50-99	10-19				
Dose-Group 4	50-99	20-49				
	50-99	50-99	84	58.8	0.3	58.4
	50-99	100-199	479	70.0	0.5	69.5
	50-99	200-299	140	87.5	0.9	86.7
	50-99	300-399	2	96.5	1.0	95.5
	50-99	400+				
	100-199	TOTAL	524	137.0	1.4	135.6
	100-199	0				
	100-199	1-5				
	100-199	6-9				
Dose-Group 5	100-199	10-19				
	100-199	20-49				
	100-199	50-99				
	100-199	100-199	79	118.0	0.9	117.0
	100-199	200-299	273	126.9	1.2	125.7
	100-199	300-399	134	159.0	1.8	157.2
	100-199	400+	38	171.3	2.4	168.9
	200-299	TOTAL	154	241.7	2.9	238.7
	200-299	0				
	200-299	1-5				
	200-299	6-9				
Dose-Group 6	200-299	10-19				
	200-299	20-49				
	200-299	50-99				
	200-299	100-199				
	200-299	200-299	13	217.4	2.2	215.2
	200-299	300-399	38	247.2	2.7	244.5
	200-299	400+	103	242.7	3.1	239.6
	300-399	TOTAL	44	342.2	4.8	337.4
	300-399	0				
	300-399	1-5				
	300-399	6-9				
Dose-Group 7	300-399	10-19				
	300-399	20-49				
	300-399	50-99				
	300-399	100-199				
	300-399	200-299				
	300-399	300-399	1	317.8	3.8	314.0
	300-399	400+	43	342.8	4.8	337.9
	400+	TOTAL	85	539.0	8.5	530.5
	400+	0				
	400+	1-5				
	400+	6-9				
Dose-Group 8	400+	10-19				
	400+	20-49				
	400+	50-99				
	400+	100-199				
	400+	200-299				
	400+	300-399				
	400+	400+	85	539.0	8.5	530.5

Cancer-Rate versus Dose : Significance Tests
Cancer Difference Method of Chapter 13

Chi-square analysis is used here to ascertain whether or not observed differences in cancer-rates (Chapter 13) are significant. Comparisons are made for various levels of exposure contrasted with the Reference-Class. The four-fold table for determination of Chi-Square is demonstrated below for the contrast between Low-Dose Exposed (Group 3) and the Reference-Class (Group 1+2). The same type of table and equation is used for all other contrasts. The contrasts are all summarized in Table 27-A.

Demonstration

Low-Dose Exposed (Group 3) versus Reference-Class. All data are from Table 13-A.

	Reference-Class	Low-Dose Exposed	
	a	b	a+b
Cancer Deaths	4297.08	1063.97	5361.05
	c	d	c+d
Persons	66028	14943	80971
	a+c	b+d	N
	70325.08	16006.97	86332.05

$$\text{Chi-square} = \frac{(N)[(ad-bc)^2]}{(a+b)(a+c)(b+d)(c+d)}$$

$$= \frac{3.15010E+18}{4.88651E+17} = 6.45$$

Degrees of freedom	Chi-square	p value	
1	6.45	p < 0.02	(Two-tailed test)
		p = 0.01	(One-tailed test)

Table 27-A :

Significance Tests for Elevation of Cancer-Rates at Different Levels of Exposure
Cancer Difference Method of Chapter 13

Reference-Class (Dose-Group(1+2)): T65DR Dose = 0.659 cSv ; DS86 Dose = 0.875 cSv. versus following dose-classes:

Dose-Group Contrasted	T65DR in cSv	DS86 in cSv	Persons	Cancer Deaths	Chi-Square	Two-tailed Test	One-tailed Test
Low-Dose: Group 3	10.994	14.564	14943	1063.97	6.45	p < 0.02	p < 0.01
Group (3+4)	16.365	20.309	19168	1369.74	8.50	p < 0.01	p < 0.01
All:(3+4+5+6+7+8)	41.673	47.388	25203	1918.67	30.46	p << 0.01	p << 0.01
Mid-Dose: (4+5)	50.653	54.924	7353	567.36	13.54	p < 0.01	p < 0.01
High-Dose:(5+6+7+8)	122.056	133.397	6035	548.93	50.58	p << 0.01	p << 0.01
Groups (6+7+8)	176.662	197.054	2907	287.34	43.50	p << 0.01	p << 0.01

NOTES ----

1. All data are from Table 13-A. Data set is normalized. Persons are unchanged
   from raw values. Cancer deaths, normalized, insure age distribution and
   sex-ratio are identical across all dose-classes studied.
   Normalization procedure has changed the number of cancer deaths so little that
   influence on Chi-Square testing is negligible. In general, normalization
   has operated to make it more difficult, not less, to prove significance.
---
2. Two-tailed test evaluates probability that the null hypothesis of no difference
   in cancer death-rate between Exposed-Class and Reference-Class can be rejected.
---
3. One-tailed test evaluates probability that the null hypothesis of no higher
   cancer death-rate in Exposed-Class can be rejected.
---
4. Preston and co-workers (Pr86, TABLE A3-7) state that the testing for higher
   cancer death-rate in Dose-Group 3 versus Dose-Group 1 gives a p = 0.0152 for
   a one-tailed test. This is in good agreement with the findings presented
   here for Low-Dose Exposed (Dose-Group 3) for the same follow-up period,
   1950-1982.

Conclusions: Since the T65DR organ-dose for Dose-Group 3 is 10.994 cSv,
it can be stated that it has been proved that there is a significant
increase in cancer death-rate for 10.994 cSv in this dosimetry.

Since the DS86 organ-dose for Dose-Group 3 is 14.564 cSv, it can
be stated that it has been proved that there is a significant increase
in cancer death-rate for 14.564 cSv dose in this dosimetry.

90% Confidence Limits for Minimum and Lifetime Fatal Cancer-Yields

In Chapter 13 the Minimum and Lifetime Fatal Cancer-Yields were estimated for the overall A-Bomb Survivor Study, including both cities, both sexes, and all five age-bands, using the Cancer Difference Method. In this Chapter the method for determination of the 90% confidence limits on those Cancer-Yields will be described, and the results presented in Table 27-B.

The Cancer Difference Method uses the following equation in comparing two dose-classes (e.g. The Low-Dose Exposed (Group 3) and the Reference-Class):

$$\text{Minimum Fatal Cancer-Yield} = \frac{\text{Difference in Cancer-Rates between Dose-Classes}}{\text{Difference in Organ-Dose between Dose-Classes}}$$

The most important determinant of the 90% confidence limits for the Fatal Cancer-Yield rests upon the magnitude of the sampling error in the numerator of this equation, namely, upon the error in the difference in cancer-rates. The error in the denominator is very small by comparison, and will not be taken into account here in determination of the confidence limits.

We shall approach the magnitude of the error in the difference in cancer-rates by a pair-wise comparison of the ratio of cancer-rates. The method will be developed using the data for Low-Dose Exposed Group and the Reference-Group. Then the method can be applied for the other dose-group comparisons.

From Chapter 13 (Table 13-A) we have the following data:

Dose-Classes	Persons	Cancer-Deaths	T65DR Dose (cSv)	DS86 Dose (cSv)
REFERENCE-CLASS (Dose-group 1+2)	66028	4297.08	0.659	0.875
LOW-DOSE EXPOSED: Group 3	14943	1063.97	10.994	14.564
GROUPS (3+4)	19168	1369.74	16.365	20.309
ALL: (3+4+5+6+7+8)	25203	1918.67	41.673	47.388
MID-DOSE: (4+5)	7353	567.36	50.653	54.924
HIGH-DOSE:(5+6+7+8)	6035	548.93	122.056	133.397
GROUPS (6+7+8)	2907	287.34	176.662	197.054

The 90% Confidence Limits on Ratio of Cancer-Rates

A cancer-rate is a proportion. When n = population size; $\bar{p}$ = fraction dying of cancer; and $\bar{q}$ = fraction not dying of cancer, then we can write (Run85) :

$$\text{Estimated standard error of proportion} = \left[\frac{(\bar{p})(\bar{q})}{n}\right]^{0.5} \quad \text{Equation(1)}$$

For simplicity in notation, we shall use p for $\bar{p}$ (p-bar), and q for $\bar{q}$ (q-bar).

===

For Low–Dose Exposed versus Reference–Class, Equation (1) yields ;

Dose– Class	Persons	Cancer– Deaths	p	q	S.E. of p
Low–Dose Exposed	14943	1063.97	0.071202	0.928798	0.002104
Reference	66028	4297.08	0.065080	0.934920	0.000960

Since p is the "cancer–rate per person," it follows that the ratio of cancer–rates (Low–Dose Exposed / Reference) = the ratio of p values.

Cancer–rate ratio = 0.071202 / 0.065080 = 1.094073

We need the standard error of this ratio, and this is obtained in terms of the fractional errors of the numerator and denominator. We obtain this S.E. with Equation (2), (Lie60) .

Equation (2) follows:
Fractional S.E. of quotient = [(Fract. S.E. of numerator)^2 + (Fract. S.E. of denominator)^2]^0.5

The fractional S.E. is the (S.E. of p) / p, so for the ratio of cancer–rates, (0.071202 / 0.065080), we use the tabulation above to find that :

Fract. S.E. (numerator) =	0.002104 / 0.071202 =	0.029546
Fract. S.E. (denominator)=	0.000960 / 0.065080 =	0.014750

Fract. S.E. of ratio = [(0.029546)^2 + (0.014750)^2]^0.5 =   0.033023

But we need the absolute error of the ratio of cancer–rates.
Since the ratio of cancer–rates = 1.094073, it follows that
Absolute S.E. of cancer–rate ratio = (0.033023)(1.094073) =   0.036130

The 90% confidence limits are obtained from use of (1.645 x S.E.).
Therefore,
 High 90% Confidence Limit = 1.094073 + (1.645)(0.036130) =   1.153506
 Low 90% Confidence Limit = 1.094073 – (1.645)(0.036130) =   1.034640

Now we can convert our cancer–rates per person (p values) to the
familiar terms of Chapter 13, namely cancer–rates per 10,000 persons.
For the Reference–Class; 10000 x p = 10000 x 0.065080 =   650.7966
For the Low–Dose Exposed; 10000 x p = 10000 x 0.071202 =   712.0190
Difference in cancer–rates = 712.012 – 650.7966 =   61.222

For the High 90% confidence limit , the cancer–rate for the
Low–dose Exposed Class = 1.153506 x 650.7966 =   750.698
Difference in cancer–rates (for High 90% confidence limit) =
Low–dose Exposed – Reference = 750.698 – 650.7966 =   99.901

For the Low 90% confidence limit, the cancer–rate for the
Low–dose Exposed Class = 1.034640 x 650.7966 =   673.340
Difference in cancer–rates (for Low 90% confidence limit) =
Low–dose Exposed – Reference = 673.340 – 650.7966 =   22.543

To obtain the Minimum Fatal Cancer Yields, the Difference in Cancer Rates must be divided by the Difference in doses between classes compared.

===

Difference in doses for Low–Dose Exposed minus Reference (data above);

	In T65DR Dosimetry Neutron RBE = 2	In DS86 Dosimetry Neutron RBE = 20
Dose Difference	10.335 cSv	13.689 cSv

Minimum Fatal Cancer Yields and 90% Confidence Limits: T65DR Dosimetry
----

    Minimum Fatal Cancer–Yield = 61.222 / 10.335 =   5.92
    High 90% Limit, Cancer–Yield = 99.901 / 10.335 =   9.67
    Low 90% Limit, Cancer–Yield = 22.543 / 10.335 =   2.18

Minimum Fatal Cancer Yields and 90% Confidence Limits: In DS86 Dosimetry
----

    Minimum Fatal Cancer–Yield = 61.222 / 13.689 =   4.47
    High 90% Limit, Cancer–Yield = 99.901 / 13.689 =   7.30
    Low 90% Limit, Cancer–Yield = 22.543 / 13.689 =   1.65

===

   The results just obtained are transferred to Table 27–B. The method used to obtain 90% confidence limits for the Cancer–Yields is precisely the same for other exposed dose categories as it was above for the Low–Dose Exposed (Group 3). All the final results are transferred to Table 27–B.

===============================

Table 27-B

Cancer-Yields at Different Levels of Exposure, and Their 90% Confidence Limits

Basis: A-Bomb survivors, 1950-82. (Cities, sexes, ages, and all cancer-sites combined. Leukemia excluded.)
Cancer Difference Method of Chapter 13 provides the Cancer-Yields.

Cancer-Yields are radiation-induced cancer-deaths among 10,000 persons of mixed ages, per cSv of whole-body internal organ-dose. The 90% High and Low Confidence Limits are calculated as described in text.

A	B	C	D	E	F	G	||	H	I	J	K	L	M
	[---- Fatal Cancer-Yield -----] T65DR Dosimetry, Neutron RBE = 2.						||	[---- Fatal Cancer-Yield ----] DS86 Dosimetry, Neutron RBE = 20					
Basis for Cancer-Yield / Row	Ref. vs. 11 cSv	Ref. vs. 16 cSv	Ref. vs. 42 cSv	Ref. vs. 51 cSv	Ref. vs. 122 cSv	Ref. vs. 177 cSv	||	Ref. vs. 15 cSv	Ref. vs. 20 cSv	Ref. vs. 47 cSv	Ref. vs. 55 cSv	Ref. vs. 133 cSv	Ref. vs. 197 cSv
1 MINIMUM FATAL CANCER-YIELD "IN THE BOX"	5.92	4.06	2.69	2.42	2.13	1.92	||	4.47	3.28	2.38	2.24	1.95	1.72
High 90% C.L.	9.67	6.30	3.50	3.51	2.67	2.45	||	7.30	5.09	3.09	3.24	2.44	2.20
Low 90% C.L.	2.18	1.82	1.89	1.33	1.60	1.38	||	1.65	1.47	1.66	1.23	1.46	1.24
2 MINIMUM FATAL CANCER-YIELD IN THE BOX" Corrected for Underascert.	7.29	5.00	3.31	2.97	2.62	2.36	||	5.50	4.04	2.92	2.75	2.40	2.12
High 90% C.L.	11.89	7.75	4.31	4.32	3.28	3.01	||	8.98	6.26	3.80	3.99	3.00	2.71
Low 90% C.L.	2.68	2.24	2.32	1.64	1.97	1.70	||	2.03	1.81	2.04	1.51	1.80	1.53
3 LIFETIME FATAL CANCER-YIELD	13.17	9.03	5.99	5.37	4.74	4.26	||	9.94	7.30	5.28	4.97	4.34	3.83
High 90% C.L.	21.50	14.00	7.78	7.80	5.94	5.45	||	16.23	11.32	6.87	7.20	5.42	4.89
Low 90% C.L.	4.85	4.05	4.20	2.96	3.56	3.07	||	3.67	3.27	3.69	2.73	3.25	2.76
4 LIFETIME FATAL CANCER-YIELD Corrected for Underascert.	16.20	11.11	7.37	6.61	5.83	5.25	||	12.23	8.98	6.50	6.11	5.34	4.71
High 90% C.L.	26.44	17.23	9.57	9.60	7.30	6.70	||	19.96	13.92	8.45	8.86	6.67	6.02
Low 90% C.L.	5.96	4.98	5.17	3.64	4.37	3.77	||	4.51	4.02	4.54	3.36	3.99	3.39

1. The basic input data for calculation of Cancer-Yields and for calculation of 90% confidence limits are provided in Table 13-A of Chapter 13.

2. The Minimum and Lifetime Fatal Cancer-Yields of this table are taken from Table 13-B of Chapter 13. Those Yields were calculated by the Cancer Difference Method.

3. The procedure used to calculate high and low 90% confidence limits is that described in the text of this chapter.

4. The central values above represent the best estimates from the Cancer Difference Method, prior to regression analysis. There is, of course, sampling variation in every database. The 90 % confidence-limits on the values above are calculated here. It is neither scientifically nor socially responsible to select the lowest value in a confidence-range for use, or the highest value either. The appropriate value to use is the one most likely to be right: The obtained value.

Estimated Spontaneous Cancer–Mortality in the A–Bomb Reference Group, for a Completed Lifespan Follow–Up

At any stage of a lifespan follow-up, there necessarily exists some ratio between the cumulative cancer death-rate in an irradiated population and the cumulative spontaneous rate in an unexposed Reference Group. Whether or not the risk-ratio of (exposed rate / spontaneous rate) is constant for the entire follow-up, or variable, is one of the important questions which the A-Bomb Study is going to answer by the time it is complete, decades from now.

Meanwhile, analysts can examine the evidence at hand from the incomplete follow-up. Having done that in Chapter 17, we find that the risk-ratio of (exposed rate over spontaneous rate) is approximately constant so far, even in age-bands where the spontaneous rate has been tripling, six-folding, ten-folding. Therefore, we will make the assumption that the risk-ratio will continue to be approximately constant, since the evidence in this study so far justifies no other.

Of course, this assumption about the future becomes useful in estimating exposed rates only when one has an estimate of the corresponding SPONTANEOUS rates. The purpose of this chapter is to use existing observations, by age-sex subsets in the A-bomb Reference Group, in order to estimate how many spontaneous cancer deaths are likely to occur in the Reference Group by the time the full lifespan follow-up is complete.

The Input Data and Key Assumption about Spontaneous Rates :
==

Table 28-A describes the relevant observations in the Reference Group from 1950-1982. It should be noted that each age-sex subset entered the follow-up, in 1950, five years older than the age at the time of bombing (ATB). And, at the end of the 1950-82 follow-up, survivors in each group were 32 years older than they had been in 1950.

Our approach is to ask, how many additional spontaneous cancer deaths will occur in each age-sex subset during the NEXT 32-year follow-up period, from 1982-2014, and for the final follow-up period beyond? Our key assumption will be that those entering the 1982-2014 follow-up period at a specific age, say 41 years of age, will show the same mortality rates during the current 32-year follow-up period as those who entered the 1950-1982 follow-up at age 41.

Obviously, it is not possible for anyone to know what all the future trends will be, by birth cohort, in mortality rates. Our approach shares the general uncertainties. Only time will tell whether tying our estimate to the experience of the A-bomb survivors will make it better, or worse, than an estimate tied to the general Japanese population.

We shall use the males who were 0-9 years old ATB to demonstrate our method. Their mean age as they enter the 1982-2014 follow-up is 9 years (Table 28-A, Column C) plus 32 years, or 41 years old. Column C shows that no male age-band had a mean age of 41 at entry to the 1950-1982 follow-up. Therefore, we have no ready-made pattern to copy, but interpolation from the existing observations can provide it. The needed information is in Table 28-B (for males) and Table 28-C (for females).

Summary :
==

The same method has been used to estimate the number of spontaneous cancers which will occur in the other nine age-sex subsets of the A-bomb Reference Group, by the time the lifespan follow-up is complete.

Table 28-D, Column G, shows the estimated fraction of each age-band which will die of cancer after 1950. These fractions apply to the A-bomb population from 1950 onwards, not to any groups from birth onwards. These are the values we want, since the issue to be analyzed is the effect on spontaneous cancer-rates of irradiation not at BIRTH, but rather at various older ages.

Table 28-D, Row 13, Column G, suggests that -- for the group as a whole -- the fraction of all deaths beyond 1950 which will be spontaneous cancer-deaths is 14.5 percent.

Demonstration follows on next page.

===

DEMONSTRATION OF THE CALCULATIONS FOR MALES 0-9 YEARS ATB :
===

October 1950 – October 1982

We start the 1950–82 follow–up with 6818 persons (Table 28–A, Col.D).
For the 1950–82 interval, Table 28–B incorporates Table 28–A:

Total deaths =	0.0484 of the starting number in 1950.	
Cancer deaths =	0.07576 x deaths in the 1950–82 interval.	

Therefore, total deaths = 0.0484 x 6818 =   329.9912   (1950–82).
And, cancer deaths = 0.07576 x 329.9912 =   25.00013   (1950–82).

Survivors: 6818 – 329.9912 =   6488.008   persons alive in 1982.

October 1982 – October 2014

The mean age of this group, as it enters the 1982–2014 follow–up, is
about 9+32 = 41 years. (This is approximately correct, but not
exactly so, because of differential death–rates within the group's
age–span.)

For age 41 years, we get from Table 28–B, the following for 1982–2014:
          Total deaths =   0.477944 of the starting number in 1982.
          Cancer deaths =   0.247752 x deaths in the 1982–2014 interval.
Total deaths = 0.477944 x 6488.008   =   3100.904   (1982–2014).
And, cancer deaths = 0.247752 x 3100.904 =   768.2551   (1982–2014).

Survivors: 6488.008 – 3100.904 =   3387.104   persons alive in 2014.

Late 2014 and Beyond

In 2014, the mean age of the group is about 41+32 = 73 years.
For age 73 years at "entry," we get the following from Table 28–B:
          Total deaths =   ALL of the persons in the next 32 years.
          Cancer deaths =   0.0893 x deaths in the interval.
Therefore, total deaths = 3387.104 x 1.0 =   3387.104
Cancer deaths =   0.0893 x 3387.104   =   302.4683

The Sum of Estimated Cancer–Deaths

Now we add up all the cancer–deaths for the entire period (during
which all of the initial persons have died of one cause or another).

Total cancer deaths =   25.00013 + 768.2551 + 302.4683 =   1095.723
And since there were 6818 persons at the start, the fraction dying of
cancer = 1095.723 / 6818 =   0.160710 .

The total cancer deaths (1095.723) and the fraction dying of cancer
(0.16071) are transferred to Table 28–D, Columns C and D, as entries
for the original 0–9 year old males ATB.

Table 28-A
Total Deaths and Cancer-Deaths in the Reference Group, Cumulative from 1950 Through 1982.

Col.A Age-Band ATB	Col.B True Mean Age ATB	Col.C Mean Age at Entry in 1950	Col.D Initial Persons in 1950	Col.E All Deaths 1950-82	Col.F Fraction Dead of All Causes	Col.G Persons Still Alive, 1982	Col.H Cancer Deaths	Col.I Cancer over Total Deaths	Col.J Cancer-Deaths per10K Initial Persons
MALES				**MALES**			**MALES**		
0 - 9	4.16	9 years	6818	330	0.048401	6488	25	0.07575	36.67
10-19	13.95	19 years	6378	748	0.117278	5630	113	0.15106	177.17
20-34	28.04	33 years	3293	884	0.268448	2409	224	0.25339	680.23
35-49	42.61	48 years	5999	3967	0.661276	2032	963	0.24275	1605.27
50+	58.14	63 years	5097	4957	0.972532	140	747	0.15069	1465.57
FEMALES				**FEMALES**			**FEMALES**		
0 - 9	4.08	9 years	6935	193	0.027829	6742	38	0.19689	54.79
10-19	14.90	20 years	7403	476	0.064298	6927	116	0.24369	156.69
20-34	26.69	32 years	9260	1233	0.133153	8027	396	0.32116	427.65
35-49	41.71	47 years	8838	3950	0.446933	4888	925	0.23417	1046.62
50+	59.05	64 years	6007	5623	0.936074	384	608	0.10812	1012.15

NOTES -----

1. The data for the Reference Group in Columns B, D, E, and H above are taken from male Table 11-B and female Table 11-D, Rows 17-21. As usual, we treat the combination of Dose-Groups 1+2 as if it were completely unexposed by the bombs, in order to gain the greater stability from larger numbers. We could use either raw or normalized data for this table; by choosing the raw data, we avoid some fractional persons until the final table (Table 28-D).

2. Col.C entries = (Col.B plus the 5-year interval from 1945 to 1950).
   Col.F entries = (Col.E / Col.D).
   Col.G entries = (Col.D minus Col.E).
   Col.I entries = (Col.H / Col.E).
   Col.J entries = (Col.H / Col.D) x (10,000). Column J is included merely as a reminder of the very great impact of age during a follow-up on the cumulative cancer-rates which will be observed in an UNexposed group.

Table 28-B :
Males : Average Fraction Dead and Average Ratio of Cancer–Deaths to Total Deaths
(For A 32–Year Period with Entry into Follow–Up at Listed Age).

Male A-Bomb Reference Group (Part 1)				Male A-Bomb Reference Group (Part 2)		
Age at Entry into Follow-Up	Fraction Dead 32 Years Later	Cancer- Deaths / Total Deaths		Age at Entry into Follow-Up	Fraction Dead 32 Years Later	Cancer- Deaths / Total Deaths
9	0.0484	0.07576 ***		43	0.53033	0.24634
10	0.05529	0.083294		44	0.556523	0.245634
11	0.06218	0.090828		45	0.582716	0.244928
12	0.06907	0.098362		46	0.608909	0.244222
13	0.07596	0.105896		47	0.635102	0.243516
14	0.08285	0.11343		48	0.6613	0.2428 ***
15	0.08974	0.120964		49	0.682046	0.23666
16	0.09663	0.128498		50	0.702792	0.23052
17	0.10352	0.136032		51	0.723538	0.22438
18	0.11041	0.143566		52	0.744284	0.21824
19	0.1173	0.1511 ***		53	0.76503	0.2121
20	0.128092	0.158407		54	0.785776	0.20596
21	0.138884	0.165714		55	0.806522	0.19982
22	0.149676	0.173021		56	0.827268	0.19368
23	0.160468	0.180328		57	0.848014	0.18754
24	0.17126	0.187635		58	0.86876	0.1814
25	0.182052	0.194942		59	0.889506	0.17526
26	0.192844	0.202249		60	0.910252	0.16912
27	0.203636	0.209556		61	0.930998	0.16298
28	0.214428	0.216863		62	0.951744	0.15684
29	0.22522	0.22417		63	0.9725	0.1507 ***
30	0.236012	0.231477		64	0.993246	0.14456
31	0.246804	0.238784		65	1	0.13842
32	0.257596	0.246091		66	1	0.13228
33	0.2684	0.2534 ***		67	1	0.12614
34	0.294593	0.252694		68	1	0.12
35	0.320786	0.251988		69	1	0.11386
36	0.346979	0.251282		70	1	0.10772
37	0.373172	0.250576		71	1	0.10158
38	0.399365	0.24987		72	1	0.09544
39	0.425558	0.249164		73	1	0.0893
40	0.451751	0.248458		74	1	0.08316
41	0.477944	0.247752		75	1	0.07702
42	0.504137	0.247046				

1. Entries marked with (***) are observed data from Table 28-A.
   All other entries are obtained by interpolation between the observed entries.

2. Cancer-fraction entries, beyond 63 years of age at entry to the follow-up, are extrapolated by using the rate of decline between 48 and 63 years of age at entry. This may tend to underestimate the cancer-fraction of total deaths at very advanced ages.

Table 28–C

Females : Average Fraction Dead and Average Ratio of Cancer–Deaths to Total Deaths
(For A 32–Year Period with Entry into Follow–Up at Listed Age).

Age at Entry into Follow–Up	Fraction Dead 32 Years Later	Cancer–Deaths / Total Deaths		Age at Entry into Follow–Up	Fraction Dead 32 Years Later	Cancer–Deaths / Total Deaths
9	0.02783	0.1969 ***		43	0.363251	0.257378
10	0.031145	0.201154		44	0.384169	0.251579
11	0.03446	0.205408		45	0.405087	0.24578
12	0.037775	0.209662		46	0.426005	0.239981
13	0.04109	0.213916		47	0.446933	0.234177 ***
14	0.044405	0.21817		48	0.475706	0.226763
15	0.04772	0.222424		49	0.504479	0.219349
16	0.051035	0.226678		50	0.533252	0.211935
17	0.05435	0.230932		51	0.562025	0.204521
18	0.057665	0.235186		52	0.590798	0.197107
19	0.06098	0.23944		53	0.619571	0.189693
20	0.064298	0.243697 ***		54	0.648344	0.182279
21	0.070048	0.250152		55	0.677117	0.174865
22	0.075798	0.256607		56	0.70589	0.167451
23	0.081548	0.263062		57	0.734663	0.160037
24	0.087298	0.269517		58	0.763436	0.152623
25	0.093048	0.275972		59	0.792209	0.145209
26	0.098798	0.282427		60	0.820982	0.137795
27	0.104548	0.288882		61	0.849755	0.130381
28	0.110298	0.295337		62	0.878528	0.122967
29	0.116048	0.301792		63	0.907301	0.115553
30	0.121798	0.308247		64	0.936074	0.108127 ***
31	0.127548	0.314702		65	0.964751	0.100713
32	0.133153	0.321167 ***		66	0.993428	0.093299
33	0.154071	0.315368		67	1	0.085885
34	0.174989	0.309569		68	1	0.078471
35	0.195907	0.30377		69	1	0.071057
36	0.216825	0.297971		70	1	0.063643
37	0.237743	0.292172		71	1	0.056229
38	0.258661	0.286373		72	1	0.05
39	0.279579	0.280574		73	1	0.05
40	0.300497	0.274775		74	1	0.05
41	0.321415	0.268976		75	1	0.05
42	0.342333	0.263177				

Female A–Bomb Reference Group (Part 1) | | Female A–Bomb Reference Group (Part 2)

1. Entries marked with (***) are observed data from Table 28–A.
   All other entries are obtained by interpolation between the observed entries.

2. Cancer–fraction entries, beyond 64 years of age at entry to the follow–up, are extrapolated by using the rate of decline between 47 and 64 years of age at entry. This may tend to underestimate the cancer–fraction of total deaths at very advanced ages.

Table 28-D

Estimated Spontaneous Cancer Mortality Beyond 1950 in the Reference Group, for a Completed Lifespan Follow-Up.

Row No.	Col.A Age- Band (Years) ATB	Col.B [------- RAW DATABASE Initial Persons Entering in 1950	Col.C Lifetime Spont. Ca-Deaths beyond 1950	Col.D -------] Fraction of Init. Persons Dying of Canc.	Col.E [---------- NORMALIZED Initial Persons Entering in 1950	Col.F DATABASE Lifetime Spont. Ca-Deaths beyond 1950	Col.G -----------] Fraction of Init. Persons Dying of Canc.	Col.H Spont. Cancer- Deaths 1950-82
MALES		**MALES**			**MALES**			
1	0 - 9	6818	1095.723	0.160710	4976.25	799.735	0.160710	18.25
2	10-19	6378	1104.859	0.173230	5312.07	920.208	0.173230	94.11
3	20-34	3293	557.441	0.169281	6644.57	1124.797	0.169281	451.98
4	35-49	5999	1064.814	0.177499	6341.76	1125.653	0.177499	1018.02
5	50+	5097	754.003	0.147931	4310.36	637.635	0.147931	631.71
6		27585			27585.01	4608.028		2214.08
FEMALES		**FEMALES**			**FEMALES**			
7	0 - 9	6935	849.648	0.122516	6935	849.648	0.122516	38
8	10-19	7403	1064.396	0.143779	7403	1064.396	0.143779	116
9	20-34	9260	1234.162	0.133279	9260	1234.162	0.133279	396
10	35-49	8838	1169.435	0.132319	8838	1169.435	0.132319	925
11	50+	6007	627.055	0.104387	6007	627.055	0.104387	608
12		38443			38443	4944.696		2083
13	Totals	66028			66028.01	9552.724	0.144677	4297.08

14   Ratio of estimated Lifetime Spontaneous over 1950-82 Spontaneous: (9552.724 / 4297.08) = 2.223 .

1. The ratio found in Row 14 suggests, for the Reference Group as a whole, that 2.223-fold more spontaneous cancers will occur, between 1950 and COMPLETION of the lifespan follow-up, than the number already observed between 1950 and late 1982. This forward projection is an estimate based on observations internal to the A-Bomb Study itself (see text).

2. The ten entries in Col.C were each calculated as demonstrated in the text of this chapter.

3. The corresponding entries in Col.F differ from those in Col.C only for males, since the Female Reference Group was unchanged by normalization (it provided the standard). The male entries in Col.C are normalized for Col.F in the usual way: (new persons / old persons) x (old value). Thus the entry in Col.F, Row 1, is (4976.25 new persons from Col.E / 6818 old persons from Col.B) x (1095.723 old value from Col.C).

4. The entries in Col.H come from Tables 11-C and 11-E, Rows 72-78. Because this is the Reference Group, the sums in this column (entries H-6, H-12, H-13) persist in Tables 11-G and 11-H.

5. The fractions in Cols.D and G (which do not differ) are all below 20 % .

CHAPTER 29

Curvilinear Regression and Equations of Best Fit

This chapter is arranged in three parts:

1. Raising a Single Dose-Term to a Series of Powers, p.2
2. Plotting Best-Fit Curves as Graphs; Construction of Table 14-D, p.3
3. Testing the Significance of Differences between Regressions, p.3
Then tables.

Introduction:

Because we use curvilinear regression repeatedly in our analyses of dose-response in the A-Bomb Study, this chapter shows the method once in detail. Each dose-response curve, described or depicted in the A-bomb chapters, has been derived in the manner shown in this chapter.

Part 3 of this chapter shows the method for determining whether or not one curve fits the observations SIGNIFICANTLY better than another curve.

Finding the shape of the dose-response relationship, for cancer-rate versus radiation dose, is one of the truly important goals of epidemiological investigation. On a practical basis, knowledge of dose-response shape enables prediction of response (cancer-rate) where interpolation of dose between observations is necessary. Also, knowledge of dose-response may rule out certain proposed mechanisms concerning radiation carcinogenesis itself.

The shape of dose-response is a reality of nature which only the data themselves can reveal. It is not an issue for pre-judgment. The technique of curvilinear regression enables analysts to determine the most probable dose-response shape given the available observations.

"Power Polynomials"

Hayek and Cheetham (Hay87) have provided a very useful discussion of the technique of curvilinear regression and have presented the program for carrying through such regressions in the Lotus 123 spreadsheet.

One commonly used technique of attempting to find the "best fit" curve to a set of datapoints is that of "power polynomials." In this method, one starts with a linear regression of cancer-rate upon dose in cSv, and one determines the value of R-squared (the correlation coefficient squared) for the best linear fit for the relationship of cancer-rate versus dose.

Next, unless the R-squared value is extremely close to 1.000, one may wish to examine whether the true relationship is curvilinear, and not linear. One adds a term in dose-squared (Dose^2) to the regression study, and again performs the regression analysis; details are given by Hayek and Cheetham (Hay87). If there is significant curvilinearity to the relationship, it will be found that R-squared (after adding the dose-squared term to the regression analysis) is significantly increased over what it was when only the linear term was present. If there has been a significant increase in R-squared, we know that the true relationship deserves at least a quadratic term, and so the whole relationship now encompasses a linear term in dose and a squared term in dose.

Next, one adds a term in dose-cubed (Dose^3) to the regression analysis, and determines the R-squared value obtained when all three terms -- Dose^1, Dose^2, and Dose^3 -- are involved in the regression analysis. If R-squared has not been significantly increased by adding the Dose^3 term in the regression analysis, we know that we are not going to get a better fit than that provided by two terms: Dose^1 and Dose^2. On the other hand, if R-squared were significantly increased by the addition of the Dose^3 term, we would go on to test out the regression with a term in Dose^4, etc.

A variety of other methods can also be used to fit curves to observed datapoints. For instance, in Chapter 23, we show that a single basic equation containing both a Dose^1 term and and Dose^2 term can be progressively altered by an exponential modifier (applying to both terms) until the one basic equation manages to produce curves which fit dose-response data having very different shapes indeed.

The point is that there are numerous devices and systems available to analysts in their search for the equation which best fits a set of actual observations.

1. Raising a Single Dose-Term to a Series of Powers

In our study of the dose-response shape for cancer-rate versus dose, we have found it very useful to do a series of regressions for which we systematically change the exponent for dose. In this technique (which will be demonstrated in detail), the dose-term is raised to a series of various powers, from fractional exponents through to powers greater than 1.0.

If in going from one exponent to the next chosen, the R-squared value DECREASES, we know that the goodness-of-fit is poorer than for the previous exponent, and there is no merit in going to even further changes of the exponent in the same direction. On the other hand, if R-squared is increasing with further changes in exponent, we have not yet reached the exponent giving the best fit to the data.

Of course, very small changes in R-squared often are not provably significant. So if there is a slight increase in R-squared as we go from Dose^0.8 to Dose^0.75, and if the increase in R-squared is not provably significant (we shall demonstrate how this can be tested), then we cannot say that Dose^0.75 provides a provably better fit than Dose^0.8.

But in the case of radiation induction of cancer, analysts are intensely interested in testing bigger distinctions. We want to know, for instance, if Dose^2 is truly a poorer choice than Dose^0.7, or truly a better choice. Dose^2 represents the "pure" quadratic choice. Dose^1 represents the "pure" linear choice, and Dose raised to a power less than 1.0 represents a "supra-linear" choice.

A dose raised to a power between 1.0 and 2.0 is for a relationship which is somewhere between purely linear and purely quadratic. Figure 14-C shows that Dose^1.4, for example, gives a dose-response curve whose concave-upward shape is closely similar to shapes which are obtained from using "power polynomials" with a linear term and a positive quadratic term. Thus it is appropriate for us to refer to curves resulting from regression upon Dose^1.4 as equivalent to customary "linear-quadratic" curves for dose-response.

However, when the power polynomial technique is used to fit curves to available observations, a linear-quadratic dose-response can also be concave-DOWNWARD in shape, if the coefficient of the quadratic term turns out to be negative (see Figure 23-H). By contrast, no such ambiguity surrounds the technique of using equations with only one term for dose. The size of the exponent immediately reveals the direction of any bend. If the exponent is greater than 1.0, the curve will be bent concave-upward, and if the exponent is smaller than 1.0, the curve will be bent concave-downward (supra-linear).

Regression Step 1: Assigning Weighting-Factors for Datapoints

Since it is obvious from Table 13-A that the low-dose points are represented by much larger numbers of cancer-deaths than the high-dose observations, it is necessary to give added weight to the low-dose datapoints in determining which equation best fits the data. A reasonable, conservative approach is to calculate the square root of the number of cancer-deaths which give rise to a dose-group's cancer-rate, and to do this for each of the dose-groups (or combined dose-groups). Then the datapoints for cancer-rate can be weighted according the relative size of those square roots.

The appropriate weighting factors, which are the same for both the T65DR and DS86 dosimetries, are determined at the top of Table 29-A. The weighting factor determines the number of entries which a dose-group receives in the input of the regression (Step 2).

Not all regression analyses require Step 1, but weighting is called for if some datapoints are obviously far more reliable than others. (See Gui56, p.425.)

Step 2: Preparing Regression Inputs for Various Dose-Exponents

Table 29-A provides the input data to do nine separate regressions -- one each for nine exponents of dose -- separately for the T65DR and DS86 dosimetries.

For all the regressions, the input for the y-range (the dependent variable) is the column showing the observed cancer-rates.

The input for the x-range is one column of dose-values per regression. In Table 29-A, the column for Dose^1 contains the true dose-values, from Table 13-A. All the other columns of dose-values are simply the true dose raised to the power indicated.

Step 3: Comparing Regression Outputs for the Best Fit of All

Table 29-B provides the output for each of the nine

regression analyses, for the T65DR dosimetry with neutron RBE = 2, in the format provided by the Lotus 123 "Data Regression" commands. Table 29-C provides the equivalent information for the DS86 dosimetry.

In each dosimetry, the maximum value of R-squared is found to occur at an exponent of 0.75, which means that the best fit of all is most likely associated with this exponent. The R-squared values of 0.9831 (T65DR) and 0.9825 (DS86) are very high and indicate a very good fit to the input datapoints. Indeed, these R-squared values are provably different from the R-squared values produced by Dose^1.0, Dose^1.16, Dose^1.4, and Dose^2, as shown by Table 29-D.

Of course, the exponent 0.75 is not provably different from either 0.80 or 0.70, but nonetheless, the best-fitting regression analysis is most likely to be associated with the highest R-squared value. Therefore, from the regression of cancer-rate on Dose^0.75, we extract the X-Coefficient and the Constant to make the equation of best fit.

Equation of best fit for T65DR with neutron RBE = 2 (Table 29-B) :

$$\text{Cancer-Rate} = (7.053)(\text{Dose}^{0.75}) + (649.544).$$

Equation of best fit for DS86 with neutron RBE = 20 (Table 29-C) :
$$\text{Cancer-Rate} = (6.579)(\text{Dose}^{0.75}) + (647.693).$$

Using Best-Fit Equations for Interpolation and Graphing :

With an equation of best fit, one can estimate or predict the most likely cancer-rate at ANY dose within a given dose-range. Readers will see this illustrated in Tables 14-A and 14-B. Then one can use the calculated or predicted datapoints, of course, to plot or graph a smooth curve of best fit. Readers will see this depicted in Figures 14-E and 14-F.

2. Plotting Best-Fit Curves As Graphs; Construction of Table 14-D

Analysts in this field often want to convert a set of regression analyses to graphs which display both the predicted cancer-rates and the observed cancer-rates. For instance, we want to depict the fit between the observed cancer-rates and the dose-response curves proposed by the regressions on Dose^0.75, Dose^1, Dose^1.4, and Dose^2 in the T65DR dosimetry with neutron RBE = 2. To do that, we need to assemble the input shown in Table 14-D. Here are the steps:

1. From Table 29-B, we extract the X-Coefficient and the Constant in order to create the equation of best fit:

$$\text{Cancer-Rate} = (7.0528)(\text{Dose}^{0.75}) + 649.544.$$

2. DOSES FOR THE X-RANGE: From Table 13-A, Rows 1 through 6 we extract the six true dose-points where we have observed cancer-rates. To this list, we could add some or all of the dose-values which we added in Table 14-A, but for brevity, we have added only one: 130 cSv, which fills the large gap between 71.308 and 176.662. These seven doses are the entries for the graph's x-range.

3. For each dose in the list, we calculate the value of Dose^0.75, which is needed for use in the right side of the equation.

4. PREDICTED CANCER-RATES FOR THE Y-RANGE: Using the equation, we calculate the predicted (or estimated) cancer-rates which correspond with the list of seven doses. The calculated cancer-rates are one set of entries for the y-range of the graph, and will be designated by the uninterrupted curve in Figure 14-A.

5. OBSERVED CANCER-RATES FOR THE Y-RANGE: Returning to Table 13-A, we copy the six observed cancer-rates from Rows 1 through 6. They are the second set of entries for the y-range of the graph, and will be designated by the boxy symbol in Figure 14-A.

6. When the equivalent steps are done for Dose^1, Dose^1.4, and Dose^2, we have assembled all the input shown in Table 14-D. The input for Figures 14-A, 14-B, 14-C, and 14-D is the same except for the calculated cancer-rates, which come from four different best-fit equations. It should be noted that in all the graphs, the unit of the x-axis is cSv because we want to see Cancer-Rate versus Dose. If we had wanted to see Cancer-Rate vs. Dose^Power, the input in Step 2 for the x-ranges would have been the columns to the right of the true dose in Table 14-D, the unit for the x-axis would have been (serially) cSv^0.75, cSv^1, cSv^1.4, cSv^2, and all the plots of calculated cancer-rate vs. Dose^Power would have been straight lines.

3. Testing the Significance of Differences Between Regressions

Hayek and Cheetham (Hay87) present a simple

format for testing whether a particular change in regression parameters provides a significant improvement in the goodness-of-fit to the observed data. Their method uses the Student's t test, with the formula presented in our Table 29-D.

The important item of information resides in the values of R-squared for the two regressions being compared. If we are to choose one regression as a superior fit to the observed data compared with another regression, there must be a significant increase in the value of R-squared in going from one regression to the other.

Table 29-D compares the regression for Dose^0.75 serially with the regressions for Dose^2, Dose^1.4, Dose^1.16, and Dose^1. These comparisons correspond with a supra-linear dose-response versus pure quadratic, linear-quadratic (Q-positive), and linear dose-responses. The method of Table 29-D is used to do all such testing in this book.

===================

Table 29-A

Input for Nine Separate Regressions of Cancer-Rate upon Dose. Output Is in Tables 29-B and 29-C .

Weighting Factors for Regression Input, for Both Dosimetries

Dose-Group	Cancer-Rate per 10,000	Number of Cancer-Deaths	Square Root of Number of Cancers		Ratio of Square Roots	Input Weighting Factor
1	649.31	2413.68	49.129		3.0376	3
2	651.89	1881.04	43.371		2.6816	3
3	712.02	1063.97	32.619		2.0168	2
4	723.72	305.77	17.486		1.0812	1
5	836.27	261.58	16.174	Lowest	1.0000	1
6+7+8	988.45	287.34	16.951		1.0481	1

INPUT DATA for Regression Analysis in the T65DR Dosimetry, Neutron RBE = 2.0. Dose^1 in cSv (rems)

Cancer-Rate	T65DR Dose^1	Dose^2	Dose^1.4	Dose^1.16	Dose^0.85	Dose^0.80	Dose^0.75	Dose^0.70	Dose^0.65
649.31	0.000	0.000	0.000	0.000	0.000	0.000	0.000	0.000	0.000
649.31	0.000	0.000	0.000	0.000	0.000	0.000	0.000	0.000	0.000
649.31	0.000	0.000	0.000	0.000	0.000	0.000	0.000	0.000	0.000
651.89	1.511	2.282	1.782	1.614	1.420	1.391	1.363	1.335	1.308
651.89	1.511	2.282	1.782	1.614	1.420	1.391	1.363	1.335	1.308
651.89	1.511	2.282	1.782	1.614	1.420	1.391	1.363	1.335	1.308
712.02	10.994	120.867	28.682	16.134	7.673	6.806	6.038	5.356	4.751
712.02	10.994	120.867	28.682	16.134	7.673	6.806	6.038	5.356	4.751
723.72	35.361	1250.432	147.212	62.560	20.713	17.331	14.501	12.133	10.152
836.27	71.308	5084.879	393.004	141.138	37.598	30.375	24.539	19.824	16.016
988.45	176.662	31209.54	1399.591	404.284	81.297	62.765	48.457	37.411	28.883

INPUT DATA for Regression Analysis in the DS86 Dosimetry, Neutron RBE = 20. Dose^1 in cSv (rems)

Cancer-Rate	DS86 Dose^1	Dose^2	Dose^1.4	Dose^1.16	Dose^0.85	Dose^0.80	Dose^0.75	Dose^0.70	Dose^0.65
649.31	0.089	0.008	0.034	0.061	0.128	0.145	0.163	0.184	0.208
649.31	0.089	0.008	0.034	0.061	0.128	0.145	0.163	0.184	0.208
649.31	0.089	0.008	0.034	0.061	0.128	0.145	0.163	0.184	0.208
651.89	1.890	3.573	2.439	2.093	1.718	1.664	1.612	1.562	1.513
651.89	1.890	3.573	2.439	2.093	1.718	1.664	1.612	1.562	1.513
651.89	1.890	3.573	2.439	2.093	1.718	1.664	1.612	1.562	1.513
712.02	14.564	212.115	42.521	22.357	9.745	8.524	7.455	6.521	5.703
712.02	14.564	212.115	42.521	22.357	9.745	8.524	7.455	6.521	5.703
723.72	40.625	1650.398	178.777	73.485	23.306	19.366	16.091	13.371	11.110
836.27	74.238	5511.223	415.790	147.885	38.907	31.369	25.291	20.391	16.440
988.45	197.054	38830.29	1630.870	458.901	89.207	68.496	52.594	40.384	31.008

The input for the y-range of the nine regressions is always the cancer-rate column.
The input for the x-range is one column of dose-values per regression.
Entries for the cancer-rate column come from Table 13-A, or from the top of this Table 29-A.
 An entry is made extra times, according to its weighting-factor from the top of this table.
Entries for the Dose^1 column come from Table 13-A (Columns B and C).
Entries in the additional dose-columns are Dose (the true dose) raised to the power indicated.

Table 29-B
T65DR Dosimetry, Neutron RBE = 2: Output for Nine Regression Analyses. Input Is in Table 29-A.

Regression of Ca-Rate on Dose^1.0
Regression Output:

Constant	661.1535
Std Err of Y Est	21.6951
R Squared	0.9630
No. of Observations	11
Degrees of Freedom	9
X Coefficient(s) 1.9474	
Std Err of Coef. 0.1273	

Regression of Ca-Rate on Dose^2
Regression Output:

Constant	680.0481
Std Err of Y Est	45.9220
R Squared	0.8342
No. of Observations	11
Degrees of Freedom	9
X Coefficient(s) 0.0105	
Std Err of Coef. 0.0016	

Regression of Ca-rate on Dose^1.4
Regression Output:

Constant	671.9217
Std Err of Y Est	34.2138
R Squared	0.9080
No. of Observations	11
Degrees of Freedom	9
X Coefficient(s) 0.2422	
Std Err of Coef. 0.0257	

Regression of Ca-Rate on Dose^1.16
Regression Output:

Constant	666.2839
Std Err of Y Est	27.1627
R Squared	0.9420
No. of Observations	11
Degrees of Freedom	9
X Coefficient(s) 0.8479	
Std Err of Coef. 0.0701	

Regression of Ca-Rate on Dose^0.85
Regression Output:

Constant	654.8536
Std Err of Y Est	16.7058
R Squared	0.9781
No. of Observations	11
Degrees of Freedom	9
X Coefficient(s) 4.2250	
Std Err of Coef. 0.2110	

Regression of Ca-Rate on Dose^0.80
Regression Output:

Constant	652.3288
Std Err of Y Est	15.4410
R Squared	0.9813
No. of Observations	11
Degrees of Freedom	9
X Coefficient(s) 5.4614	
Std Err of Coef. 0.2516	

Regression of Ca-Rate on Dose^0.75
Regression Output:

Constant	649.5441
Std Err of Y Est	14.6569
R Squared	0.9831
No. of Observations	11
Degrees of Freedom	9
X Coefficient(s) 7.0528	
Std Err of Coef. 0.3082	

Regression of Ca-Rate on Dose^0.70
Regression Output:

Constant	646.4655
Std Err of Y Est	14.5872
R Squared	0.9833
No. of Observations	11
Degrees of Freedom	9
X Coefficient(s) 9.0975	
Std Err of Coef. 0.3956	

Regression of Ca-Rate on Dose^0.65
Regression Output:

Constant	643.0565
Std Err of Y Est	15.4274
R Squared	0.9813
No. of Observations	11
Degrees of Freedom	9
X Coefficient(s) 11.7191	
Std Err of Coef. 0.5395	

Each of the nine regression analyses above (all for T65DR, RBE=2) proposes an equation having the form:
    CANCER-RATE = (X-Coefficient) times (Dose raised to the indicated power) + (a Constant).

The equation proposed by each regression analysis is the equation of best fit for the regression's own particular constraints -- namely, its own input from Table 29-A. While all nine regressions had the same input for the y-range (the observed cancer-rates), each had a different input for the x-range (Dose^power), so each regression analysis produces its own value for the X-Coefficient and for the Constant (which is the y-intercept, or cancer-rate when dose = 0).

The number of observations and degrees of freedom are values used later to determine the significance of differences in R-Squared values, between one regression analysis and another (Table 29-D).

For each regression analysis, R-Squared (the correlation coefficient squared) is a measure of how well the input datapoints are fitted by the equation. The closer R-Squared is to 1.00, the better is the fit between the input and the equation. The maximum value is reached, above, with the dose-exponent of 0.75 (if two dose-exponents have the same R-Squared value after R-Squared is rounded to the third decimal place, we use the higher dose-exponent). Thus,

---

(Best-fit equation is):   CANCER-RATE = (7.0528)(Dose^0.75) + (649.544).

Table 29-C
DS86 Dosimetry, Neutron RBE = 20: Output for Nine Regression Analyses. Input Is In Table 29-A.

Regression Output:			Regression Output:			Regression Output:	
Constant	660.5057		Constant	680.6983		Constant	672.1875
Std Err of Y Est	22.6388		Std Err of Y Est	47.5206		Std Err of Y Est	35.8134
R Squared	0.9597		R Squared	0.8224		R Squared	0.8991
No. of Observations	11		No. of Observations	11		No. of Observations	11
Degrees of Freedom	9		Degrees of Freedom	9		Degrees of Freedom	9
X Coefficient(s)	1.7595		X Coefficient(s)	0.00837		X Coefficient(s)	0.20795
Std Err of Coef.	0.1202		Std Err of Coef.	0.00130		Std Err of Coef.	0.02322

Regression of Ca-Rate on Dose^1.16			Regression of Ca-Rate on Dose^0.85			Regression of Ca-Rate on Dose^0.80	
Regression Output:			Regression Output:			Regression Output:	
Constant	666.0985		Constant	653.5907		Constant	650.7975
Std Err of Y Est	28.4603		Std Err of Y Est	17.2294		Std Err of Y Est	15.8237
R Squared	0.9363		R Squared	0.9767		R Squared	0.9803
No. of Observations	11		No. of Observations	11		No. of Observations	11
Degrees of Freedom	9		Degrees of Freedom	9		Degrees of Freedom	9
X Coefficient(s)	0.7506		X Coefficient(s)	3.8911		X Coefficient(s)	5.0619
Std Err of Coef.	0.0653		Std Err of Coef.	0.2005		Std Err of Coef.	0.2391

Regression of Ca-Rate on Dose^0.75			Regression of Ca-Rate on Dose^0.70			Regression of Ca-Rate on Dose^0.65	
Regression Output:			Regression Output:			Regression Output:	
Constant	647.6933		Constant	644.2209		Constant	640.3063
Std Err of Y Est	14.9092		Std Err of Y Est	14.7215		Std Err of Y Est	15.4417
R Squared	0.9825		R Squared	0.9830		R Squared	0.9813
No. of Observations	11		No. of Observations	11		No. of Observations	11
Degrees of Freedom	9		Degrees of Freedom	9		Degrees of Freedom	9
X Coefficient(s)	6.5793		X Coefficient(s)	8.5437		X Coefficient(s)	11.0840
Std Err of Coef.	0.2925		Std Err of Coef.	0.3750		Std Err of Coef.	0.5107

Each of the nine regression analyses above (all for DS86) proposes an equation having the form:
    CANCER-RATE = (X-Coefficient) times (Dose raised to the indicated power) + (a Constant).

The equation proposed by each regression analysis is the equation of best fit for the regression's own particular constraints -- namely, its own input from Table 29-A. While all nine regressions had the same input for the y-range (the observed cancer-rates), each had a different input for the x-range (Dose^power), so each regression analysis produces its own value for the X-Coefficient and for the Constant (which is the y-intercept, or cancer-rate when dose = 0).

The number of observations and degrees of freedom are values used later to determine the significance of differences in R-Squared values, between one regression analysis and another (Table 29-E).

For each regression analysis, R-Squared (the correlation coefficient squared) is a measure of how well the input datapoints are fitted by the equation. The closer R-Squared is to 1.00, the better is the fit between the input and the equation. The maximum value is reached, above, with the dose-exponent of 0.75 (if two dose-exponents have the same R-Squared value after R-Squared is rounded to the third decimal place, we use the higher dose-exponent). Thus,

---

    (Best-fit equation is): CANCER-RATE = (6.5793)(Dose^0.75) + (647.693).

Table 29-D

T65DR : Significance Tests for Difference In Best-Fit Curves, and Conclusions about Shape of Dose-Response.

The fundamental relationship we use in testing is the following equation (Hay87):

Student's t value = [(increase in R-Squared)(degrees of freedom) / (1 - R-Squared)]^0.5

Once the Student's t value is obtained, it is compared with a standard statistical Student's
t-distribution table to ascertain the level of statistical significance of the findings.

===

Results In the T65DR Dosimetry, Neutron RBE = 2. Input from Table 29-B.

===

COMPARISON OF DOSE^0.75 WITH DOSE^2.0 (Supra-Linear vs. Pure Quadratic Dose-Response).
Conclusion from below: Dose^0.75 provides a highly significant improvement in fit contrasted with Dose^2.

REGRESSION COMPARED	R-Squared	Increase in R-Squared	Student's t	Degrees of Freedom	p value
Dose^2	0.8342				
Dose^0.75	0.9831	0.1489	8.9078	9	<<0.01

===

COMPARISON OF DOSE^0.75 WITH DOSE^1.4 (Supra-Linear vs. Linear-Quadratic Dose-Response).
Conclusion from below: Dose^0.75 provides a significant improvement in fit contrasted with Dose^1.4 .

REGRESSION COMPARED	R-Squared	Increase in R-Squared	Student's t	Degrees of Freedom	p value
Dose^1.4	0.9080				
Dose^0.75	0.9831	0.0752	6.3278	9	< 0.01

===

COMPARISON OF DOSE^0.75 WITH DOSE^1.16 (Supra-Linear vs. Linear-Quadratic Dose-Response).
Conclusion from below: Dose^0.75 provides a significant improvement in fit contrasted with Dose^1.16 .

REGRESSION COMPARED	R-Squared	Increase in R-Squared	Student's t	Degrees of Freedom	p value
Dose^1.16	0.9420				
Dose^0.75	0.9831	0.0411	4.6808	9	< 0.01

===

COMPARISON OF DOSE^0.75 WITH DOSE^1.0 (Supra-Linear vs. Pure Linear Dose-Response).
Conclusion from below: Dose^0.75 provides a significant improvement in fit contrasted with Dose^1.

REGRESSION COMPARED	R-Squared	Increase in R-Squared	Student's t	Degrees of Freedom	p value
Dose^1	0.9630				
Dose^0.75	0.9831	0.0201	3.2740	9	0.01

Table 29-E

DS86 : Significance Tests for Difference In Best-Fit Curves, and Conclusions about Shape Of Dose-Response.

The fundamental relationship we use in testing is the following equation (Hay87):

Student's t value = [(increase in R-Squared)(degrees of freedom) / (1 - R-Squared)]^0.5

Once the Student's t value is obtained, it is compared with a standard statistical Student's t-distribution table to ascertain the level of statistical significance of the findings.

===

Results In the DS86 Dosimetry, Neutron RBE = 20. Input from Table 29-C.

===

COMPARISON OF DOSE^0.75 WITH DOSE^2.0 (Supra-Linear vs. Pure Quadratic Dose-Response).

Conclusion from below: Dose^0.75 provides a highly significant improvement in fit contrasted with Dose^2.

REGRESSION COMPARED	R-Squared	Increase in R-Squared	Student's t	Degrees of Freedom	p value
Dose^2	0.8224				
Dose^0.75	0.9825	0.1601	9.0792	9	<<0.01

===

COMPARISON OF DOSE^0.75 WITH DOSE^1.4 (Supra-Linear vs. Linear-Quadratic Dose-Response).

Conclusion from below: Dose^0.75 provides a significant improvement in fit contrasted with Dose^1.4 .

REGRESSION COMPARED	R-Squared	Increase in R-Squared	Student's t	Degrees of Freedom	p value
Dose^1.4	0.8991				
Dose^0.75	0.9825	0.08	6.5522	9	< 0.01

===

COMPARISON OF DOSE^0.75 WITH DOSE^1.16 (Supra-Linear vs. Linear-Quadratic Dose-Response).

Conclusion from below: Dose^0.75 provides a significant improvement in fit contrasted with Dose^1.16 .

REGRESSION COMPARED	R-Squared	Increase in R-Squared	Student's t	Degrees of Freedom	p value
Dose^1.16	0.9363				
Dose^0.75	0.9825	0.0462	4.8780	9	< 0.01

===

COMPARISON OF DOSE^0.75 WITH DOSE^1.0 (Supra-Linear vs. Pure Linear Dose-Response).

Conclusion from below: Dose^0.75 provides a significant improvement in fit contrasted with Dose^1.

REGRESSION COMPARED	R-Squared	Increase in R-Squared	Student's t	Degrees of Freedom	p value
Dose^1	0.9597				
Dose^0.75	0.9825	0.0228	3.4280	9	0.01

29-empty, after tables.
==

Dose–Response with Cancer–Rates Expressed in Cancer Deaths per 10,000 Person–Years

As mentioned in Chapter 14, Part 1, analysis of dose versus response can be done with the cancer-response expressed as cancer-deaths per 10,000 person-YEARS rather than cancer-deaths per 10,000 initial persons.

In this chapter, we do the analysis of response in the A-bomb survivors exactly as we did it in Chapter 29, with the sole exception of expressing the response in cancer-deaths per 10,000 person-YEARS (cumulated for the 1950-82 period).

Results and Comparison :
==================================

The tables in this chapter are self-explanatory, and follow the tables in Chapter 29 in detail. Examination of Tables 30-A through 30-E makes it apparent that the same shape is obtained from this database when person-years are used as the shape obtained when initial persons are used. See also the FIGURES 30-A,B and 14-E,F.

Muirhead and Butland, of the National Radiological Protection Board (NRPB, Britain), have commented on our finding of supra-linearity in the A-Bomb Study, after we reported it (with the use of initial persons) in a letter to HEALTH PHYSICS (Go89a). Muirhead and Butland suggest in their own letter (Mu89) that our finding might be due to our use of cancer-deaths per 10,000 initial persons rather than cancer-deaths per 10,000 person-YEARS. In addition, Muirhead and Butland claim that the best-fit equation -- with cancer-rate expressed as deaths per 10,000 person-YEARS -- has a dose-exponent of 1.16 (Mu89), rather than a supra-linear exponent below 1.0. They use only the DS86 sub-cohort (1950-1985) to reach their conclusion of slight upward curvature.

In our rebuttal-letter (Go89b), we point out that the concave-downward shape of the dose-response relationship is the SAME when we use person-years as when we use initial persons. Chapters 29 and 30 show the basis for our statement. Moreover, in these chapters, we added Dose^1.16 to our analyses, and have shown that supra-linearity provides a better fit to the data than does Dose^1.16.

Since our analyses include the DS86 dosimetry, handled with the "constant-cohort, dual-dosimetry" approach, the disparity between our findings and the finding of Muirhead and Butland cannot be explained by the revised DS86 dose-estimates any better than by "person-years."

"Why Do Experts Disagree ?"
======================================

We have explained step-by-step how we arrive at supra-linearity as the best description of dose-response curvature in the A-Bomb Study. We do not know how Muirhead and Butland arrive at slight upward curvature. We do not rule out the possibility that the additional cancer-deaths in 1983, 84, and 85, actually could convert the shape from concave-downward to concave-upward. However, since the shape has been turning out supra-linear for three consecutive 4-year follow-ups, this should not be anyone's "best bet."

We, and others, have to worry that the explanation of the Muirhead-Butland finding lies in the meaning of "DS86 sub-cohort." This special new group, used not only by Muirhead and Butland but also by RERF (TR-5-88) and UNSCEAR-88, is a group from which one-sixth of the initial 91,231 persons have been removed, and a group in which the remaining 75,991 initial persons and their cancer-deaths have been shuffled into new cohorts. Does this handling introduce a change in shape?

If the dose-response relationship for an identical period (1950-1985) and for an identical dosimetry (DS86) were to be one way with exclusions and shufflings, and another way without exclusions and shufflings -- namely, with "constant-cohort, dual-dosimetry" analysis -- this would raise very serious questions about a potential decision not to FIND OUT.

This is a matter of profound scientific importance, and it is addressed further in Chapter 25, Part 3, "First Crisis for the A-Bomb Study."

The requirement for resolving the mystery is the provision of the cancer-death results for the 1982-85 follow-up period -- FOR THE ORIGINAL 91,231 PERSONS GROUPED IN THE SAME COHORTS USED BY RERF IN ITS FOLLOW-UP REPORT THROUGH 1982, NAMELY TR-1-86. We hope to obtain these data from RERF.

Table 30-A

Input for Nine Separate Regressions of Cancer-Rate upon Dose. Output Is in Tables 30-B and 30-C.

Cancer-Rates Expressed as Cancer-Deaths per 10,000 Person-Years (PYRS).

Weighting Factors for Regression Input, for Both Dosimetries

Dose-Group	Cancer-Rate per 10,000 Pers-Yrs	Number of Cancer-Deaths	Square root of Number of Cancers		Ratio of Square Roots	Input Weighting Factor
1	24.06	2413.68	49.129		3.0376	3
2	24.25	1881.04	43.371		2.6816	3
3	26.36	1063.97	32.619		2.0168	2
4	26.75	305.77	17.486		1.0812	1
5	31.22	261.58	16.174	Lowest	1.0000	1
6+7+8	37.55	287.34	16.951		1.0481	1

==

INPUT DATA for Regression Analysis in the T65DR Dosimetry, Neutron RBE = 2.0. Dose^1 is in cSv (rems).

Cancer-Rate	T65DR Dose^1	Dose^2	Dose^1.4	Dose^1.16	Dose^0.85	Dose^0.80	Dose^0.75	Dose^0.70	Dose^0.65
24.06	0	0	0	0	0	0	0	0	0
24.06	0	0	0	0	0	0	0	0	0
24.06	0	0	0	0	0	0	0	0	0
24.25	1.511	2.28202	1.7817	1.6137	1.4200	1.3910	1.3626	1.3348	1.3075
24.25	1.511	2.28202	1.7817	1.6137	1.4200	1.3910	1.3626	1.3348	1.3075
24.25	1.511	2.28202	1.7817	1.6137	1.4200	1.3910	1.3626	1.3348	1.3075
26.36	10.994	120.8674	28.6825	16.1339	7.6733	6.8065	6.0376	5.3556	4.7506
26.36	10.994	120.8674	28.6825	16.1339	7.6733	6.8065	6.0376	5.3556	4.7506
26.75	35.361	1250.432	147.2116	62.5597	20.7134	17.3310	14.5010	12.1331	10.1518
31.22	71.308	5084.879	393.0035	141.1376	37.5984	30.3747	24.5389	19.8243	16.0155
37.55	176.662	31209.54	1399.591	404.2841	81.2966	62.7646	48.4571	37.4111	28.8831

==

INPUT DATA for Regression Analysis in the DS86 Dosimetry, Neutron RBE = 20. Dose^1 is in cSv (rems).

Cancer-Rate	DS86 Dose^1	Dose^2	Dose^1.4	Dose^1.16	Dose^0.85	Dose^0.80	Dose^0.75	Dose^0.70	Dose^0.65
24.06	0.089	0.00798	0.03398	0.06068	0.12831	0.14479	0.16338	0.18435	0.20801
24.06	0.089	0.00798	0.03398	0.06068	0.12831	0.14479	0.16338	0.18435	0.20801
24.06	0.089	0.00798	0.03398	0.06068	0.12831	0.14479	0.16338	0.18435	0.20801
24.25	1.890	3.57306	2.43853	2.09297	1.71808	1.66424	1.61209	1.56158	1.51265
24.25	1.890	3.57306	2.43853	2.09297	1.71808	1.66424	1.61209	1.56158	1.51265
24.25	1.890	3.57306	2.43853	2.09297	1.71808	1.66424	1.61209	1.56158	1.51265
26.36	14.564	212.1152	42.5207	22.3569	9.7453	8.5237	7.4553	6.5208	5.7034
26.36	14.564	212.1152	42.5207	22.3569	9.7453	8.5237	7.4553	6.5208	5.7034
26.75	40.625	1650.398	178.7772	73.4855	23.3064	19.3658	16.0915	13.3708	11.1101
31.22	74.238	5511.223	415.7896	147.8849	38.9072	31.3689	25.2911	20.3909	16.4401
37.55	197.054	38830.29	1630.870	458.9010	89.2067	68.4965	52.5943	40.3840	31.0085

==

The input for the y-range of the nine regressions is always the column of cancer-rates / 10,000 PYR.
The input for the x-range is one column of dose-values per regression.
Entries for the cancer-rate column come from Table 11-H, Column Q (also at the top of this table).
  An entry is made extra times, according to its weighting-factor from the top of this table.
Entries for the Dose^1 column come from Table 11-H, Cols.D,E (also Table 13-A, Cols.B,C).
Entries in the additional dose-columns are Dose (the true dose) raised to the power indicated.

Table 30-B

T65DR Dosimetry, Neutron RBE = 2: Output for Nine Regression Analyses. Input Is in Table 30-A. Cancer-Rates Expressed as Cancer Deaths per 10,000 Person-Years (PYRS).

Regression of Ca-Rate on Dose^1.0 Regression Output:		Regression of Ca-Rate on Dose^2 Regression Output:		Regression of Ca-rate on Dose^1.4 Regression Output:	
Constant	24.4852	Constant	25.2208	Constant	24.9034
Std Err of Y Est	0.7513	Std Err of Y Est	1.6924	Std Err of Y Est	1.2273
R Squared	0.9713	R Squared	0.8545	R Squared	0.9235
No. of Observations	11	No. of Observations	11	No. of Observations	11
Degrees of Freedom	9	Degrees of Freedom	9	Degrees of Freedom	9
X Coefficient(s)	0.0769	X Coefficient(s)	0.00042	X Coefficient(s)	0.00961
Std Err of Coef.	0.0044	Std Err of Coef.	0.00006	Std Err of Coef.	0.00092

Regression of Ca-Rate on Dose^1.16 Regression Output:		Regression of Ca-Rate on Dose^0.85 Regression Output:		Regression of Ca-Rate on Dose^0.80 Regression Output:	
Constant	24.6842	Constant	24.2414	Constant	24.1438
Std Err of Y Est	0.9541	Std Err of Y Est	0.5895	Std Err of Y Est	0.5611
R Squared	0.9538	R Squared	0.9823	R Squared	0.9840
No. of Observations	11	No. of Observations	11	No. of Observations	11
Degrees of Freedom	9	Degrees of Freedom	9	Degrees of Freedom	9
X Coefficient(s)	0.0336	X Coefficient(s)	0.16659	X Coefficient(s)	0.21517
Std Err of Coef.	0.0025	Std Err of Coef.	0.00744	Std Err of Coef.	0.00914

Regression of Ca-Rate on Dose^0.75 Regression Output:		Regression of Ca-Rate on Dose^0.70 Regression Output:		Regression of Ca-Rate on Dose^0.65 Not needed.	
Constant	24.0363	Constant	23.9175		
Std Err of Y Est	0.5570	Std Err of Y Est	0.5838		
R Squared	0.9842	R Squared	0.9827		
No. of Observations	11	No. of Observations	11		
Degrees of Freedom	9	Degrees of Freedom	9		
X Coefficient(s)	0.2776	X Coefficient(s)	0.35782		
Std Err of Coef.	0.0117	Std Err of Coef.	0.01583		

Each of the nine regression analyses above (all for T65DR, RBE=2) proposes an equation having the form:
    CANCER-RATE = (X-Coefficient) times (Dose raised to the indicated power) + (a Constant).

The equation proposed by each regression analysis is the equation of best fit for the regression's own particular constraints -- namely, its own input from Table 30-A. While all nine regressions had the same input for the y-range (the observed cancer-rates), each had a different input for the x-range (Dose^power), so each regression analysis produces its own value for the X-Coefficient and for the Constant (which is the y-intercept, or cancer-rate per 10,000 person-years when dose = 0).

The number of observations and degrees of freedom are values used later to determine the significance of differences in R-Squared values, between one regression analysis and another (Table 30-D).

For each regression analysis, R-Squared (the correlation coefficient squared) is a measure of how well the input datapoints are fitted by the equation. The closer R-Squared is to 1.00, the better is the fit between the input and the equation. The maximum value is reached, above, with the dose-exponent of 0.80 (if two dose-exponents have the same R-Squared value after R-Squared is rounded to the third decimal place, we use the higher dose-exponent).

Thus, best-fit equation is : CANCER-RATE = (0.2152) x (Dose^0.80) + (24.144)

Table 30-C

DS86 Dosimetry, Neutron RBE = 20: Output for Nine Regression Analyses. Input Is in Table 30-A. Cancer-Rates Expressed as Cancer-Deaths per 10,000 Person-Years (PYRS).

Regression of Ca-Rate on Dose^1.0		Regression of Ca-Rate on Dose^2		Regression of Ca-rate on Dose^1.4	
Regression Output:		Regression Output:		Regression Output:	
Constant	24.4595	Constant	25.2462	Constant	24.9136
Std Err of Y Est	0.7918	Std Err of Y Est	1.7580	Std Err of Y Est	1.2939
R Squared	0.9682	R Squared	0.8430	R Squared	0.9150
No. of Observations	11	No. of Observations	11	No. of Observations	11
Degrees of Freedom	9	Degrees of Freedom	9	Degrees of Freedom	9
X Coefficient(s) 0.06953		X Coefficient(s) 0.00033		X Coefficient(s) 0.00825	
Std Err of Coef. 0.00420		Std Err of Coef. 0.00005		Std Err of Coef. 0.00084	

Regression of Ca-Rate on Dose^1.16		Regression of Ca-Rate on Dose^0.85		Regression of Ca-Rate on Dose^0.80	
Regression Output:		Regression Output:		Regression Output:	
Constant	24.6766	Constant	24.1916	Constant	24.0836
Std Err of Y Est	1.0089	Std Err of Y Est	0.6125	Std Err of Y Est	0.5782
R Squared	0.9483	R Squared	0.9809	R Squared	0.9830
No. of Observations	11	No. of Observations	11	No. of Observations	11
Degrees of Freedom	9	Degrees of Freedom	9	Degrees of Freedom	9
X Coefficient(s) 0.0297		X Coefficient(s) 0.1534		X Coefficient(s) 0.1994	
Std Err of Coef. 0.0023		Std Err of Coef. 0.0071		Std Err of Coef. 0.0087	

Regression of Ca-Rate on Dose^0.75		Regression of Ca-Rate on Dose^0.70		Regression of Ca-Rate on Dose^0.65	
Regression Output:		Regression Output:		Regression Output:	
Constant	23.9636	Constant	23.8294	Constant	23.6782
Std Err of Y Est	0.5690	Std Err of Y Est	0.5912	Std Err of Y Est	0.6473
R Squared	0.9836	R Squared	0.9822	R Squared	0.9787
No. of Observations	11	No. of Observations	11	No. of Observations	11
Degrees of Freedom	9	Degrees of Freedom	9	Degrees of Freedom	9
X Coefficient(s) 0.2590		X Coefficient(s) 0.3360		X Coefficient(s) 0.4355	
Std Err of Coef. 0.0112		Std Err of Coef. 0.0151		Std Err of Coef. 0.0214	

Each of the nine regression analyses above (all for DS86, RBE=20) proposes an equation having the form:
    CANCER-RATE = (X-Coefficient) times (Dose raised to the indicated power) + (a Constant).

The equation proposed by each regression analysis is the equation of best fit for the regression's own particular constraints -- namely, its own input from Table 30-A. While all nine regressions had the same input for the y-range (the observed cancer-rates), each had a different input for the x-range (Dose^power), so each regression analysis produces its own value for the X-Coefficient and for the Constant (which is the y-intercept, or cancer-rate per 10,000 person-years when dose = 0).

The number of observations and degrees of freedom are values used later to determine the significance of differences in R-Squared values, between one regression analysis and another (Table 30-E).

For each regression analysis, R-Squared (the correlation coefficient squared) is a measure of how well the input datapoints are fitted by the equation. The closer R-Squared is to 1.00, the better is the fit between the input and the equation. The maximum value is reached, above, with the dose-exponent of 0.75 (if two dose-exponents have the same R-Squared value after R-Squared is rounded to the third decimal place, we use the higher dose-exponent).

Thus, best-fit equation is: CANCER-RATE = (0.2590) x (Dose^0.75) + (23.964).

Table 30–D

Significance Tests for Difference in Best–Fit Curves, and Conclusions about Shape of Dose–Response. Cancer–Rates Expressed as Cancer–Deaths per 10,000 Person–Years (PYRS).

The fundamental relationship we use in testing is the following equation (Hay87):

$$\text{Student's } t \text{ value} = [(\text{increase in R-Squared})(\text{degrees of freedom})/(1 - \text{R-Squared})]^{0.5}$$

Once the Student's t value is obtained, it is compared with a standard statistical Student's t–distribution table to ascertain the level of statistical significance of the findings.

===

RESULTS IN THE T65DR DOSIMETRY, NEUTRON RBE = 2. INPUT FROM TABLE 30–B.

===

COMPARISON OF DOSE^0.80 WITH DOSE^2.0 (Supra-Linear vs. Pure Quadratic Dose-Response).
Conclusion from below: Dose^0.80 provides a highly significant improvement in fit contrasted with Dose^2.

REGRESSIONS COMPARED	R-Squared	Increase in R-Squared	Student's t	Degrees of Freedom	p value
Dose^2	0.8545				
Dose^0.80	0.9840	0.1295	8.54	9	<<0.01

===

COMPARISON OF DOSE^0.80 WITH DOSE^1.4 (Supra-Linear vs. Linear-Quadratic Dose-Response).
Conclusion from below: Dose^0.80 provides a significant improvement in fit contrasted with Dose^1.4 .

REGRESSIONS COMPARED	R-Squared	Increase in R-Squared	Student's t	Degrees of Freedom	p value
Dose^1.4	0.9235				
Dose^0.80	0.9840	0.0605	5.84	9	< 0.01

===

COMPARISON OF DOSE^0.80 WITH DOSE^1.16 (Supra-Linear vs. Linear-Quadratic Dose-Response).
Conclusion from below: Dose^0.80 provides a significant improvement in fit contrasted with Dose^1.16 .

REGRESSIONS COMPARED	R-Squared	Increase in R-Squared	Student's t	Degrees of Freedom	p value
Dose^1.16	0.9538				
Dose^0.80	0.9840	0.0303	4.13	9	< 0.01

===

COMPARISON OF DOSE^0.80 WITH DOSE^1.0 (Supra-Linear vs. Pure Linear Dose-Response).
Conclusion from below: Dose^0.80 provides a significant improvement in fit contrasted with Dose^1.

REGRESSIONS COMPARED	R-Squared	Increase in R-Squared	Student's t	Degrees of Freedom	p value
Dose^1	0.9713				
Dose^0.80	0.9840	0.0127	2.67	9	0.05 > p > 0.01

Table 30-E

Significance Tests for Difference in Best–Fit Curves, and Conclusions about Shape of Dose–Response. Cancer–Rates Expressed as Cancer–Deaths per 10,000 Person–Years (PYRS).

The fundamental relationship we use in testing is the following equation (Hay87):

$$\text{Student's } t \text{ value} = \left[\frac{(\text{increase in R-Squared})(\text{degrees of freedom})}{(1 - \text{R-Squared})}\right]^{0.5}$$

Once the Student's t value is obtained, it is compared with a standard statistical Student's t–distribution table to ascertain the level of statistical significance of the findings.

==

RESULTS IN THE DS86 DOSIMETRY, NEUTRON RBE = 20. INPUT FROM TABLE 30-C.

==

COMPARISON OF DOSE^0.75 WITH DOSE^2.0 (Supra-Linear vs. Pure Quadratic Dose-Response).
Conclusion from below: Dose^0.75 provides a highly significant improvement in fit contrasted with Dose^2.

REGRESSION COMPARED	R-Squared	Increase in R-Squared	Student's t	Degrees of Freedom	p value
Dose^2	0.8430				
Dose^0.75	0.9836	0.1405	8.7706	9	<<0.01

==

COMPARISON OF DOSE^0.75 WITH DOSE^1.4 (Supra-Linear vs. Linear-Quadratic Dose-Response).
Conclusion from below: Dose^0.75 provides a significant improvement in fit contrasted with Dose^1.4 .

REGRESSION COMPARED	R-Squared	Increase in R-Squared	Student's t	Degrees of Freedom	p value
Dose^1.4	0.9150				
Dose^0.75	0.9836	0.0686	6.1275	9	< 0.01

==

COMPARISON OF DOSE^0.75 WITH DOSE^1.16 (Supra-Linear vs. Linear-Quadratic Dose Response).
Conclusion from below: Dose^0.75 provides a significant improvement in fit contrasted with Dose^1.16 .

REGRESSION COMPARED	R-Squared	Increase in R-Squared	Student's t	Degrees of Freedom	p value
Dose^1.16	0.9483				
Dose^0.75	0.9836	0.0353	4.3929	9	< 0.01

==

COMPARISON OF DOSE^0.75 WITH DOSE^1.0 (Supra-Linear vs. Pure Linear Dose-Response).
Conclusion from below: Dose^0.75 provides a significant improvement in fit contrasted with Dose^1.

REGRESSION COMPARED	R-Squared	Increase in R-Squared	Student's t	Degrees of Freedom	p value
Dose^1	0.9682				
Dose^0.75	0.9836	0.0154	2.9033	9	0.05 > p > 0.01

Figure 30–A

T65DR Dosimetry: Best–Fit Curve for Cumulative Cancer–Deaths per 10,000 Person–Years vs. Dose.

For the atomic-bomb survivors, this plot shows cumulative cancer-deaths (1950-1982) per 10,000 person-years, versus mean whole-body internal organ-dose in the T65DR dosimetry (RBE = 2). Figure 30-A can be compared with Figure 14-E, which depicts the best-fit curve when cancer-response is expressed as cancer-deaths per 10,000 initial persons.

● -- The boxy symbols, which show the observed cancer death-rate per 10,000 person-years versus dose, come from Table 11-H, Columns D and Q.

● -- Points along the best-fit curve are calculated from the equation of best fit, obtained in Table 30-B and shown again below.

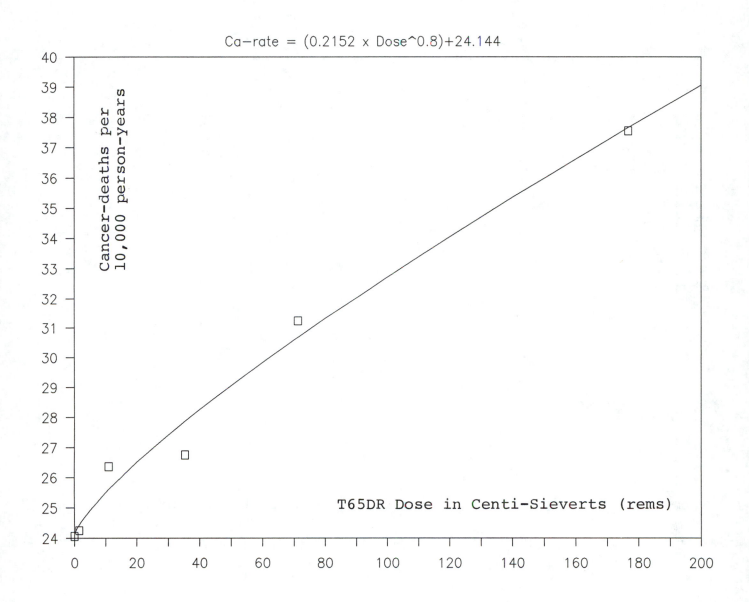

Ca−rate = (0.2152 x Dose^0.8)+24.144

Figure 30-B

DS86 Dosimetry: Best–Fit Curve for Cumulative Cancer–Deaths per 10,000 Person–Years vs. Dose.

For the atomic-bomb survivors, this plot shows cumulative cancer-deaths (1950-1982) per 10,000 person-years, versus mean whole-body internal organ-dose in the DS86 dosimetry (RBE = 20). Figure 30-B can be compared with Figure 14-F, which depicts the best-fit curve when cancer-response is expressed as cancer-deaths per 10,000 initial persons.

● -- The boxy symbols, which show the observed cancer death-rate per 10,000 person-years versus dose, come from Table 11-H, Columns E and Q.

● -- Points along the best-fit curve are calculated from the equation of best fit, obtained in Table 30-C and shown again below.

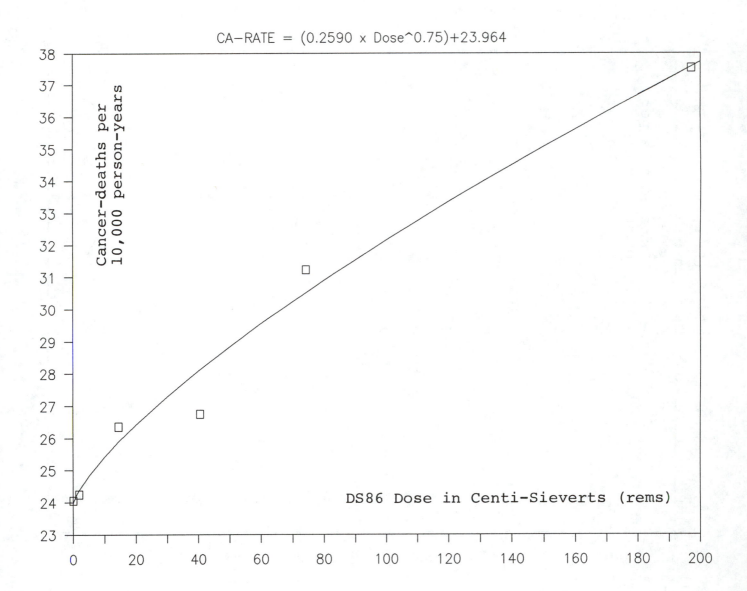

CA–RATE = (0.2590 x Dose^0.75)+23.964

Figure 30-B

CHAPTER 31

Dose–Increment for Small Body–Size in Age–Band 0–9 Years ATB

In Chapter 15 it was pointed out that the organ-doses in Table 26 A,B,C,D do not include any correction for the small body-size of the 0-9 year olds ATB. Such a correction is required before calculations of cancer-risk from K-values is made for those who were 0-9 years old ATB. As we shall see, these corrections prevent us from an over-estimation of the cancer-risk in those very young at the time of irradiation. This chapter presents the detailed method of making the appropriate corrections.

Three types of adjustment factors needed
===================================

In going from kerma dose to organ-dose, we must deal with three adjustment factors;

(a) factor converting gamma kerma to gamma absorbed dose,
(b) factor converting neutron kerma to direct neutron absorbed dose,
(c) factor converting neutron kerma to absorbed dose from gammas produced by the neutron, gamma reaction in tissue.

These adjustments are made in Table 9-C for T65DR and in Table 10-E for DS86 dosimetry. It is these adjusted organ doses that are subject to correction in those individuals who are 0-9 years of age ATB.

In Chapter 8 (Organ Dosimetry), of the book , DS86 Dosimetry, Kaul and co-authors (Kau87) provide tables which permit a reasonable approach to the calculation of appropriate factors for comparison of organ doses for children versus those for adults. Calculations were made there for transmission factors (expressed as Organ Kerma divided by Free-Field Kerma) for the three types of radiation we must consider, based upon the use of Japanese phantoms for adults (55 kg) and children (19.8 kg). The authors indicate that the "adult" phantom is valid for ages 12 and older, whereas the "child" phantom is valid for ages 3 to 12 years of age. We shall make the reasonable approximation that we can use data for the child phantom for our age-group 0-9 years ATB.

Transmission factors are provided for numerous organs, and in some listings, for different postures of the individual. However, since we are studying all cancers (except leukemia), we continue with our practice of using the intestinal dose as the surrogate for the various organs which are the major contributors to "all cancers, leukemia excepted". Tables 68 through 79 (Chapter 8, DS86 Dosimetry) provide the data necessary for our analyses.

The transmission factors presented there are for "the DS86 organ data base at 1500 meters from the hypocenter, standing phantom, facing hypocenter." We recognize that the A-bomb survivors will have had varying positions, and were not all facing the hypocenter. Moreover, we shall be dealing with some dose-groups definitely not at 1500 meters from the hypocenter. So we do not have perfect data to make all the transmission factor calculations. However, it seems reasonable to expect that the RATIO of transmission factors (child / adult) will only have second-order corrections needed to cover all orientations and all distances from the hypocenter. If we keep in mind the limitations, it is reasonable to expect that these factors will permit a good approximation to organ-doses for those 0-9 years old ATB.

The data in the tables provide transmission factors for prompt and delayed neutrons, for prompt and delayed gamma rays, and for the three interactions listed above. A summary of these values, from Tables 68-79, is presented in Table 31-A (this chapter), together with an average value in each instance for the two cities.

It will be noted that the ratio of transmission factors, child / adult, is not always in the same direction. The factors for gamma rays produced in tissue by the neutron, gamma reaction are lower in children than they are in adults. Kaul and his co-authors point out that this is due to the fact that with increasing phantom size there are more chances for radiative capture of neutrons in the larger phantoms.

For our purposes in obtaining an estimate of the factor by which we should increase doses to take account of smaller body size, it is sufficient to combine the factors for prompt and delayed neutron effects, and, separately, for prompt and delayed gamma effects. We have the following average factors for the three major sources of radiation, as a best estimate for both cities, making averages of values from Table 31-A.

===

Radiation Type	Ratio of Trans-mission-Factors Child / Adult	Factors averaged to give result
Neutrons,		
overall	1.771	
prompt		1.487
delayed		2.055
Gammas,		
overall	1.109	
prompt		1.104
delayed		1.114
Gammas, from		
n, gamma reaction		
overall	0.802	
prompt		0.761
delayed		0.843

The fact that the three kinds of factors are so different from each other makes it evident that the final overall conversion from adult dose to child dose will depend on the particular mixture of neutrons and gamma rays making up the total radiation for a particular situation.

The reader may wonder why the ratio of Child to Adult Transmission factors is the appropriate factor. From DS86 Dosimetry we get Child Organ Kerma / Free-Field Kerma, and for Adults we have Adult Organ Kerma / Free-Field Kerma. But Free-Field Kerma for child and adult are the same, and hence cancel out, leaving Child Organ Kerma / Adult Organ Kerma.

Application of the Ratio of Child / Adult Transmission Factors

=======================================

In Chapters 15 and 16 we evaluate cancer-risks by individual age-bands, and we do so for both sexes separately. We do combine the results for both cities, for each age-sex grouping. We need a "best factor" to convert the dose in cSv for each dose-category from the calculated dose for adults to what it would be after making the correction for smaller body-size in the 0-9 year olds ATB.

We have the material for determining this "best factor" for T65DR dosimetry in Table 9-C, where the three components of dose, neutron, (n,gamma), and gamma, are available for an overall population essentially of adults. And we have the similar material in Table 10-E for the DS86 dosimetry.

We shall demonstrate the procedure for determination of these "best factors" in the T65DR dosimetry. The only difference in the DS86 Dosimetry is that the data entries are from Table 10-E instead of Table 9-C. All the final results of such calculations are provided in Table 31-B.

Illustrative calculation in the T65DR Dosimetry, Neutron RBE = 2.0.

===

We will use Dose-Group 2 for illustrative purposes.
    From Table 9-C we have the following results for Hiroshima and Nagasaki organ doses, and from the discussion above we have the ratio of transmission factors (child / adult):

Organ-dose	Values for adults Hiroshima	Nagasaki	Ratio of transmission factors (child/adult)
Neutrons	0.352	0.000	1.771
N,gammas	0.056	0.000	0.802
Gammas	1.250	1.300	1.109

For Hiroshima the doses to the 0-9 year olds ATB would be:
    For neutrons,   (1.771)(0.352) =   0.623 cSv
    For n,gammas,   (0.802)(0.056) =   0.045 cSv
    For gammas,   (1.109)(1.250) =   1.386 cSv

    Total dose, for 0-9 year olds =   2.055 cSv (Sum of 0.623+0.045+1.386)
    Total dose,adults, Hiroshima   =   1.658 cSv (Sum of 0.352+0.056+1.250)
                                                           (Slight rounding difference in 0-9 yr olds)
For Dose-Group 2, Hiroshima, "Best" conversion from adult dose to that
for 0-9 year olds ATB = (2.055) / (1.658) =   1.239

For Nagasaki the doses to the 0–9 year olds ATB would be:

For neutrons,   (1.771)(0)   =   0 cSv
For n,gammas,   (0.802)(0)   =   0 cSv
For gammas,   (1.109)(1.300) =   1.442 cSv

Total dose, for 0–9 year olds   =   1.442 cSv (Sum of 0+0+1.442)
Total dose, adults, Nagasaki   =   1.300 cSv (Sum of 0+0+1.300)

For Dose-Group 2, Nagasaki, "Best" conversion from adult dose to that
for 0–9 year olds ATB = (1.442)/(1.300) =   1.109

In application, we will be combining Hiroshima with Nagasaki persons, so we need the weighted "Best" conversion factor separately for males and for females of the 0–9 year olds ATB.

From Table 26 A,B,C,D we have the following number of persons in Hiroshima and Nagasaki for Dose-group 2, males and females separately, in the 0–9 year olds ATB :

City	Males	Females
Hiroshima	1446	1519
Nagasaki	1585	1574

Weighted "Best" conversion factor, from adults to 0–9 year olds, for males of both cities combined =

[(1446)(1.239)+(1585)(1.109)] / (1446+1585) =   1.171

Weighted "Best" conversion factor, from adults to 0–9 year olds, for females of both cities combined =

[1519)(1.239)+(1574)(1.109)] / (1519+1574) =   1.173

Since this description of method is perfectly general, it is applied serially for all 8 dose-groups in the T65DR dosimetry with RBE for neutrons = 2.0, and then for all 8 dose-groups in the DS86 dosimetry with RBE for neutrons = 20. The final "Best" conversion factors for going from adult organ-doses to organ-doses for 0–9 year olds ATB are assembled in Table 31–B. The reader who wishes to, can check any entry by going through the steps just demonstrated above.

The direct application of the conversion factors for estimating organ-doses for 0–9 year olds in the Cancer-Rate Ratio method of analysis is demonstrated in Table 15–A of Chapter 15.

Table 31–A

Transmission Factors (Organ Kerma / Free–Field Kerma) for Adult and Child

Col.A Type of Radiation	Col.B City	Col.C Adult	Col.D Child	Col.E Child / Adult	Col.F Source of data
Prompt Neutrons	Hiroshima	0.192	0.291	1.516	Table 68
Prompt Neutrons	Nagasaki	0.229	0.334	1.459	Table 74
Prompt Neutrons	Average			1.487	Calc.
Delayed Neutrons	Hiroshima	0.090	0.186	2.067	Table 71
Delayed Neutrons	Nagasaki	0.091	0.186	2.044	Table 77
Delayed Neutrons	Average			2.055	Calc.
Prompt Gammas	Hiroshima	0.802	0.891	1.111	Table 69
Prompt Gammas	Nagasaki	0.823	0.903	1.097	Table 75
Prompt Gammas	Average			1.104	Calc.
Delayed Gammas	Hiroshima	0.820	0.906	1.105	Table 70
Delayed Gammas	Nagasaki	0.811	0.911	1.123	Table 76
Delayed Gammas	Average			1.114	Calc.
Prompt Neutrons yielding gamma rays in tissue					
n, gamma reaction	Hiroshima	0.311	0.244	0.785	Table 72
n, gamma reaction	Nagasaki	0.240	0.177	0.737	Table 78
n, gamma reaction	Average			0.761	Calc.
Delayed Neutrons yielding gamma rays in tissue					
n, gamma reaction	Hiroshima	0.809	0.680	0.841	Table 73
n, gamma reaction	Nagasaki	0.836	0.706	0.844	Table 79
n, gamma reaction	Average			0.843	Calc.

Notes ----

1. Column C and Column D entries are transmission factors taken directly from the designated tables of Ch.8 in DS86 Dosimetry .

2. Column E entry is always Column D entry / Column C entry .

3. Column F entries are the source tables of Ch.8 in the book, DS86 Dosimetry, from which the transmission factors are obtained . (Kau87.)

4. Organ kerma can be considered equal to organ absorbed dose.

Table 31-B

Conversion Factors from Adult Dose to Dose in 0-9 Year olds ATB

| T65DR Dosimetry; Neutron RBE = 2.0 | | | | DS86 Dosimetry; Neutron RBE = 20 | | |
Dose-Group	Both cities Males	Females		Dose-Group	Both cities Males	Females
1	1.000	1.000		1	1.074	1.074
2	1.171	1.173		2	1.128	1.128
3	1.179	1.178		3	1.138	1.138
4	1.175	1.173		4	1.162	1.161
5	1.173	1.181		5	1.169	1.173
6	1.172	1.177		6	1.179	1.183
7	1.186	1.189		7	1.192	1.194
8	1.182	1.176		8	1.203	1.199

NOTES ----

1. These tabulated conversion factors are to be used directly when one wishes to convert an adult dose for a particular dose-group to what it would be for 0-9 year olds ATB. These tables are for combined Hiroshima plus Nagasaki groups, either males or females.

2. The application of these conversion factors is demonstrated in Table 15-A, where the factors are used for the first time. It is to be emphasized that the adjustment of doses for the 0-9 year olds ATB is to INCREASE the the doses and hence to reduce the cancer-risk per unit dose, since the cancer-rates themselves are not affected by the dose increase.

31-empty, after tables.
==

Calculation of Primary Electrons per Photon, and Their Energies

We consider irradiation by various classes of photons, including the following:

A. 30 KeV photons -- these represent the photons of average energy associated with medical x-rays with peak energy of 90 KeV. These are the photons commonly employed in medical diagnostic radiation.

B. 596 KeV photons -- these photons have the average energy of photons associated with Radium-226 and its daughter products.

C. 662 KeV photons -- these represent the photons of energy associated with Cesium-137. They are actually emitted in the transition from Barium-137m to Barium-137. Cesium-137 is a major source of worldwide dose from the Chernobyl accident (see Chapters 24 and 36).

D. 1608 KeV photons -- these represent photons of an average energy estimated for the Hiroshima bomb from data of Kerr and co-workers (Kerr87b). We shall explain the derivation of this average energy at the end of this chapter.

Since our interest is in the tracks through cells and cell-nuclei produced by electrons set in motion as a result of photon interaction with tissue, we must necessarily learn about the electrons thus set in motion. The processes which produce electrons traveling at high speed in tissue are the following:

A. The photoelectric process.
B. Incoherent scattering---the Compton Effect.
C. Pair production for gamma energies above
    1.02 MeV. (Not estimated here.)

The treatment of the various processes for setting electrons in motion as given by Paretzke (Par87) is highly informative, and we shall make extensive use of information from that reference.

The Photoelectric Process:
In the photo-electric process the photon is completely absorbed and an electron is ejected from the atom which absorbs the photon. The electron has a kinetic energy which is equal to the difference between the energy of the initial photon and the binding energy of the emitted electron. For matter of low atomic number, the binding energy is of the order of only about 500 eV, so that we can neglect the binding energy term, and say

that the photo-electric process produces a sharp energy spectrum of photo-electrons which carry essentially all the photon energy. Some secondary processes occur which can use some of the energy to produce very low energy Auger electrons and low-energy photons. We shall make the approximation of considering only the photo-electrons here.

For matter of low atomic number, e.g. for biological tissue, the photo-electric process dominates at photon energies below 40 KeV, and we can consider this process to be the only process of consequence for the 30 KeV photons we listed above. Therefore, as a practical matter, we shall state that the absorption of photon energy in tissue for 30 KeV photons sets electrons in motion with an energy of 30 KeV.

The Compton Process:
For photons of energy above 40 KeV, the Compton process becomes increasingly dominant over a very wide range of energies, whereas the photo-electric process becomes less and less prominent as energy of the photons increases.

However, the situation becomes complicated for photons in the energy range where the Compton process dominates. One reason is that for such photons, electrons are set in motion, with energies varying from near zero up to nearly the entire energy of the photon, and new photons are created carrying off the energy not carried off by the electrons set in motion by the Compton process. A second reason is that we must consider not only the transfer of energy from the initial photon to electrons, but also the transfer of energy from the photons produced in each of the successive Compton processes and the final photo-electric processes which follow the initial Compton event.

Borrowing some of the data presented so well by Paretzke, we can develop a reasonable approximation for treating the electrons set in motion by various Compton processes. We need such approximations for the three photon classes listed above, the 596 KeV photons, the 662 KeV photons, and the 1608 KeV photons. We can now turn to that approximation.

1. Development of Method for Treating Compton Electrons

Step 1: For any specific energy of the photon which undergoes the Compton process, the energy of the electrons produced ranges essentially from zero energy up to a calculable maximum energy (to which we shall return). Paretzke (Par87) shows in his Figure 3.6a that the mean energy of the electrons produced (for a specific energy of the photon) is very close to one-half of the maximum energy of the electrons produced. And this is true for a large range of photon energies, a range which covers all the photons with which we shall have to deal.

Therefore, we write the following equation:

Mean energy of electrons produced
                        = Maximum Energy / 2.

Step 2: Next we must learn what the maximum energy is for electrons produced in the Compton process for photons of any specific energy. Based on Paretzke (Par87, p.96) ,we have the following:

Let m = the mass of the electron.
Let hv = the energy of the original photon,
    where h = Planck's constant,
    and v = the frequency of the photon radiation.
Let E = the kinetic energy of electron produced in the Compton process.

We have shown above that the binding energy of an electron set in motion in the photo-electric process is negligible compared with the energy of the photons we are considering. When this is true, and it is true here, we can write the following:

Let hv' be the energy of the photon available after the Compton collision.

Then,   hv' = hv – E

We now define a function, alpha, as follows:

$$\text{alpha} = \frac{hv}{\text{(mass of electron at rest)} \times \text{(velocity of light)}^2}$$

But, from general physics, the denominator of this expression is the energy equivalent of an electron at rest, and this equals 511 KeV.

Therefore, we write

alpha = hv / 511, if hv is expressed in KeV .

Paretzke (p96) gives the following for the maximum energy that can be transfered to the ejected electron in Compton collisions;

$$\text{Emax} = \left[\frac{2 \times \text{(alpha)}}{1 + (2) \times \text{(alpha)}} \right] \times [\, hv \,]$$

So now we have both items needed, (a) the mean energy of Compton electrons if we know the maximum energy of Compton electrons, and (b) the maximum energy of the Compton electrons.

Since we can neglect the small binding energy of the electrons, we can say that the mean energy of the photons after collision will be:

Original photon energy MINUS
        mean energy of electrons ejected.

We can now apply the information in these relationships to a specific case, the 596 KeV photons associated with Radium-226.

alpha = hv / 511 and hv = 596   (Both in KeV)
alpha = 596 / 511 = 1.16634

And substituting in the equation for Emax, we have

$$\text{Emax} = \left. \frac{2 \times 1.16634}{1 + (2)(1.16634)} \right] \times [\, 596 \,]$$

Emax =   417.1649 Kev
Emin =   0 Kev

And we have shown above that Emean = 0.5 x Emax .

Therefore, mean energy of Compton electrons =
        417.1649 / 2, or 208.5824 KeV.

And, the photon energy after Compton collision was shown above to be:
    Original photon energy MINUS
        mean energy of Compton electrons.

Therefore, hv', the photon energy after Compton collision = 596 minus 208.5824 = 387.4176 KeV

But we are concerned about the electrons produced when all of the energy of the original photon is absorbed in the tissue. Therefore, we must consider the fate of the residual photons of 387.4176 KeV energy. Since this energy is still in the region where the Compton process

===

dominates, we must go through iteration after iteration to produce Compton electrons and photons of successively lower energy. We have chosen, as a reasonable approximation, to continue the iterations until the residual photon has an energy equal to or less than 100 KeV, and then assign this energy to a photo-electric process which produces electrons of this residual energy.

We can best show this entire calculation process in a tabulation which serves in a compact manner to show all the steps in the iterative procedure (See Tables 32-A and 32-B for 596 and 662 KeV photons.) All the equations needed to evaluate items in the tabulation have been presented above. The initial photon energy for the iterative steps is always the residual mean photon energy after the immediately preceding Compton process.

Table 32-C presents the similar calculations for Hiroshima gamma rays. The derivation of the mean energy for those gamma rays is presented in the following section of this chapter.

2. Determination of Average Gamma Ray Energy for A-Bomb Survivors

Our objective is a determination of the average energy of gamma rays for exposure of A-Bomb survivors. We shall use the data for Hiroshima as a reasonable source of information. Data are provided by Kerr and co-workers (Kerr87b) for the fluences of prompt gamma rays in Chapter 3, Table 11 and for the average energies of 22 groups of gamma rays in Chapter 3, Table 10.

From Table 10 we obtain the upper bound of energies in MeV for each of the 22 energy-groups. And from these data the average energy of gamma rays is readily determined for each energy-group.

From Table 11 fluences of gamma rays, for each energy-group, are obtained for two distances from the hypocenter of the explosion. We use the data for 5 meters and 2000 meters. "Fluence" describes the number of gamma rays of any particular energy passing through a unit area -- at various distances from the hypocenter of the explosion. The fluences are given in terms of a number of gamma rays per cm^2 per kiloton yield of explosive. The reader will note in Table 32-D that the units of fluence are cm^-2 and kt^-1. These are the appropriate units for expression of "per cm^2" and "per kiloton of yield."

We next multiply the fluence by the average energy for each gamma-ray energy-group, and finally take the sum of all those products. Then we take the sum of the fluences for all 22 energy-groups. And finally we divide the sum of (the products of fluence by average energy) by the sum of fluences to obtain the average gamma ray energy for all 22 energy-groups combined.

We shall use, for our estimations, the mean of the average energy at 5 meters and the average energy at 2000 meters, to obtain an average energy of gamma rays for exposure at Hiroshima, to be used in estimation of a reasonable value for average gamma ray energies for A-bomb survivors. Since our purpose in making these estimates is to obtain an estimate of the order of magnitude of gamma ray energy for A-bomb survivors as compared with gamma ray energy for radium-226, cesium-137, and medical x-rays, we do not feel it is essential to go through the same procedures for Nagasaki separately.

Table 32-D provides all the input data and the calculations which lead to the final estimation of average gamma ray energy for exposure of A-bomb survivors. The table is self-explanatory.

Table 32-A

Tabular Calculation of Compton Electron Energies and Residual Final Photo-Electron Energy

For 596 KeV Photons of Radium-226 And Daughters

(All energies are expressed in KeV)

Row	Col.A INITIAL PHOTON ENERGY	Col.B ALPHA	Col.C MAXIMUM COMPTON ELECTRON ENERGY	Col.D MEAN COMPTON ELECTRON ENERGY	Col.E POST-COMPTON PHOTON ENERGY	Col.F TYPE OF ELECTRON	Col.G ENERGY OF ELECTRON
1	596	1.166340	417.16500	208.58250	387.4174	COMPTON	208.58250
2	387.4174	0.758155	233.45502	116.72751	270.6899	COMPTON	116.72751
3	270.6899	0.529726	139.25211	69.626058	201.0639	COMPTON	69.626058
4	201.0639	0.393471	88.545549	44.272774	156.7911	COMPTON	44.272774
5	156.7911	0.306832	59.626470	29.813235	126.9779	COMPTON	29.813235
6	126.9779	0.248489	42.155092	21.077546	105.9003	COMPTON	21.077546
7	105.9003	0.207241	31.031758	15.515879	90.38449	COMPTON	15.515879
8	90.38449					PHOTO	90.384494
							SUM = 596

The sum of energies of all electrons should be equal to the original gamma ray energy. We find the sum to be 596 KeV, in perfect agreement with the 596 KeV for the original gamma ray energy.

NOTES---

1. In Row 1 the initial photon energy is the input energy for Radium-226 photons, which is 596 KeV. For all other rows, the initial photon energy is the value in Col.E of the row above it.

2. In all rows, the value of ALPHA is the value in Col.A divided by 511.

3. The value of maximum Compton electron energy is from the equation:
Emax = (Initial photon energy) x (2xALPHA) / (1 + 2xALPHA)

4. The mean Compton electron energy is one-half the maximum Compton electron energy.

5. The post-Compton photon energy is the initial photon energy minus the mean Compton electron energy. Col.E = (Col.A minus Col.D)

6. In all rows but the last row, the mean Compton electron energy is repeated in Col. G. But when the initial photon energy falls below 100 KeV, we approximate that this energy all goes into a final photo-electron. Thus, in the last row the initial photon energy in Col. A is also the the final photo-electron energy of Col.G.

Table 32-B

**Tabular Calculation of Compton Electron Energies
and Residual Final Photo-Electron Energy**

For 662 KeV Photons of Cesium-137

(All energies are expressed in KeV)

Row	Col.A INITIAL PHOTON ENERGY	Col.B ALPHA	Col.C MAXIMUM COMPTON ELECTRON ENERGY	Col.D MEAN COMPTON ELECTRON ENERGY	Col.E POST-COMPTON PHOTON ENERGY	Col.F TYPE OF ELECTRON	Col.G ENERGY OF ELECTRON
1	662	1.295499	477.65013	238.82506	423.1749	COMPTON	238.82506
2	423.1749	0.828130	263.86273	131.93136	291.2435	COMPTON	131.93136
3	291.2435	0.569948	155.14186	77.570930	213.6726	COMPTON	77.570930
4	213.6726	0.418146	97.311717	48.655858	165.0167	COMPTON	48.655858
5	165.0167	0.322929	64.754934	32.377467	132.6393	COMPTON	32.377467
6	132.6393	0.259568	45.326989	22.663494	109.9758	COMPTON	22.663494
7	109.9758	0.215216	33.092968	16.546484	93.42932	COMPTON	16.546484
8	93.42932					PHOTO	93.429329
							SUM = 662

The sum of energies of all electrons should be equal to the original gamma ray energy. We find the sum to be 662 KeV, in perfect agreement with the 662 KeV for the original gamma ray energy.

NOTES---
1. All notes are as for the Radium-226 calculations of Table 32-A except that here the entry for initial photon energy in row 1 is the 662 KeV for Cesium-137.

Table 32–C

Tabular Calculation of Compton Electron Energies and Residual Final Photo–Electron Energy

For 1608 KeV Photons of Hiroshima Gamma Rays

(All energies are expressed in KeV)

Row	Col.A INITIAL PHOTON ENERGY	Col.B ALPHA	Col.C MAXIMUM COMPTON ELECTRON ENERGY	Col.D MEAN COMPTON ELECTRON ENERGY	Col.E POST- COMPTON PHOTON ENERGY	Col.F TYPE OF ELECTRON	Col.G ENERGY OF ELECTRON
1	1608	3.146771	1387.5309	693.76549	914.2345	COMPTON	693.76549
2	914.2345	1.789108	714.54225	357.27112	556.9633	COMPTON	357.27112
3	556.9633	1.089947	381.81192	190.90596	366.0574	COMPTON	190.90596
4	366.0574	0.716355	215.58431	107.79215	258.2652	COMPTON	107.79215
5	258.2652	0.505411	129.82766	64.913831	193.3514	COMPTON	64.913831
6	193.3514	0.378378	83.289862	41.644931	151.7064	COMPTON	41.644931
7	151.7064	0.296881	56.518893	28.259446	123.4470	COMPTON	28.259446
8	123.4470	0.241579	40.214519	20.107259	103.3397	COMPTON	20.107259
9	103.3397	0.202230	29.760110	14.880055	88.45973	COMPTON	14.880055
10	88.45973					PHOTO	88.459732
							SUM = 1608

The sum of energies of all electrons should be equal to the original gamma ray energy. We find the sum to be 1608 KeV, in perfect agreement with the 1608 KeV for the original gamma ray energy.

NOTES---

1. All notes are as for the Radium-226 calculations of Table 32-A except that here the entry for initial photon energy in row 1 is the 1608 KeV for Hiroshima gamma rays.

2. Even though the mean energy of the gamma rays is above 1.02 MeV, we shall neglect the contribution of pair-production here. Paretzke's Figure 3.4, p.95, provides good justification for this decision. For a mean gamma ray energy of 1608 KeV the cross-section for pair-production is quite low compared with that for the Compton process.

Table 32-D

Input Data and Calculations Leading to Determination of Average Gamma Ray Energy for Hiroshima A-Bomb Survivors

(Fluences are given per unit yield (cm^-2 kiloton^-1)
at one meter above ground at 5 meters and 2000 meters)
(Energies are in MeV)

	COL.A	COL.B	COL.C	COL.D	COL.E	COL.F
GAMMA ENERGY GROUP	UPPER LIMIT GAMMA ENERGY	AVERAGE GAMMA ENERGY	FLUENCE AT 5 METERS	(B x C) FLUENCE X AVG. ENERGY	FLUENCE AT 2000 METERS	(B x E) FLUENCE X AVG. ENERGY
1	14	13	1420000	18460000	3020	39260
2	12	11	7.12E+09	7.832E+10	11400000	125400000
3	10	9	4.16E+09	3.744E+10	7160000	64440000
4	8	7.5	1.090E+10	8.175E+10	6930000	51975000
5	7	6.5	1.350E+10	8.775E+10	9000000	58500000
6	6	5.5	4.010E+10	2.206E+11	23800000	130900000
7	5	4.5	2.410E+10	1.085E+11	17900000	80550000
8	4	3.5	3.140E+10	1.099E+11	20000000	70000000
9	3	2.5	1.240E+10	3.100E+10	10700000	26750000
10	2.5	2.25	7.030E+10	1.582E+11	12300000	27675000
11	2	1.75	3.000E+10	5.250E+10	14400000	25200000
12	1.5	1.25	2.890E+10	3.612E+10	18600000	23250000
13	1	0.85	2.650E+10	2.253E+10	15700000	13345000
14	0.7	0.67	4.860E+10	3.256E+10	28900000	19363000
15	0.45	0.37	4.730E+10	1.750E+10	26200000	9694000
16	0.3	0.22	1.130E+11	2.486E+10	62700000	13794000
17	0.15	0.125	8.770E+10	1.096E+10	50800000	6350000
18	0.1	0.085	7.830E+10	6.66E+09	47500000	4037500
19	0.07	0.067	6.500E+10	4.36E+09	42800000	2867600
20	0.045	0.037	1.400E+10	518000000	9510000	351870
21	0.03	0.025	770000000	19250000	517000	12925
22	0.02	0.015	6770000	101550	3530	52.95
SUMS			7.54E+11	1.12E+12	4.37E+08	7.54E+08

Average Gamma Energy =

$$\text{Average Gamma Energy} = \frac{\text{Sum of (Fluence x Energy) Products}}{\text{Sum of Fluences}}$$

Average Gamma Energy

At 5 meters	1.12E+12 / 7.54E+11 =	1.4879	MeV
At 2000 meters	7.54E+08 / 4.37E+08 =	1.7272	MeV
Average Gamma Energy, Overall		1.608	MeV
Average Gamma Energy, Overall		1608	KeV

The average gamma energy in KeV is transferred to Table 32-C.

32-empty, after tables.
===

Calculation of Range for Each High–Speed Electron

This chapter is arranged in three parts:

1. The Range in Biological Tissue for Electrons Produced by Low–LET Photons, p.1
2. The Consequences of Escape of Some Post–Compton Photons, p.6
3. The Agreement between Our Estimates of Nuclear Traversals per cGy (Rad) and the Estimates of Four Other Workers, p.7

1. The Range in Biological Tissue for Electrons Produced by Low–LET Photons

In Chapter 32 calculations are made of the ENERGIES of electrons, (photo-electrons and Compton electrons), produced in the interaction of photons of various energies with biological tissue. Those calculations are based upon the approximation that once an initial photon is absorbed in tissue, the total photon energy is ultimately delivered to the tissue in the form either of Compton electrons or photo-electrons. That approximation is very reasonable for the case of a large block of tissue uniformly irradiated with photons (e.g., whole-body irradiation in a uniform field of gamma rays.)

In such irradiation circumstances we have a situation which can be described as a quasi-equilibrium. A post-Compton photon originating at one point has the same probability of being absorbed at a second point as a post-Compton photon originating at the second point has of being absorbed at the first point. Effectively, then, this means we get the correct result by saying that a high proportion of post-Compton photons are absorbed in the tissue and are not lost.

Those calculations represents a step on the way toward determination of the number of cell-traversals and nuclear-traversals per cGy (rad) which would occur with the absorption of energy from various sources of photon irradiation.

The first step in such calculations is a determination of the ranges in tissue of electrons of various energies. Such determinations are made in this chapter.

Martell has provided basic data which are extremely useful in the determination of electron ranges in tissue. The data from his Table IV are provided here (Marte89). We have checked an independent source of estimate of ranges for electrons of various energies (CRC Handbook of Radiation Measurement and Protection), edited by Brodsky (Brod78), and find the values in excellent accord with those of Martell. Martell's estimates are on page 2 of this chapter.

We shall use the Martell tabulations to develop equations with which electron ranges can be estimated for the photo-electrons and Compton electrons of various energies derived from the analyses of Chapter 32, where we ascertained such energies for the photons of interest in our calculations concerning the number of primary ionization tracks per nucleus per cGy for various radiation sources.

No single equation fits the entire range of data. In order to obtain a useful fit for the relationship of range of electrons in tissue to mean energy of electrons, we shall do separate linear-quadratic regression analyses for three segments of the entire data set provided by Martell. It is not essential that every entry from Martell be used; rather we want to be sure that the entire range is represented in the calculations.

Electron Range–Energy Relationship

Electron energies are average energies in MeV:
(From Martell, Table IV)

Radioisotope Source	Average Energy	Range in tissue (micrometers)
234–Th	0.052	48
234–Th	0.026	13
234mPa	0.87	3600
234mPa	0.54	1900
228Ac	0.4	1200
228Ac	0.8	3200
228Ac	0.65	2100
228Ra	0.013	3 (approx.)
214Pb	0.19	380
214Pb	0.21	470
214Bi	1.3	5800
214Bi	0.54	1900
214Bi	0.33	880
212Bi	0.85	3400
208Tl	0.66	2200
208Tl	0.55	2000
210Pb	0.016	4 (approx.)
210Pb	0.004	1 (approx.)
212Pb	0.094	110
212Pb	0.18	340
87Rb	0.075	84
40K	0.59	2100

Martell cites Evans, 1955 (Ev55) as the source of the equations used in calculation of the ranges in tissue for these electrons.

===

A. The very low energy region: energies between 0.016 and 0.094 MeV

Energy	Energy^2	Observed Range in Tissue	Regression of Range on E and E^2 Regression Output:		
0.016	0.000256	4	Constant		-15.9307
0.026	0.000676	13	Std Err of Y Est		2.4271
0.052	0.002704	48	R Squared		0.9986
0.075	0.005625	84	No. of Observations		5
0.094	0.008836	110	Degrees of Freedom		2
			X Coefficient(s)	1115.083	2507.964
			Std Err of Coef.	199.822	1808.437

The correlation-squared is 0.998568, which is excellent.
Equation (1) follows, for calculation of ranges in micrometers:

$$Range = (1115.083 \times Energy) + (2507.964 \times Energy^2) - 15.9307$$

Applying Equation (1) we calculate tissue ranges for comparison with Martell's values (for lowest energy group). The agreement is close.

Energy (MeV)	Energy^2	Calculated Range	Observed Range
0.016	0.000256	2.5528	4 (Approx.)
0.026	0.000676	14.7569	13
0.052	0.002704	48.8353	48
0.075	0.005625	81.8079	84
0.094	0.008836	111.0476	110
0.03	0.0009	19.7791	No observed data

The range for electrons of 0.03 MeV energy is calculated above since we have extensive interest in such electrons in connection with studies of persons exposed to such electrons produced in the photo-electric process with photons of this same energy (from medical X-rays).

Aside from some disagreement for the very lowest energy electrons, for which the observed ranges are only approximations, there is excellent agreement between observed and calculated ranges. Therefore, we shall use this relationship to calculate ranges of electrons in the energy region up to 0.094 MeV.

B. The intermediate energy region: energies 0.075 to 0.21 MeV

Energy	Energy^2	Observed Range in Tissue	Regression of Range on E and E^2 Regression Output:		
0.075	0.005625	84	Constant		88.47800
0.094	0.008836	110	Std Err of Y Est		1.38348
0.18	0.0324	340	R Squared		0.99997
0.19	0.0361	380	No. of Observations		5
0.21	0.0441	470	Degrees of Freedom		2
			X Coefficient(s)	-1080.63	13780.78
			Std Err of Coef.	137.1292	486.9323

==

Excellent correlation is found for this regression.
Equation (2) follows, for calculation of ranges in micrometers:

Range = (-1080.62 x Energy) + (13780.77 x Energy^2) + 88.478

Energy (MeV)	Energy^2	Calculated Range	Observed Range
0.075	0.005625	84.9371	84
0.094	0.008836	108.6525	110
0.18	0.0324	340.4363	340
0.19	0.0361	380.6175	380
0.21	0.0441	469.2483	470

Equation (2) provides an excellent fit to the observed data and we shall use the equation for calculations of ranges for energies between 0.095 and 0.21 MeV. Equation (1)had already provided ranges for electron energies up through 0.094 MeV.

C. The high energy region: energies from 0.18 through 1.3 MeV

Energy (MeV)	Energy^2	Observed Range in Tissue		Regression of Range on E and E^2 Regression Output:		
0.18	0.0324	340		Constant		-279.879732
0.19	0.0361	380		Std Err of Y Est		121.2807851
0.21	0.0441	470		R Squared		0.9954
0.33	0.1089	880		No. of Observations		11
0.54	0.2916	1900		Degrees of Freedom		8
0.55	0.3025	2000				
0.59	0.3481	2100		X Coefficient(s)	3288.126	1072.438
0.65	0.4225	2100		Std Err of Coef.	408.3467	284.9669
0.66	0.4356	2200				
0.85	0.7225	3400				
1.30	1.69	5800				

Excellent correlation is noted.
Equation (3) follows, for calculation of ranges in micrometers:

Range = (3288.126 x Energy) + (1072.438 x Energy^2) - 279.879

Energy (MeV)	Energy^2	Calculated Range	Observed Range
0.18	0.0324	346.731	340
0.19	0.0361	383.580	380
0.21	0.0441	457.922	470
0.33	0.1089	921.991	880
0.54	0.2916	1808.432	1900
0.55	0.3025	1853.003	2000
0.59	0.3481	2033.431	2100
0.65	0.4225	2310.508	2100
0.66	0.4356	2357.438	2200
0.85	0.7225	3289.865	3400
1.30	1.69	5807.105	5800

Equation (3) provides a good fit to the observed data and will be used for calculations of range in the electron energy region 0.22 through 1.30 MeV.

===

Calculation of Ranges in Tissue for the Electrons in the Tables of Chapter 32

===

In making the calculations we must convert the energies in the tables of Chapter 32 to MeV from KeV, since our equations are for energies in MeV.

In making the calculations for each electron energy, the appropriate one of the three equations will be used, depending on the energy of electrons.

Data from Table 32-A

Electrons produced from interaction of 596 Kev Photons of Ra-226

(All energies are converted to MeV)

In our cuboidal model (see Chapter 20) we use a dimension of 11.4 micrometers as an edge of a cuboidal cell. Therefore, if we divide the range of the electron by 11.4, we obtain the number of cells traversed, for the case of electrons normal to a cell face.

Electron energies in MeV

Electron Energy	Energy^2	Calculated Range (in micrometers)	Equation Used	Cells Traversed
0.2086	0.043507	462.6348	(2)	40.5820
0.1167	0.013625	150.1072	(2)	13.1673
0.0696	0.004848	73.8662	(1)	6.4795
0.0443	0.001960	38.3533	(1)	3.3643
0.0298	0.000889	19.5425	(1)	1.7143
0.0211	0.000444	8.6874	(1)	0.7620
0.0155	0.000241	1.9748	(1)	0.1732
0.0904	0.008169	105.3433	(1)	9.2406

Sum of cell traversals if all post-Compton photons
are absorbed in biological tissue.   75.4833

Data from Table 32-B

Electrons produced from interaction of 662 Kev Photons of Cs-137

(All energies are converted to MeV)

Electron energies in MeV

Electron Energy	Energy^2	Calculated Range (in micrometers)	Equation Used	Cells Traversed
0.2388	0.057037	566.5767	(3)	49.6997
0.1319	0.017406	185.7767	(2)	16.2962
0.0776	0.006017	85.6586	(1)	7.5139
0.0487	0.002367	44.2622	(1)	3.8827
0.0324	0.001048	22.8021	(1)	2.0002
0.0227	0.000514	10.6293	(1)	0.9324
0.0165	0.000274	3.2062	(1)	0.2812
0.0934	0.008729	110.1429	(1)	9.6617

Sum of cell traversals if all post-Compton photons
are absorbed in biological tissue.   90.2680

===

Data from Table 32-C
Electrons produced from interaction of 1608 Kev Photons (Hiroshima)
(All energies are converted to MeV)

Electron Energy	Energy^2	Calculated Range (in micrometers)	Equation Used	Cells Traversed
0.6938	0.481310	2517.483	(3)	220.8318
0.3573	0.127643	1031.762	(3)	90.5055
0.1909	0.036445	384.4227	(2)	33.7213
0.1078	0.011619	132.1162	(2)	11.5891
0.0649	0.004214	67.0220	(1)	5.8791
0.0416	0.001734	34.8566	(1)	3.0576
0.0283	0.000799	17.5833	(1)	1.5424
0.0201	0.000404	7.5043	(1)	0.6583
0.0149	0.000221	1.2171	(1)	0.1068
0.0885	0.007825	102.3349	(1)	8.9767

Sum of cell traversals if all post-Compton photons
are absorbed in biological tissue.   376.8686

Ranges and cell traversals are all transferred to Table 20-FG.

2. The Consequences of Escape of Some Post-Compton Photons

While we consider total absorption of Post-Compton photons to represent the most reasonable description of what actually occurs, we can consider the extreme possibility that ALL Post-Compton photons are lost from the tissue, and that the delivery of 1 cGy of energy to the tissue all comes from the electrons set in motion by the first Compton process involving the original photon incident on tissue.

For this purpose, we can consider the case of the gamma rays from radium-226 and its daughters. The physics demands that the first process is a Compton process, since the cross-section for photon absorption for gamma rays of 596 KeV is far higher than that for any other possible process. The data from Table 32-A show that the average energy of the Compton electrons is 0.2086 MeV, and therefore that the Post-Compton photons have an average energy = 0.596 - 0.2086, or 0.3874 MeV. If those Post-Compton photons are totally lost from the tissue, then only 0.2086 MeV are absorbed per original photon.

Our interest is in the calculation of the number of nuclear traversals per nucleus at 1 cGy absorbed dose. In order to absorb 1 cGy under these circumstances we would have to increase the number of original photons by a factor of 0.596/0.208582, or 2.857389 . And instead of 40.582 cell traversals being produced by the first Post-Compton electron, we would have 2.857389 x 40.582, or 115.9585 cell traversals per 1 cGy. In the data for Table 32-A, we saw that total absorption of all the Post-Compton photons leads to 75.483 cell traversals at a dose of 1 cGy.

Cell traversals at 1 cGy would therefore be increased by a factor of (115.9585 / 75.483), which is 1.53622. Number of nuclear traversals is proportional to the number of cell traversals, so nuclear traversals would likewise be increased by a factor of 1.53622.

In Chapter 20, it was demonstrated that with total absorption of all Post-Compton photons, the number of nuclear traversals per nucleus at 1 cGy would be 2.9370 (from Table 20-K in Chapter 20.) If this number were increased by a factor of 1.53622, the number of nuclear traversals per nucleus at 1 cGy would be 1.53622 x 2.9370, or 4.806. Even this wildly extreme case of loss of all Post-Compton photons leads to a value of nuclear traversals per nucleus at 1 cGy which would not meaningfully alter our considerations in these discussions of disproof of a safe threshold.

==

Since the extreme assumptions are certainly not correct, and since most Post-Compton photons will be absorbed, we can hardly be off in our discussions by our approximation that all Post-Compton photons will be absorbed.

3. The Agreement between Our Estimates of Nuclear Traversals per cGy (Rad) and the Estimates of Four Other Workers

Even though some committees, such as UNSCEAR-88, hardly make any use of considerations of the crucial importance of ionization track analysis in assessing problems such as that of a "safe dose with respect to cancer induction by radiation," workers other than us are showing a keen interest in this approach. It is of great interest to us to ascertain whether or not reasonable agreement exists between workers in this field concerning the number of nuclear traversals per cGy in tissue for various low-LET radiations.

A. The Estimates of Rossi

Rossi (Rossi84) presented estimates of nuclear track traversals per unit dose of radiation for two types of radiation (a) ortho-voltage X-rays (tube operated at 250 kilo-volts peak) and (b) gamma rays from Cobalt-60. Rossi based his calculations on cells with a nuclear diameter of 5 microns, and indicated (correctly) that the calculation would be different for nuclei of some other diameter. We presented the method for converting nuclear traversals per unit dose for one cell-size to the value for another cell-size (Go86, p.46). Since others may wish to do such calculations for cells of varying nuclear and cellular diameter, we shall demonstrate how the conversions are to be made.

We shall start the comparison of our evaluation with that of Rossi by showing what answer we would get for cells with a nuclear diameter of 7.1 micro-meters. And since we suspect strongly that he must have converted all the photon energy for Cobalt-60 gamma rays to photo-electrons (which we do not consider to be the correct approach), we shall make this conversion just for the purpose of seeing how well we agree with Rossi in general method. For the X-rays, the conversion of all the photon energy to photo-electrons is reasonable, and we ordinarily do use this conversion in the calculations of Chapter 32. We start with consideration of the X-rays.

(a) X-rays from operation at 250 kilo-volts peak.
In Table 20-"O" the detailed calculations are made for nuclear traversals per cGy for the 83.3 KeV photo-electrons created by the photons of same average energy when 250 Kvp sources are used. The value presented there is 2.28 nuclear traversals per nucleus for a dose of one cGy. This value, of course, is what we calculate for a nuclear diameter of 7.1 micrometers.

(b) photons from Cobalt-60
We are here making the approximation (with which we disagree) that only PHOTO-electrons of an energy of 1173 KeV are produced.

The range in tissue from such electrons is calculated from the equation developed earlier in this chapter.

$$Range = (3288.126 \times Energy) + (1072.438 \times Energy^2) - 279.879$$

Energy in MeV	Energy^2	Range microns	Cuboidal Cell Traversals per Electron (for cells 11.4 microns across)
1.173	1.3759	5052.691	443.2185

Now, for the Cobalt-60 source, we go through the various steps required to obtain the number of nuclear traversals per nucleus for one cSv of dose.

Item C: Number of photons required to deliver a dose of 1 cGy.
The energy delivery must be 6.24E+10 KeV per gram of tissue.

Photon Energy in KeV	Number of photons required for 1 cGy delivered
1173	53196930.94 (5.32E+07 in exponential notation)

    (Since, for this calculation, all photon energy is converted to
photo-electrons, the number of electrons = number of photons.)

Item H: Total cell traversals for 1 cSv

Electron Energy in KeV	Electrons Required for 1 cGy	Cell Traversals per Electron	Total Cell Traversals
1173	5.32E+07	443.2185	2.36E+10

Item I: Total nuclear traversals per nucleus at 1 cSv

Electron Energy in KeV	Total Nuclear Traversals equals (Cell Traversals x 0.25)
1173	5.89E+09

Item J: Earlier (Chapter 20) we calculated the number of nuclei per
gram of cells to be 6.75E+08 per gram, for cuboidal cells of thickness
of 11.4 microns.

Item I / Item J: Nuclear traversals per nucleus for 1 cGy

Electron Energy in KeV	Nuclear Traversals per Nucleus
1173	8.733046

    This would be our answer IF we used the conversion of all photon energy to photo-electron
energy, without considering the Compton process for the 1173-KeV photons.

    Rossi assigned cells a nuclear diameter of 5 microns. We must now see what factor must be applied to
his answers if he were to use cells with a nuclear diameter of 7.1 microns. The nuclear diameter enters the
calculation in two ways. We shall assume our convention of taking cell diameter as twice the nuclear
diameter.

    Cell volume goes up as the cube of diameter, so if we go from a nuclear diameter of 5 to one of 7.1
microns, we have cell volume going up by a factor of $(7.1 / 5)^3$. And this means that cells per gram of
cellular material will go down, and the factor of decrease will be $(5 / 7.1)^3$. Nuclei per gram equal cells per
gram, so nuclei per gram would decrease by that same factor.

    Cell traversals will go down with increase in cellular (or nuclear) diameter by the factor, 5 / 7.1. This will
also be true of nuclear traversals.

==

Now, nuclear traversals per nucleus = $\dfrac{\text{Total nuclear traversals}}{\text{Nuclei per gram of cells}}$

If we convert Rossi's values of nuclear traversals per nucleus to what they would be for a nuclear diameter of 7.1 instead of 5.0 microns, we would multiply the numerator by a factor (5 / 7.1), and we would multiply denominator by (5 / 7.1)^3. This means that overall we would be multiplying Rossi's values by a factor of (1)/(5 / 7.1)^2, which is the same as multiplying the Rossi value by a factor of (7.1 / 5)^2.

Rossi reported his value of nuclear traversals per nucleus at 1 cGy(rad) to be 5 for the Cobalt-60. Therefore, adjusted to nuclear diameter of 7.1 microns, his value becomes:

$$5 \times (7.1 / 5)^2 = 5 \times 2.0164 = 10.082 \text{ nuclear}$$
$$\text{traversals per nucleus.}$$

We have calculated (above) a value of 8.733 nuclear traversals per nucleus. So if both Rossi's and our own calculations were based on total conversion of the 1173-KeV photon energy to photo-electrons, we find our calculated values only 13 % apart. We do not consider it correct to convert all the photon energy to photo-electrons, because the physics of the situation states that the energy must be converted to Compton electrons. But the agreement of Rossi's estimate (after an adjustment of Rossi's value to a nuclear diameter of 7.1 microns) and our own calculation to within 13 % indicates that all the other elements of the calculation must be in close agreement.

For the case of 83.33 KeV photons, Rossi's value is 1 nuclear traversal per nucleus at 1 cGy. If we adjust this for a nuclear diameter of 7.1 microns instead of 5 microns, we multiply as follows:

$$1 \times (7.1 / 5)^2 = 1 \times 2.0164 = 2.0164 \text{ nuclear traversals}$$
$$\text{per nucleus at 1 cGy (rad).}$$

Our value (above) is 2.28 nuclear traversals per nucleus at 1 cGy (rad). The difference between our value and Rossi's value is about 15 %, which is very close agreement. In this case we consider the values as the correct values, since it is appropriate to approximate, for photons of this energy, that total conversion to photo-electrons is correct.

Overall, therefore, it appears that we are in agreement with Rossi about the major dimensions of calculation of the nuclear traversals per nucleus at one cGy (rad), for two low–LET radiations widely separated in energy per primary electron.

B. The estimate of Brackenbush and Braby

Brackenbush and Braby (Brack88,p.252) state: "On the other hand, a gamma–ray exposure of 30 mGy produces an average of 24 events per cell nucleus." Since they are referring to a cell nucleus (spherical) of diameter of 7 micrometers, we are in agreement with respect to size of cell nucleus. Their calculation is for Cobalt-60 gamma rays, for which the energy is 1.173 MeV (1173 KeV).

A dose of 30 mGy is the same as 3 rads. This would mean their estimate of nuclear tracks per nucleus is 8 events per cGy (rad).

Unfortunately, Brackenbush and Braby provide no details about how they arrived at their estimate of nuclear tracks per nucleus.

We showed above that IF we used the conversion of 1173-KeV gamma rays totally to photo-electrons, we would get a value of 8.733 nuclear traversals per nucleus, which is exceedingly close to the Brackenbush-Braby estimate of 8 nuclear traversals per nucleus at one cGy. It is this close agreement which makes us believe that they must have used total energy conversion to photo-electrons for Cobalt-60 photons.

===

C. The Estimate of Goodhead

Goodhead (Good87, p.237, Figure 5a) states: " A dose of 1 Gy corresponds to approximately 1000 tracks." We found that his Figure evaluates to a nuclear diameter of ~7.5 micrometers. Goodhead provides no energy value for the gamma rays, other than to say that the gamma rays represent low-LET radiation. Nor are any details whatever given as to how the estimate of nuclear tracks is made. If there are 1000 tracks per nucleus for 1 Gy, this would correspond to 10 tracks in each nucleus for one cGy. Since Goodhead uses a nuclear diameter of 7.5 microns, his nuclear tracks per nucleus would be corrected by a factor of $(7.1 / 7.5)^2$, or 0.896177. His estimate of nuclear tracks per nucleus at one cGy would become 8.96. Our estimate assuming total conversion of photon energy to photo-electrons yielded a corresponding value of 8.73 tracks. However, since Goodhead does not tell us the energy of his assumed photons, we cannot usefully pursue the comparison any further.

The comparison of our approach with the approaches of four other investigators indicates that all of us must be in reasonable general agreement as to how the estimate of nuclear traversals per nucleus should be made. I consider the estimates in Table 20-K to be reliable, within the explicit approximations made.

Comments on Range Measurement and Path Length of Electrons

All of the measurements of the electron's travel through tissue are based upon what is known as the "extrapolated range." Electrons suffer severe deflections as they pass through tissue. As a result the true total path length traversed is not identical with the range, which is a penetration distance in a single direction.

If one studies the decrease in number of electrons transmitted through absorbers, one observes a progressive decrease in transmission with increasing absorber thickness even though the electrons are monoenergetic. If one extrapolates this transmission-decrease curve to the point of intersection with "background" (the measurement without any radiation source added), a reproducible entity is obtained, known as the "extrapolated range."

For very low energy electrons (e.g. 19.6 KeV electrons), the "extrapolated range" is less than the mean path length actually traveled by electrons (in oxygen, a medium of low atomic number close to the atomic number of tissue) by approximately 20 % (Ev55). The fractional difference between "extrapolated range" and path length actually traveled decreases with increasing energy of the electron. Thus, for electrons of 30 KeV, set in motion by the photo-electric process by medical X-rays, we may be underestimating the true distance traveled per electron, on the average, by somewhere between 0 and 15 %. We have not endeavored to correct for this difference between "extrapolated range" and true distance traveled.

For most of the electrons set in motion by the photo-electric and Compton effects in our studies, the energies are high enough so that the fractional difference between "extrapolated range" and distance traveled is negligible. For the low-energy electrons produced in Compton processes, the contribution to total cell traversals is negligible for these electrons, even if their true distance traveled deserves a correction for the difference between the "extrapolated range" and true distance traveled.

======

CHAPTER 34

Allusions to the Possible Existence of Safe Doses and Dose-Rates

At the beginning of Chapter 18, we asserted that there are influential supporters in the radiation community for the idea that safe doses or dose-rates of ionizing radiation are a realistic possibility.

The purpose of this chapter is to back up our assertion with documentation, and to show that safe-dose speculations appear in some very influential publications. Because this is the chapter's purpose, and because the scientific substance of the threshold issue has been presented elsewhere in this book, we are keeping our own comments to a minimum here.

The entries in this chapter illustrate the nature and dissemination of safe-dose speculations. The sampling is arranged in alphabetical order. Affiliations of persons generally refer to their affiliations when they made the statements. The following names have entries in this chapter:

Alexander, 1988.
Anspaugh, Catlin, and Goldman, 1987 and 1988.
BEIR-3 Committee, 1980.
Department of Energy Report, 1987.
Evans, Wennberg, and McNeil, 1986.
Gilbert, 1985.
Goldschmidt and Sherwin, 1985.
Hickey, 1981 and 1988.
Loken, 1987.
Nuclear Regulatory Commission, 1985.
Rasmussen, 1989.
Ray, 1986 and 1987.
Southwood, 1987.
Taylor, 1980.
UNSCEAR Committee, 1986.
Upton, 1987 and 1989.
Wagner and Ketchum, 1989.
Webster, 1982 and 1987.
Wolfe, 1986.
Yalow, 1980-1989.

The Evans, Hickey, and Southwood entries include suggestions that "repair" may deliver a threshold below which doses are safe. The Gilbert, Hickey, Rasmussen, Wolfe, and Yalow entries include suggestions that low doses may be good for health -- a topic examined by us in Chapter 35. The Upton entries are "mixed," as readers will see for themselves.

● -- *Alexander, 1988 :*

=======================================

Robert E. Alexander identifies himself (Alex88a; Alex88b) as the 1988-89 President of the Health Physics Society, official with U.S. Nuclear Regulatory Commission, and member of a panel assisting the Veterans' Administration in adjudicating claims of service-related radiogenic cancer. The panel was organized by the White House Office of Science and Technology Policy, Committee on Interagency Radiation Research and Policy Coordination (Alex88b, p.592).

Referring to estimates of cancer and genetic consequences from nuclear power accidents, Alexander states that "the probability of zero effects [is] a highly significant probability at low doses" (Alex88a, p.144).

Referring to the Department of Energy's 1987 report which estimated cancer fatalities from the Chernobyl accident (Doe87), Alexander says, "... a recent study sponsored by the U.S. Department of Energy published an estimate of 28,000 fatalities. This report repeatedly states that it is possible that no delayed deaths will occur... The DOE report makes it clear that ... very low lifetime doses would likely produce no additional radiological risk, and that there are no direct data confirming that a few random ionizations in tissue will cause fatal cancers" (Alex88a, p144).

Still using the DOE report as the authority on such matters, Alexander points out that the DOE report repeatedly states, with respect to radiation-induced cancer, that "The possibility of zero health effects at very low doses and dose rates cannot be excluded" (Alex88a, p.145). He continues, "Many health physicists are dismayed by the now-common practice of including extremely low doses in health effects estimates. When doses obtained in this manner are multiplied by risk coefficients valid at best for doses exceeding 10 rads and dose rates exceeding 1 rad / yr, the results can be alarming and misleading, and they may have a detrimental influence on decision-makers. If individual doses below 10 rads and dose rates below 1 rad / yr for a lifetime are excluded from the 28,000 estimated cancer deaths, only the evacuees are affected and the theoretical result is 410" (Alex88a, p.145).

Alexander's views are quoted at much greater length

in Chapter 24, Parts 9 and 10, and so readers will be in a position to make their own interpretations.

● -- Anspaugh, Catlin, and Goldman, 1987 and 1988 :

===

Lynn R. Anspaugh is an analyst in environmental sciences at DOE's Livermore National Laboratory, and a new member of the 1988 UNSCEAR radiation committee. Robert J. Catlin is an advisor to the Radiation Studies Program of the Electric Power Research Institute (EPRI). Marvin Goldman is Professor of Radiobiology at the University of California School of Veterinary Medicine at Davis.

Anspaugh, Catlin, and Goldman are three of the five principal authors of DOE's report on Chernobyl (Doe87), and they are the three authors named on the report's revised and condensed version, which appeared as a very widely quoted article in the journal SCIENCE (Ansp88).

Both the long and short versions of the report are filled with allusions to the possible existence of safe doses and dose-rates (as noted by Alexander, above), and both repeatedly cite this lower limit on risk. For instance, allusions to zero-risk can be found in the DOE report even in the Executive Summary (p.xi twice, p.xiii), and then throughout the chapters relating to cancer-risk (for instance, at pages 7.5, 7.8, 7.10, 7.13, 7.14, 7.22, 7.29, J.3, J.7, J.8).

Within the six-page SCIENCE version of the DOE report, the authors assert ten times that there may be NO Chernobyl-induced cancers beyond the immediate vicinity of the accident. On the final page (Ansp88, p.1518), they state: "The numbers we derive are increments in a probability distribution, and are not the certainty frequently reported in the media. Thus we reiterate that these risk estimates do not rule out zero as a possibility." Of course, this feature of their article was widely reported by the mass media.

Readers will find additional safe-dose allusions from these authors quoted in Chapter 24, Part 8. These authors make no analysis of the threshold issue on their own; they rely as follows on the NCRP and BEIR-3 Committees:

"As noted in NCRP Report No. 64 (1980), there are no direct data that confirm that a few random ionizations in tissue cause fatal cancers. Moreover, the BEIR Committee noted that for low dose and dose rates, the likelihood of zero deleterious effects is not precluded" (Doe87, p.7.5).

● -- BEIR-3 Committee, 1980 :

===

The BEIR radiation committee was described in Chapter 1. The BEIR-3 Report of 1980 is the one which preceded the BEIR-5 Report of 1990. (The BEIR-4 Report concerned only radon and other alpha-emitting radionuclides.) Authors of the BEIR Reports are acknowledged in our Chapter 37.

In BEIR-3, following a discussion of equations which might describe cancer as a function of dose, the following statement alludes to the issue of a threshold (safe dose):

"The mathematical functions discussed above assume that there is no threshold dose below which there is no excess risk. On statistical grounds, however, the existence or non-existence of a threshold dose is practically impossible to determine ..." (Beir80, p.22).

Later, at page 139: "It is by no means clear whether dose rates of gamma or x radiation of about 100 mrads/yr are in any way detrimental to exposed people; any somatic effects would be masked by environmental or other factors that produce the same types of health effects as does ionizing radiation."

Shortly thereafter, BEIR-3 states that it will make estimates of radiogenic cancer-risk for three situations: (1) A single exposure of a representative population to 10 rads, (2) a continuous, lifetime exposure of a representative population to one rad per year, and (3) adult exposure to one rad per year as if it were occupational exposure.

Then BEIR-3 makes the following statement (Beir80, p.144): "Below these doses, the uncertainties of extrapolation of risk were believed by some members of the Committee to be too great to justify calculation."

Later, BEIR-3 explicitly leaves open the possibility of a threshold below which doses would be safe (Beir80, p.181): "There are a number of possible dose-response functions, but there is no compelling evidence of the validity of any one. Although none can be proved to be inapplicable to carcinogenesis, in its estimates of low-dose risk the Committee chose not to include the class of functions with a threshold, i.e., functions in which the cancer risk is zero up to some positive value on the dose-scale."

And referring back to its three types of risk-estimates, BEIR-3 again speculates about existence of a completely safe dose (Beir80, p.193): "Selection of dose increments for which cancer-risk estimates are made was guided by existing maximal permissible dose limits, information on occupational exposure recorded in recent surveys, concern for a hypothetical situation in which some part of the general population might be exposed to a single dose of 10 rads, and uncertainty as to whether a total dose of, say, 1 rad would have any effect at all."

● -- *Department of Energy, 1987, 1988 :*
=======================================

See Anspaugh.

● -- *Evans, Wennberg, and McNeil, 1986 :*
=======================================

John S. Evans, at the Harvard School of Public Health, Department of Environmental Sciences, is one of the three principal authors of the Nuclear Regulatory Commission's 1985 report (Nrc85), which is used by Anspaugh (in the DOE report) and others to make their central estimates of cancer-risk from radiation exposure. John E. Wennberg is at the Dartmouth Medical School, Department of Community and Family Medicine. Barbara J. McNeil is at the Harvard Medical School, Department of Radiology. Wennberg and McNeil were NOT the other co-authors of Nrc85.

Evans, Wennberg and McNeil are co-authors of an article in the NEW ENGLAND JOURNAL OF MEDICINE on the risk of breast-cancer and leukemia from diagnostic radiography (Evans86). They provide "central, lower, and upper estimates of risk" and then they allude to the possibility of a completely safe dose, based on "repair" (Evans86, p.814):

"Nonetheless, it is possible that the true risk is either zero [Jab80] or perhaps even higher than our upper estimates. Values may be lower than ours if cellular repair processes are rapid enough to reverse damage caused by the low doses employed in diagnostic studies."

● -- *Gilbert, July 1985 :*
=======================================

Ethel S. Gilbert, an analyst at Battelle Pacific Northwest Laboratories, was not one of the three principal authors of Nrc85, but she is named as author of its key chapter with respect to radiogenic cancer ("Late Somatic Effects"). Discussing estimated cancer-consequences of accidental exposure, she inserts an allusion to a possible threshold AND possible benefit from low-dose exposure:

"It is noted that although the possibility that an effect

might not be detrimental (in fact, it might even be beneficial) cannot be excluded at very low doses and dose rates, these possibilities have not been incorporated into the calculation of the lower bound estimates" (Nrc85, page II: 93).

● -- *Goldschmidt and Sherwin, 1985 :*
=======================================

Herbert Goldschmidt and William K. Sherwin are co-authors of the chapter on "Dermatologic Radiation Therapy" in a widely used dermatology textbook. They allude to the possibility of a safe-dose when they say (Goldsc85, p.2062):

"In contrast to the effects of large radiation doses, there is no unequivocal evidence of injury in man from doses of the order of those received during LOW-DOSE medical treatments (including properly administered dermatologic radiotherapy), particularly for doses below 0.5 Gy (50 rad)."

● -- *Hickey, 1981 and 1988 :*
=======================================

Richard J. Hickey is Professor Emeritus of Statistics, Ecological Statistics Group, University of Pennsylvania Wharton School, Philadelphia. Our Chapter 21, Part 2, discusses one of Hickey's studies (Hic81), which appeared in HEALTH PHYSICS in 1981. The study is a "Denver-Type" study which cannot address the threshold issue. Nonetheless, Hickey and co-workers interpret their study as evidence for a safe dose:

"This preliminary work suggests ... that models implying important long-term deleterious effects of low levels of ionizing radiation on humans may be invalid" (Hic81, p.625).

Hickey et al suggest that the no-threshold hypothesis is no more credible than the following hypothesis: "... adaptive mechanisms have evolved which cope with ambient radiation ... although ionizing radiation is damaging at elevated levels and rates of exposure, there is a level of radiation exposure below which health effects at the level of the organism are negligible or beneficial" (Hic81, p.625).

They assert that their "... preliminary observations are not compatible with models that assert that all levels of radiation, no matter how low, are damaging" (Hic81, p.635).

They suggest: "The hypothesis may be considered that under ecologically realistic conditions of exposure to low levels of radiations, DNA-repair (and other defense mechanisms) are stimulated to such an extent that efficiency is elevated above the level necessary to repair low-level radiation damage" (Hic81, p.637).

In the years since 1981, Hickey appears not to have changed his views. In a letter entitled "Health and Nuclear Power Plants," published in CHEMICAL AND ENGINEERING NEWS (Hic88, p.2), Hickey makes the following statements (parentheses are his own):

"The linear, no-threshold hypothesis (ideology?) must be considered to be scientifically invalid on the ground that it is incompatible with observed data. It is also incompatible with extensive evidence on the reality of the biophysical phenomenon of radiation hormesis, as discussed in depth by T.D. Luckey [Luc80] ... and by R.J. Hickey and E. J. Bowers ..." (Hic88, p.2).

Hickey's letter reveals that he and Bowers had the opportunity to write about hormesis in the 1986 edition of PHYSICS IN MEDICINE AND BIOLOGY ENCYCLOPEDIA, Volume 1, p.387, which we have not seen. Luckey's book is briefly described in our Chapter 35.

Hickey's letter also criticizes newspapers for reporting statements "alleging that all levels of ionizing radiation are hazardous to health (usually based on the linear, no-threshold 'theory,' which is erroneous) ..." (Hic88, p.47).

Hickey ends this letter by warning against extrapolations "which are speculative and possibly influenced by ideology" (Hic88, p.47).

● -- *Loken, 1987 :*
==

Merle K. Loken is at the Division of Nuclear Medicine, University of Minnesota Hospitals, Minneapolis, and is a member of the American Medical Association's Committee on Non-Military Radiation Emergencies. In an invited "Commentary" article entitled "Physicians' Obligations in Radiation Issues," featured in the JOURNAL OF THE AMERICAN MEDICAL ASSOCIATION, Loken states (emphasis in the original):

"...effects, whether genetic or somatic, have been clearly demonstrated ONLY after exposures to relatively large doses of radiation (usually >1 Gy or 100 rads). To address the possibility of biologic effects of low-level radiation exposure, it is necessary to extrapolate from the data points obtained at relatively high doses toward zero dose. This permits ESTIMATES OF RISK to be made, but in the final analysis, NO DATA FROM HUMANS EXIST THAT SHOW THAT LOW-LEVEL RADIATION EXPOSURES PRODUCE MEASURABLE BIOLOGIC EFFECTS" (Loken87, p.673).

Later on the same page, he asserts "... it is reasonable to conclude that there is no proved body of fact that establishes an increase in human cancer after low doses of ionizing radiation (such as those received environmentally, occupationally, or for medical diagnostic procedures), that is, radiation levels below about 0.1 Gy (10 rad)." At the end of this sentence, Loken offers one citation to support his assertions. He cites Webs81.

[We interrupt to identify Webster. Edward Webster was a member of the BEIR-3 Committee, and is a member of the 1988 UNSCEAR Committee. A more recent Webster paper (Webs87) is discussed in our Chapter 24, Part 9. Also, we remind readers that even in 1981, there was good human evidence of radiation carcinogenesis below ten rads; we refer to the dates of some studies cited in Chapter 21, Part 1.]

● -- *Nuclear Regulatory Commission, 1985 :*
==

See Gilbert.

● -- *Rasmussen, 1989 :*
==

Norman C. Rasmussen is a nuclear engineer at the Massachusetts Institute of Technology (MIT). He was director in 1974 of the (U.S.) Atomic Energy Commission's famous $3 million study, in fourteen volumes, AN ASSESSMENT OF ACCIDENT RISKS IN U.S. COMMERCIAL NUCLEAR POWER PLANTS, WASH-1400, widely called "the Rasmussen Report" (Ras74). Recently, Rasmussen has spoken to a vast readership via the NATIONAL GEOGRAPHIC magazine. Rasmussen says:

"There is a lot of evidence that low radiation doses not only don't cause harm but may in fact do some good. After all, humankind evolved in a world of natural low-level radiation" (Ras89, p.411).

● -- *Ray, 1986 and 1987 :*
==

Dixy Lee Ray is a biologist, former Chairperson of the U.S. Atomic Energy Commission, and former governor of Washington state.

In 1986, in the course of reviewing the book UNDER THE CLOUD: THE DECADES OF NUCLEAR TESTING,

Ray charges "anti-nuclear activists" with disregarding "the extensive and growing evidence that even chronic exposure to low levels of radiation causes no damage" (Ray86).

In 1987, she uses the phrase "safe levels" directly. In remarks distributed to Congress on the first anniversary of the Chernobyl accident and quoted by the SEATTLE POST-INTELLIGENCER , April 30, 1987 (Ray87):

"Reindeer meat contamination is well below safe and permissible levels," "there were no fatalities or hospitalizations among the general public," radiation effects outside the Soviet Union "were negligible," and the most important lesson from Chernobyl is "how poorly we communicate scientific information to the American public."

[We interrupt to remind readers that Table 24-B offers a set of realistic estimates of radiation effects inside and outside the Soviet Union from Chernobyl.]

● -- *Southwood, 1987 :*

==

Sir Richard Southwood is chairman of Britain's National Radiological Protection Board (NRPB), and co-editor with Jones of the 1987 book RADIATION AND HEALTH: THE BIOLOGICAL EFFECTS OF LOW-LEVEL EXPOSURE TO IONIZING RADIATION (Jones87). In this book, Southwood says that there is no way to know the dose-response shape below 50 cSv (his figure 2), and then he adds speculations which include the possibility of a completely safe dose somewhere in this allegedly mysterious region:

"The problem arises in determining what happens at lower levels. Should the line be projected as a straight linear line to zero or is there some non-linear relationship of enhanced or reduced sensitivity at lower levels or perhaps, related to the body's repair mechanisms, a threshold?" (South87, p.5).

● -- *Taylor, 1980 :*

==

Lauriston Taylor, now retired, is a physicist and was for many years the president of the National Council on Radiation Protection (NCRP, USA). His 1980 Sievert Lecture, "Some Non-Scientific Influences on Radiation Protection Standards and Practice," was published in HEALTH PHYSICS (Tay80) and quoted by Hic85 (p.949) as follows -- with the brackets provided by Hickey:

"Let us stop arguing about the people who are being injured by exposures to radiation at levels far below those where any effects can be found. The fact is, the [harmful] effects are not found despite over 40 years of [searching]. The theories about people being injured have still not led to the documentation of injury, and though considered as fact by some, must only be looked upon as figments of the imagination."

● -- *UNSCEAR Committee, 1986 :*

==

The United Nations Scientific Committee on the Effects of Atomic Radiation (UNSCEAR) refers to the absence of any safe doses and dose-rates as "a working hypothesis" which no one has proven:

"The absence of a threshold dose is assumed by the Committee as a working hypothesis for the moment" (Un86, p.13, Para.46-C).

"Although absence of the threshold is often assumed, this has not been proved for any form of radiation-induced malignancy and must be regarded as a working hypothesis... Proving or disproving a threshold below the levels of direct observation may be impossible, due to statistical fluctuations of the spontaneous level and of the presumably induced response ..." (Un86, p.166, Para.3).

[Readers are reminded that these problems can be overcome when young adults receive a HIGH total dose via a series of small doses, and when an appropriate control group is available; Chapters 18 and 21.]

● -- *Upton, 1987 and 1989 :*

==

Arthur C. Upton is Chairman of the current BEIR-5 Committee. In earlier times, he did radiation studies, sponsored by the Atomic Energy Commission, with experimental animals at the Oak Ridge National Laboratory, Biology Division. Upton has been a member of almost all the radiation committees (see Chapter 37), and has also been director of the National Cancer Institute.

In 1987, Upton wrote a paper entitled "Prevention of Work-Related Injuries and Diseases: Lessons from Experience with Ionizing Radiation," which was published in the AMERICAN JOURNAL OF INDUSTRIAL MEDICINE (Up87). In this paper, Upton makes a statement which encourages threshold speculations, while at the same time he acknowledges that human evidence supports the hypothesis that no such threshold exists. We shall quote the passages verbatim (from Up87, p.300-301), except that we shall put his citations into the form used in our own reference list.

"... the dose-incidence data in irradiated human populations, although available over a relatively wide range of doses (Un77; Beir80), do not suffice to define precisely the dose-incidence relationship for carcinogenesis in the low dose domain or to exclude the possibility of a threshold.

"Several lines of epidemiological evidence support the hypothesis that there may be no threshold in the dose-incidence relationship (Beir80; Nih85). Perhaps the strongest lines of evidence are 1) the excess of leukemia and other cancers in children exposed prenatally to diagnostic X radiation at dose levels as low as 10-50 mGy (Mon84; Har85); 2) the excess of thyroid tumors that is associated with an average dose of only 60-80 mGy to the thyroid gland from X irradiation of the scalp for tinea capitis in childhood (Modan77; Sho80); 3) the dose-dependent excess of leukemia in A-bomb survivors, which is detectable at doses as low as 0.25 Gy (Beir80; Nih85); and 4) the dose-dependent excess of breast cancer (Fig. 3), which is of similar magnitude per unit dose in a) women exposed to A-bomb radiation, b) women given therapeutic irradiation for postpartum mastitis, c) women subjected to multiple fluoroscopic examinations of the chest during the treatment of pulmonary tuberculosis with artificial pneumothorax, and d) women exposed occupationally to external gamma radiation in the painting of luminous clock and instrument dials (Boice79; Beir80; Bav81). The similarity of the dose-incidence relationships in all four groups of women, in spite of marked differences among the groups in duration of exposure, implies that the carcinogenic effect of a small dose on the breast is largely irreparable and that the effects of successive doses are additive (Beir80; Un82)."

In a publication which reaches many more people, namely THE NATIONAL GEOGRAPHIC, April 1989, an interview with Upton on the safe-dose topic is related as follows (Up89, p.418, p.420). The narrative is presented within the double quotation-marks, and specific statements by Upton are presented within the single quotation-marks:

"Is there a threshold below which radiation will have no effect? Few scientists think so any more. Said Dr. Arthur C. Upton, chairman of the New York University Medical Center Department of Environmental Medicine: 'Any radioactive track can, in principle, deposit enough energy to cause a mutation.' But, Dr. Upton stressed, at low levels 'it would be a prodigious task to prove' what the biological effect is ... Said Dr. Upton: 'There is no proof that a millirem does or does not do anything.

One is in the position of making guesses.'"

[A careful track-analysis is the opposite of making guesses. And it is the careful track-analysis in Chapters 20, 32, and 33 which has shown that below a few HUNDRED millirems of total tissue-dose, virtually no further reduction in dose at the level of cell-nuclei is even POSSIBLE -- as discussed in Chapter 20, Part 3.]

● *-- Wagner and Ketchum, 1989 :*

==

Henry N. Wagner, Jr., is Director of the Divisions of Nuclear Medicine and Radiation Health Sciences at the Johns Hopkins University School of Medicine. Linda E. Ketchum is medical editor and writer at ProClinica, Inc. in New York. The University has published their book, LIVING WITH RADIATION (Wag89).

In this book, Wagner and Ketchum devote about two pages (Wag89, pp.41-43) directly to the threshold issue. We will quote (in sequence) as much context as we can.

"In the past, scientists made a significant assumption ... and many many scientists still accept it today -- namely, that the harmful effects from high doses of radiation also occur at low doses of radiation, even if such effects have never been observed and cannot be observed. This is known as the no-threshold hypothesis" (Wag89, p.41).

"If the no-threshold hypothesis is not true for acute lethality, can it be true for cancer? ... This may be true, but it is impossible to test the hypothesis, because so many people develop cancer from other causes" (Wag89, p.41-42).

"In their efforts to ensure safety in the absence of direct experimental evidence, international and national organizations whose responsibility it is to establish standards of acceptable radiation levels have adopted the 'linear dose-effect extrapolation with no threshold' hypothesis ... Although this assumption provides a generous margin of safety for avoiding the possible harmful effects of ionizing radiation, it has also led at times to excessive caution in the use of radiation" (Wag89, p.42).

[We interrupt to note that (A) the linear model UNDERestimates risk and provides NO margin of safety if the dose-response is supra-linear, and (B) the radiation committees have NOT been using the linear model when they recommend REDUCING risk-estimates by factors of 1.5 to 10 for low and slow exposures. See Chapters 14, 22 and 23.]

"For example, because of fear of radiation, some developing (and developed) countries have chosen to reject nuclear power as a source of electricity when, in fact, nuclear power might have been the best and safest choice. The no-threshold hypothesis can also impede public acceptance of even the minimal risk posed by small amounts of radiation. This hypothesis has led some people to believe that any level of radiation, no matter how small, carries some risk, even if that risk is not measurable. An alternative approach is to assume that a threshold exists unless one can prove with measurements that it does not" (Wag89, p.42).

"Acceptance of the no-threshold linear hypothesis has created a mindset in the public -- and even among many radiation experts -- that radiation at the millirem level of exposure is harmful and is a cause for concern, despite the fact that the no-threshold hypothesis has never been proved and cannot be proved. With doses of radiation in the millirem range, as in diagnostic X-rays and nuclear medical procedures, harmful effects, if they occur, are too infrequent to be observed" (Wag89, p.42).

"The 1980 report of the National Academy of Sciences' Committee on the Biological Effects of Ionizing Radiations, which examined all the data published up to that time, concluded that it is impossible to determine whether any risk to health is associated with radiation at doses of less than 10,000 millirems (10 rems)" (Wag89, p.43).

Setting the Record Straight :

Elsewhere in the same book, Wagner and Ketchum purport to tell readers about my estimate of radiation-induced cancer from diagnostic X-rays. They are wrong by 30-fold in stating my estimate. These authors assert (Wag89, p.99):

"... he [Gofman] has claimed that every year in the United States more than 1.5 million people die as a result of unnecessary medical radiation."

With minimal effort, they could have been accurate. My estimate is derived, step-by-step, in Chapter 17 of Go85. My estimates's time-frame is stated explicitly (Go85, p.14, 365, 369) as 30 years -- one generation -- not one year. The estimate does not concern dying -- it explicitly relates to cancer INCIDENCE (Go85, p.368). My estimate does not concern medical irradiation in general -- it explicitly includes only the unnecessarily high portion of doses received from diagnostic medical and dental X-rays, and excludes nuclear medicine and therapeutic irradiation (Go85, p.369).

We will set the record straight, here. My estimate is that unnecessary overdosing in diagnostic X-ray exams is inducing cancer at the rate of 50,000 unnecessary cases per year in the United States. Realistic reductions in dose -- without giving up a single exam -- would prevent 1.5 million unncessary cases of cancer PER 30 YEARS -- one generation (Go85, p.14, p.369).

Wagner and Ketchum also make false statements about my summers spent in commercial salmon fishing, but such misinformation is unimportant by comparison with their grossly incorrect statement about my cancer-estimate from diagnostic X-rays.

● -- Webster, 1982 and 1987 :
=======================================

Edward W. Webster, at the Division of Radiological Sciences, Massachusetts General Hospital (MGH), was an author of the BEIR-3 and UNSCEAR 1988 reports (see Chapter 37).

Webster has been talking about the hormetic speculation for quite a while. For instance, he and I and Edward Radford (Chairman of the BEIR-3 Committee) participated in a three-way "roundtable" discussion for the NEW YORK TIMES in 1982. In the discussion of a no-effect threshold, I said, "I do not believe that there is any dose at this time that has been shown to be without effect. Moreover, I think it is public health irresponsibility to assume that such a dose exists when one is not absolutely certain." In response to my statement, Webster made the following comment.

Dr. Webster (Webs82, p.EY 19): "I would disagree with that. I would say that there is considerable uncertainty. There are some interesting examples of increased lifespan at very low doses in animal populations. In fact, there's a whole body of thought which is developing called hormesis, which means that maybe a little bit of radiation could be beneficial. I'm not saying that I agree with this, but it's a school of thought which is the exact antithesis of saying that all low doses of radiation are bad."

[Evidence on longevity in irradiated animals is explored in Chapter 35, Part 2. Indeed, the 1988 UNSCEAR Committee, of which Webster was a member, concludes that "At the doses of greatest interest for practical purposes ... and down to the smallest doses and dose rates, evidence showed overwhelmingly (Un82) that irradiated animals live, on the average, fewer years than non-irradiated controls" (Un88, p.22, para.129). The reason for the observed life-shortening: Radiation-induced malignancies in the animals (Un88, p.22, para.130).]

In the years since 1982, Webster appears to have maintained his view that low doses, slowly delivered, may be without any carcinogenic effect at all. For instance, this is his position in a 1987 article (Webs87, last paragraph), an article from which we quote several passages in Chapter 24, Part 9.

[In Webs87, Webster invokes a "Denver-Type" study from China and the Holm radio-iodine study from Sweden for support. The irrelevance of both, to the threshold issue, is shown in our Chapter 21, Part 2, and in Chapter 22, Part 5.]

● -- Wolfe, 1986 :
===

In 1986, Bertram Wolfe was President of the American Nuclear Society. After the Chernobyl accident, he received space in THE DENVER POST to to tell the readership that there may be safe doses of radiation, or even doses which are good for people ("Maybe those who take mineral baths, which usually have elevated radioactivity levels, are on to something").

Wolfe begins his article by saying that public concern ("almost panic in some cases") about fallout from the Chernobyl and Three Mile Island accidents demonstrates "... that we nuclear scientists have failed to provide a common-sense view of health effects from radiation" (Wolfe86).

Then he procedes to speculate that there may be an undiscovered threshold:

"There is an increased risk of future cancer for doses of 100 Rem and above ... At much lower, more common radiation exposures, no clear effects on health have been found despite more than 40 years trying to find them. If there are any effects, they are so small they are masked by normal variations in health unconnected with radiation ... Nevertheless ... a collective dose of 10,000 Rem spread among many people is assumed to produce one cancer among them regardless of how small the individual doses are. When applied to aspirin, this assumption says that if a hundred aspirin will kill a person, then one person will die if 100 people each take one aspirin. There is no evidence that this assumption is truer for low doses of radiation than for low doses of aspirin ..." (Wolfe86).

"As a matter of prudence it is wise to avoid any unnecessary exposure. But at inadvertent exposures of a few Rem, and at natural background levels which are a tenth or two-tenths of a Rem per year, the effects -- whether harmful, beneficial, or absent -- are so

insignificant that they are masked by normal variations in health ... predictions of many thousands of future cancer deaths in Russia, as reported in the media, are derived from the exposure of 75 million Russians to levels of radiation comparable to that in Denver" (Wolfe86).

[In the absence of a safe dose or dose-rate, the unavoidable "background" doses are inducing cancers everywhere, and ADDING to the background doses adds still further to the radiation-induced number of cancers.]

● -- Yalow, 1980-1989 :
===

Rosalyn S. Yalow, who earned her doctorate in nuclear physics in 1945, is is senior medical investigator at the Veterans Administration Medical Center in the Bronx, New York. She won a Nobel Prize in 1977 for developing the radio-immunoassay technique for measuring substances in blood.

Yalow is a frequent critic of what she calls the public's "radiation hysteria" and "radiophobia." In 1985, she was selected to be one of nine members of the National Institutes of Health (USA) committee to quantify radiation hazards ("Working Group to Develop Radioepidemiological Tables"); see Nih85. Some of her statements are quoted in chronological order below.

1980: In her article entitled "Science: Our Hope, Not Our Foe" (Ya80), she says, "People are now urging that Congress spend money to re-examine the problem of low-level radiation effects. But on the basis of work over the past 50 years we can anticipate that this will provide no new information worth the cost because we already have a tremendous amount of knowledge in the field." In the same article, she implies a safe dose when she states "There is no scientific reason to expect that radioactive hospital wastes are potentially harmful."

1981, quoted in a newspaper (Ya81): "People have always been exposed to radioactivity and can withstand exposures to levels up to the kinds produced by nature."

1982: In her essay on "Psychology Tomorrow" (Ya82), she begins: "An interesting problem for psychology to investigate is what I call the almost phobic fear of radiation. Psychologists should be able to help people deal more reasonably in terms of real risk rather than perception of risk. Why do people have almost phobic reactions, when scientific analysis says there is no real risk?"

1983: Yalow is cited by Hickey (Hic85, p.950) as having written that "... probably a better case can be made for low-level radiation as an asset than the reverse" (Ya83).

1984: Yalow is also quoted by Hickey (Hic85, p.949) as having said, "To date, no proven body of evidence has established an increase in either malignancies or other harmful effects from low-level radiation" (Ya84).

1985: On ABC-Television's network program "Nightline," Yalow referred to "radiation hysteria" in the public (June 6, 1985).

1988: Yalow received space in THE SCIENTIST (which calls itself "the newspaper for the science professional") to write an article entitled "Unwarranted Fear about the Effects of Radiation Leads to Bad Science Policy" (Ya88). After referring to the A-Bomb Study, and to "studies in experimental animals," and to one leukemia study on hyperthyroid patients, she asserts that, "The overwhelming conclusion of these studies -- and others that could be cited -- is that doses under 10 rem, particularly when given at a low dose-rate, are not demonstrably carcinogenic" (Ya88, p.11).

She ends the article by scolding the National Institutes of Health (NIH) for undertaking a new survey of cancer-rates around nuclear facilities. "It is regrettable that the NIH has yielded to political pressure by beginning a new study rather than affirming the scientific conclusions reached in its own report [Nih85]. By this action, a disservice is done, not only to science, but to the U.S. populace as well. It contributes to and reinforces the radiation phobia that interferes not only

with our ability to employ the safest means for generating electricity but even with our ability to make optimal use of radiation in medicine" (Ya88, p.12).

1989: Yalow received the guest-editorial space in MEDICAL PHYSICS to write about "The Contributions of Medical Physicists to Radiation Phobia" (Ya89).

Early in her article, Yalow mistakenly asserts that I use an exaggerated risk-coefficient to assess the leukemia consequences from the Chernobyl accident -- although in fact the risk-coefficient to which she refers (from Go85 and Go86) is in good agreement with RERF's 1988 value -- as shown in Chapter 24, Part 3.

But this mistake of hers is a small matter compared with her embrace of inconclusive studies like the Holm radio-iodine study (Ya89, p.160), and compared with the "model" which she uses in speculating about a safe dose and dose-rate (Ya89, pp.160-161). This "model" is discussed in Chapter 19, Part 3; the nature of inconclusive studies in Chapter 21, Part 2; and the Holm Study in Chapter 22, Part 5.

Yalow concludes her editorial by stating that radiation phobia "is based on the concept that any amount of ionizing radiation delivered at any rate is hazardous to human health. Such fears impact on the beneficial role of radiation in diagnosis and therapy, nuclear medicine, and nuclear power."

==============

34-empty, after 34-9
===

| Hormesis : The Nature of Speculations about Undemonstrated "Beneficial Effects" |

This chapter is arranged in nine parts:

1. Introduction

The speculation, that some beneficial health effects from low-doses of ionizing radiation may be discovered, is referred to as "radiation hormesis," and those who do the speculating can be called the "hormetics." A few are quoted in our Chapter 34.

The formal definition of hormesis in medicine is: "The stimulating effect of subinhibitory concentrations of any toxic substance on any organism" (Dor51). However, a segment of the radiation community has decided to equate stimulation with net benefit, and to use the term to suggest that low doses of ionizing radiation may be GOOD for people.

Sheldon Wolff has recently put the issue clearly (Wolff89):

"The orginal definition of the once obsolete word hormesis came to us from pharmacology, and meant a stimulation brought about by a low-level exposure to a substance that was toxic at high levels. In recent times, however, the word has been resurrected and the definition has been modified to refer not only to a stimulatory effect but also to a beneficial effect. In other words, hormesis now connotes a value judgment whereby a low dose of a noxious substance is supposedly good."

A Thousand Studies ?

Dr. Thomas Luckey seems to have been the first really serious radiation hormetic. In his 1980 book (Luc80), he assembled over 1,000 citations of studies purporting to have found measurable non-cancer effects from ionizing radiation upon microbes, seeds, plants, animal species and animal cells of many types. Purported effects have an immense variety:

● -- "Chickens matured faster when irradiated with 500 roentgens" (at p.91).

● -- "Rat brain is stimulated into activity by as little as 1 mR/min; after short-term irradiation, as little as 72 R/hr will make them move" (p.91).

● -- Low-level irradiation, 50-400 R, make female finches produce pigmented feathers..." (p.115).

Like the examples above, many of Luckey's thousand-plus citations were not studies of LOW-dose effects at all. And conspicuously missing were studies demonstrating protection AGAINST human cancer. In a later paper (Luc82, p.776), Luckey cites Hickey's 1981 paper and other "Denver-Type" studies as if they were evidence in favor of protection AGAINST human cancer by low doses. We have already shown the fallacy of that position (Chapter 21, Part 2).

The Issue of Human Cancer-Induction :

In prior chapters of this book, the case has been made that harm, in the form of excess human cancer, occurs at all doses of ionizing radiation, down to the lowest conceivable dose and dose-rate.

It follows that, if radiation hormesis occurs, the health benefit must occur in some aspect of health OTHER than the induction of human cancer. Moreover, the postulated health benefit will have to be greater than the adverse carcinogenic effect for the same level of exposure, for otherwise it would be highly misleading to suggest that exposure to ionizing radiation might be good for people.

The human epidemiological evidence AGAINST hormesis, with respect to radiation-induced cancer, does not rule out the possibility that some hypothetical beneficial effect from exposure to low-dose radiation -- perhaps on the immune system, for instance -- might reduce the risk of serious or fatal diseases OTHER than cancer (Go88a).

We certainly would welcome any credible evidence of a benefit -- which would mean either a reduced or an absent net hazard from low-dose ionizing radiation, or better yet, a net benefit. Who would NOT?

However, since self-delusion about a proven and ubiquitous carcinogen is so very likely to get many millions of people killed over time, all of us need to be rigorous about sorting real evidence from mere conjecture and from wishful thinking.

Natural Hope, Predictable Search :

It is hardly unexpected that those in charge of (or dependent upon) an enterprise will always hope that by-products or products of the enterprise will be innocuous, with respect to creation of hazards to health.

Entrepreneurs and other sponsors of potentially menacing enterprises, and their dependents, are not trying to find ways to stop their enterprises -- quite obviously the opposite is true. Thus, we find repeatedly that they go through a period of denial, before evidence of harm from a product or by-product is overwhelming. Then they go through a period of hoping that the harm, observed at moderate and high doses, will not be present at "low doses" of the product or by-product. Indeed, this is how the concept of "low doses" probably gets invented. It may be a moving target, but nonetheless, for many, the "low dose" is the ephemeral dose which produces no harm.

It is certainly true that some chemical substances can produce a beneficial effect biochemically in the human in a particular dose-range. Yet, if the dose is increased greatly, beneficial effects can be overtaken by serious, even fatal, adverse effects. Some vitamins, some trace minerals, some metal ions, some pharmaceutical agents, show this type of behavior.

Therefore, it is neither surprising nor inherently "wicked" that the radiation community should seek to find out whether ionizing radiation might, at some low dose, have some health benefits big enough to compensate for radiation carcinogenesis. On the other hand, since the radiation community has a stake in the outcome, its search cannot be disinterested, by definition.

An Intensified Effort :

By 1985, an effort was underway to present "possible beneficial effects" from low-dose radiation as a reputable hypothesis. For instance, we find the (U.S.) Nuclear Regulatory Commission hinting at unspecified "beneficial" effects in Nrc85 (see our Chapter 34, p.3). And in August 1985, parts of the radiation community held the "Conference on Radiation Hormesis" in Oakland, California.

According to the Conference chairman (Cohen87, p.519), it was sponsored by: The Northern California Section of the American Nuclear Society, the Northern California Chapter of the Health Physics Society, the Electric Power Research Institute (Palo Alto, California), the U.S. Department of Energy, EG&G-Idaho, Inc. (a major player in the nuclear weapons program), and the General Electric Company (a major supplier of nuclear power systems). The entire May 1987 issue of HEALTH PHYSICS (Volume 52, Number 5) was devoted to that conference and its topic.

Also in May, 1987, a workshop, "Low-Dose Radiation and the Immune System," was held at Dreieich-Frankfurt, Federal Republic of Germany. This was jointly organized by: The Electric Power Research Institute (EPRI), the U.S. Department of Energy, the Commission of the European Communities, and the Kernforschungsanlage Julich. The Proceedings of this Workshop became a "Special Issue" of the INTERNATIONAL JOURNAL OF RADIATION BIOLOGY, Volume 53, Number 1, January, 1988.

By August 1989, the editors of the journal SCIENCE had invited EPRI's Dr. Leonard Sagan to tell its worldwide readership about radiation hormesis in the journal's "Policy Forum" section (Sag89). The Forum also presented a contrasting point of view, by Dr. Sheldon Wolff (Wolff89). From there, the medical journal LANCET picked up the story and put the idea, that radiation may be good for people, into even wider dissemination (Lanc89).

Hormesis is enjoying a great wave of popularity in parts of the radiation community, with multiple large-scale conferences organized to facilitate the presentation and publication of papers. A natural consequence is the propagation of hormetic speculations also through the mass media -- for instance, in a letter-to-the-editor headlined "Radiation Exposure: A Little Might Be Good," in the WALL STREET JOURNAL, September 26, 1989 (Hogue89).

Sampling of the Latest Findings :

Since the Electric Power Research Institute (EPRI) helps to sponsor hormetic research and conferences, it can be regarded as one of the private sector's "prime movers" in the search for benefits.

Therefore, a good place to begin a sampling of the latest findings, produced by the search for hormesis, is with the evidence cited by EPRI's main spokesman on this topic, Dr. Leonard Sagan. Sagan was the special "Guest Editor" of the HEALTH PHYSICS issue (May 1987) which was devoted entirely to hormesis. Also, as we mentioned above, Sagan was recently invited to present the "pro-hormesis" position in the "Policy Forum" section of the journal SCIENCE (Sag89).

Sagan is asking the scientific community to take radiation hormesis seriously, and so we will evaluate the type of evidence he offers. His greatest emphasis is on radiobiological studies -- an emphasis with many scientific pitfalls, as we have already shown in Chapter 23.

The Three Lines of Inquiry Cited by Sagan :

According to Sagan:

"Three lines of inquiry have recently raised the surprising possibility that very low doses of ionizing radiation may not be harmful after all or may even have net benefits, a phenomenon known as hormesis" (Sag89, p.574).

Using the evidence which Sagan recommends, we shall examine each of these "three lines of inquiry" -- by which Sagan seems to mean the following:

(1) Effects on Longevity in Laboratory Animals.
(2) Effects on Injury of Genetic Material.
   (A) Thymidine Kinase and DNA.
   (B) Priming Doses and Chromosomes.
   (C) Rates of DNA Synthesis.
(3) Effects on the Immune System.

2. Sagan's First Line of Inquiry : Effects on Longevity in Laboratory Animals

Sagan states the following on this topic, in his "Policy Forum" case (Sag89, p.574):

"Many studies (but not all) show that laboratory animals exposed to low doses of radiation outlive

unexposed animals (1). How could this happen? DNA damage occurs commonly as a result of normal metabolic processes as well as from environmental mutagens. Whether the outcome is harmful depends on the dynamic balance between damage and repair processes. A net benefit can result when protective responses to low-grade exposure more than compensate for the harmful effects of the radiation. For example, a major cause of radiation injury at high doses is thought to result from the production of free radicals. Feinendegen et al. have shown that free radical scavengers increase after low-dose radiation, possibly to a greater extent than that necessary to to neutralize the radicals produced by the radiation (2). The increased production of scavengers might increase cell defenses against free radicals that result from exposure to other environmental mutagens or those produced by normal oxidative metabolism."

Speculations abound in that brief quotation: "could", "net benefit can result", "possibly to a greater extent", "might increase cell defenses." For substance, we must turn to the references which Dr. Sagan cites to support the plausibility of his speculations.

Sagan's reference (1) is to Congdon's 1987 paper entitled "A Review of Certain Low-Level Ionizing Radiation Studies in Mice and Guinea Pigs" (Cong87). Sagan's reference (2) is to Feinendegen's 1987 paper entitled "Intracellular Stimulation of Biochemical Control Mechanisms by Low-Dose, Low-LET Radiation" (Fein87).

We shall defer examination of the Feinendegen paper until Part 3 of this chapter. First, we must examine Sagan's premise -- that exposure to low-doses of radiation extends the lifespan of laboratory animals. Sagan cites Cong87 as his support for this claim.

The Lorenz Experiments :

Congdon produced a quite thoughtful paper. His paper suggests to me that what Dr. Sagan did not tell us, about the studies of radiation and longevity, might be far more important than what Sagan did tell us. Congdon's paper is largely focused on the frequently cited work done by Egon Lorenz in the 1940s and 1950s.

Lorenz' initial experiment involved exposure of 45 mice to gamma radiation at 0.11 roentgen per eight-hour day from about two months of age until natural death. There were 54 control mice. Mean survival time in the exposed group, after the beginning of the exposure, was 761 days, so the total mean entrance-dose for the mice must have been about 75 rads. At 0.11 R per day, the macroscopic dose-rate must have been more than 100-times ambient rates, but at the level of the cell-nuclei, dose-rate must have been less than one track per day, per nucleus (see Table 20-M).

Congdon states, "Table 1 shows that the experimental group had a slightly longer mean survival time by nearly 2 mo compared to the control group. This difference was not statistically significant. A repeat of this experiment was then performed with a much larger number of LAF1 mice [Lor55]. The results, given in Table 2, again show longer mean survival time in the exposed group compared to the control" (Cong87, p.593). Congdon himself is a co-author of Lor55. In the larger experiment, 111 male and 120 female mice were exposed, with a total of 226 controls.

Commentary :
=======================================

There are several points to be made about this larger experiment -- points which cast real doubt upon the validity of using this work as supportive evidence for radiation hormesis.

Point 1, Male vs. Female Response :
While there was a difference in longevity for males at the $p = 0.01$ level of significance, no significant difference was found for females, in an experiment with nearly equal numbers of animals. The difference in life-span for irradiated versus control females was approximately 2 % (820 days versus 803 days).

Of course, a real biological effect might actually differ between the two sexes, but the difference does raise a flag of warning with regard to speculation about the cause. No sex-difference is fit into the following hypothesis, which Congdon labels as "the Lorenz et al. speculation" (Cong87, p.594):

"In more general terms, the Lorenz et al. speculation can be rephrased to interpret higher ionizing radiation exposure as a situation where repair or compensation processes cannot keep up with the continuing injury processes in radio-sensitive tissues. At some lower level, repair processes and continuing injury could be in balance. At still lower levels of exposure, repair processes could rebound, over-shoot or out-distance continuing minimal injury in very radiosensitive tissues such as bone marrow and the small intestine. This regenerative hyperplasia, rebound repair or over-shoot in bone marrow and lymphatic tissues, could then create

a larger mass of tissues devoted to defense mechanisms against intercurrent lethal infections. These infections are hypothesized to cause death in a few young animals in control groups but not in the 'better defended' experimental ones."

The reasoning reported by Congdon seems plausible. But the experimental basis for it seems thin indeed. This leads directly to our POINT 2, which deals with the experimental basis for the conclusions.

Point 2, Need to Replace the Control Group :
Congdon points out that for the male mice (the only group showing the increased longevity), the following happened: "The control group, unfortunately, in this experiment [Lor55] had to be replaced 1 yr into the study because the original group developed dermatitis" (Cong87, p.593).

A "new" control group -- chosen a year later -- hardly represents a real control group. Moreover the fact that the "dermatitis" singled out the control group may say a lot about a lack of comparability of the controls and the experimental groups. And where infection is at issue, as the major suspected cause of death-rate differences, comparability of groups means everything. Under the circumstances, the only scientifically appropriate response is to disregard the results of this experiment, because they lack credibility.

We are not suggesting that such experiments are easy to accomplish well; they are definitely very difficult. And this is all the more reason for avoiding sweeping hormetic conclusions from experiments which are demonstrably faulted, as was this one.

Subsequent Experiments :

Point 3, Confounding Variables :
Congdon mentions work published in the 1960s by Sacher and colleagues (Sa64, Le65, Ru66), and says that "This work essentially confirmed the Lorenz results" (Cong87, p.595). Despite this statement, Congdon seems to warn readers on the very next page against placing their confidence in alleged life-lengthening hormetic effects reported in the past. Congdon, who worked with Lorenz himself, says (Cong87, p.596):

"Of course, continued investigation of these hormetic effects in mice would be done with contemporary animal husbandry techniques and in pathogen-free animals. One hypothesis is that these median life span and possibly body weight changes of the hormetic type will

===

not be found with use of state-of-art animal husbandry and mice free of parasites and the common mouse pathogens."

And of exceedingly great interest is the fact that Dr. Congdon provides a footnote giving the source of this hypothesis. The footnote states: "Personal communication (1985) with D. Grahn, Argonne National Laboratory, Argonne, Il. 60439." Dr. Douglas Grahn, it may be noted, devoted a significant share of his research career to this subject of radiation and longevity, and he is a co-author of each of the "confirmatory" studies cited above (Sa64, Le65, Ru66).

None of these problems is mentioned by Sagan, who presents longevity as firmly established in many "low dose" experiments. But the one source he cites in support of his claim, Congdon, seems to consider the claim to be far from established. Moreover, Congdon indicates that Grahn, also, sees legitimate room for doubt. If, someday, the longevity claim is finally established for mice or other laboratory animals, still no one will know if it occurs or not in HUMANS.

Another Aspect Not Mentioned by Sagan :

Point 4, the Cancer-Price :

Dr. Sagan did not mention another aspect of the experiments on radiation and alleged life-extension. But Dr. Congdon does fill us in on this issue. He points out that, in the same experiments where the increase in longevity supposedly occurred, an excess of cancer was also observed. We quote Congdon (Cong87, p.595):

"In Lorenz's experiments, there was an increase in neoplasia at the low-level exposure of 0.11 R [per day]. Ovarian, lung, mammary, and lymphatic tissue tumors were more frequent than in the control mice [Lor55]. This type of pathologic growth at a hormetic level of exposure was compatible with the linear hypothesis of radiation injury."

Readers are reminded that this radiogenic cancer in mice occurred from doses giving less than one track per nucleus per day. It would seem a reasonable guess that persons currently enthusiastic, about the supposed hormetic effect of radiation at such doses, might be a bit less enthusiastic if they were told that the experimental data showed more cancer as the price of less infection. Their enthusiasm might cool even further if they realized that, at total doses lower than the experimental total doses, one might get the linear increase in cancer, but little or no benefit in terms of longer average lifespan. The two dose-responses (if the longevity-effect occurs at all) do not

necessarily share the same shape within a single species, or across species either.

Sagan's First Line of Inquiry :

On Sagan's first line of inquiry, we have reviewed the evidence which he cites. We have shown, above, that Sagan's suggestion of "net benefits" from "very low doses" is just speculation -- unsupported, even for laboratory animals, by the evidence he cited. By contrast, UNSCEAR 1988 says (p.22, para.129) " ... evidence showed overwhelmingly that irradiated animals live ... fewer years than non-irradiated controls" (full quote in Chapter 34, Webster).

3. Sagan's Second Line of Inquiry (A): Thymidine Kinase and DNA

We begin by returning, as promised, to the latter part of the Sagan statement (Sag89, p.574) quoted in our Part 2:

"A net benefit can result when protective responses to low-grade exposure more than compensate for the harmful effects of the radiation. For example, a major cause of radiation injury at high doses is thought to result from the production of free radicals. Feinendegen et al. have shown that free radical scavengers increase after low-dose radiation, possibly to a greater extent than that necessary to neutralize the radicals produced by the radiation (2). This increased production of scavengers might increase cell defenses against free radicals that result from exposure to other environmental mutagens or those produced by normal oxidative metabolism."

Sagan's reference (2) is Feinendegen and co-workers' 1987 paper entitled "Intracellular Stimulation of Biochemical Control Mechanisms by Low-Dose, Low-LET Radiation" (Fein87).

In addition, in an effort to tie Sagan's speculation with some substance, we have examined a later paper by Feinendegen and co-workers on their work: "Biochemical and Cellular Mechanisms of Low-Dose Effects" (Fein88).

The Feinendegen Experiments :
==
In both papers, Feinendegen and co-workers base suggestions of possible hormesis on certain biochemical studies of thymidine and thymidine kinase.

Thymidine kinase is an ubiquitous enzyme which catalyzes the phosphorylation of thymidine to produce

===

thymidine mono-phosphate. This latter, with two additional phosphorylations, provides a part of the cell's supply of thymidine tri-phosphate, which is one of the four tri-phosphates needed to synthesize cellular DNA. Thymidine is only part of the source of thymidine triphosphate, with the remainder coming from other biochemical transformations. The thymidine in serum is regarded as that provided by "salvage" pathways, meaning thymidine left over after death and destruction of cells. Some part of this thymidine is metabolized in the liver; some part is used toward DNA synthesis.

Essentially the Feinendegen studies center around this "salvage" pathway for thymidine incorporation ultimately into DNA. Since the catalysis of phosphorylation is by the enzyme, thymidine kinase, the studies center around the activity measurements of this enzyme, plus two other measurements:

1. The measurement of serum thymidine (mouse). The logic of this measurement is that if thymidine kinase activity is suppressed, thymidine will not be used as rapidly to make thymidine phosphate, and hence the serum levels of thymidine itself will increase. The converse is also expected -- if thymidine kinase activity is increased, the serum level of thymidine will fall, due to its increased rate of utilization to form thymidine phosphate.

2. The measurement of the rate of incorporation (in vitro) of radioiodine-labeled iododeoxyuridine into bone marrow cells taken from irradiated animals. The logic of this is that iododeoxyuridine is an analogue chemically of thymidine, and hence its uptake (as measured using the iodine-125 label) is an indicator for uptake of thymidine by those cells.

These workers studied whole-body irradiation of mice with cesium-137 gamma radiation over the dose-range from 0.1 cGy through 1.0 Gy (some sporadic data are given for 0.01 cGy). In particular, the studies included measurements of change in activity of TDr-kinase (the common abbreviation for thymidine kinase), serum thymidine levels, and incorporation-rates of iododeoxyuridine into bone marrow cells taken from irradiated mice.

The Experimental Findings :

===

Both papers present the same data concerning effects of gamma radiation on these three parameters. The claims follow, although in my opinion, the data do not really support the claims.

1. TDr-kinase activity drops to ~ 65 % of its

pre-irradiation level at 4 hours post-irradiation with 1 cGy, and separate experiments show about the SAME extent of decline in activity-level with 10 cGy and with 100 cGy -- doses 10-fold and 100-fold higher (their Figure 3, p.666). The experimental points for 100 cGy are really just one point -- at 4 hours post-irradiation (Figure 2, p.665). Below 1 cGy, their Figure 3 suggests a lesser reduction (to about 85 % of values in the controls), with no clear dose-response.

2. Serum thymidine levels rise appreciably at 4 hours post-irradiation following either 10 cGy or 100 cGy, (their Figure 2). No data are presented for 1 cGy, as a function of time after irradiation. Serum concentrations at 4 hours post-exposure are dose-dependent (their Figure 3).

3. Iododeoxyuridine incorporation falls appreciably at 4 hours post-irradiation following 10 or 100 cGy of gamma radiation (their Figure 2). No data are presented for 1 cGy, as a function of time after irradiation. Incorporation is dose-dependent (their Figure 3).

The workers take the findings to be internally consistent in suggesting that a peak reduction in TDr-kinase activity is achieved at 4 hours post-irradiation. By an additional 6 hours, the TDr-kinase activity is back to pre-irradiation levels (their Figure 2).

Several studies suggested to these workers that radiation-induced free radicals might be involved in the depression of thymidine kinase activity. To confirm this suspicion, mice were placed on a vitamin E deficient diet for four weeks. They found that thymidine kinase activity after induction of Vitamin-E deficiency was reduced, to a degree similar to that observed 4 hours after gamma radiation. Further, as a test of "the activity of the intracellular radical removal system," the concentration of non-protein-bound glutathione was measured, and both in the irradiated mice and the Vitamin-E deficient mice, there was a comparable rise in glutathione level.

For the authors, these results justified the following conclusions (Fein87 p.664):

"These data strengthen the hypothesis that (a) intracellular radicals are indeed involved in the depression of thymidine kinase activity and (b) the enzyme responds independent of the cause of radical formation."

There are many very good reasons for skepticism about some of these conclusions, but for now we can accept the authors' own conclusions in order to see if

==

the authors can FORGE A LINK, between their interpretations of the biochemical findings and hormesis from low-dose radiation.

Interpretations in the 1987 Paper :
==

Following are some of the conclusions which the authors appear to derive from their biochemical data, in this 1987 paper. In their abstract, they state (Fein87, p.663):

"A reduction of cellular thymidine kinase activity is expected to cause a temporary reduction of DNA synthesis and may be of advantage to the cell. Such a response may be regarded as an instance of radiation hormesis in the sense that such a compensatory response to the stimulus of irradiation may confer protection against a repeated increase in free radical concentration whether by renewed radiation exposure or by metabolism in general. An improvement of the efficiency of repair or an increased level of free radical detoxification should be of benefit to both the individual cell and to the organism as a whole."

In the paper's section, "Introduction," the authors state: "The response in question involves an enzyme which is thought to react with free radicals and may represent a process enabling cells to acquire means of protection against the detrimental effects of continued perturbation of the intracellular milieu. The foregoing considerations may lend support to the hormesis hypothesis, i.e. that a small amount of irradiation (or other stress) stimulates the metabolism of a living system so as to react in a compensatory manner to reestablish normal function. This effect may be beneficial as long as the degree of stress remains well below an irreversibly damaging limit" (Fein87, p.663).

Commentary on the 1987 Paper :
==

We shall examine this cascade of hormetic speculations -- speculations which are barely tied at all to any of the paper's biochemical findings.

Temporary Reduction in DNA Synthesis :
These workers have not shown that this occurs at all. They claim a 15 % to 35 % reduction in the enzyme-activity of ONE pathway for producing thymidine monophosphate. The major pathway for producing this nucleotide is from uridine monophosphate, a pathway which uses the enzyme thymidylate synthetase. The partial closing of the less important pathway, for a few hours, may not result in ANY delay in DNA synthesis.

Alleged Benefit from Delay :
Let us assume, however, that a temporary delay DOES occur in unscheduled DNA synthesis, in the hours after irradiation. Would it follow that a delay "may be of advantage to the cell" (Fein87, p.663) ? When radiation-induced DNA lesions are types which are inherently unrepairable, it is self-evident that delaying the repair "effort" cannot matter at all. And when the radiation-induced DNA lesions are types which ARE repairable, delay in unscheduled DNA synthesis might just be the opposite of beneficial -- by providing time for the injury to become transformed into a permanently fixed lesion. The suggestion by Feinendegen and co-workers, of an "advantage to the cell," is a speculation which seems to deserve some symmetry.

Improvement of the Efficiency of Repair :
The authors have demonstrated exactly nothing about improved efficiency of DNA repair, so there is no basis for a hormetic claim on that score.

Doses Below an Irreversibly Damaging Limit :
Feinendegen et al mention protection against free radical production by "metabolism in general" and protection against "the detrimental effects of continued perturbation of the intracellular milieu," protection which they seem to suggest might be provided by radiation "as long as the degree of stress remains well below an irreversibly damaging limit" (Fein87, p.663). Sagan is more explicit. He suggests that low-dose irradiation might help protect people "against free radicals that result from exposure to other environmental mutagens or those produced by normal oxidative metabolism" (Sag89, p.574).

Their "low-dose" hormetic suggestions above are seriously faulted on both epidemiological and plain logical grounds.

The Epidemiological Difficulty :

The epidemiological evidence already shows that excess cancer arises in humans from radiation exposures which deliver an average of only one or a few primary ionization tracks per cell-nucleus (Table 21-A).

Let us suppose, for the moment, that the same exposures which induced the excess cancers in those nine studies ALSO temporarily inhibited thymidine kinase activity. Then the excess cancers observed are the ones which occur "anyway" -- despite the speculative benefits (delayed DNA repair, scavenging of free radicals) supposedly associated with the temporary inhibition of the enzyme.

In other words, radiation doses -- which were as low at the cellular level as they could ever be -- were still not low enough to be "below an irreversibly damaging limit." Indeed, they killed some people with fatal cancer.

The key point, acknowledged by Sagan himself (see Part 1), is that support for the hormetic hypothesis requires the demonstration of NET benefits from low-dose irradiation. In terms of fatal cancer-rates, the humans received a real INJURY from exposures in the very low dose-range.

But was it a NET injury? Does the Feinendegen work suggest that those who escaped the fatal radiation-induced cancers may have had a meaningful benefit from their exposure? The answer is explored by the logic below.

The Logical Difficulty :

The thymidine-related measurements, reported by Feinendegen and co-workers, peaked at four hours post-irradiation and returned to pre-irradiation levels by about ten hours after the mice were exposed (Fein87, Figure 2). Thus, in order for mice (or people) to receive more than a fleeting benefit -- if any benefit at all exists -- they must receive new doses about twice a day, along with the risk of fatal radiation-induced cancer associated with each new dose.

That's where the logical difficulty arises.

In order for "the stimulus of irradiation" to "confer protection against a repeated increase in free radical concentration whether by renewed radiation exposure or by metabolism in general" (Fein87, p663), each cell would have to experience the stimulation of at least one primary ionization track per exposure, twice a day.

Doses which can put an average of one primary ionization track through each cell-nucleus have been estimated in our Table 20-M for various sources of radiation. The range is 0.3 to 0.7 rad. Thus, to achieve the postulated protection against "free radicals that result from exposure to other environmental mutagens or those produced by normal oxidative metabolism" (Sag89, p.574), one has to start talking about total doses in the ballpark of ONE HUNDRED RADS OR MORE PER YEAR, per person.

In short, the logic leads straight into conflict -- between the reality-based evidence on radiation CARCIN-OGENESIS and the rosy speculations about "net benefits" -- if any benefits are ever demonstrated at all.

Additions from the 1988 Paper :
==

In case Feinendegen and co-workers might have been more explicit elsewhere, about how their findings support the hormetic hypothesis, we also examined their 1988 paper on additional experiments (Fein88, p.23):

" ... mice were acutely exposed to 0.01 or 0.1 Gy and again exposed to the same dose at different times up to 12 h after the first exposure. At regular time intervals after the second exposure bone marrow cells were obtained and thymidine kinase activity was studied by various assays. The results indicate that the first acute irradiation conditioned the cells in such a way that the second acute irradiation produced either an enhanced inhibition and recovery of thymidine kinase activity, or no effect at all was seen, when the second irradiation was given between about 3 and 8 h after the first irradiation. From 8 to 12 h after the first irradiation the cells apparently resumed their original state, so that the second irradiation produced effects quite similar to those seen after a single irradiation in unconditioned cells."

The authors continue: "Thus, acute low-dose irradiation producing few radiation absorption events per exposed cell induces a biochemical alteration that is indeed related to some kind of defense system in such a way that the cells become temporarily conditioned to tolerate the same dose a second time without reaction."

This statement, beginning with "Thus ...", is hard to interpret. Without explanation, the authors appear to neglect the "enhanced" response reported in the previous paragraph and to emphasize only the ABSENCE of response ("without reaction"). And previously, the PRESENCE of the response was interpreted as beneficial (hormetic) and presumed to be a function of radical-removal, and now its absence ALSO seems to be interpreted as beneficial -- "related to some kind of defense system in such a way that the cells become temporarily conditioned to tolerate the same dose a second time without reaction."

We seem to end up with a report that, if mice are acutely irradiated a second time within three to eight hours after the first acute exposure, further inhibition of thymidine kinase activity may or may not be observed, whereas the inhibition is observed in previously unirradiated ("unconditioned") cells and in cells previously irradiated at least eight hours earlier.

The authors refer to the inhibition as

==

"radiation-induced temporary resistance of thymidine kinase activity against single radiation absorption events."

The Cancer-Issue :

In the end, the authors state (Fein88, p.36):

"For the time period of induced resistance, damage to the DNA from intracellular radicals may be temporarily decreased, irrespective of the mechanism by which radicals are produced, and perhaps also the risk of a 'spontaneous malignant transformation' may be reduced."

The speculation, that radiation might REDUCE the rate of spontaneous cancer, is already invalidated by solid human epidemiological data that exposure to ionizing radiation -- at any dose or dose-rate -- ELEVATES the cancer mortality-rate above its spontaneous rate (see Chapter 21).

The 1988 paper does not seem to explain any more than the 1987 paper, how the Feinendegen work can possibly be interpreted as support for hormetic "net benefits" from low-dose exposure. On the contrary. The 1988 paper confirms that the speculated benefit has disappeared within eight hours, and cannot possibly provide any "protection" against chronic production of free radicals by normal metabolism or environmental mutagens.

Speculation -- The Forging of Hormetic Links :

==

Feinendegen and co-workers report that, in irradiated mice, there is a temporary biochemical response involving the enzyme, thymidine kinase. No one knows whether the response has any health significance at all -- good or bad -- for mice or humans.

With unlimited speculation, therefore, the response could be "linked" with either benefit or with injury. The speculations of these workers are directed exclusively toward possible benefit.

The possibilities are not exhausted. Hundreds or thousands of other enzymes may also show some response of unknown significance (if any), when mouse or man is irradiated.

If such responses, persisting for only a few hours, were presumed beneficial, then the presumed benefit would require frequent re-dosing -- with truly awesome cancer-consequences. Even the very first dose carries

an extra risk of fatal cancer.

4. Sagan's Second Line of Inquiry (B): Priming Doses and Chromosomes

Also in this second line of inquiry, Dr. Sagan refers to "evidence that DNA repair may be enhanced by low doses of radiation (3)" (Sag89, p. 574).

Sagan's reference (3) is Sheldon Wolff and co-workers' 1988 paper (from the Frankfurt workshop mentioned in Part 1), entitled "Human Lymphocytes Exposed to Low Doses of Ionizing Radiations Become Refractory to High Doses of Radiation As Well As to Chemical Mutagens That Induce Double-Stranded Breaks in DNA" (Wolff88).

Sagan goes on to say: "This suggests another means of protection, namely, that radiation-exposed DNA may be more readily repaired after subsequent exposures to mutagens."

It appears that here again, Dr. Sagan has misinterpreted the evidence as being supportive of the concept of hormesis. A decreased level of genetic damage following additional insult (radiation or other) cannot be considered the equivalent of a net benefit. There is still net INJURY from both the first and second insults. We shall return to this point, after relating what Wolff himself says about his own work.

Wolff's Own Description of his Work :

==

In Wolff's "Policy Forum" presentation (Wolff89, p.575), he describes the work cited by Sagan:

"The other experiments consist of the repeatable adaptation of human lymphocytes (5-10) and V79 Chinese Hamster cells (11) to low-level radiations from tritiated thymidine or x-rays, which then makes the cells less susceptible to the induction of chromosomal damage by subsequent high doses of x-rays. This phenomenon lasts for up to three cell cycles after the cells have been preexposed to doses as little as one-half rad (0.5 cGy). The response is induced by radiation and other agents, such as alkylating agents, bleomycin, or oxidative radicals, that produce breaks in DNA, and is negated by the inhibition of poly(ADP-ribosyl)ation, which is itself induced by DNA breaks. This adaptive response has been attributed to the induction of a hitherto unknown chromosomal break repair mechanism that, if in place when the cells are subsequently exposed to high doses of radiation, can repair much of the initial damage and leave the cells with only approximately one-half as much cytogenetic damage as expected. The response has also been found to take 4 to 6 hours after the preexposure to become fully operational, and it can be inhibited by the protein synthesis inhibitor, cycloheximide, if it is present for this 4- to 6-hour period. Presumably, the enzymes are being synthesized at this time and, indeed, two-dimensional gel analysis of protein extracts from lymphocytes exposed to 1 cGy of x-rays shows that certain proteins are absent in all control cultures, but are reproducibly present in all irradiated cultures. These proteins are excellent candidates for being the induced enzymes needed for the repair of the cytogenetic damage."

Warning from Wolff :

Wolff continues directly: "Nevertheless, the fact that a protein (enzyme) involved in repair can be induced by very low doses of radiation does not necessarily mean that these doses are in and of themselves 'good' or hormetic. Several new proteins were found to have been induced, which indicates that the metabolism of the cells had been changed. Some of these proteins might have a metabolic effect of their own, and could possibly lead to a cascade effect whereby subsequent metabolic steps unrelated to the induced repair would be altered. To call this beneficial would be premature, indeed."

Additional Findings by Wolff et al :

Wolff and co-workers did their experiments with human lymphocytes which had been induced to go into the active cell cycle of division by the stimulant, phytohemagglutinin M (PHA-M).

The research group (Shad87b) did attempt to get the induction of the repair capacity in unstimulated lymphocytes (said to be in the G-zero phase of the cell cycle). They found that administration of the priming dose of X-rays (1 cGy to 5 cGy) failed to give any reduction in chromatid breaks if given even immediately before adding the PHA mitogenic stimulant to the lymphocyte culture. But when the priming dose was given four or more hours after PHA addition, significantly fewer chromatid breaks were observed.

The effect of stimulating this chromosomal repair system has a limited duration. Shadley et al (Shad87b, p.514) reported that the effect of a priming dose could be detected at 66 hours in culture, but not at 90 or 114 hours. And since most cells were (by 66 hours) in the 3rd or later cell-division, it was concluded that this is about the limiting duration of effectiveness of a priming dose.

Without the prior presence of the special stimulant (PHA-M), however, the priming dose appears not to operate at all -- in terms of lessened vulnerability of genetic material in lymphocytes to radiation injury.

Increased Damage From Subsequent MMS :

One experimental finding, not commented upon by Dr. Wolff in "Policy Forum," is that the lessened vulnerability to chromosomal aberrations was not observed for all kinds of lesions introduced. For example, when Wolff and co-workers challenged the irradiated cells with the alkylating agent, methyl methanesulfonate (MMS), which can produce single-strand breaks in DNA, approximately twice as much damage was found as was induced by MMS alone. We quote Wolff on this (Wolff88, p.39):

"The results indicate that prior exposure to 0.01 Gy of X-rays reduces the number of chromosome breaks induced by double-strand breaks, and perhaps even by cross-links, in DNA, but has the opposite effect on breaks induced by the alkylating agent MMS. The results also show that the induced repair mechanism is different from that observed in the adaptive response that follows exposure to low doses of alkylating agents."

Additional Comments by Wolff :
==

Before making some comments of our own on the work by Wolff and co-workers (including Oli84, Wien86, Shad87a, Shad87b), we think it is important here to note two more comments by Wolff himself (both from Wolff89, p.575).

1. "The usual experiment on the genetic effects of ionizing radiation, however, has shown the effects induced, rather than being hormetic with a beneficial effect, are deleterious (1). This has been shown in innumerable experiments in mutation in which it has been found that radiation-induced mutations themselves, unlike spontaneous ones, are, indeed, usually deleterious. That this should be so is not surprising, in that all living organisms are the result of eons of evolution in which they have been selected to fit their proper ecological niches. Any random mutational change then would be expected to change this fine balance and decrease fitness. With ionizing radiation, in which most of the induced mutations are deletions, this is even more likely."

2. And in a lesson which needs to be emphasized

==

and re-emphasized concerning the ease of misuse of science in the service of politics, Dr. Wolff points out:

"The field of hormesis is replete with sporadic reports of unrepeatable beneficial effects being brought about by irradiation. Perhaps the greatest profusion of these reports came out of the Soviet Union in the late 1940s to early 1950s, in the era of Lysenko, during which there was a severe repression of modern Mendelian genetics. For reasons of political ideology whereby the State could change the environment and thus ameliorate man's (and other organisms') condition, the whole basis of modern genetics was suppressed."

My own opinion is, sadly, that this Soviet experience with the misuse of science in the service of "politics" (broadly construed) will not be the last instance of its kind. Only eternal vigilance and early counter-action can possibly prevent recurrence of this anti-human behavior, and its high-priced consequences for people everywhere.

Chromatid Breaks from the Initial Dose Itself :
======================================

Shadley and Wolff (Shad87a, p.95, Table II) have reported on the chromatid and isochromatid breaks associated with PHA stimulation plus just the initial acute dose:

Treatment (rad)	Chromatid and isochromatid breaks in 200 cells.
0	6
1	9
5	11
10	18
20	30
30	40
40	46
50	54
150	83

There is one difference about the point (above) at 150 rads. The radiation was delivered at 48 hours after PHA stimulation, whereas all other doses were delivered at 32 hours after PHA stimulation. In their calculations, the authors treat the doses in the same manner, in spite of this difference in time of dose-delivery.

We have plotted the data above, in Figure 35-A. The dose-response is clearly supra-linear. Regression analysis (as demonstrated in Chapter 29) indicates that the best fit is associated with Dose^0.5. Readers can see for themselves that the R-Squared values are much better for supra-linearity than linearity. The data are provided with Figure 35-A.

It is self-evident that the damage from the initial radiation dose is marked, in and of itself, under the conditions required for the presumed benefit. Sagan does not mention any of this.

Yet it is the so-called priming dose itself which is the real issue, in speculations about low-dose radiation hormesis. There is nothing at all in the experiments reported by Wolff and co-workers to suggest that such doses constitute a net benefit. By contrast, real-world human epidemiology already shows that, even from minimal track-rates at the cellular level, the non-speculative result is excess cancer (Chapter 21).

No Support for Hormetic Speculations :
==

The reduction in total chromatid deletions, found in the human lymphocyte experiments, is clearly not an illustration of hormesis. It is, as Wolff states, a reduction in the deletions found from a high dose of radiation (and certain other insults), if a low priming dose is used during the (induced) active cell cycle of division, compared with the deletions found for that same high dose when NO priming dose or pre-exposure is used.

But the net effect is certainly not a net benefit. On the contrary, the net effect is genetic injury -- some from the priming dose itself, plus some more from the subsequent insult (radiation or other).

Moreover, these workers report (as mentioned above, but not by Sagan) that pre-exposure to ionizing radiation INCREASED the genetic damage by almost two-fold from subsequent exposure to the alkylating agent, MMS.

The "Policy Forum" (Wolff89) is not the only place where Wolff himself has warned against misuse of his work by the hormetics. After SCIENCE published an earlier paper by himself and co-workers (Oli84), in which priming doses were chronic rather than acute, Wolff said (Wolff84):

"This does not mean that a little radiation is good for you. The chronic low-level radiation still causes chromosome damage, but there is considerably less damage from subsequent irradiation."

5.   Sagan's Second Line of Inquiry (C): Rates of DNA Synthesis

In connection with citing the work of the Wolff research group, Sagan states (Sag89, p.574):

"This suggests another means of protection, namely, that radiation-exposed DNA may be more readily repaired after subsequent exposure to mutagens. One study demonstrates that enhanced DNA repair exists in workers occupationally exposed to radiation (4)."

Sagan's reference (4) is Tuschl and co- workers' 1980 paper entitled "Effects of Low-Dose Radiation on Repair Processes in Human Lymphocytes" (Tusc80).

The Population Samples :

This is a study of the speed of unscheduled DNA synthesis, following exposure to ultra-violet light, in lymphocytes of some persons occupationally exposed to ionizing radiation versus controls. The same paper also compares the rate of semi-conservative DNA synthesis or routine DNA synthesis, in the absence of any ultra-violet insult, in the lymphocytes of the occupationally exposed sample versus the controls.

Persons working intermittently (two to four hours per day) in a former gold mine, with high radon levels and an air temperature of 41 degrees Centigrade (about 106 degrees Fahrenheit) and a relative humidity of about 95 percent, were compared with persons living in areas of Austria with normal background radioactivity.

Apparently part of the former gold mine is now used as a medical therapy center referred to as "Bad Gastein," with a "thermal gallery" -- a hot, humid inhalation room for treating "rheumatic and vascular diseases as well as metabolic and endocrine disorders" (Tusc80, p.2). Thus, it is explained, "miners inspecting the gallery, train-leaders driving patients into the mine, and accompanying physicians stay about 2 to 4 hours a day within the gallery" (Tusc80, p.2).

According to Tuschl et al, among the gallery-exposed workers, the "mean blood dose calculated from alpha emission and external gamma radiation varied from 400 to 800 mrad in half a year" (Tusc80, p.2). Of course, this means we are dealing with a mixed exposure, to low-LET and high-LET radiations. This is the "exposed" group in the discussion below.

Experimental Findings and Interpretations :

Unscheduled DNA Synthesis :

Tuschl and co-workers exposed lymphocytes, taken from gallery-exposed workers and from controls, to ultra-violet radiation. Using tritiated thymidine, these workers found that the rate of unscheduled DNA synthesis -- in response to the ultra-violet insult -- was significantly elevated in lymphocytes from the exposed group compared with lymphocytes from the controls. The experiment was terminated at 90 minutes.

Sagan appears to equate speedier DNA synthesis with "enhanced DNA repair" (Sag89, p.574). If "enhanced" is meant to imply "better," this would require proof that a faster rate of DNA synthesis reduces the fraction of DNA lesions which becomes MISrepaired. Sagan does not deal with this at all.

One has to wonder why Sagan says, in 1989, that "One study [1980, Tuschl] demonstrates that enhanced DNA repair exists in workers occupationally exposed to radiation." Where are the confirming studies? If the effect is real -- and not an artefact of some confounding variables in the Tuschl study -- the effect must be demonstrable in occupationally exposed workers generally. As we shall see in Part 8 of this chapter, "hormetic" findings reported in the literature, and cited by radiation committees, cannot always be replicated in the next attempt.

Sagan's use of the 1980 Tuschl paper in "Policy Forum" may be another example of unsymmetrical speculation. A biological response of unknown health consequence (if any) is observed. With unlimited speculation, it could be interpreted as either beneficial or harmful -- and the hormetics speculate in only the rosy direction.

This even leads to internal inconsistency. In Part 3 of this chapter, DELAY (not acceleration) in unscheduled DNA synthesis was speculated to be "of advantage to the cell" (Fein87, p.663).

For the sake of exploration, let us speculate (as Sagan does) that speedier DNA synthesis is "good." The objective analyst must nonetheless ask, "What about the harm induced -- in the form of increased carcinogenic risk -- in order to get exposed persons into the state where their rate of unscheduled DNA synthesis is speedier in response to DNA insults? Why do we presume the net effect is benefit, when it might be serious harm?"

===

Semi-Conservative DNA Synthesis :

The other finding reported by Tuschl et al is that the level of semi-conservative (routine) DNA synthesis -- in lymphocytes NOT exposed to the ultra-violet insult -- was significantly lower in lymphocytes from the occupationally exposed group compared with lymphocytes from the controls. The only comment from the authors is:

"The reduced thymidine incorporation into DNA in cells of exposed persons indicates an alteration in the the kinetics of semiconservative DNA synthesis."

This is not an explanation of anything; it is, rather, a re-statement in words of the observations themselves. Whether this finding is beneficial, neutral, or deleterious is simply up in the air.

In a balanced approach to the hormetic hypothesis, we might expect analysts to look as hard for dismal possibilities as for rosy ones. For instance, here we might expect a speculation that this finding (lower level of routine DNA synthesis in lymphocytes) could be an indication that occupational exposure might WEAKEN the vitality of the immune system.

The Search for Net Benefits :
===========================

The paper cited by Sagan, on rates of DNA synthesis, provides no evidence whatsoever of any net benefits from low-dose irradiation -- as we have shown above. The Tuschl paper provides as much basis for speculation about previously unrecognized harm, as about previously unrecognized benefit.

Indeed, Sagan provides no assurance that the findings in the Tuschl paper are real (repeatable, experimentally).

6. *Sagan's Third Line of Inquiry :*
   Effects on the Immune System

Sagan states the following on this topic, in his "Policy Forum" presentation (Sag89, p.574):

"Third, radiation-induced cell death stimulates cell reproduction as a homeostatic mechanism that maintains cell compartment size. Accordingly, Kondo has suggested another possible response to low-level stimulation, namely, that immune cell production may be enhanced by low-dose radiation (5)."

Sagan's reference (5) is to Sohei Kondo's 1988

paper (from the Frankfurt workshop) entitled "Altruistic Cell Suicide in Relation to Radiation Hormesis" (Kondo88).

Kondo in his Own Words :

Kondo's paper deals with the concept that   "... the high radiosensitivity of undifferentiated primordial cells can be described as a manifestation of the suicide of injured cells for the benefit of an organism as a whole if their suicide stimulates proliferation of healthy cells to replace them, resulting in COMPLETE elimination of injury [the emphasis is Kondo's]." He credits the pioneer work of Bergonie and Tribondeau of 1906 for some of this.

Early in the paper, Kondo prepares the ground for his hypothesis (Kondo88, p.95):

"Why are undifferentiated primordial cells hypersensitive to killing by radiation and radiomimetic chemicals? Recent developments in biology have provided an answer to this question. Very great replication of DNA and extensive gene expression are required for differentiation from primordial cells to specialized cells during development from embryos to adult animals, or for maintenance of physiological functions by cell renewal systems. Therefore, intracellular anomalies induced in primordial cells due to inherent errors in DNA replication and gene expression would be greatly amplified unless they were COMPLETELY eliminated. DNA repair is rarely complete (Kondo 1975). This can be seen from the fact that frequency-vs-dose curves for mutations induced by various mutagens in various organisms do not usually show threshold effects. One of the simplest ways for COMPLETE elimination of an endogenously or exogenously induced anomaly in a cell is suicide of the cells on recognition of the anomaly ... Thus the high radiation sensitivity of undifferentiated cells of embryos may be assumed to be a manifestation of the ability of cells with lesions to commit suicide for the benefit of the whole animal. This altruistic suicide of cells will stimulate proliferation of healthy pluripotent cells to replace them. This repair is named 'cell-replacement repair' (Kondo et al. 1984) to distinguish it from DNA repair."

Of course, Kondo is not suggesting a willful action on the part of the cells in such "altruistic" death, but rather he is suggesting that some genetic programming allows recognition of injury and sets in motion an action -- for example, synthesis of a protein -- which selectively inhibits proliferation of the injured cell.

Kondo states that if this is correct, programmed cell death (altruistic cell death) may be an important defense mechanism in the human body. (Obviously not a perfect one.)

Forging A Link to Radiation Hormesis:

A link with hormesis is proposed as follows (Kondo88, p96): "Here I propose the hypothesis that the inactivation of radiosensitive cells by low-dose irradiation of a growing or slowly renewing organ stimulates proliferation of healthy primordial cells. The resulting increase in cell proliferation may lead, at least for a limited period, to an increase in the functional activity of the organ."

Kondo's concept of low-dose radiation bears no resemblance to environmental or occupational doses. He refers to semi-acute whole-body irradiation of mice in the dose-range of 5 to 80 rads as low-dose.

For instance, citing Anderson (And88), Kondo describes an experiment in which mice were given 5 to 25 whole-body rads five days before, up to immediately before, inoculation with a tumor. Kondo characterizes the result as "significantly retarded tumor growth" and "augmented antitumor responses" (Kondo88, p.99).

In some other studies which Kondo cites, alterations in certain lymphocyte classes were reported in mice, after whole-body irradiation at levels of one to four cGy per day for 20 days -- which means whole-body doses of twenty to eighty rads (James88).

Kondo makes the following statement (Kondo88, p99): "The observed antitumor effects of low-dose radiation are probably due to selective deletion of highly radiosensitive, primordial cells that develop into suppressor cells." (Earlier on the same page, Kondo has said that, under ordinary circumstances, tumor inoculation evokes effector T-cells, which have anti-tumor effectiveness, but they become over-whelmed by another class of T-cells, the suppressor cells, which interfere with the anti-tumor action.)

And Kondo continues directly (Kondo88, p.99): "If the immune system in animals can be augmented by low-dose radiation, as suggested from studies in mice by James and Makinodan (1988), and if the up-regulated immunity can be maintained spontaneously or by continuous irradiation at a very low dose rate, then the animals would acquire the trait of increased resistance to progression of spontaneous tumors, provided that the tumor cells possess tumor-specific antigens (Naor 1987)."

Comments on Kondo's Paper :

Many of Kondo's speculations about undifferentiated cells, and about the immune system, seem quite thoughtful and reasonable, and we do not wish to denigrate them in any way. Nor do we wish to challenge the possible effectiveness of high-dose radiation therapies against cancer.

However, as readers have probably already noted, Kondo does not address the question of the HARM produced by the doses of radiation used to obtain some of the presumed "up-regulation" of immune-responses.

Perhaps some of the hormetic researchers are just unaware of the non-speculative epidemiological evidence, that excess cancer is induced in humans right down to the lowest doses and dose-rates. (Chapter 34 illustrates how this could happen.) Unawareness might explain how they can still be speculating that biochemical or physiological effects of radiation -- upon the immune system, for example -- may prevent cancer from occurring at low doses.

Kondo suggests, for instance, that radiation- induced "up-regulation" of the immune system in "animals" might confer "increased resistance to progression of spontaneous tumors" -- presumably a lower spontaneous cancer-rate. He suggests that this benefit might follow even if chronic irradiation were given in ADDITION to an initial jolt -- which was 20 to 80 whole-body rads in James88.

Such a regime, if applied to human animals, would be a very effective way to INCREASE cancer-rates above their spontaneous levels.

The conclusive reality-based human evidence is that excess cancer -- above the spontaneous rate -- follows irradiation, no matter how low or slow the radiation dose. And the observed excess is what occurs, NET, after the immune system and the repair system have received the competing ANTI-cancer benefits (if any) from the same exposure.

7. Sagan's Allusion to Human Epidemiological Evidence

Sagan, in his "Policy Forum" presentation (Sag89, p.574), does not omit human epidemiological studies from his claims. On the contrary, he makes a sweeping and erroneous claim:

"Epidemiological studies of human populations exposed to relatively low doses of ionizing radiation have not shown the existence or absence of low-dose effects. For example, the studies of populations living in areas of high natural background have not shown any increase in adverse health effects (9)."

Sagan's reference (9) is to Liu and co-workers' 1987 paper (from the Hormesis Conference in Oakland) entitled "Radiation Hormesis: Its Expression in the Immune System" (Liu87).

The Liu paper relies on what we refer to as "Denver-Type studies," in our Chapter 21, Part 2. But Sagan cites Liu without hinting that such studies are inherently unable, scientifically, to address either the threshold issue or the hormesis issue (see our Chapter 21, Part 2).

Sagan's Treatment of the Conclusive Evidence:

Moreover, Sagan's claim is far, far broader than natural background studies. He has claimed that no low-dose effects -- good or bad -- have been shown in "epidemiological studies of human populations exposed to relatively low doses of ionizing radiation."

Sagan does not evaluate and does not even mention the conclusive human epidemiological studies, described in Chapter 21, which definitely DO show the presence of carcinogenic effects at minimal doses and dose-rates of ionizing radiation (one or very few primary ionization tracks per cell-nucleus per exposure).

Nor does he mention the conclusive low-dose evidence from the A-Bomb Study itself. When he happily cites mouse studies in which whole-body doses from 5 to 80 rads are characterized as "low-dose" exposures, he is obliged to treat the A-Bomb Study as a low-dose study too.

When Sagan has been prodded (Go87) to mention the topic of radiation-induced CANCER, in his public speculations about "net benefits" from irradiating people, his response has been to call the topic "this increasingly tiresome debate regarding low-dose carcinogenesis" (Sag87, p.680).

Comments on the Liu Paper :

The Liu paper cited by Sagan comes from the People's Republic of China, and it attempts to explain the alleged protection AGAINST cancer provided to people living in the so-called HNR (High Natural Radioactivity) area of Guangdong Province of China. The authors cite reports that cancer mortality is lower in Guangdong's HNR area than in the control area.

Readers are reminded of our warning in Chapter 24, Part 9, specifically about the Chinese high-background studies.

Moreover, such reports -- regardless of their origin -- are inherently inconclusive Denver-Type reports which we discussed in Chapter 21, Part 2. These studies do not and cannot control for variables other than radiation -- variables which profoundly alter cancer-rates wholly aside from any radiation effect.

Therefore, Denver-Type studies are scientifically meaningless citations in support of the hormetic hypothesis.

8. Two Multi-Center Chromosome Studies Which Produce Differing Results

We will describe an experiment in which exposure of human lymphocytes in vitro to 0.4 rad of ionizing radiation was reported to REDUCE chromosome aberrations in comparison with unirradiated samples. This experiment was cited without criticism by the 1986 UNSCEAR Report (Un86, p.92, para.440, and p.97, para.472).

Another group which is re-doing the work has obtained very different findings. We shall discuss both the positive study (Poh83) and the negative study (Lloyd88).

Chromosome Studies of Irradiated Cells :

Because of evidence relating chromosomal alterations with human cancer, many cell-culture studies in radiation research evaluate chromosomal aberrations in relation to radiation dose. This is a valid and interesting approach.

However, one needs to be cautious in interpreting results, because for the study of chromosomes, human lymphocytes in peripheral blood culture are artificially stimulated to undergo mitosis (see, for instance, Part 4 of this chapter). The results obtained may or may not be readily generalizable to natural biological conditions.

The frequency of chromosome aberrations detectable under the microscope is spontaneously quite low, and increases in frequency with low doses of radiation are also relatively small. All of this means that investigation of even a few limited questions requires the study of many tens of thousands of cells in mitosis, if statistically significant results are to be obtained.

One approach to this problem is to organize a multi-institutional study, using blind-coded slides, where the labor of seeking the chromosome aberrations is divided among many laboratories. Obviously, careful controls are needed to insure that biases are not introduced.

Pohl-Ruling's Positive Report :

One such study was carried out under the auspices of the International Atomic Energy Agency (Vienna, Austria), by Pohl-Ruling and seventeen collaborators. Published in 1983, the reported findings were as follows (Poh83, p.71-72):

1. The frequencies of all types of chromosome aberrations at 0.4 rad are significantly lower than the control values.

2. There is no increase in the frequencies of dicentrics up to 2 rad, and no increase in the frequencies of terminal deletions up to 5 rad.

3. The mean frequencies of all aberrations considered together are not significantly different from one another at 1, 2 and 3 rad (P = 0.05).

4. Over the entire dose range, the dose-effect relationship is clearly non-linear. A fit of these data to a linear quadratic model (E(D) = c + alpha x D + beta x D^2) showed that the total aberration frequencies at doses 1, 2, 3, and 5 rad are below the curve defined by the model.

The authors venture the following opinion:

"The deviations can be explained by an altered kinetics of aberration production at very low doses probably due to DNA repair mechanisms operating in these cells."

Findings at Variance with Epidemiology :

The Poh83 findings might be important, if real (repeatable) or relevant to in vivo (realistic) conditions.

Immediate skepticism was appropriate on several grounds, however. For instance, the second finding above indicates that there may be a dose below which chromosome damage does not occur, whereas chromosome damage has been observed from in vivo occupational radiation doses and dose-rates.

Epidemiological evidence is the reality-check on artificial conditions.

Modern occupational doses (below 5 rems per year) and dose-rates are such that a cell-nucleus experiences only one primary ionization track at a time, and then many weeks pass before the same nucleus experiences another track. (In the Baverstock studies of luminizers, annual doses were far higher.)

In 1979, Evans and co-workers reported on a ten-year prospective study of chromosome aberrations in occupationally exposed workers (Eva79). We will use Evans' own words (from Eva87, p.185) to describe the study and its findings:

" [It was] a large ten years' study on a group of occupationally exposed dockyard workers who were exposed to radiations, largely gamma-rays, within the occupational limits of 5 rads per annum. We took blood samples from over 200 men before they were ever occupationally exposed to radiation, and then sampled blood cells from them at six-monthly intervals over a period of ten years. All the slides were coded and scored blind and the total analysis was not performed until the study had run for ten years.

"We scored a very large number of cells and the results [Eva79] show that with increasing accumulated dose there is a detectable increase in aberration yield (Figure 5) -- although no workers were exposed above occupational limits. If we consider just the dicentrics and ring aberrations we see: (i) that there is no threshold, (ii) that there is an approximately linear dose response and (iii) that we observe significant increases in aberration frequency at doses clearly well below the accepted occupational limits" (Eva87, p.185).

The three findings stated by Evans above are clearly in conflict with all four findings reported by Poh83.

We will discuss Pohl-Ruling's remarkable first finding in more detail, below, under "Comments."

Nature of the Experiment (Poh83) :

In terms of in vitro irradiation, the 1983 Pohl-Ruling paper appears to be the first to suggest that a BENEFICIAL effect of radiation has been achieved with respect to chromosome injury in human lymphocytes. It is not only that a "safe" dose below 2 rads acute radiation is suggested -- but much more is claimed. It is claimed that old and established chromosome aberrations are being "cured" by an acute dose of 0.4 rad. ("Cure" is our term.)

The experiment used blood from two donors. Blood was divided into samples, each of which received (except for the control) one acute radiation exposure from a 250 kVp X-ray machine (which means photons with an average energy of about 83.3 KeV). The dose-groups were 0 rad, 0.4 rad, 1 rad, 2 rad, 3 rad, 5 rad, 10 rad, and 30 rad, and the mitogenic stimulant was introduced after exposure.

From Table 2 of the Pohl-Ruling paper, we ascertain that 60,685 metaphases in all were scored, distributed among the eight sub-groups of exposure. Five of the sub-groups had 9000-10000 metaphases scored, and three of the subgroups had 4000-5000 metaphases scored. The difficulty of this type of study is reflected by the fact that the error bands are still relatively large, even when so many metaphases are analyzed.

There are some disturbing details about the procedure. For instance, the 2 and 5 rad values were derived from one blood donor, whereas all other values were pooled from the data from both the donors. Also the authors admit that "As the slides for 2 rad were not scored by all participants, these aberration frequencies were corrected to fit the overall means." In a well-designed multi-center study, it should not have been possible that certain participants could possibly have avoided scoring the 2 rad slides.

We shall not dwell on these details, but rather shall go on to consider the purported results.

Comments on the 1983 Paper :

It is widely considered that chromosome lesions are essentially permanently fixed in a matter of several hours -- certainly in less than one day -- after the aberrations are established. Thus when the bloods for this study were drawn, the "spontaneous" aberrations which were scored reflected aberrations which had been present for days, weeks, months, years, and even decades. Such aberrations may well cause the cells to be selected against in cell divisions, but despite any force of selection, studies have established that radiation-induced aberrations are still detectable in humans, after in vivo irradiation, for many years post-irradiation (for instance, see Eva79 and Sas68). I am unaware that it has ever been considered likely that the aberrations can be un-done.

But un-doing is precisely what would have had to happen to explain the first finding above, since the same blood is the source for the 0 rad dose-sample and the 0.4 rad dose-sample.

The apparent "cure" occurred only at 0.4 rad of acute dose. It was gone by 1.0 rad. The dose of 0.4 rad happens to be the dose at which cell-nuclei each receive an average of about one primary ionization track per nucleus (from our Table 20-"O"), which means about 37 % of nuclei experience no track at all, about 37 % experience exactly one track, and about 26 % experience two or more tracks (our Table 20-N, top). All the effects -- good or bad -- have to arise from the microzones of reactivity created by these tracks, as described in our Chapter 19.

We have two comments.

(1) Flatness from 1-3 Rads :

If we suppose for the moment that the finding -- the "cure" -- is real (repeatable), we can imagine that dose-dependent "good" effects are competing with dose-dependent "bad" effects, and we can postulate that the "good" dominates at the acute dose of 0.4 rad, and that when acute dose has been changed to 1.0 rad in this experiment, then "good" and "bad" cancel each other to produce approximately no net effect. In other words, this speculation rests on a dose-dependent change (which means a track-dependent change) in the relative strength of "good" versus "bad" effects.

But Pohl-Ruling's third finding above is that the aberration-frequencies are not significantly different from each other at 1.0, 2.0, and 3.0 rads. How could there be no further dose-dependent change when the acute dose is changed from 1.0 rad to 2.0 rads (meaning twice as many tracks per nucleus as at 1.0 rad)? And how could there still be no detectable change, even when the acute dose is 3.0 rad? If the consequence of changing dose from zero to 0.4 rad, and from 0.4 rad to 1.0 rad is detectable, why does the even bigger change from 1.0 to 3.0 rads produce no detectable change in the frequency of chromosome aberrations?

(2) Occupational Evidence :

If we put aside all doubts about the finding itself -- a bigger "cure" of old, established lesions by an acute dose of 0.4 rad than induction of new lesions by the same exposure -- what might it imply about hormesis from occupational or environmental exposures?

In the 1979 Evans study described above (Eva79, Eva87), the cell-nuclei in slowly exposed dockyard workers were very rarely experiencing more than one primary ionization track at a time. Although Table 20-M suggests that, at a total gamma dose of 5 rads, a single nucleus would experience about 15 tracks, in the dockyard workers these tracks would be spread out over a year. Nonetheless, these workers accumulated more and more chromosome aberrations in a dose-dependent fashion. (The dose-response was approximately linear.) The finding means that the passage of a new track through a nucleus, every few weeks, did not cause any net decrement ("cure") of such aberrations within the nucleus.

This epidemiological finding may suggest that the "cure" in Poh83 -- if real at all -- had to be occurring exclusively in the 26 % of nuclei which were receiving multiple tracks SIMULTANEOUSLY in those experiments.

If this were the case, then there would be no conceivable protective benefit with respect to chromosome injury, from doses received by people at environmental and occupational rates -- rates at which multiple, simultaneous tracks almost never occur in the same cell-nucleus.

The Possibility of a Lab Mistake :

Instead of speculating at length to explain the Pohl-Ruling finding for lymphocytes irradiated in vitro at an acute dose of 0.4 rad, an outsider might think it more reasonable to await some confirmation that the laboratory result is real (repeatable).

But Pohl-Ruling et al do not think so. They state the following (Poh83, p.80):

"The lower value at 0.4 rad could derive from erroneous scoring but it is not very probable that all the laboratories made an error at this particular dose and for all the different types of chromosome aberrations. If we regard the low values at 0.4 rad as a casual event, then it is strange that it occurs in the same manner for both donors. Even if the irradiation was for any reason lower or higher than 0.4 rad, it remains a remarkable deviation, being lower than the controls. Therefore we favor the view that this deviation is real and that the most probable explanation is a modified mechanism of chromosome aberrations at very low doses which could be a result of repair processes. The inducible repair enzymes might be stimulated at a certain amount of damage, as it occurs also with other inducible enzymes."

It should be pointed out that the same finding in both donors and all labs is not an argument at all against spurious results. If a technical error had been made in labeling, so that the zero and the 0.4 rad groups were mislabeled (for instance), then the erroneous answer is built-in before the scoring is even begun.

Lloyd's Negative Report :

Recently a separate study of the same question has been reported by D.C. Lloyd, of the (U.K.) National Radiological Protection Board, and eight collaborators (Lloyd88). The findings were completely at variance with those of the Pohl-Ruling Study.

The Lloyd Study is on-going, but the results reported in the Lloyd88 paper are based already upon an even larger number of scored metaphases than in the Pohl-Ruling study. Lloyd's 1988 preliminary database is about 1.5 times larger than Pohl-Ruling's 1983 database. The total metaphases in Lloyd88 were 95068, distributed at 11500-12000 per dose-group, for doses of 0 rads, 0.3 rad, 0.6 rad, 1 rad, 2 rad, 3 rad, 5 rad, and 30 rad.

The summary of findings reported by Lloyd and colleagues is as follows (Lloyd88, p.49) :

"Preliminary data are presented from a large experiment by six laboratories in which the low dose-response for X-rays has been re-examined. The plateau in the dose-response relationship, if it exists, does not extend to doses above ~10 mGy [one cGy]. No irradiated cells yielded aberration levels significantly below the control. Over the range 0-300 mGy [0-30 cGy] the response can be fitted to a linear regression. There are, however, variations in sensitivity between cells from different donors. An unexpected finding was that some lymphocytes contained >1 exchange aberrations. This may indicate a small subset of cells that are especially susceptible to the induction of aberrations by low doses."

The "Cure" at 0.4 Rad Not Found :

With respect to the reported lowering of chromosome aberrations at 0.4 rad in the Pohl- Ruling Study (what we have called the "cure" of long-standing aberrations), Lloyd and co-workers did not find it. They state (Lloyd88, p.52) :

"Irradiated cells show no significant decrease in the aberration yield below the level for zero dose controls, and this contrasts with the dip noted at 4 mGy by Pohl-Ruling et al (1983)."

Lloyd and co-workers suggest the following

===

explanation for the Pohl-Ruling observation at 0.4 rad (Lloyd88, p.50):

"A surprising observation [in Poh83] was that at the lowest dose used (4 mGy) the yield of aberrations was significantly below the control level. This was considered to be a real effect, and not a chance effect, because it was consistent for cells from both donors, and it was not the product of an odd scoring result from just one or two of the collaborating laboratories. However, examination of the data shows that the control levels of aberrations were somewhat higher than usual (e.g. 2.8 dicentrics per 1000 cells). Had more typical control values been found, say, 0.5 - 1.5 dicentrics per 1000 cells (Lloyd et al. 1980), this would have removed the significance of the dip at the lowest dose."

One should indeed worry about the unusually high value in the "control" samples.

Additional Differences from the 1983 Paper :

Unlike Poh83, Lloyd et al find a significant increase in the aberration yields at doses of 20 mGy (2 cGy) and above. Pohl-Ruling et al had claimed no significant rise in the frequencies of dicentrics up to 2 rad and in those of terminal deletions up to 5 rad.

Also in contrast with Poh83, Lloyd et al report (Lloyd88, p.52): "Whether a very low-dose plateau exists is debatable in view of the statistical uncertainties on the data. If it exists it appears to extend only up to the 10 mGy point [1 rad]."

Moreover, Lloyd et al state (Lloyd88, p.52) that "... the data fit well over the range 0-50 mGy [0-5 cGy] to the linear model."

Comments on the 1988 Paper :

The 1988 Lloyd paper is at variance with the 1983 Pohl-Ruling paper on almost every key finding.

The on-going study by Lloyd et al already has a larger database (by 1.5-fold) than the Pohl-Ruling database. This gives the Lloyd Study the greater scientific credibility -- quite aside from the procedural flaws acknowledged in the Pohl-Ruling paper.

Even without the Lloyd Study, and even without invalidating the Pohl-Ruling findings, the human epidemiological evidence shows that the Pohl-Ruling Study is irrelevant as any support for PROTECTIVE action against human carcinogenesis. If 0.4 rad (an average of 0.91 primary ionization track per nucleus) were able to "cure" lesions important for human carcinogenesis without inducing even more new ones, the people irradiated in-utero and in adulthood would have had LESS cancer than the controls in Studies 5, 6, 7, and 8 of our Chapter 21. But they had MORE cancer.

In summary, there are powerful and multiple reasons for rejecting the Pohl-Ruling Study as any support for the hormetic hypothesis.

9.   The Bottom Line on Radiation Hormesis

We have sampled the types of evidence cited by Sagan, perhaps the world's leading hormetic, as support for his speculation that "... very low doses of ionizing radiation may not be harmful after all or may even have net benefits ..." (Sag89, p574).

In the evidence we examined, there is nothing to support the hormetic hypothesis, as we have shown.

However, we would REJOICE if someday the hypothesis were well supported by evidence. We do not enjoy the role of bearer of bad news. We would love it if the cancer-evidence were to melt away, or if there were some greater compensating benefit.

We have no antipathy whatsoever toward an objective search for a net benefit. We, too, hope it exists. We favor more research, as we have stated elsewhere (Go88a).

But we will always have a quarrel if speculations are misrepresented as fact. Such behavior can produce literally deadly policies.

It is sad to find suggestions -- usually made with some vague protective caveat -- that radiation hormesis is a reality instead of a chain of conjectures very loosely attached (and NOT always objectively) to observations which themselves are quite possibly irrelevant and maybe even spurious.

In addition, we have another objection not yet mentioned specifically in this chapter. It is the excessive subdivision of data.

The Excessive Subdivision of Data :

In the study of radiation-induced cancer, it has become customary for analysts to do "site-specific" division of data, notwithstanding the data's sparsity even while they remain combined. There is a real hazard of generating biologically meaningless datapoints, whose subsequent "interpretation" will be badly misleading -- as pointed out in Go79.

Such site-specific analyses could even lead to claims that, while radiation CARCINOGENESIS occurs at organ X, radiation HORMESIS occurs at organ Y. With sampling variation and the artificially intensified small-numbers problem, it is inevitable that exposed persons will have a lower rate than controls of some cancers, and a higher rate than controls of other cancers, after the division of one disease into 5, 10, 20, 50, or more parts.

Likewise, excessive subdivision of data by dose-classes can also create such a small-numbers problem that NOTHING remains statistically significant. An entire database can be rendered meaningless this way.

Readers who look again at Figures 13-A and 13-B will see, for instance, that even after 32 years of follow-up, the datapoints in the A-Bomb Study are still jagged when Dose-Groups are NOT subdivided or are partially COMBINED. Moreover, in Chapter 8, Part 4, we explained how residual radioactivity makes the dosimetry in the two lowest Dose-Groups permanently uncertain. Further subdivision would just increase the chance for spurious results. The appropriate handling is to COMBINE them -- which has been commonly done.

It was predictable, however, that sooner or later the OPPOSITE approach to low-dose subdivisions of the A-Bomb Study would be explored in the hormetic context.

Additional Subdivision of the A-Bomb Study :

At the Hormesis Conference in Oakland, Kato et al (Kato87) presented a finer subdivision of the 1950-1978 (note, not 1950-1982) findings in Dose-Groups 1, 2, and 3. The three groups became ten. The data were presented for Hiroshima separately from Nagasaki, and in five dose-groups for each city.

It is interesting that in what we would call Dose-Group 2-B, the relative risk is higher than Dose-Group 1 in Nagasaki, and lower than Dose-Group 1 in Hiroshima (Kato87 Figures 1 and 2). Yet no one would suggest that low-dose exposure is hormetic in Hiroshima and carcinogenic in Nagasaki. Such data are just meaningless.

Kato and co-workers appropriately commented (Kato87, p.651): "In general, it is difficult to determine the effects of ionizing radiation directly among subjects exposed to low doses of radiation; huge sample sizes are required if the estimates are to have reasonable stability and small differences are to be detected (Land80b). Moreover, extraneous sources of variation which may vary among dose groupings become more important than at higher doses, and at these levels of exposure the actual doses may not be as reliably ascertained as would obviously be desirable ..."

It is not clear why they undertook to subdivide the data nonetheless.

They conclude (Kato87, p.651): "The frequency of events so far observed among the five dose-groups varied, but haphazardly, and there were no statistically significant differences among them."

There is simply no doubt -- it is in the very nature of numbers -- that every database will become inconclusive if it is increasingly subdivided.

Dose-Group 1 versus Dose-Group 2 :

Nonetheless, comparison of Dose-Group 1 (unexposed) with Dose-Group 2 (internal organ-dose of only 1.5 to 1.9 cSv) is now treated by some as meaningful in a hormetic context. For instance, at the hormesis conference in Frankfurt, Kusunoki and co-workers cite the Kato87 paper, in which Dose-Group 2 is identified by its KERMA dose-range of 1 up to 10 rads -- see our Table 26-E. They cite Kato in the following context (Ku88, p.196):

"Kato et al recently reported that leukemia and cancer mortality appears to be lower in atomic bomb survivors exposed to low doses of radiation (1-10 cGy) than in the control group (Kato et al 1987)."

And again on the next page: "In addition, it is of interest to determine if there is a relationship between the apparently decreased cancer mortality (Kato et al. 1987) and the level of immune competence of survivors after low-dose irradiation. These investigations will be carried out more extensively in the future."

It might be noted that Kato87 used the 1950-1978 database. In the 1950-1982 database, we do NOT find the cancer death-rate to be lower in Dose-Group 2 than

===

in Dose-Group 1, though we find them to be very close -- as they should be. See Table 13-A, Columns A, B, C and F.

If we had found Dose-Group 2 to be lower, however, we would not regard it as biologically meaningful, in view of the very small difference in the estimated doses and in view of the permanent uncertainty about those doses (Chapter 8, Part 4).

One of the Questionable Practices :

As we stated earlier, we are emphatically in favor of a disinterested search for radiation hormesis. However, we cannot applaud practices like excessive subdivision which can inadvertently and innocently interfere with extracting biological meaning from databases. The sad thing is that -- even though databases grow steadily more reliable, from addition of new observations over time, and grow increasingly able to yield important and solidly based information for society -- the gain can be lost due to excessive new subdivision.

Closing Remarks
on Hormetic Speculations :
==

The search for radiation hormesis will surely go on. And it will generate a profusion of new radiobiological experiments.

Certain "findings" are predictable. For instance, studies in experimental animals and cell-studies have produced almost any dose-response one can imagine or desire, so a "J" shape (hormetic shape) is bound to show up now and then in the search for hormesis.

The problem is, of course, that differences among non-human species are so great that it is impossible to know which findings (if any) might correctly predict the human response.

Even when HUMAN cells are irradiated in the laboratory, they do not reliably predict the response of cells irradiated in whole, living humans (for instance, see Eva87), or cells irradiated in other laboratories (for instance, see Lloyd88).

Solid evidence on net human health-effects can come from the reality-check of human epidemiology, but that, too, can be exquisitely difficult. Very few studies are capable of addressing extremely low-dose questions, for the reasons discussed in Chapter 21.

At this time, what can we responsibly say about low-dose radiation hormesis?

First: The possible benefits from low-dose radiation are highly speculative, whereas the radiation-induced cancers are NOT speculative. They are real.

Second: The observed cancer-excess is a NET effect which has been observed despite beneficial effects (if any) from low-dose radiation upon the immune system or the repair system.

Third: It is reasonable to conclude that the human evidence already invalidates any speculation that low-dose radiation might help to protect anyone against cancer. Low-dose exposure helps to INCREASE the frequency of cancer.

Fourth: Sponsorship of the search for hormesis is not always disinterested, and therefore the public would be prudent to develop an independent way to verify any rosy claims. Error in this field carries the prospect of unnecessary cancer-misery for hundreds of millions of people over time -- plus a presently unquantifiable amount of misery from heritable unrepaired genetic damage.

===================================

Figure 35–A

Plot of Chromatid and Isochromatid Breaks versus X–Ray "Priming" Dose, in Rads.

The data plotted below (transferred from this chapter, Part 4) come from Shadley and Wolff (Shad87a).

The dose-response is clearly supra-linear. In fact, the equation of best fit for the data above has a dose-exponent of 0.5. The equation is: Breaks per 200 cells = (6.789 x Dose^0.5) + 1.325. (Readers can review the method in Chapter 29. The regression-input, and part of the output, are shown.)

The dose-point at 150 rads may not really belong in the series. See text, Part 4. Without that point, the dose-response is approximately linear, and is clearly NOT concave-upward.

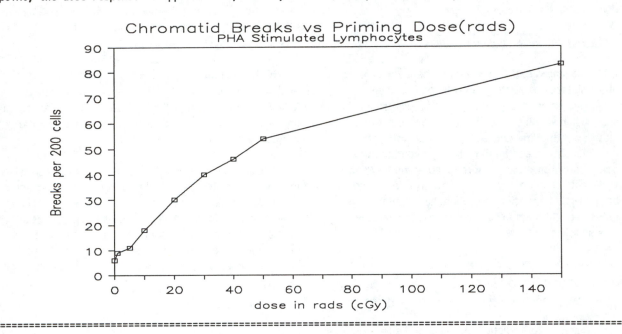

Chromatid Breaks vs Priming Dose(rads)
PHA Stimulated Lymphocytes

A test of curvilinear regression on these data:

Breaks	Dose	D^0.9	D^0.8	D^0.7	D^0.6	D^0.5	Dose^0.4
6	0	0.0000	0.0000	0.0000	0.0000	0.0000	0.0000
9	1	1.0000	1.0000	1.0000	1.0000	1.0000	1.0000
11	5	4.2567	3.6239	3.0852	2.6265	2.2361	1.9037
18	10	7.9433	6.3096	5.0119	3.9811	3.1623	2.5119
30	20	14.8227	10.9856	8.1418	6.0342	4.4721	3.3145
40	30	21.3506	15.1949	10.8140	7.6961	5.4772	3.8981
46	40	27.6601	19.1270	13.2264	9.1461	6.3246	4.3734
54	50	33.8122	22.8653	15.4625	10.4564	7.0711	4.7818
83	150	90.8829	55.0647	33.3629	20.2141	12.2474	7.4206

Regression on Dose^1			Regression on Dose^0.5		
Regression Output:			Regression Output:		
Constant	15.7588		Constant		1.3247
Std Err of Y Est	9.6408		Std Err of Y Est		3.9277
R Squared	0.8744		R Squared		0.9792
No. of Observations	9		No. of Observations		9
Degrees of Freedom	7		Degrees of Freedom		7
X Coefficient(s)	0.5071		X Coefficient(s)	6.7891	
Std Err of Coef.	0.0726		Std Err of Coef.	0.3743	

For the reasons given in Chapter 24, our September 1986 estimate of the radiation-induced cancers to come from Chernobyl is reproduced here in its original form, exactly as presented. The calculations and estimate were part of a longer paper. Only the sections relating specifically to the Chernobyl accident are reproduced here.

==

ASSESSING CHERNOBYL'S CANCER CONSEQUENCES:[*]

APPLICATION OF FOUR "LAWS" OF RADIATION CARCINOGENESIS

John W. Gofman, M.D., Ph.D.

Department of Biophysics and Medical Physics

102 Donner Laboratory

University of California at Berkeley

Berkeley, California 94720

Presentation at the 192nd National Meeting

The American Chemical Society

Anaheim, California

September 9, 1986

Symposium On Low-Level Radiation
Division of Chemical Health and Safety

For contacting author

P.O. Box 11207
San Francisco, California 94101

Telephone:
415-776-8299

September 7 - 10:

Hotel, 714-774-7817, or via
Press Office of the
American Chemical Society

Tel: (714) 740-4529
at the Anaheim Hilton,
Monterey Room, Concourse Level

* Country-by-Country Summary Page 39

(Page 36-19 in this book).

Because the analysis of cancer consequences from the Chernobyl accident begins with Section 4, we have omitted Sections 1, 2, 3, and Technical Appendix 1. The omissions make the original page numbers irrelevant, so we have added appropriate page numbers in parentheses.

Table Of Contents

==

----

(4) THE CANCER-DOSE FOR MIXED AGES

The Whole-Body Cancer-Dose is a ratio: a whole-body dose in person-rads per one fatal radiation-induced cancer. Gofman[3] has demonstrated extensively how the Whole-Body Cancer-Dose is derived for each sex and at various ages from the existing human evidence. As Generalization 3 indicates, the Cancer-Dose is far lower for children than for adults, and is very high for adults age 50 and older. The range (Gofman[3], 1981, Tables 21 and 22) is from about 65 whole-body person-rads for newborns to about 20,000 whole-body person-rads at age 55.

Risk Possibly Underestimated: Up to the 40th year following exposure to low LET radiation, there is evidence that the observed / expected ratio for solid cancers is increasing[3, 9, 30, 61]. There are as yet no studies with follow-up for longer periods. But we have data for leukemia, where the O/E ratio peaks about 7.5 years following a single exposure and then declines. Using this decline as a model, we have included in the Whole-Body Cancer-Dose the assumption that the O/E ratio for solid cancers from low LET exposures will also begin declining after it peaks. This assumption may underestimate the risk from such exposures.

● THE CANCER-DOSE FOR A MIXTURE OF AGES

Following a situation like the Chernobyl accident, the world is interested in assessing the overall excess number of cancer fatalities and non-fatal cancer cases for populations in which all ages are present.

A Cancer-Dose for mixed ages is available (Gofman[3]).We simply took account of the distribution of persons by age and sex in a population (the U.S. population

was used) and then weighted the Whole-Body Cancer-Dose for each age by the
fraction of the population at that age. In a population of constant size,
the distribution also remains virtually constant. The error introduced by
this approximation is trivial except in a population with age distributions
grossly and permanently different from the U.S. (details in Gofman[3],1981).
The result obtained from such weighting gave the following Whole-Body Cancer-
Dose for a population of mixed ages (both sexes included) (Gofman[3],1981,p.294):

> 268 whole-body person-rads per fatal cancer, or
>
> 268,000 whole-body person-millirads per fatal cancer.

● LEUKEMIA-DOSE FOR A POPULATION

There is unanimous agreement on treating leukemia separately from the solid
cancers, because leukemia behaves differently with respect to speed of appearance,
duration of radiation effect, loss of life-expectancy, and the absence of a
definitive age-trend with risk-per-rad. The Whole-Body Leukemia-Dose for a mixed-
aged population is estimated at 6,500 person-rads, or 6,500,000 person-millirads
per leukemia case (Gofman and O'Connor, 1985)[46] .

(5) THE CHERNOBYL ACCIDENT: CANCER-LEUKEMIA CONSEQUENCES

● ELEMENTS OF THE CALCULATION

If in each country, we knew the whole-body radiation dose received by each
person and if we added up those doses for the entire population, we would know
the total person-rads or person-millirads received in that country. For illustration, suppose we had a country with 10^8 person-millirads of whole-body dose.
Then,

Fatal cancers = 10^8 person-millirads / 268,000 person-millirads per cancer

= 373 fatal cancers from the Chernobyl accident.

Since there will be approximately one non-fatal cancer induced by radiation for
each fatal cancer, there would be an additional 373 non-fatal cancers.

Leukemia cases = 10^8 person-millirads / 6.5 x 10^6 person-millirads per leukemia

= 15 leukemia cases.

● SOURCES OF DOSE FROM A NUCLEAR POWER ACCIDENT

There are several sources of exposure in areas where fallout occurs:

(1) Direct radiation of the whole body from gamma rays in the cloud of
radionuclides passing over a population;

(2) Inhalation of radioactive substances from the passing cloud and from radionuclides re-suspended after deposition on the ground;

(3) Direct external radiation of the whole body by gamma rays emitted from radionuclides deposited on the ground;

(4) Internal exposure by ingestion of radionuclides with milk, water, meat, fruits, and vegetables.

One or another source of exposure will dominate, according to the type of accident and where a population is located with respect to the event.

● RADIOCESIUM AS THE DOMINANT MENACE

In most countries receiving fallout from the Chernobyl accident, it is clear that the major doses will come from gamma rays emitted from radionuclides deposited on the ground, and from internal radiation via food and water.

Fallout measurements show that a large quantity of radioactive cesium did come out of the Chernobyl reactor. The dose received from cesium-137 ($T_{1/2}$ =30.2 years) and cesium-134 ($T_{1/2}$ = 2.3 years) will be the most important part of the whole-body exposures. Of course, we do not deny additional doses from other nuclides. Even without the incremental dose they inflict, we can reach a good appreciation of Chernobyl's cancer and leukemia consequences if we are able to calculate the doses delivered by the cesium-137 and cesium-134, both from direct gamma radiation from the ground and from these nuclides in the food chain.

(6) THE SOURCES OF FALLOUT DATA

There are two major sources of multi-nation information available. The first is a series of reports from the World Health Organization (WHO)[48] in Copenhagen, and the second is a series of reports from the United States Environmental Protection Agency (EPA) [49] in Washington, D.C. The organizations issued their last reports, respectively, on June 12 and June 30, 1986.

These reports rely upon measurements provided by the various reporting countries. Some countries reported data rather professionally. Others, such as East Germany, reported none at all. The Soviet Union, in spite of its assurances of being forthcoming with data, provided no cesium-137 or cesium-134 measurements at all, until the Soviet report in late August[65].

In addition to the WHO and EPA reports, there are reports for some single countries, most particularly Finland[50, 51] and the United Kingdom[52].

We will describe below the kinds of measurements available, and their
use in estimating doses from cesium-137 and cesium-134. In this paper's
Technical Appendix, dose data are described country-by-country.

• Opportunity for Future Measurements

We can state at the outset that all the requisite measurements for a
perfect assessment of Chernobyl's cancer consequences are far from available.
To match existing measurements with exact population distribution would require a grid over each country with measurements of both the population within
a particular grid-location and the cesium-137 and cesium-134 deposition in
that same grid-location. It is regrettable that society is not set up to provide such information on a timely basis. However, if the will exists to obtain
such data, the opportunity has not been lost (see Section 8).

• THREE KINDS OF AVAILABLE DATA AND THEIR HANDLING

• (1) The Best Type of Data

Here the country reports the integrated deposition of cesium-137 and
cesium-134 up through the entire period of significant fallout. Among the
reports, this occurs relatively rarely. Some countries provide the deposition
values for a very limited period of the fallout, so that the true total deposition
must be higher than the values reported.

• (2) The Next Best Type Of Data

Here the country reports the values for gamma-ray exposure from the
deposition of all radionuclides on the ground for a specified date following the
accident. These data can be used effectively to obtain indirectly what the
cesium-137 and cesium-134 depositions were at the same locations.

The basis for such conversion from external gamma-ray dose to cesium values
resides in the provision by the Finnish Centre for Radiation and Nuclear Safety
of values for the percent of the total gamma-ray dose which is to be assigned to
cesium-137. In the Finns' first report[50], they provide the datum that 1.8%
(1.7% - 1.9%) of the total gamma-ray dose for April 29, 1986 is to be assigned to
gamma-rays from cesium-137's decay (via barium-137m). In their second report[51],
they provide the datum that 11% of the total gamma-ray dose for May 6-7, 1986 is
to be assigned to gamma-rays from cesium-137. By using the daily decay curve of
of gamma-ray dose for Uusikaupunki for the first two weeks, it is possible to
interpolate and extrapolate the percent of the gamma-dose to be assigned to

cesium-137 for dates others than those for which data are provided directly. These assignments are listed in Table 5.

Table 5:

Percent Of Gamma-Ray Dose Assigned To Cesium-137 Gamma-Rays

Date Of Gamma-Ray Measurement	Percent Of Measured Dose Assigned To Cesium-137
April 29,1986	1.8%
April 30,1986	4.1%
May 1,1986	4.9%
May 2,1986	5.8%
May 3,1986	6.8%
May 4,1986	8.0%
May 5,1986	9.1%
May 6,1986	10.2%
May 7,1986	11.7%
May 8,1986	12.9%
May 9,1986	14.4%
May 10,1986	16.0%
May 11,1986	17.3%
May 12,1986	18.8%

The reason for the rising percent of the gamma-ray dose assigned to cesium-137 is that the cesium-137 hardly changes its output of gamma-rays during this brief period of about two weeks, whereas many of the short-lived nuclides are decreasing their output due to substantial decay during the same time period.

● (3) The Last Type Of Data

Here we are not provided either with gamma-ray dose measurements or with radiocesium deposition measurements, but we are provided with iodine-131 deposition measurements. From analysing other data where both I-131 and Cs-137 deposition data are available, we are able to estimate Cs-137 deposition indirectly from I-131 deposition data.

(7) METHOD: ILLUSTRATIVE USE OF THE DATA

● METHOD 1: BEST TYPE OF DATA (DENMARK)

Cesium-137 integrated deposition is available. Denmark did provide such data.
Denmark provided (WHO June 5, 1986 Report)[48] the following data (from 10 stations
for May 15 through May 27) for countrywide contamination in Becquerels/m^2 of surface soil:

	Mean	S.D.	Max
Cs-137	1075	758	2943
Cs-134	602	424	3477

These reports note that the above values are corrected with respect to cesium-137
still present from weapons-test fallout.

For Cs-137: (1075 Bq/m^2) x (27 Picocuries/Bq) = 29025 pCi/m^2.

For Cs-134: (602 Bq/m^2) x (27 Picocuries/Bq) = 16254 pCi/m^2.

● Cesium-137 Dose, Method 1

From data for worldwide fallout from weapons testing, described by UNSCEAR[4]
and summarized in Gofman[3](1981, p.548), we calculate that the total absorbed dose
commitment is 0.66 millirads for each 1000 pCi/m^2. This includes
the dose commitment both from external radiation from Cs-137 gamma rays coming
from the ground, adjusted by UNSCEAR for weathering to an average depth of 3 cm,
for body-shielding, and for time spent indoors, and from internal radiation from
Cs-137 ingested via the food chain.

Internal doses vary by soil type, and here we are using average
values observed from weapons fallout. Unfortunately for people in the Ukraine,
UNSCEAR[4] estimates that a much larger internal dose will be received from cesium
there than in most areas, due to special soil characteristics there. But for
average conditions, of the 0.66 millirads total dose commitment from each 1000 pCi/m^2,
UNSCEAR's estimate is that 70 % is from external dose and 30 % from internal dose.

For Denmark, therefore, we can make the following calculation of dose.

External Cs-137 Dose Commitment

External dose = (total deposition) x (dose per unit of deposition) x
(external share) = (29025 pCi/m^2) x (0.66 mrads per 1000 pCi/m^2) x (0.70)
=13.4 millirads.

==

<u>Internal Cs-137 Dose Commitment</u>

The internal share changes to 30 %, and therefore internal dose = (29025 pCi/m^2) x (0.66 mrads per 1000 pCi/m^2) x (0.30) = <u>5.7 millirads.</u>

● <u>Cesium-134 Dose, Method 1</u>

<u>External Cs-134 Dose Commitment</u> : There are two factors to consider in evaluating the dose from Cs-134 for the <u>same</u> number of picocuries/m^2 as for Cs-137.

(a) The total <u>average</u> gamma-ray energy per disintegration for each nuclide.
    Ratio of gamma-ray energy Cs-134 / Cs-137 = 2.52
(b) The mean life of Cs-134 atoms versus Cs-137 atoms (mean life = half life / 0.693).
    Ratio of mean life Cs-134 / Cs-137 = 0.076

<u>Relative Dose-Effectiveness:</u> The relative dose-effectiveness of Cs-134 versus Cs-137 per pCi/m^2 deposition is the product of factors (a) and (b).
Dose-effectiveness Cs-134 / Cs-137 = (2.52) x (0.076) = 0.19.

<u>Calculation of Dose:</u> The external dose commitment from Cs-134 is:
(Relative Deposition Cs-134/Cs-137) x (Dose-Effectiveness Factor) x (External

Cs-137 Dose). For Denmark, we have therefore Cs-134 external dose = (16254 pCi per square meter / 29025 pCi per square meter) x (0.19) x (13.4 millirads) =
<u>1.4 millirads.</u>

<u>Internal Cs-134 Dose Commitment:</u> There are two factors to consider.
(a) The average peak <u>beta</u> energy of Cs-134 versus that of Cs-137; the predominant source of <u>internal</u> dosage is from disintegrations via beta particles.

Ratio of beta-particle energy Cs-134 / Cs-137 = 0.65 / 0.51 = 1.275. (Note that some handbooks give 1.17 MEV as the Cs-137 beta energy. This is true for only 8 % of the disintegrations; 92 % go via the 0.51 MEV disintegration pathway.)
(b) The ratio of mean-life, calculated above to be 0.076.

<u>Relative Dose-Effectiveness:</u> This factor is the product of (a) and (b).
Dose-effectiveness Cs-134 / Cs-137 = (1.275) x (0.076) = 0.097

<u>Calculation of Dose:</u> The internal dose commitment from Cs-134 is

(Relative Deposition of Cs-134 / Cs-137) x (Dose-Effectiveness Factor) x (Internal Cs-137 Dose). For Denmark we have, therefore, Cs-134 internal dose = (16254 pCi per m^2 / 29025 pCi per m^2) x (0.097) x (5.7 millirads) = <u>0.3 millirads.</u>

● Combined Cs-137 and Cs-134 Doses, Method 1

The combined external and internal doses from both nuclides, in Denmark =
(13.4 + 5.7 + 1.4 + 0.3) millirads = <u>20.8 millirads</u>.

● Cancer and Leukemia Consequences, Denmark

$$\underline{\text{Fatal Cancers}} = \frac{(\text{Population Size}) \times (\text{Dose in millirads})}{(268{,}000 \text{ person-millirads per fatal cancer})}$$

$$= \frac{(5.1 \times 10^6 \text{ persons}) \times (20.8 \text{ millirads})}{(268{,}000 \text{ person-millirads per fatal cancer})}$$

= 396 fatal cancers, which we round off to 400, in Denmark.

<u>Non-fatal Cancers</u>, additional = 400 cases.

$$\underline{\text{Leukemias}} = \frac{(5.1 \times 10^6 \text{ persons}) \times (20.8 \text{ millirads})}{(6{,}500{,}000 \text{ person-millirads per leukemia})}$$

= 16.3 leukemias, rounded off to 16 cases.

This completes the analysis for Denmark, based upon what we are calling the best type of data, namely, integrated Cs-137 and Cs-134 deposition on the ground, averaged over the country.

● METHOD 2: NEXT BEST TYPE OF DATA (POLAND)

Gamma-ray exposure from deposition of all radionuclides on the ground is provided. Poland reports data usable for this illustrative example. The WHO[48] report of May 30, 1986, provides gamma-ray exposure from the ground for "all Poland" for the very early period, April 29, 1986, which is ideal since the 1.8 % factor for the contribution by cesium-137 applies correctly. Although we would much prefer to have separate gamma-ray measurements and population distributions for each part of Poland, such data are not supplied. The measurement supplied is, for "all Poland", a range of 20-1000 micro-roentgens per hour, or 20-1000 μR/hr. Subtracting 12 μR/hr for background, we have 8-988 μR/hr as the range, outdoors, free-in-air. So we use Criterion II (see Technical Appendix 2) to derive a gamma dose for Poland of 249 μR/hr.

===

● Cesium-137 Dose, Method 2

Since cesium-137's contribution to the gamma dose is 1.8%, the Cs-137 gamma dose = (0.018) x (249 μR/hr) = 4.48 μR/hr. We are interested in calculating the Cs-137 dose for the whole first year, and thereafter for the entire mean-life of the Cs-137 atoms. That mean-life is $T_{\frac{1}{2}}$ / 0.693, or about 43.5 years. The first-year dose is only 2.3 % of the total dose commitment. The total dose is 43.5 times the first year dose.

If all the deposited Cs-137 were to remain right on the surface for the first year (and thereafter), the calculation would simply involve multiplication of the early deposition dose by the number of hours in a year, 8760 hours per year. But the cesium-137 has been found to work its way into the soil during the first year, with the result that the average external dose is appreciably lower than it would be if the Cs-137 had all remained on the surface. How much lower?

Devell and co-workers[53] have given a value for external dose one meter above the ground of 0.0811 mR/yr per 1000 pCi/m^2 --- provided the Cs-137 remains on the surface of the earth for the entire period of one year.

Beck's work is cited by UNSCEAR[4] as leading to the conclusion that the cesium-137 works its way into soil, with the establishment of an exponential profile for the Cs-137 , with a mean depth of 3 cm. For the average dose in the first year, UNSCEAR gives a value of 0.033 mR/yr per 1000 pCi/m^2. The cesium apparently stabilizes at this distribution in soil, and the average value for the first year can be used for all the subsequent years in estimation of dose commitment over the mean-life of the Cs-137.

Therefore, the value we would get for external dose one meter above the ground for deposited Cs-137 is too high if we use the very early dose. The correction factor is 0.0811 / 0.033, or 2.46.

In our analysis, we have, for Poland, an external dose of 4.48 μR/hr. This must be divided by 2.46, yielding 1.821 μR/hr as the appropriate external dose per hour for the hours in the first year. Therefore, for the first year the total dose will be (8760 hrs) x (1.821 μR/hr), or 15,952 μR in the first year. And for the total dose commitment over the mean-life, we have (43.5 yrs) x (15,952 μR/yr), or 6.939 x 10^5 μR.

● Correction of the External Cs-137 Dose Commitment

The UNSCEAR[4] recommendation is that the external dose in μR should be reduced by a factor of 0.32 μrads/μR to take into account back scattering, shielding by the body itself, and time spent indoors, on the average. Therefore, the whole-body

==

absorbed dose from external Cs-137 = (0.32 μrads/μR) x (6.939 x 10^5 μR) , or
2.22 x 10^5 μrads. Thus, external Cs-137 dose = (2.22 x 10^5 μrads) x (1 mrad/1000 μrads),
or <u>222 millirads</u>.

● Internal Cs-137 Dose Commitment

Given the usual distribution of Cs-137 dose (70% external and 30 % internal),
we must multiply the external dose by (0.3 / 0.7) or 0.43 to obtain the internal Cs-137
dose. Therefore, internal dose from Cs-137 = (222 mrads) x (0.43) = <u>95.5 millirads.</u>

● Cesium -134 Dose, Method 2

Poland provides no data for the Cs-134 / Cs-137 ratio of deposition. We use the
average value calculated from many other data in the WHO[48] and EPA[49] reports. Since the
ratio is fixed in the reactor, use of the average ratio from such measurements is
fully justified in the absence of actual measurements in a particular country. The
average deposition ratio , Cs-134 / Cs-137 = 0.76.

● External Cs-134 Dose Commitment

The external Cs-134 dose is the (deposition ratio) x (dose-effectiveness factor)
x (external Cs-137 dose). Borrowing the dose-effectiveness factor of 0.19 from
Method 1, we calculate the external Cs-134 dose = (0.76) x (0.19) x (222 mrads) =
<u>32.1 mrads.</u>

● Internal Cs-134 Dose Commitment

This is the (deposition ratio) x (dose-effectiveness factor) x (internal Cs-137
dose). Borrowing the appropriate dose-effectiveness factor of 0.097 from Method 1,
we calculate the internal Cs-134 dose = (0.76) x (0.097) x (95.5 millirads) =
<u>7.0 mrads.</u>

● Combined Cs-137 and Cs-134 Doses, Method 2

Total cesium dose, from above, = 222 + 95.5 + 32.1 + 7.0 = <u>356.6 millirads.</u>

● Cancer and Leukemia Consequences, Poland

$$\text{Fatal Cancers} = \frac{(\text{Population Size}) \times (\text{Dose in mrads})}{268,000 \text{ person-mrads per fatal cancer}} = \frac{(36.9 \times 10^6 \text{ persons}) \times (356.6 \text{ mrads})}{268,000 \text{ person-mrads per fatal cancer}}$$

= 49,099 fatal cancers. This is rounded off to <u>49,000 fatal cancers.</u>

Non-fatal cancers, additional, are <u>49,000 cases.</u>

$$\text{Leukemias} = \frac{(36.9 \times 10^6 \text{ persons}) \times (356.6 \text{ mrads})}{6,500,000 \text{ person-mrads per leukemia}} = \underline{2025 \text{ leukemias}} \text{ (rounded off.)}$$

● METHOD 3: LAST TYPE OF DATA (ITALY)

This type of analysis is based upon Iodine-131 deposition on the ground, with conversion of such data to Cesium-137 deposition on the ground. Fortunately, there were few instances where this method had to be used. Italy was such a case. The EPA report of May 12, 1986,[49] provides values for I-131 deposition in five separate regions. The average is 269 nanocuries/m^2, or 269,000 pCi/m^2.

From excellent Swedish data on the ratio of I-131 to Cs-137 depositions,[49] daily, in the early days of the accident, we obtain a factor of 0.202 for converting from Iodine-131 deposition to Cesium-137 deposition. Therefore, average Cs-137 deposition in Italy = (0.202) x (269,000 pCi/m^2) = 54338 pCi/m^2. This value is used as if it were Type (1) data, (see especially EPA Report, May 12,1986).

● Cs-137 External and Internal Doses

Total Cs-137 dose = (0.66 mrads per 1000 pCi/m^2) x (54338 pCi/m^2) = 35.9 millirads. External share is 70%, or 25.1 millirads. Internal share is 30 %, or 10.8 millirads.

● Cs-134 External and Internal Doses

Using the deposition ratio from Method 2 and the dose-effectiveness ratio from Method 1, we obtain:

External Cs-134 dose = (0.76) x (0.19) x (25.1 mrads) = 3.6 millirads.

Internal Cs-134 dose = (0.76) x (0.097) x (10.8 mrads) = 0.8 millirads.

● Combined Cs-137 and Cs-134 Doses, Method 3

Total cesium dose, from above, = (25.1 + 10.8 + 3.6 + 0.8) millirads = 40.3 millirads.

● Cancer and Leukemia Consequences, Italy

$$\text{Fatal Cancers} = \frac{\text{(Population size) x (Dose in Millirads)}}{\text{(268,000 person-millirads per fatal cancer)}}$$

$$= \frac{(5.624 \times 10^7 \text{ persons}) \times (40.3 \text{ millirads})}{\text{(268,000 person-millirads per fatal cancer)}}$$

= 8457 fatal cancers, rounded off to 8450 fatal cancers.

Non-fatal Cancers, additional = 8450 cases.

$$\text{Leukemias} = \frac{(5.624 \times 10^7 \text{ persons}) \times (40.3 \text{ millirads})}{\text{(6,500,000 person-millirads per leukemia)}}$$

= 350 leukemias, rounded off.

● UNIFORM REDUCTION OF "FIRST-STEP" VALUES

The dose commitments from cesium derived above are not the final values used to assess the cancer consequences; they are "first-step" values. The final values are the entries in Table 6, which are lower.

We are confident that Methods 1, 2, and 3 provide very reasonable dose commitments from cesiums in the localities where some measurements were reported. But we could not know how representative those localities were for the whole country. For instance, the localities measured may sometimes have been the arbitrary locations of permanent monitoring equipment, or may often have been localities where rainfall produced much greater concern and much more fallout. The variability of fallout within some countries was illustrated by Poland, where gamma doses ranged from 8 μR/hour to 988 μR/hour on the same date. Therefore, before calculating "first-step" dose commitments, we tried to correct for such variability by using the two criteria stated at the beginning of Technical Appendix 2.

After obtaining "first-step" dose commitments for each country by Methods 1, 2 and 3, we obtained reasonable factors by which all "first-step" values could be reduced uniformly. We shall call these the "lowering factors."

● BASIS OF THE LOWERING FACTORS

The "first-step" dose commitments from cesiums correspond to "first-step" deposition-values for cesiums. These were easily obtained in picocuries per meter^2 for cesium-137 with a single equation. Because in Methods 2 and 3 the ratio is constant for the deposition of Cs-134 to Cs-137, the ratio of the dose commitment from each nuclide is likewise constant. The share of the nuclides' combined dose commitment which is contributed by the Cs-137 is always 0.89. And because a Cs-137 deposition of 1,000 pCi/m^2 gives an absorbed dose commitment of 0.66 millirads (see Method 1), the following equation can be applied for all countries where Methods 2 and 3 were used. Cesium-137 deposition in units of 1,000 pCi/m^2 = (0.89) x (dose commitment Cs-137 + Cs-134 in mrads) / 0.66 mrads per 1,000 pCi/m^2.

With this equation, we obtained average "first-step" values for cesium-137 deposition in pCi/m^2 for every country in Table 6. We multiplied by each country's area in meters^2 to get "first-step" values for total cesium-137 deposition in each country.

The sum of those "first-step" values was 2.73×10^6 curies of cesium-137 deposited in all the countries combined. By comparing this value with some conservative estimates of total cesium-137 released by the accident, we obtained two appropriate lowering factors which we applied to the "first-step" dose commitments.

● Cesium: Amount Released and Initial Inventory

Several groups have attempted to estimate the total quantity of cesium-137 released from the Chernobyl reactor. Knox [54] suggested a value of 3.0×10^6 curies. The Imperial College Group [55] in England suggested a much lower value of 1.4×10^6 curies released. It is hard to know whether one of these values is better than the other.

The initial inventory of Cs-137 at the time of the accident depends on the length of operation and refueling schedule. Estimates for the Chernobyl reactor have been offered [54, 56], based on approximately two years of operation, which place its cesium-137 inventory at 5.8×10^6 and 6.0×10^6 curies. However, because our objective is to determine a credible lower-limit on the cancer-consequences from the accident, we have used the much lower value of 3.53×10^6 curies as the cesium-137 inventory, which corresponds with one year's full-power operation.

From this minimal value, we are going to derive and apply (separately) two lowering factors. Their results are in good agreement with the Soviet report[65]; see foot of Table 6.

● FACTOR FOR CESIUM-137 DEPOSITION OF 1,990,000 CURIES

For one factor, we have assumed that 75% of the minimal cesium-137 inventory was released at the temperatures and disruption which occurred at the reactor: $(3.53 \times 10^6$ curies$) \times (0.75) = 2.65 \times 10^6$ curies released. After we assumed that 25% of this amount was deposited on lands and waters not considered in the areas of Table 6, the cesium-137 deposition was reduced to $(2.65 \times 10^6$ curies$) \times (0.75) = 1.99 \times 10^6$ curies. This compares with our "first-step" value of 2.73×10^6 curies deposited. Therefore this lowering factor for all the "first-step" dose commitments is $(1.99 / 2.73) = 0.729$.

● FACTOR FOR CESIUM-137 DEPOSITION OF 1,330,000 CURIES

For the other factor, we have assumed that 50% of the minimal cesium-137 inventory was released: $(3.53 \times 10^6$ curies$) \times (0.50) = 1.77 \times 10^6$ curies

released.   Then this value was reduced for the 25% "loss" in areas not
considered: $(1.77 \times 10^6 \text{ curies}) \times (0.75) = 1.33 \times 10^6$ curies deposited.
Comparison with our "first-step" value of 2.73×10^6 curies leads to the
lowering factor of $(1.33 / 2.73) = 0.487$.

● FINAL ENTRIES IN TABLE 6

After a dose commitment is lowered by one of the factors, it is
multiplied by the country's population to obtain person-millirads, and then
person-millirads are divided by 268,000 person-millirads per fatal cancer
and 6,500,000 person-millirads per leukemia to obtain the entries for Table 6,
as explained in Section 5 of this paper.

The two sets of entries for malignancies in Table 6 correspond to
cesium-137 depositions of 1,990,000 curies and 1,330,000 curies respectively
(Technical Appendix 2-B illustrates the country-by-country calculation).   The
lower value of 1.3 million curies is very close to the estimate by the
Imperial College Group[55] .   It may be much too low, especially if the initial
Cs-137 inventory was about 6 million curies instead of the 3.53 million
curies used in this paper.

Unfortunately, scientists must be skeptical about the validity of any
Soviet statements concerning cesium-137 inventory or percentage released.
Indeed, one must wonder how much the Soviets can know about the percentage
released when the condition of their reactor is hidden under tons of sand,
lead, and boron, and when the explosion rendered worthless any measurements
at normal vents.

Moreover, the Soviets have an obvious interest in underestimating the amount
of cesium released, and this interest is powerfully shared by many nuclear experts
in other countries which have nuclear power plants, or plan to have them.

===

===

(8) RESULTING ASSESSMENT OF CHERNOBYL'S CANCER CONSEQUENCES

===

Table 6 shows that the Chernobyl accident will cause between 634,200 and 951,000 total cases of radiation-induced cancer, and between 13,100 and 19,500 cases of radiation-induced leukemia. (Table 6 is on page 39.) Which end of the range is the more credible?

● REALITY-CHECK ON TABLE 6's ASSESSMENT

For reasons of compassion, we would much prefer that the lower values from Table 6 be the true ones. On the other hand, we must recognize that it is the higher estimate which corresponds more closely with the "first-step" values derived from actual measurements (see Section 7 of this paper). And although we did not tabulate the results if the cesium-137 inventory was 6,000,000 curies instead of 3,530,000 curies, anyone can see by simple proportion that the total cancers would rise to a range of 1,000,000 to 1,600,000 from the same analysis.

In the absence of additional measurements, we will use the lower range based on the lower inventory.

A way does exist for the scientific community to make a reality-check on Table 6's assessment. The cesium-137 and cesium-134 are going to remain as fallout in the various regions for a long period of time. Even though cesium-137 measurements, made retroactively without "trays" to collect only fresh fallout, are complicated somewhat by residual Cs-137 from weapons-testing, the solution is still easy. An independent team of scientists could go to all the affected countries and measure the cesium-134 contamination, making samples which are coded and split before analysis whenever possible. There is no significant cesium-134 left from weapons-testing. From such measurements, reliable values of the Cs-137 fallout from Chernobyl could be obtained. The Soviet Union would necessarily have to agree to such testing by independent scientists. Whether that will ever come to pass in not known. But there can be no doubt that a correct final assessment of the cancer consequences from the Chernobyl accident can be validated if the will for such assessment exists.

Meanwhile, Table 6 reveals that a credible lower-limit on the cancer-consequences from the Chernobyl accident is: 317,100 fatal cancers
                                                      317,100 additional non-fatal cancers
                                                       13,100 leukemias.
                                                      ─────────────────────
                                                      647,300 malignancies.

It must be noted that the number 647,300 excludes cancers from the following

===

additional sources of exposure:

- (a) from external gamma-dose delivered from the ground by deposited radionuclides
  other than the radio-cesiums. This dose will add approximately 3% to each
  of the totals for malignancies in Table 6.

  For the lower estimate, the sum would become

  647,300 + 19,400 = 666,700 malignancies.

  For the higher estimate, the sum would become

  970,500 + 29,100 = 999,600 malignancies.

- (b) from inhalation and ingestion of the radio-iodines, which concentrate in
  the thyroid gland and can cause thyroid cancers and abnormalities;

- (c) from internal dose (via food, water, and inhalation) delivered from
  radionuclides other than radio-cesiums and radio-iodines;

- (d) from the passing radioactive cloud, which irradiated people directly with
  gamma rays.

- THE DISTRIBUTION OF DOSES OVER TIME

Exposure from Chernobyl's radioactive cloud occurred only once, but exposure
from Chernobyl's cesium fallout extends through time, because of the 2.3 year
half-life of cesium-134 and the 30.2 year half-life of cesium-137. Calculation
shows (Technical Appendix 2-C) that approximately 50% of all the dose ever to be
received from the cesiums from the accident will have been received in a little
over ten years. About 2/3 of the dose ever to be received will have been received
by about the 25th year after the accident. About 75% of the dose ever to be
received will have been received by the 40th year.

The delivery of about 50% of the dose commitment during the first ten years
after the accident means that about 50% of the cancers in Table 6 will result from
that part of the exposure. However, the malignancies will definitely not appear
simultaneously. Even if the dose had occurred in an instant instead of gradually
over ten years, the leukemias would be spread over 25 years (with the peak excess
about 7.5 years after the exposure), and the cancers would be spread over the

Table 6:

Cancer and Leukemia Tolls From the Chernobyl Nuclear Power Plant Accident
(Based Upon Dose Commitments In Millirads From Cesium-137 Plus Cesium-134)

Country or Region	Population	Method (see text)	Corresponding To Deposition Of 1,990,000 Curies Of Cesium-137				Corresponding To Deposition Of 1,330,000 Curies Of Cesium-137			
			Dose Commit. mrads	Fatal Cancers	Addit'l Non-fatal Cancers	Leuke-mias	Dose Commit. mrads	Fatal Cancers	Addit'l Non-fatal Cancers	Leuke-mias
Albania	2,500,000	(2)	12	110	110	5	8	73	73	3
Austria	7,600,000	(2)	174	4,900	4,900	200	116	3,300	3,300	135
Belgium	10,000,000	(1)	2	75	75	3	1.3	50	50	2
Bulgaria	8,600,000	(2)	172	5,500	5,500	225	115	3,700	3,700	150
Canada	22,125,000	(3)	0.4	33	33	1	0.3	22	22	1
*Czechosl.	15,500,000	(2)	52	3,000	3,000	125	35	2,000	2,000	83
Denmark	5,100,000	(1)	15	280	280	12	10	190	190	8
**Finland	4,800,000	(2)	249	4,450	4,450	180	166	3,000	3,000	120
France	54,540,000	(2)	58	11,800	11,800	480	39	7,900	7,900	320
Germany,W	61,400,000	(2)	172	39,400	39,400	1,600	115	26,300	26,300	1,100
Germany,E	17,100,000	(2)	201	12,800	12,800	530	134	8,600	8,600	350
Greece	9,700,000	(1)	3	110	110	5	2	72	72	3
Hungary	10,600,000	(2)	41	1,620	1,620	65	27	1,080	1,080	43
Ireland	3,100,000	(2)	1.3	15	15	1	0.9	10	10	0
*Italy	56,200,000	(3)	29	6,100	6,100	250	17	4,000	4,000	165
*Japan	119,500,000	(3)	0.8	360	360	15	0.5	240	240	10
S.Korea	33,900,000	(3)	0.6	75	75	3	0.4	50	50	2
Luxemb'rg	350,000	(2)	12	16	16	1	8	11	11	0
Nether'ds	14,400,000	(2)	12	640	640	26	8	430	430	17
Norway	4,130,000	(1)	86	1,300	1,300	55	57	880	880	37
***Poland	36,900,000	(2)	259	35,700	35,700	1,470	173	23,800	23,800	980
Romania	22,900,000	(2)	770	66,000	66,000	2,700	513	44,000	44,000	1,800
Spain	38,200,000	(2)	2.6	370	370	15	1.7	250	250	10
***Sweden	8,300,000	(1)	496	15,400	15,400	630	331	10,200	10,200	420
Switzer'd	6,500,000	(2)	236	5,700	5,700	240	157	3,800	3,800	160
Turkey	48,000,000	(2)	100	18,000	18,000	740	67	12,000	12,000	490
United K.	56,000,000	(2)	65	13,600	13,600	560	43	9,100	9,100	370
U.S.A.	235,000,000	(3)	0.05	44	44	2	0.03	29	29	1
*U.S.S.R.										
Ukraine	50,700,000	(2)	936	177,000	177,000	7,300	624	118,000	118,000	4,900
Byelor'a	9,900,000	(2)	714	26,400	26,400	1,100	476	17,600	17,600	730
Moldavia	4,080,000	(2)	125	1,900	1,900	80	83	1,300	1,300	55
Baltic R.	7,660,000	(2)	104	3,000	3,000	120	69	2,000	2,000	80
Moscow	8,400,000	(2)	40	1,250	1,250	50	27	830	830	35
Lening'd	4,700,000	(2)	148	2,600	2,600	110	100	1,700	1,700	75
Yugoslav.	23,000,000	(2)	185	15,900	15,900	650	123	10,600	10,600	430
Sum (all countries) (Rounded off)				475,500	475,500	19,500		317,100	317,100	13,100
			Total Malignancies = 970,500				Total Malignancies = 647,300			

*Czechoslovakia, Italy, Japan, USSR: The values in Table 6 are probably too low; details in Technical Appendix 2-A. We have no data for the area close to Chernobyl, and none for the Russian SSR except for Moscow and Leningrad.
**Finland: There have been serious inconsistencies in the Finnish data; details in Technical Appendix 2-A.
***Poland and Sweden:
Poland reported extremely high gamma-dose rates in Warsaw during the early days of the accident, but these values were later deleted from EPA reports as "too high" without any explanation (compare EPA reports of May 12 and 14 with the EPA report of June 4, 1986).
Sweden reported extremely high gamma measurements in Uppsala for April 29, but these high values simply disappeared from later reports without explanation (compare EPA reports of May 8 and 9 with EPA reports of May 12 and thereafter).
In epidemiological science, authorities cannot select only high measurements for checking; unless low measurements are checked for error with exactly the same amount of diligence, the net result is to create a bias toward lowering a whole set of measurements. Such practice is not acceptable in science.

August 22, 1986: The Soviets are estimating 1,000,000 curies of cesium-137 deposition within their own european regions [65]. Table 6 matches extremely well with the Soviet value. The higher estimate of dose and malignancies corresponds with cesium-137 deposition of 991,874 curies in european regions of the Soviet Union; see Technical Appendix 2-B. The lower estimate in Table 6 corresponds with 2/3 of that value, or 661,458 curies.

remaining lifespans of the irradiated population (with the peak excess occurring
between 30-40 years after exposure).

● THE DISTRIBUTION OF IMPACT BY AGE

     The third "law" of radiation carcinogenesis (Section 1 of this paper) means
that children will be the most affected by the cesium fallout. Not only will
they experience more fatal cases per 100,000 exposed individuals than will adults,
but each cancer fatality means a far greater loss of lifespan for those
irradiated young than for those irradiated at older ages. This point is
demonstrated by considering three ages: newborn, age 25, and age 45 at irradiation.

     When newborn males are irradiated, among those who do develop fatal
radiation-induced cancer, the average loss of life expectancy is about 22.3 years.
Half of those cases die before reaching age 54.5 years, and half die later.

     By comparison, if irradiation occurs at age 25, among those who do develop
fatal radiation-induced cancer, the average loss of life expectancy (for males)
is 12.8 years. Half of such cases die before reaching age 67.5 years, and
half die later.

     And if irradiation occurs at age 45, among those who do develop fatal
radiation-induced cancer, the average loss of life expectancy is about 8.7 years.
Half of such cases die before reaching age 75.2 years, and half die later.

     The calculations leading to the statements about loss of life expectancy
are based upon Tables 21 and 56 in Gofman[3] .

==
----
                    (9) DISCUSSION AND CONCLUSIONS

==

● THE SINGLE MOST SERIOUS INDUSTRIAL ACCIDENT EVER

     It is correct to say that a single event --- the Chernobyl accident --- has
caused between 600,000 and a million cases of cancer and leukemia. The
radio-cesiums are on the ground, and humans are committed to receive the doses
from them. To the extent that a share of the dose has already been received,
a share of the malignancies is already underway, even though they will not
become manifest, clinically, for years.

     The Chernobyl accident obviously represents the most serious industrial
tragedy in the history of mankind, and by a very large factor.

● THE QUALITY OF EVIDENCE

With respect to the proven human carcinogens, the <u>existing</u> quantitative evidence of human carcinogenesis by ionizing radiation is second to none (UNSCEAR[4], BEIR[6], GOFMAN[3], N.I.H.[11]). The data on ionizing radiation may be the strongest of all, and they cover virtually every site of human cancer. Moreover, several studies examine very low doses --- a total of 250 millirads in one series[25]; even the A-bomb survivors provide a large subset of people who received less than 20 rads of exposure[18]. In addition, studies of occupationally and medically exposed populations have contributed much evidence at low doses.

Coupled with the quantitative human evidence hard-won over the past half-century, the three generalizations described in this paper provide a very good assessment of the cancer consequences of the Chernobyl accident. The real problem we have in making such an assessment is simply the acquisition of <u>dose</u> data. The problem <u>does not have to do</u> with any mystery about consequences, once the doses are known.

● WHAT WE NEED, AND DO NOT NEED, TO ASSESS CHERNOBYL ACCIDENTS

On June 6, 1986, Mr. Stuart Loory, broadcasting from Moscow to many nations on the Cable News Network, reported that an agreement had been reached between Dr. Robert Gale of the U.S.A. and the Soviet Government to arrange for a lifetime study of the approximately 100,000 persons who received high doses from Chernobyl and were finally evacuated from the nearby area. Mr. Loory added that such a study might determine for radiation and cancer what we already know for cigarette smoking and cancer.

We can imagine nothing further from the truth than the suggestion that science has not yet firmly established a causal relationship between radiation exposure and human cancer. If the follow-up study of the Soviet high-dose group is promoted as necessary to establish this relationship, it will represent a cruel deception of mankind concerning the massive body of existing evidence which already demonstrates in quantitative detail the production of cancer by radiation, and at very low doses.

● A PREDICTION

We can predict with high confidence that an honest study of the proposed population sample will simply confirm --- but decades from now --- the magnitude of radiation production of cancer, a magnitude we know quite well prior to such

==

a study.

The existing human evidence provides a solid basis for assessing the Chernobyl toll. The credible lower-limit of malignancies from the cesium fallout is approximately 640,000 cases, and a credible upper-limit is probably 1,600,000 malignancies. Only additional and reliable measurements of cesium fallout, made by independent scientists, can narrow the range.

● IMPLICATIONS FOR MEDICAL, DENTAL, AND OCCUPATIONAL IRRADIATION

The findings in Section 2 of this paper that there cannot be a safe threshold dose of ionizing radiation with respect to human carcinogenesis, and that linearity cannot exaggerate the carcinogenic effect at very low doses, disprove the "hormetic" notion that exposure at low doses may protect humans against malignancies [62].

Also the findings of Section 2 have daily applicability for medical, dental, and occupational exposures. Although lip-service is generally paid to the absence of any safe dose, in reality the hazard at low doses is often dismissed as "purely theoretical." The findings presented here show why the hazard is not imaginary --- it is real.

The aggregate dose each year from diagnostic radiology is sufficient to cause about 78,000 radiation-induced cancers per year in the United States alone (Gofman-O'Connor [46], pp.365-70). Occupational exposures, in their aggregate, add another large number. The findings in Sections 2 and 3 of this paper provide ample evidence that measures to reduce individual doses would constitute a scientifically sound method of achieving large reductions in the human cancer-rate.

TECHNICAL APPENDIX 2
The Basis Of Table 6

Part A of this Technical Appendix shows the handling of fallout data, country by country.

Part B provides the area of each country and demonstrates how the 1,990,000 curies of cesium-137 are distributed country-by-country.

Part C shows the calculations supporting the statement that 50% of the dose commitment from the cesiums will occur during the first ten years after the Chernobyl accident.

● (A) TYPES, DATES, AND HANDLING OF FALLOUT MEASUREMENTS, BY COUNTRY

● General Criteria

Examination of all the fallout data from the various reporting countries shows that there is a high degree of variability of results within a single country. This is wholly expected, largely because rainfall can grossly increase deposition of radionuclides, and also because cloud plumes seldom cover a country uniformly.

In our endeavor to obtain the best representation of the average dose received by residents of any region, we have established some criteria for handling the limited quantity of fallout data provided from the various countries.

● Criterion I: Any country can be divided into four quadrants. When data are presented for each of the quadrants, we shall use the data as presented. When data are provided for three quadrants, we shall assign a zero value for the fourth quadrant, and then shall average all four values. When data are provided for two quadrants, we shall assign a zero value for the two remaining quadrants before averaging the four values. When data are provided for a single quadrant, we shall assign a zero value to each of the remaining quadrants before averaging. This set of procedures provides a cautious method of estimation.

● Criterion II: Some data are reported as a range of values. If values are provided within the range and if all four quadrants are represented, we shall average the values given. Where only the outer limits of the range are provided, we shall take these to represent two of the four quadrants of the country, and shall assign zero values to two other quadrants, and then average all four values.

● CONVERSION OF UNITS

There are 10^9 picocuries per millicurie.

There are 27 picocuries per Becquerel.

There are 100 rads per Gray.

There are 100 rems per Sievert.

There is 1 rem per rad, for gamma and for X-rays.

===

COUNTRY	SOURCE	COMMENTS
Albania	WHO Report June 12, 1986	Data are given for only one site. Therefore, three zeroes were assigned to other sites. The final result is 1/4 the value given for the one site. Date for the direct gamma dose was not given. Therefore, Cesium-137 % is taken as 1.8%, the lowest possible value. This effectively minimizes the fallout estimate.
Austria	EPA Report June 11, 1986	Excellent data are provided for the direct gamma dose. The average dose is based upon reports from 322 stations. The peak value for direct gamma dose was almost always for May 2, 1986. Therefore, the appropriate Cesium-137 % is 5.8% of the total gamma dose.
Belgium	WHO Report June 5, 1986	Data are given as a range for Cs-137 deposition, for May 9, 1986. Therefore, two zeroes were assigned, and the average of these plus the range limits were used to obtain average Cs-137 deposition.
Bulgaria	WHO Report June 5, 1986	Data for the direct gamma dose are given for five separated sites. The average of these is taken. Values are for May 8, 1986. The appropriate Cs-137 % is 12.9% of the total gamma dose.
Canada	EPA Report June 11, 1986	Data are given for Iodine-131 deposition on the ground for nine widely separated locations-- a reasonable representation of Canada. Most deposition values given were for May 12 or May 13. The conversion factor (in Method 3) for conversion from Iodine-131 to Cs-137 takes these dates into account appropriately.
Czecho-slovakia	WHO Report June 5, 1986	A single peak value of 200 uR/hr is given for the direct gamma dose. Three additional values of zero were assigned, giving an average value of 50 μR/hr for use in Method (2) calculation. Since the only indication for the date of this one reading was that it was before May 6, 1986, caution requires using the lowest Cs-137 %, the value of 1.8% of the total gamma dose. The effect is to make the cancer estimate given here too low, if the true date were later than April 29, 1986.
Denmark	WHO Report June 5, 1986	Excellent data are provided. The mean value for the integrated Cs-137 and Cs-134 depositions on the ground are provided for the period between May 7 and May 27, 1986. The data were obtained as a mean for 10 separate locations, labeled as "countrywide". It is not clear whether there may have been additional depositions before the May 7, 1986 date. If there were additional depositions, the Cs-137 and Cs-134 deposition totals here are too low, and the cancer estimates are also too low.
Finland	WHO Report May 30, 1986 and WHO Report June 5, 1986 plus Communication with Finnish Authorities. Also Finnish Reports: STUK-B-VALO 44 STUK-B-VALO 45	In the May 30, 1986 WHO report, the statement is made that "the deposition of Cs-137 varied between 100 and 1300 kBq/m^2." These values would lead to an extremely high cancer rate compared with the ones in Table 6 of this paper. In the June 5, 1986 WHO report, these data have just disappeared and the following data, bearing no resemblance, are presented for the cesiums: "Contamination of surface soil in kBq/m^2 (in-situ measurements) 6-7 May in Southern Finland was as follows: Cs-137 3 to 40 kBq/m^2; Cs-134 0.9 to 24 kBq/m^2." Inquiry produced from the Finnish Centre For Radiation and Nuclear Safety the reply that "WHO made an obvious error in their first figures from Finland. We straightened out that mistake, but why WHO did not inform in their next report about their misprint, I do not know." The letter, dated July 16, 1986, was signed by Olli Paakkola, Acting Director of the Surveillance Dept., Finnish Center for Radiation and Nuclear Safety. In the same letter, it is stated that "only half the country was affected by Chernobyl fallout," which is the basis for using half the area in Technical Appendix 2-B. Finnish authorities are designating one-third of the gamma-dose measured for Uusikaupunki as representative of Finnish exposures (STUK-B-VALO 45)[51]. That value is the basis for Method 2 calculations for Finland, and for the entries in Table 6.
France	EPA Report June 11, 1984	Only a single value is given for the direct gamma dose rate. It is for Paris for May 4, 1986. Three additional values were assigned as zero, and hence the average is 1/4 of the value for the Paris datum. The appropriate value for Cs-137 % of gamma dose rate is 8.0%. It is remarkable that France, a sophisticated nation in the field of nuclear power, provides so little data to WHO and the EPA.
Germany, East	No data provided	East Germany provided no data at all to the World Health Organization. Since it lies between Poland and West Germany, it is reasonable to assign it a dose intermediate to that of Poland and West Germany. Since West Poland most probably had a lesser dose than East Poland, we have heavily weighted the West German dose twice as heavily as the Poland dose, to arrive a reasonable estimate for East Germany. It is certainly regrettable that the East German authorities saw fit to refuse to provide any measurements.
Germany, West	WHO Report May 30, 1986	The WHO Report provides an "average" value for the direct gamma dose rate for Southern Germany for May 4, 1986. A comparison of air values for many stations in Northern Germany showed that the fallout was heavier in the Southern region than the northern region. By using such comparisons, a value was estimated for Northern Germany. It appears that most of the data reviewed are for the eastern region of Southern Germany. Therefore, two additional values of zero were assigned for the western quadrants, north and south, in arriving at an appropriate value for the gamma dose rate. Since the gamma dose rate is reported for May 4, 1986, it is appropriate to take 8.0% as the Cs-137 % of the total gamma dose rate.
Greece	WHO Report May 30, 1986 and WHO Report June 5, 1986	A single value for Cs-137 deposition is given as follows: " May 9-11 0.8 kBq/m^2 " This is difficult to interpret, since the data as reported suggest that the value reflects only deposition for the period between May 9- May 11, rather than the entire surface contamination with Cs-137 on the ground. Nevertheless we have used this value here. Since only a single value is given, we have assigned a zero value to three other quadrants, giving a final value 1/4 that of the single value given. Both WHO Reports show the same inadequate statement concerning Cs-137 deposition.
Hungary	WHO Report June 5, 1986	Direct gamma dose rates are presented as a range for May 1, 1986. Therefore, the outer limits of the range plus two assigned values of zero for two other quadrants are all used. The final average is 1/2 the mid-point of the given range. This was used in Method (2) calculation of Cs-137 deposition. For May 1, 1986 measurements, the appropriate Cs-137 % of total gamma dose rate is 4.9 %.

==

COUNTRY	SOURCE	COMMENTS

Ireland — WHO Report June 12, 1986 — A single measurement is given for direct gamma dose rate for May 7, 1986. Therefore, three additional values of zero were assigned for other quadrants, giving a final value to be used in Method (2) of 1/4 the measurement given. For May 7, 1986 measurements, the appropriate Cs-137 % of total gamma dose rate is 11.7 %.

Italy — EPA Report May 12, 1986 — Data are given for Iodine-131 depositions for five separate locations in Italy, for dates ranging from May 1 through May 3, 1986. To be cautious, we are treating these values as cumulative depositions, but if they are values for single days, we are underestimating Cs-137 deposition and dose by Method (3).

Japan — WHO Report June 5, 1986 and EPA Report June 11, 1986 — Deposition of Iodine-131 is given for four separate locations in Japan. The results are given "by day", so that they may not reflect the cumulative deposition of Iodine-131. If this is true the Cs-137 deposition estimated by Method (3) is too low, and the cancer estimates presented here are also too low.

Korea (South) — WHO Report June 5, 1986 and EPA Report June 11, 1986 — No direct data are given for South Korea. However, measurement of Iodine-131 in air in Seoul, Korea is available for comparison with Iodine-131 in air in Kanagawa, Japan for the same day. So, an indirect calculation can be made based upon the Japanese deposition data plus the Korea-Japan comparison for air data.
While this is not an ideal basis for calculation, it certainly gives the order-of-magnitude level for cancers in Korea.

Luxembourg — WHO Report June 5, 1986 — A single direct gamma dose rate measurement is given for May 2, 1986. Therefore, a zero value was assigned for three additional quadrants, and the final average value used in Method (2) is 1/4 the given value. For May2, 1986 measurements, the appropriate Cs-137 % of total gamma dose rate is 5.8%.

Norway — WHO Report June 5, 1986 — Excellent data are given for Cs-137 deposition on the ground. The data are presented as the cumulative surface soil contamination by Cs-137 for the period between May 1 and May 22, 1986. The results are based upon 70 separate samples having been measured.

Netherlands — WHO Report June 5, 1986 — A direct gamma dose rate is given for May 4, 1986 and thereafter. However, since it is not clear whether this dose is for a single location or is an average, we have, for caution, assigned three additional zero values to other quadrants. The final value used in Method(2) is, therefore, 1/4 of the given value. For May 4, 1986 measurements, the appropriate Cs-137 % of total gamma dose rate is 8.0%.

Poland — WHO Report June 5, 1986 — Multiple direct gamma-dose rate measurements are provided as a range for "all Poland". The two extremes of the range are taken and an additional two zero values are assigned to two quadrants. Therefore, the final value used in Method (2) calculations is 1/4 of the midpoint of the range given. For measurments made on April 29, 1986, the appropriate Cs-137 % of total gamma dose rate is 1.8%.
Early EPA reports showed extremely high values for gamma-dose rates in Warsaw, Poland in the early period of fallout. These values were deleted in later EPA reports, as noted in Table 6. Inquiry revealed that EPA did not know the reason; "must be too high," was suggested.

Romania — WHO Report June 5, 1986 — Multiple direct gamma dose rates are given as a range for the period April 29, 1986 through May 8 ,1986. The two extremes of the range for May 1 are used and zero values are assigned for two additional quadrants. The final value for May 1 used in Method (2) calculations is 1/4 of the midpoint of the range for that date. For May 1, 1986 measurements, the appropriate value for Cs-137 % of total gamma dose rate is 4.9%.

Spain — WHO Report June 12, 1986 — Direct gamma dose rates are given as a range for the period April 29 to May 8 ,1986. The extremes of the range for April 29 are taken and zero values are assigned for two additional quadrants. Therefore, the final value used in Method (2) calculations is 1/4 of the midpoint of the range for April 29. For April 29 measurements, the appropriate value for Cs-137 % of total gamma dose rate is 1.8 %.

Sweden — WHO Report May 30, 1986 — Detailed data are provided for Cs-137 deposition on the ground for eight separate stations. Four stations report deposition for May 15, 1986 and four other stations report deposition data for April 30, 1986. While the early data may be very much too low for measuring the cumulative deposition of Cs-137, those data were averaged in with the data for May 15.
It is puzzling that Sweden did not continue reporting measurements after April 30 at four of the stations. Also it is puzzling that very high gamma-doses reported from Uppsala on April 29, in the EPA reports of May 8 and 9, simply disappeared as noted in Table 6. EPA is left in its May 12 report and thereafter with a single value for Uppsala (1,000 uR/hr on May 4) and no other data at all for that city.
Since the eight stations reporting on cesium deposition were mainly in eastern Sweden, we elected to assign zero values for western Sweden. Therefore, the final value used is half the average for the eight reporting stations. This approach may underestimate radiation-induced cancers in Sweden.
The basis for using half the area of Sweden in Technical Appendix 2-B is the map on page 32 of Hohenemser[56].

Switzerland — EPA Report June 11, 1986 — Direct gamma dose rates are given for four parts of the country, central, east, west, and south. These values are for May 4, 1986. The average of these four gamma dose rates is used for indirect estimation of Cs-137 by Method (2). For May 4, 1986 measurements, the appropriate value for Cs-137 % of total gamma dose rate is 8.0 %.

Turkey — WHO Report June 12, 1986 — A range of values for the direct gamma dose rate is given for the period May 4- May 7, 1986. The two extremes of the range are taken for May 4 and a zero value is assigned to two additional quadrants. The final value used in Method (2) calculations is, therefore, 1/4 of the mid-point of the range for May 4, 1986. For May 4, 1986 measurements, the appropriate Cs-137 % of total gamma dose rate is 8.0 %.

==

COUNTRY	SOURCE	COMMENTS
United Kingdom	Report in NATURE Volume 321 [52] 15 May, 1986	Fry, F.A., Clarke, R.H., and O'Riordan, M.C. published a paper entitled "Early Estimates of UK Radiation Doses from the Chernobyl Reactor". This useful paper provides representative data for gamma dose rates, weighted by population distribution for two major regions of the United Kingdom. "South" is the description of the region with 82.1% of the UK population, and "North" is the region with 17.9 % of the UK population (including the northwest of England, North Wales, Scotland, and Northern Ireland). These dose rates for May 2 ,1986 were used here for estimation of Cs-137 deposition by the indirect method (Method (2)). For May 2, 1986 measurements, the appropriate Cs-137 % of total gamma dose rates is 5.8 %.
United States	EPA Report May 11, 1986	Deposition of Iodine-131 on the ground is reported for fifteen widely separated stations in the United States. These data are satisfactory for indirect estimation of Cs-137 deposition by Method (3). The iodine-131 deposition data are for May 5- May 8, 1986, and I-131 to Cs-137 conversion factors for those dates were used.
Yugoslavia	WHO Report June 11, 1986	Direct gamma dose rates are provided for three separate regions. Peak gamma dose rates were reached May 2 - May 3, 1986. Two of the regions were close together, so the average of these two was used as a single value. Zero values were assigned to two additional quadrants. Then an average was taken of the four values so derived. This average was used in Method (2) calculation of Cs-137 deposition. For measurements of May 2, 1986, the appropriate value of Cs-137 % of total gamma dose rate is 5.8%.

Note: The values in Table 6 are rounded off. Some may have preferred that we do not round off so as to facilitate cross-checking between column entries. Others complain that the goodness of the data do not justify keeping the number of significant figures which would be present without rounding off. This dilemma is ever-present. The reader simply needs to keep in mind that rounding has been done, when the reader makes use of Table 6.

COUNTRY	SOURCE	COMMENTS
U.S.S.R. Ukraine	WHO Report June 12, 1986	Direct gamma dose rates are reported for Oster, just north of Kiev, starting with May 9, 1986. The data for May 10 are used as a first step in the indirect estimation for Cs-137 deposition. A second usable value is that for Kishinev, Moldavia, which borders the Ukraine in the southwestern region. Therefore, we have assigned two zero values to cover the other quadrants of the Ukraine. The final average for gamma dose rate for May 10 is that obtained by averaging the values for Oster, for Kishinev, and the two assigned zero values. For May 10 measurements, the appropriate value for Cs-137 % of total gamma dose rate is 16.0 %. We should note that the Ukraine is one of the regions where Cs-137 remains available to plants through the root-soil pathway for longer periods than is the case elsewhere. As a result, our estimate of the internal dose from Cs-137 to residents of the Ukraine may be too low.
U.S.S.R. Byelo-russia	WHO Report June 12, 1986	Direct gamma dose rates are reported for Bialystok, Poland on the west border of Byelorussia. And, as mentioned above, direct gamma dose rates are available for Oster (north of Kiev, and 100 km south of the southern border of Byelorussia). It appears reasonable that the average of these two results can be used as representative of the southern 1/3 of Byelorussia. Therefore, we have assigned a zero value for each of the other 1/3 segments of Byelorussia. The final average is 1/3 of the value midway between the values for Bialystok and Oster. For measurements in Bialystok (data for April 29), the appropriate value for Cs-137 % of total gamma dose rate is 1.8 %. For Oster, as stated above (for May 10 measurements), the appropriate value for Cs-137 % of total gamma dose rate is 16.0 %. These adjustments were made before combining the Bialystok and Oster measurements.
U.S.S.R. Moldavian Republic	WHO Report June 12, 1986	Direct gamma dose rate data are provided by the Soviet Union for Kishinev, the capitol of the Moldavian Republic, starting with May 10, 1986. The data used here are for May 11, 1986. Three additional values of zero were assigned for other quadrants of Moldavia where we have no measurements. Therefore, the average value used in Method (2) calculations is 1/4 of the value for Kishinev. For measurements of May 11, 1986, the appropriate value for Cs-137 % of total gamma dose rate is 17.3 %.
U.S.S.R. Baltic Republics Latvia Lithuania Estonia	WHO Report June 12, 1986	No really useful data for Cs-137 or gamma dose rates are provided for the Baltic Republics. But, data are available for direct gamma dose rates for sites in Poland (Bialystok, Olsztyn) bordering these Republics, for Southern Finland not far from the northern part of these republics, and from Sweden to the northwest of these Republics. From all these data, a <u>minimal</u> estimate of 100 μR/hr as the peak direct gamma dose rate has been here assigned to the Baltic Republics. This appears cautious and reasonable. Further, to err on the side of underestimation of cesium dose, we shall assign this value for April 29, 1986, for which the appropriate value for Cs-137 % of total gamma dose rate is 1.8 %.
U.S.S.R. Moscow and Suburbs	EPA Report June 11, 1986	Some values for direct gamma dose rate are provided, starting with data for May 5, 1986. We shall used the May 5 data for indirect estimate of Cs-137 deposition by Method (2). For May 5 measurements, the appropriate value for Cs-137 % of total gamma dose rate is 9.1%.

===

COUNTRY	SOURCE	COMMENTS
U.S.S.R. Leningrad and Suburbs	EPA Report June 11, 1986	Direct gamma dose rates are provided for May 2- May 7, 1986. The peak gamma dose rates are reported for May 7 ,1986, and these data are used in the indirect estimate of Cs-137 by Method (2). For May 7, 1986 measurements, the appropriate Cs-137 % of total gamma dose rate is 11.7 %.
U.S.S.R. Russian Soviet Republic		No really satisfactory data are available which enable us to provide any estimates for Cs-137 deposition in this largest of the Soviet Republics, aside from the data for Moscow and Leningrad, which are described above. This is regrettable, since this Russian Republic is not only the largest geographically, but is also the most populous of the Soviet Republics.
U.S.S.R. Chernobyl Region	No data	This area very near the Chernobyl nuclear power plant had some very high doses, since radiation sickness and deaths have occurred there. Since no data have been made available for this special region, no cancer calculations have been made.
U.S.S.R. All Other Soviet Republics	No data	No data have been provided for all these other Soviet Republics, nor are there any data for regions close by from which any reasonable estimates of Cs-137 deposition can be made. We therefore refrain from making any cancer calculations for these Republics.

===

● (B) DISTRIBUTION OF 1,990,000 CURIES OF CESIUM-137, BY COUNTRY

The tabulation below corresponds with the left-hand side of Table 6.

Country	Deposition (pCi/m^2)	Area in meters^2	Deposition Total, in Curies
Albania	1.618×10^4	2.886×10^{10}	467
Austria	2.346×10^5	8.417×10^{10}	19,746
Belgium	2.697×10^3	3.063×10^{10}	83
Bulgaria	2.319×10^5	1.113×10^{11}	25,810
Canada	0.539×10^3	1×10^{13}	539
Czechoslovakia	7.012×10^4	1.284×10^{11}	9,003
Denmark	2.022×10^4	4.324×10^{10}	874
Finland (½ area)*	3.358×10^5	1.692×10^{11}	56,817
France	7.821×10^4	5.491×10^{11}	42,945
Germany, West	2.319×10^5	2.495×10^{11}	57,859
Germany, East	2.710×10^5	1.086×10^{11}	29,431
Greece	4.045×10^3	1.325×10^{11}	536
Hungary	5.529×10^4	9.340×10^{10}	5,164
Ireland	1.753×10^3	7.055×10^{10}	124
Italy	3.911×10^4	3.024×10^{11}	11,827
Japan	1.079×10^3	3.738×10^{11}	403
Korea, South	0.809×10^3	9.887×10^{10}	80
Luxembourg	1.618×10^4	2.590×10^9	42
Netherlands	1.618×10^4	4.100×10^{10}	663
Norway	1.160×10^5	1.627×10^{11}	18,873
Poland	3.493×10^5	3.139×10^{11}	109,645
Romania	1.038×10^6	2.383×10^{11}	247,355
Spain	3.506×10^3	5.067×10^{11}	1,776
Sweden (½ area)*	6.688×10^5	2.258×10^{11}	151,015
Switzerland	3.182×10^5	4.145×10^{10}	13,189
Turkey	1.348×10^5	7.836×10^{11}	105,629
United Kingdom	8.765×10^4	2.45×10^{11}	21,474
United States	0.067×10^3	7.60×10^{12}	469
Ukraine	1.262×10^6	6.032×10^{11}	761,238
Byelorussia	9.628×10^5	2.083×10^{11}	200,551
Moldavia	1.686×10^5	3.370×10^{10}	5,662
Baltic Republics	1.402×10^5	1.742×10^{11}	24,423
Yugoslavia	2.495×10^5	2.568×10^{11}	64,072

Moscow and Leningrad not computed, because area is so small

Sum of All Depositions, in Curies		1,987,784
$(0.75)(0.75)(3.53 \times 10^6) =$ ----------------------------		1,985,625

* See Technical Appendix 2-A

Comparison with cesium-137 deposition from weapons fallout:

According to UNSCEAR[4] (p.146), the deposition of cesium-137 in the temperate latitudes of the northern hemisphere from all the atomspheric nuclear bomb-tests of the United States, Soviet Union, and Britain combined was 136,000 or 1.36×10^5 picocuries per square meter.[5]

● (C) TIME-DISTRIBUTION FOR DOSE COMMITMENT FROM CESIUMS

Cesium-134 with its half-life of 2.3 years will deliver its committed dose to exposed populations very much earlier than is the case for cesium-137, with its half-life of 30.2 years. Calculations below show what fraction of the total dose commitment (over all time, from the cesiums combined) is delivered by the end of each decade following the accident. To calculate, we used the observations (from Section 7 of this paper) that

Cesium-134 (internal + external) accounts for 11% of the total dose from cesiums;
Cesium-137 (internal + external) accounts for 89% of the total dose from cesiums;
and of the 89%, the internal share is 30% and the external share is 70%.

● First Decade CESIUM-134 will deliver 94.6% of both its internal and external doses; this amounts to (0.946) x (11%) = 10.4% of the total dose from cesiums. CESIUM-137 will deliver approximately 95% of its internal dose in the first decade; this amounts to (0.95) x (0.30) x (89%) = 25.4% of the total dose from cesiums. CESIUM-137 will deliver 20.0% of its external dose in the first decade; this amounts to (0.20) x (0.70) x (89%) = 12.5% of the total dose from cesiums. COMBINED DELIVERY (%) BY THE END OF THE FIRST DECADE = 10.4 + 25.4 + 12.5 = 48.3% of total.

● Second Decade CESIUM-134 will deliver 5.4% of (11%) = 0.59% of the total dose. CESIUM-137 (internal) will deliver 5% of (0.30)(89%) = 1.34% of the total dose. CESIUM-137 (external) will deliver 16% of (0.70)(89%) = 10.0% of the total dose. COMBINED DELIVERY (%) BY THE END OF THE SECOND DECADE =

48.3 + 0.59 + 1.34 + 10.0 = 60.2% of the total dose committed.

● Third Decade The only new contribution will be from external cesium-137 because internal contributions from the cesiums are essentially over. CESIUM-137 will deliver 14% of (0.70)(89%) = 8.7%. COMBINED DELIVERY (%) BY THE END OF THE THIRD DECADE =

60.2 + 8.7 = 69% of the total dose committed from the cesiums.

● Fourth Decade Additional contribution from external CESIUM-137 is 10% of (0.70)(89%) = 6.2% of the total dose. COMBINED DELIVERY (%) BY THE END OF THE FOURTH DECADE =

69 + 6.2 = 75.2% of the total dose committed from the cesiums.

References

(1) University of California at Berkeley

(2) Gofman, J.W.; Tamplin, A.R. "Low Dose Radiation and Cancer" I.E.E.E.
    Transactions on Nuclear Science , Part 1, 1970, NS-17, 1-9.

(3) Gofman, J.W. Radiation and Human Health ; Sierra Club Books: San Francisco, 1981.

(4) UNSCEAR (United Nations Scientific Committee on the Effects of Atomic Radiation)
    1977; Sources and Effects of Ionizing Radiation Report to the General Assembly,
    with annexes. United Nations, New York.

(5) UNSCEAR 1982; Ionizing Radiation: Sources and Biological Effects Report to the
    General Assembly, with annexes. United Nations, New York.

(6) BEIR-III (The Advisory Committee on the Biological Effects of Ionizing Radiation)
    1980; (Final Report); The Effects on Populations of Exposure to Low Levels of
    Ionizing Radiation; National Academy of Sciences (Typescript Edition), Washington.

(7) Gofman, J.W. The Cancer-Leukemia Risk from Ionizing Radiation: Let's Have a
    Closer Look A.A.A.S. Symposium Presentation, Detroit, Michigan May 30, 1983.
    (Copies available from author, P.O.B 11207, San Francisco, Ca. 94101).

(8) Radford, E.P. "Radiogenic Cancer in Underground Miners" In Radiation Carcino-
    genesis: Epidemiology and Biological Significance ; Boice, J.D. Jr., J.F.
    Fraumeni, Eds.; Raven Press, New York, 1984, 225-230.

(9) Wagoner, J.K. "Leukemia and Other Malignancies Following Radiation Therapy for
    Gynecological Disorders" In Radiation Carcinogenesis: Epidemiology and Biolog-
    ical Significance ; Boice, J.D. Jr., J.F. Fraumeni, Eds. ; Raven Press, New
    York, 1984, 153-159.

(10) Radford, E.P. In A Roundtable: with radiation, how little is too much? New York
    Times, Week in Review, Section 4, p. Ey 19.

(11) Report of the National Institutes of Health Ad Hoc Working Group to Develop
    Radioepidemiological Tables; National Institutes of Health, Publication No.
    85-2748, 1985, 15.

(12) Wakabayashi, T.; Kato, H.; Ikeda,T.; Schull, W.J. " Studies of the Mortality
    of A-Bomb Survivors, Report 7, Part III. Incidence of Cancer in 1959-1978,
    Based on the Tumor Registry, Nagasaki" Radiation Research 1983, 93, 112-146.

(13) Boice,J.D. Jr.; Land, C.E.; Shore, R.E.; Norman, J.E.; Tokunaga, M. Radiology
    1979, 131, 589-597.

(14) BEIR-I; (See above re BEIR-III). This report is for 1972.

(15) Court-Brown, W.M.; Doll, R. "Mortality from Cancer and Other Causes after
    Radiotherapy for Ankylosing Spondylitis" British Medical Journal 1965,
    2, 1327-1332.

(16) Smith, P.G.; Doll, R.; "Age- and Time-dependent Changes in the Rates of Radiation-
    induced Cancers in Patients with Ankylosing Spondylitis Following a Single Course
    of X-ray Treatment" In Late Biological Effects of Ionizing Radiation, Vol 1;
    International Atomic Energy Agency: Vienna, 1979.

(17) Smith, P.G. "Late Effects of X-ray Treatment of Ankylosing Spondylitis" In
    Radiation Carcinogenesis: Epidemiology and Biological Significance; Boice, J.D.
    Jr., J.F. Fraumeni, Eds. ; Raven Press, New York , 1984, 107-118.

==

(18) Kato, H.; Schull, W.J. "Studies of the Mortality of A-Bomb Survivors .
     7. Mortality, 1950-1978: Part 1. Cancer Mortality" Radiation Research 1982,
     90, 395-432.

(19) Schull, W.J. "Atomic Bomb Survivors: Patterns of Cancer Risk" In Radiation
     Carcinogenesis: Epidemiology and Biological Significance; Boice, J.D. Jr.,
     J.F. Fraumeni, Eds. ; Raven Press, New York, 1984, 21-36.

(20) Associated Press. "Pravda Sneers at Oregon's Bill" as carried in San Francisco
     Examiner, August 10, 1986, A-16.

(21) Natarajan,A.T.; Csukas,I.; Degrassi, F.; van Zeeland, A.A.; Palitti, F.;
     Tanzarella, C.; de Salvia, R.; Fiore, M. "Influence of Inhibition of Repair
     Enzymes on the Induction of Chromosomal Aberrations by Physical and Chemical
     Agents" In Progress in Mutation Research , Vol. 4 A.T. Natarajan et al, Eds.;
     Elvesier Biomedical Press, Amsterdam, 1982, 47-59.

(22) Kihlman, B.A.; Natarajan, A.T. "Potentiation of Chromosomal Alterations by
     Inhibitors of DNA Repair" In DNA Repair and Its Inhibition Collins,A.,
     Downes, C.S., R.T. Johnson, Eds.; IRL Press, Oxford, 1984, 319-339.

(23) Riccardi, V.M.; Sujansky,E.; Smith, A.C.; Francke, U. "Chromosomal Imbalance
     in the Aniridia-Wilm's Tumor Association: 11 p Interstitial Deletion" Pediatrics,
     1978, 61, 604-610.

(24) Zellweger, H.; Simpson,J. "Chromosomes of Man" (Clinics in Developmental Med-
     icine Nos. 65/66).Spastic International Medical Publications, J.B. Lippincott,
     Philadelphia, 1977, 153-156.

(25) Cohen, A.J.; Li, F.P.; Berg, S.; Marchetto, D.J.; Tsai, S.; Jacobs, S.C.;
     Brown, R.S. : "Hereditary Renal-cell Carcinoma Associated with a Chromosomal
     Translocation" New England Journal of Medicine 1979, 301, 592-595.

(26) Croce, C.M. "Chromosomal Translocations, Oncogenes, and B-cell Tumors"
     Hospital Practice January 15,1985, 20, 41-48.

(27) Bender, M.A.; Preston, R.J. "Role of Base Damage in Aberration Formation:
     Interaction of Aphidicolin and X-rays" In Progress in Mutation Research,
     Vol. 4 A.T. Natarajan et al, Eds.; Elvesier Biomedical Press, Amsterdam, 1982,
     37-46.

(28) Preston, R.J. "The Effect of Cytosine Arabinoside on the Frequency of X-ray-
     Induced Chromosome Aberrations in Normal Human Leukocytes" Mutation Research,
     1980, 69, 71-9.

(29) Gofman, J.W.; Tamplin, A.R. "Epidemiological Studies of Carcinogenesis by
     Ionizing Radiation" In Proceedings of the Sixth Berkeley Symposium on
     Mathematical Statistics and Probability: Volume VI: Effects of Pollution on
     Health Lecam, L.M., Neyman, J., E. Scott, Eds.; University of California Press,
     Berkeley, 1970, 235-277.

(30) Baverstock, K.F.; Papworth, D.; Vennart, J. "Risk of Radiation at Low Dose
     Rates" Lancet 1981, i (Feb. 21), 430-433.

(31) Baverstock, K.F.; Vennart, J. "A Note on Radium Body Content and Breast
     Cancers in U.K. Radium Luminisers" Health Physics , 1983, 44, Suppl. No.1,
     575-577.

==

(32) Myrden, J.A.; Hiltz, J.E. "Breast Cancer Following Multiple Fluoroscopies During Artificial Pneumothorax Treatment of Pulmonary Tuberculosis" Canadian Medical Association Journal, 1969, 100, 1032-1034.

(33) Modan, B.; Ron,E.; Werner, A. "Thyroid Cancer Following Scalp Irradiation" Radiology 1977, 123, 741-744.

(34) Boice, J.D. Jr.; Monson, R.R. "Breast Cancer in Women After Repeated Fluoroscopic Examinations of the Chest" Journal of the National Cancer Institute, 1977, 59, 823-832.

(35) Stewart, A.M.; Webb, J.W.; Giles, B.D.; Hewitt, D. "Preliminary Communication: Malignant Disease in Childhood and Diagnostic Irradiation in-Utero" Lancet, 1956, 2, 447.

(36) Stewart, A.M.; Webb,J.W.; Hewitt, D. "A Survey of Childhood Malignancies" British Medical Journal 1958, 2, 1495-1508.

(37) Stewart, A.M.; Kneale, G.W. "Radiation Dose Effects in Relation to Obstetric X-rays and Childhood Cancers" Lancet, 1970, 1, 1185-1188.

(38) MacMahon, B. "Pre-natal X-ray Exposure and Childhood Cancer" Journal of the National Cancer Institute ,1962, 28, 1173-1191.

(39) Newcombe, H.B.; McGregor, J.F. "Childhood Cancer Following Obstetric Radio-Graphy" Lancet, 1971, 2, 1151-1152.

(40) Holford, R.M. "The Relation Between Juvenile Cancer and Obstetric Radiography" Health Physics, 1975, 28, 153-156.

(41) Mole, R.H. "Antenatal Irradiation and Childhood Cancer; Causation or Coincidence?" British Journal of Cancer 1974, 30, 199-208.

(42) Mole, R.H. "Radiation Effects on Pre-natal Development and Their Radiological Significance" British Journal of Radiology, 1979, 52, 89-101.

(43) Monson, R.R.; MacMahon, B. "Prenatal X-ray Exposures and Cancer in Children" In Radiation Carcinogenesis: Epidemiology and Biological Significance; Boice, J.D. Jr., J.F. Fraumeni, Eds.; Raven Press, New York, 1984, 97-106.

(44) Beebe, G.W.; Kato, H.; Land, C.E. "Studies of the Mortality of A-bomb Survivors: 6. Mortality and Radiation Dose, 1950-1974" Radiation Research 1978, 75, 138-201.

(45) Tokunaga, M.; Land, C.E.; Yamamoto, T.; Asano, M.; Tokuoka,S.; Ezaki, H.; Nishimori,I. "Breast Cancer in Japanese A-Bomb Survivors" Lancet 1982, ii, (Oct.23), 924.

(46) Gofman, J.W.; O'Connor, E. X-rays: Health Effects of Common Exams; Sierra Club Books, 1985 , 282-297.

(47) Hoffman, D.A.; Radford, E.P. A Review of the Carcinogenic Effects of Low Doses of Ionizing Radiation; Three-Mile Island Public Health Fund, Philadelphia, 1985(April), Table 2, p.124.

(48) World Health Organization " Updated Background Information on the Nuclear Reactor Accident,(Chernobyl) USSR" 1986, (1) May 30, 1986, (2) June 5, 1986, (3) June 12, 1986. Copenhagen, Denmark. Contact Person: J.I. Waddington.

(49) United States Environmental Protection Agency "Chernobyl Radiation Data Summary" 1986, A series issued between May 8, 1986 and June 30, 1986. Contact Person: H. Michael Mardis, Environmental Studies and Statistics Branch, ASD (ANR-461), Office of Radiation Programs, U.S.E.P.A., Washington,D.C. 20460.

===

(50) Finnish Centre For Radiation and Nuclear Safety "Interim Report on Fallout
     Situation in Finland from April 26 to May 4, 1986" STUK-B-VALO 44, May, 1986.
     PL- P.O. Box 268, SF-00101 Helsinki 10, Finland.

(51) Finnish Centre For Radiation and Nuclear Safety "Second Interim Report on
     Radiation Situation in Finland from 5 to 16 May 1986" STUK-B-VALO 45, May,
     1986. Address as in Reference (50).

(52) Fry, F.A.; Clarke, R.H.; O;Riordan, M.C. "Early Estimates of UK Radiation
     Doses" Nature, 1986, 321, 193-195.

(53) Devell, L.; Tovedal, H.; Bergstrom, U.; Appelgren, A.; Chyssler,J.; Anderson,L.
     "Initial Observations of Fallout from the Reactor Accident at Chernobyl"
     Nature, 1986, 321, 192-193.

(54) Knox, J.B. "Description of ARAC I-131 and Cs-137 Deposition and Dose Calcula-
     tions: Preliminary" May 7, 1986. From Livermore National Laboratory, California.

(55) Apsimon,H.M.; Wilson, H.N. "Preliminary Analysis of Dispersion of the Chernobyl
     Release", Paper given at the (U.K.) Nuclear Inspectorate on 20th May, 1986
     and Helen ApSimon , letters to Frank von Hippel, June 19, 22, 1986. (Cited in
     von Hippel, F. ; Cochran, T.B in an article in press , September, 1986, Bulletin
     of the Atomic Scientists.)

(56) Hohenemser, C.; Deicher, M.; Ernst,A.; Hofsass, H.;, Linder, G.; Recknagel,E.
     "Chernobyl: An Early Report" Environment 1986, 28, (June) 6-43.

(57) Hammersen, F. Sobotta/Hammersen Histology; Color Atlas of Microscopic Anatomy;
     Urban and Schwarzenberg, Baltimore, 1985.

(58) Elias, H.; Pauly, J.E.; Burns,E.R. Histology and Human Microanatomy ; John
     Wiley & Sons; New York, 1978.

(59) Gardner, D.L.; Dodds, T.C. Human Histology: An Introduction to the Study of
     Histopathology; Churchill Livingstone, Edinburgh, 1976.

(60) Johannessen, J.V. (Editor); Electron Microscopy in Human Medicine; In 12 Volumes,
     through 1985; McGraw-Hill International Book Co., New York.

(61) Tokunaga, M.; Land, C.E.; Yamamoto, T.; Asano, M.; Tokuoka, S.; Ezaki, H.;
     Nishimora, I.; Fujikura, T. "Breast Cancer Among Atomic Bomb Survivors" In
     Radiation Carcinogenesis: Epidemiology and Biological Significance; Boice,
     J.D. Jr., J.F. Fraumeni , Eds.; Raven Press, New York, 1984, 45-56.

(62) Luckey, T.D. "Physiological Benefits from Low Levels of Ionizing Radiation"
     Health Physics , 1982, 43, 771-789.

(63) Loewe, W.E.; Mendelsohn, E. "Neutron and Gamma Ray Doses at Hiroshima and
     Nagasaki" Nuclear Science and Engineering,1982, 81, 325-350.

(64) McGregor, D.H.; Land, C.E.; Choy, K.; Tokuoka, S.; Liu, P.I.; Wakabayashi, T.;
     Beebe, G.W. "Breast Cancer Incidence Among Atomic Bomb Survivors, Hiroshima
     and Nagasaki, 1950-1969" Journal of the National Cancer Institute, 1977, 59,
     799-811.

(65) State Committee For Using the Atomic Energy Of the U.S.S.R. The Accident At
     the Chernobyl AES and Its Consequences; Data Prepared For the International
     Atomic Energy Agency Expert Conference 25-29 August 1986 in Vienna.

36-empty, after 36-33.

==

CHAPTER 37

Membership on Various Radiation Committees

We have repeatedly mentioned the reports of various radiation committees, without giving recognition to the many individuals whose names are provided inside those reports. In compiling the following list from those reports, we have included only those individuals associated with a report's entirety or with its sections on cancer-induction.

The following abbreviations are used (full citations are in the Reference list):

● -- Beir72, Beir80, Beir90
These reports are commonly called BEIR-1, BEIR-3, and BEIR-5, and they are prepared by the Committee on the Biological Effects of Ionizing Radiations, National Academy of Sciences, National Research Council, Washington, D.C.

Beir80 Compromise is a special category. There was a large disagreement in the Committee after the release of the first version of the section on Somatic Effects. As a result, some members of the committee participated in preparing a compromise report for the Somatic Effects section. These members are designated as "Beir80 Compromise Group."

● -- Doe87
This is the report issued by the (U.S.) Department of Energy following the Chernobyl nuclear power accident (its report DOE/ER-0332).

● -- Icrp77, Icrp86
Icrp77 refers to the 1977 recommendations of the International Commission on Radiological Protection (its publication 26). Icrp86 refers to the 1986 membership of ICRP. A new report is expected.

● -- Ncrp80
Ncrp80 refers to the 1980 report of the (U.S.) National Council on Radiation Protection and Measurements (its Report 64). This report was prepared by NCRP's Scientific Committee 40, and was approved by the full Council (p.201).

● -- Nih85
Nih85 refers to the 1985 report of the (U.S.) National Institutes of Health Ad Hoc Working Group to Develop Radioepidemiological Tables (its publication NIH 85-2748).

● -- Nrc85
Nrc85 refers to the 1985 report of the (U.S) Nuclear Regulatory Commission (its report NUREG/CR-4214).

● -- Unsc77, Unsc82, Unsc86, Unsc88
These abbreviations refer to the series of reports issued (1977, 1982, 1986, 1988) by the United Nations Scientific Committee on the Effects of Atomic Radiation.

ABRAHAMSON, Seymour -- Beir 72, full Committee. Icrp85-89, Member, Committee on Radiation Effects. Beir80, full Committee. Ncrp80, member, Scientific Committee 40. Ncrp80, member, full NCRP.

ADELSTEIN, S. James -- Ncrp80, member, full NCRP.

ALBERT, Roy E. -- Ncrp80, member, full NCRP.

ALEXAKHIN, R. -- Unsc77, Specialist Scientist, U.S.S.R. Delegation. Unsc82, Specialist Scientist, U.S.S.R. Delegation.

ALPEN, Edward L. -- Ncrp80, member, full NCRP.

ANDERSON, R.E. -- Unsc82, Specialist Scientist, United States Delegation. Unsc86, Unsc88, United States Delegation.

ANSPAUGH, Lynn -- Doe87, Interlaboratory Task Group on Health and Environmental Aspects of the Soviet Nuclear Accident. Unsc88, United States Delegation.

ARAICO, E. -- Unsc88, Mexico Delegation.

ATEN, J.T.B. -- Unsc77, Specialist Scientist, Belgium Delegation. Unsc82, Unsc86, Unsc88, Specialist Scientist, Belgium Delegation.

AUXIER, John A. -- Ncrp80, member, full NCRP.

BAIQUNI, A. -- Unsc77, Specialist Scientist, Indonesia Delegation. Unsc82, Specialist Scientist, Indonesia Delegation. Unsc86, Unsc88, Indonesia Delegation.

BAIR, William J. -- Icrp85-89, Member, Committee 2 - Secondary Limits. Ncrp80 -- member, full NCRP.

BAKER, R. -- Unsc77, Specialist Scientist, United States Delegation. Unsc82, Specialist Scientist, United States Delegation. Unsc86, Unsc88, United States Delegation.

BARENDSEN, G.W. -- Icrp85-89, Member, Committee on Radiation Effects.

BARKCHUDAROV, K.M. -- Unsc88, U.S.S.R. Delegation.

BARNES, Edgar C. -- Ncrp80, Honorary member, full NCRP.

BARTH, Delbert S. -- Beir72, Subcommittee on Environmental Effects.

BEEBE, Gilbert W. -- Beir72, Subcommittee on
Somatic Effects. Beir80, full Committee.
Beir80, Compromise Group. Beir80, Subcommittee
on Somatic Effects. Nih85, member, Ad Hoc
Working Group.

BENDER, Michael A. -- Beir80, full Committee.
Beir80, Compromise Group. Ncrp80, Consultant to
Scientific Committee 40.

BENGTSSON, G. -- Unsc88, Sweden Delegation.

BENINSON, Dan. -- Unsc77, Scientific Staff or
Consultant to UNSCEAR. Icrp77, Member of the
Main Commission of the ICRP. Unsc82, Argentina
Delegation. Icrp85-89, Chairman, Main
Commission of the ICRP. Unsc86, Unsc88,
Argentina Delegation.

BENNETT, B.G. -- Unsc77, Unsc88, Scientific Staff
or Consultant to UNSCEAR.

BERGSTROM, S. -- Unsc77, Specialist Scientist,
Sweden Delegation.

BERRY, R.J. -- Icrp85-89, Member of the Main
Commission of the ICRP.

BERTIN, M. -- Unsc88, France Delegation.

BOECKER, Bruce B. -- Beir90, member, full
Committee.

BOICE, John D., Jr. -- Ncrp80, Consultant to
Scientific Committee 40. Ncrp80, member, full
NCRP.

BOND, Victor P. -- Beir72, full Committee.
Beir72, Subcommittee on Somatic Effects.
Ncrp80, member, full NCRP.

BOOTH, A.H. -- Unsc77, Specialist Scientist,
Canada Delegation.

BOUVILLE, A. -- Unsc77, Scientific Staff or
Consultant to UNSCEAR. Unsc82, Unsc86,
Unsc88, Specialist Scientist, France
Delegation.

BOYNE, Harold S. -- Ncrp80, member, full NCRP.

BRAESTRUP, Carl B. -- Ncrp80, Honorary member,
full NCRP.

BRENT, Robert L. -- Beir80, Consultant to the
Subcommittee on Somatic Effects. Ncrp80,
member, full NCRP.

BRILL, A. Bertrand -- Beir80, full Committee.
Beir80, Compromise Group. Beir80, Subcommittee
on Somatic Effects.

BROOKS, Antone -- Ncrp80, member, full NCRP.

BROWN, J. Martin -- Beir72, full Committee.
Beir72, Subcommittee on Somatic Effects.
Beir72, Ad Hoc Committee.

BROWN, Reynold F. -- Beir80, full Committee.
Beir80, Subcommittee on Somatic Effects.
Ncrp80, member, full NCRP.

BRUES, A.M. -- Unsc77, Specialist Scientist,
United States Delegation. Ncrp80, Honorary
member, full NCRP. Unsc82, Specialist
Scientist, United States Delegation.

BRUNER, H.D. -- Unsc77, Specialist Scientist,
United States Delegation.

BRYANT, Pamela M. -- Unsc77, Scientific Staff or
Consultant to UNSCEAR.

BUSH, W.R. -- Unsc77, Specialist Scientist,
Canada Delegation. Unsc82, Unsc86, Unsc88,
Specialist Scientist, Canada Delegation.

BUTLER, G.C. -- Unsc77, Specialist Scientist,
Canada Delegation. Unsc82, Unsc86, Unsc88,
Specialist Scientist, Canada Delegation.

CALDAS, L.R. -- Unsc77, Unsc86, Unsc88,
Specialist Scientist, Brazil Delegation.

CANCIO, Dr. D. -- Unsc77, Unsc88 Specialist
Scientist, Argentina Delegation.

CARPENTER, James H. -- Beir72, Subcommittee on
Environmental Effects.

CARTER, C.O. -- Unsc82, Specialist Scientist,
United Kingdom Delegation.

CARTER, D. -- Unsc77, Specialist Scientist,
United Kingdom Delegation.

CARTER, Melvin W. -- Ncrp80, member, full NCRP.

CASARETT, Goerge W. -- Beir72, full Committee.
Beir72, Subcommittee on Somatic Effects.
Ncrp80, member, full NCRP.

CASWELL, Randall S. -- Ncrp80, member, full NCRP.

CATLIN, Robert J. -- Doe87, Interlaboratory Task
Group on Health and Environmental Aspects of the
Soviet Nuclear Accident.

CHAMBERLAIN, R.H. -- Unsc77, Specialist
Scientist, United States Delegation.

CHILTON, Arthur B. -- Ncrp80, member, full NCRP.

CLARKE, R.H. -- Icrp85-89, Member, Committee 2 -
Secondary Limits. Unsc88, U.K. Delegation.

CLEARY, Stephen F. -- Beir80, full Committee.
Beir80, Subcommittee on Somatic Effects.
Ncrp80, member, full NCRP.

CLIFTON, Kelly H. -- Beir90, member, full
Committee.

COMAR, Cyril L. -- Beir72, Chairman of the full
Committee. Beir72, Ad Hoc Committee. Beir72,
Subcommittee on Environmental Effects.
Beir80, full Committee. Beir80, Subcommittee
on Somatic Effects.

COOPER, Douglas W. -- Nrc85, Co-Principal
Investigator.

COOPER, Raymond D. -- Beir90, Senior Program
Officer, Board on Radiation Effects Research,
Commission on Life Sciences.

===

COPPOLA, M. -- Unsc82, Scientific Staff or
Consultant.

COTTRALL, M.F. -- Unsc82, Scientific Staff or
Consultant

COULON, R. -- Unsc77, Specialist Scientist,
France Delegation. Unsc82, Unsc86, Unsc88,
Specialist Scientist, France Delegation.

COWAN, Frederick P. -- Ncrp80, Honorary member,
full NCRP.

CROW, James F. -- Beir72, full Committee.
Beir72, Ad Hoc Committee.

CUDDIHY, Richard G. -- Doe87, Interlaboratory Task
Group on Health and Environmental Aspects of the
Soviet Nuclear Accident.

CZEIZEL, A. -- Unsc86, Scientific Staff or
Consultant to UNSCEAR.

DARBY, S.C. -- Unsc88, United Kingdom Delegation.

DAVIS, William E. -- Doe87, Interlaboratory Task
Group on Health and Environmental Aspects of the
Soviet Nuclear Accident.

De-CHANG, Wu -- Icrp85-89, Member, Committee on
Radiation Effects. Unsc88, China Delegation.

De GARAY, A.L. -- Unsc77, Specialist Scientist,
Mexico Delegation.

DENEKAMP, J. -- Unsc88, United Kingdom Delegation.

DENIM, V. -- Unsc88, U.S.S.R. Delegation.

DENNISTON, Carter -- Beir80, full Committee.
Beir90, member, full Committee.

DEPING, Li -- Icrp85-89, Member of the Main
Commission, ICRP. Unsc88, China Delegation.

DINGLE, John H. -- Beir72, full Committee.

DIXON, Wilfrid J. -- Beir72, consultant to the
full Committtee. Beir72, consultant to the
Subcommittee on Somatic Effects.

DODD, Gerald -- Ncrp80, member, full NCRP.

DREXLER, Gunter -- Icrp85-89, Member, Committee
2 - Secondary Limits.

DUNSTER, H.J. -- Unsc77, Specialist Scientist,
United Kingdom Delegation. Icrp85-89, Member of
the Main Commission of the ICRP. Unsc86,
Unsc88, United Kingdom Delegation.

DURBIN, Patricia W. -- Ncrp80, member, full NCRP.

DUTRILLAUX, B.H. -- Unsc77, Specialist
Scientist, France Delegation. Unsc82,
Specialist Scientist, France Delegation.
Unsc86,Unsc88, France Delegation.

ECKERMAN, Keith F. -- Icrp85-89, Member,
Committee 2 - Secondary Limits.

EDINGTON, C. -- Unsc82, Specialist Scientist,
United States Delegation. Unsc86, Unsc88,
United States Delegation.

EDVARSON, K. -- Unsc77, Specialist Scientist,
Sweden Delegation. Unsc82, Specialist
Scientist, Sweden Delegation. Unsc86, Unsc88,
Sweden Delegation.

EDWARDS, J.H. -- Unsc86, Unsc88, United Kingdom
Delegation.

EHLING, U.H. -- Unsc77, Specialist Scientist,
West Germany Delegation. Unsc82, Specialist
Scientist, West Germany Delegation.
Unsc86, Unsc88, West Germany Delegation.

EISENBUD, Merril -- Ncrp80, member, full NCRP.

EL-DIN HASHISH, S. -- Unsc86, Unsc88, Egypt
Delegation.

EL-KHARADLY, M.E.A. -- Unsc77, Specialist
Scientist, Egypt Delegation. Unsc82, Unsc86,
Unsc88, Specialist Scientist, Egypt
Delegation.

ELKIND, Mortimer -- Ncrp80, member, Scientific
Committee 40.

ELLETT, William H. -- Beir90, Study Director, Board
on Radiation Effects Research, National Research
Council.

ELLIS, R.E. -- Unsc77, Scientific Staff or
Consultant to UNSCEAR.

ELY, Thomas S. -- Ncrp80, member, full NCRP.

EPP, Edward R. -- Beir90, member, full Committee.

ERRERA, M. -- Unsc82, Specialist Scientist,
Belgium Delegation. Unsc86,Unsc88, Belgium
Delegation.

EVANS, John C. -- Beir72, Subcommittee on
Environmental Effects.

EVANS, John S. -- Nrc85, Co-Principal Investigator.

EVANS, Robley D. -- Ncrp80, Honorary member,
full NCRP.

FABRIKANT, Jacob I. -- Beir72, consultant to the
Subcommittee on Somatic Effects. Beir80, full
Committee. Beir80, Compromise Group. Beir80,
Subcommittee on Somatic Effects. Icrp85-89,
Member, Committee on Radiation Effects. Doe87,
Interlaboratory Task Group on Health and
Environmental Aspects of the Soviet Nuclear
Accident. Beir90, member, full Committee.

FAGNANI, F. -- Unsc88, Consultant to UNSCEAR.

FEARON, Thomas -- Ncrp80, NCRP Secretariat.

FERRIS, Benjamin G. -- Ncrp80, member, full NCRP.

FIELD, S.B. -- Icrp85-89, Member, Committee on
Radiation Effects.

FINKEL, Asher J. -- Ncrp80, member, full NCRP.

FLECKENSTEIN, Donald C. -- Ncrp80, member, full
NCRP.

FOSTER, Richard F. -- Ncrp80, member, full NCRP.

FRIEDELL, Hymer L. -- Ncrp80, member, full NCRP.

FRITTELLI, F. -- Unsc88, Consultant to UNSCEAR.

FRY, R.J. Michael -- Icrp85-89, Member,
    Committee on Radiation Effects. Ncrp80,
    member, Scientific Committee 40.

GARNER, R. John -- Beir72, Subcommittee on
    Environmental Effects.

GILBERT, Ethel S. -- Nrc85, Author, Vol.I,
    Chapter 2, "Late Somatic Effects."

GLADSTEIN, Arthur H. -- Ncrp80, member, full
    NCRP.

GOEPP, Robert A. -- Ncrp80, member, full NCRP.

GOLDBERG, Barry B. -- Ncrp80, member, full NCRP.

GOLDMAN, Marvin -- Ncrp80, member, full NCRP.
    Doe87, Interlaboratory Task Group on Health and
    Environmental Aspects of the Soviet Nuclear
    Accident.

GOLUBKIN, E. -- Unsc86, U.S.S.R. Delegation

GONZALEZ, A.J. -- Unsc82,Unsc88, Specialist
    Scientist, Argentina Delegation.

GOOD, Robert A. -- Beir72, full Committee.

GOPAL-AYENGAR, A.R. -- Unsc77, Specialist
    Scientist, India Delegation.

GORSON, Robert O. -- Ncrp80, member, full NCRP.

GOUSKOWA, Angelina -- Unsc77, Specialist
    Scientist, U.S.S.R. Delegation. Unsc82,
    Specialist Scientist, U.S.S.R. Delegation.
    Unsc86, Unsc88, U.S.S.R. Delegation.

GRAHN, Douglas -- Ncrp80, member, Scientific
    Committee 40. Ncrp80, member, full NCRP.
    Beir90, member, full Committee.

GROSSBLATT, Norman -- Beir80, Editor, BEIR
    Committee.

GUY, Arthur W. -- Ncrp80, member, full NCRP.

GUZMAN-ACEVEDO, C. -- Unsc77, Specialist
    Scientist, Peru Delegation. Unsc82, Specialist
    Scientist, Peru Delegation.

HAGEN, A. -- Unsc88, Consultant to UNSCEAR.

HALL, Eric J. -- Beir90, member, full Committee.

HALNAN, K.E. -- Unsc82, Specialist Scientist,
    United Kingdom Delegation. Unsc86, Unsc88,
    United Kingdom Delegation.

HARLEY. John H. -- Unsc77, Specialist Scientist,
    United States Delegation. Unsc82, Specialist
    Scientist, United States Delegation. Unsc86,
    Unsc88, United States Delegation.
    Ncrp80, member full NCRP.

HARPER, P.S. -- Unsc86, Unsc88, United Kingdom
    Delegation.

HARTL, Daniel L. -- Beir90, member, full
    Committee.

HEALY, John W. -- Ncrp80, member, full NCRP.

HEMPELMANN, Louis H. -- Beir72, Subcommittee on
    Somatic Effects. Ncrp80, member, full NCRP.

HENDRY, J. -- Unsc88, Consultant to UNSCEAR.

HERBERT, Donald E. -- BEIR90, member, full
    Committee.

HESLEP, John M. -- Ncrp80, member, full NCRP.

HICKS, Samuel P. -- Beir72, full Committee.
    Beir72, Ad Hoc Committee.

HIDAYATALLA, A. -- Unsc77, Unsc82, Specialist
    Scientist, Sudan Delegation. Unsc86,
    Unsc88, Sudan Delegation.

HILBERG, Albert W. -- Beir80, Principal Staff
    Officer of BEIR Committee.

HODGES, Paul C. -- Ncrp80, Honorary member, full
    NCRP.

HOEL, David G. -- Nih85, member, Ad Hoc Working
    Group. Beir90, member, full Committee.

HOLM, Lars-Erik -- Icrp85-89, Member, Committee on
    Radiation Effects. Unsc86, Unsc88,
    Sweden Delegation.

HOWE, Geoffrey R. -- Beir90, member, full
    Committee.

HULL, Andrew P. -- Doe87, Interlaboratory Task
    Group on Health and Environmental Aspects of the
    Soviet Nuclear Accident.

HUTCHISON, George G. -- Beir72, full Committee.
    Beir72, consultant to the Subcommittee on
    Somatic Effects. Ncrp80, member, Scientific
    Committee 40. Ncrp80, member, full NCRP.

ICHIKAWA, R. -- Unsc77, Specialist Scientist,
    Japan Delegation. Unsc82, Specialist Scientist,
    Japan Delegation. Unsc86, Japan Delegation.

ILYIN, L. -- Unsc77, Specialist Scientist,
    U.S.S.R. Delegation. Unsc86, Unsc88,
    U.S.S.R. Delegation.

INABA, J. -- Unsc86, Japan Delegation.

INGRAM. Marylou -- Beir80, full Committee.
    Beir80, Subcommittee on Somatic Effects.

ISKANDAR, O. -- Unsc86, Unsc88, Indonesia Delegation.

ITO, N. -- Unsc77, Specialist Scientist, Japan
    Delegation.

JABLON, Seymour -- Beir72, consultant to the
    Subcommittee on Somatic Effects. Ncrp80,
    member, full NCRP. Nih85, member, Ad Hoc
    Working Group. Beir90, member, full Committee.

JACOBI, Wolfgang -- Unsc77, Specialist
    Scientist, West Germany Delegation. Unsc82,
    Specialist Scientist, West Germany Delegation.
    Icrp85-89, Member of the Main Commission of the
    ICRP. Unsc86, Unsc88, West Germany Delegation.

JAMES, A. Everette -- Ncrp80, member, full NCRP.

==

JAMMET, H. -- Unsc77, Specialist Scientist, France Delegation. Icrp77, Member of the Main Commission of the ICRP. Unsc82, Specialist Scientist, France Delegation. Icrp85-89, Vice-Chairman of the Main Commission of the ICRP. Unsc86, Unsc88, France Delegation.

JAWOROWSKI, Z. -- Unsc77, Specialist Scientist, Poland Delegation. Unsc82, Specialist Scientist, Poland Delegation. Unsc86, Unsc88, Poland Delegation.

KAHN, Bernd -- Ncrp80, member, full NCRP.

KAMEYAMA, Y. -- Unsc86, Japan Delegation.

KASAI, A. -- Unsc82, Specialist Scientist, Japan Delegation. Unsc86, Unsc88, Japan Delegation.

KASTNER, Jacob -- Ncrp80, member, full NCRP.

KAUL, Alexander -- Icrp85-89, Member, Committee 2 - Secondary Limits. Unsc82, Specialist Scientist, West Germany Delegation. Unsc86, Unsc88, West Germany Delegation.

KELLERER, Albrecht M. -- Icrp85-89, Member, Committee on Radiation Effects. Unsc86, Scientific Staff or Consultant to UNSCEAR.

KENNEDY, Ann R. -- Beir90, member, full Committee.

KHOKHLOVA, D.F. -- Unsc86, Unsc88, U.S.S.R. Delegation.

KISHIMOTO, Y. -- Unsc82, Specialist Scientist, Japan Delegation.

KLIMEK, A. -- Unsc77, Unsc82, Specialist Scientist, Czechoslovakia Delegation.

KLIMEK, M. -- Unsc86,Unsc88, Czechoslovakia Delegation.

KNUDSON, Alfred G., Jr. -- Beir90, member, full Committee.

KOBAYASHI, S. -- Unsc82, Specialist Scientist, Japan Delegation.

KRIEGEL, H. -- Unsc77, Specialist Scientist, West Germany Delegation. Unsc82, Specialist Scientist, West Germany Delegation. Unsc86, Unsc88, West Germany Delegation.

KUMATORI, T. -- Unsc82, Unsc86, Unsc88, Specialist Scientist, Japan Delegation.

KUZIN, A.M. -- Unsc77, Specialist Scientist, U.S.S.R. Delegation. Unsc82, Specialist Scientist, U.S.S.R. Delegation.

LAFUMA, Jacques. -- Unsc77, Specialist Scientist, France Delegation. Icrp85-89, Member, Committee on Radiation Effects. Unsc82, Specialist Scientist, France Delegation. Unsc86, Unsc88, France Delegation.

LAND, Charles E. -- Beir80, full Committee. Beir80, Subcommittee on Somatic Effects. Beir80, Compromise Group. Icrp85-89, Member, Committee on Radiation Effects. Nih85, member, Ad Hoc Working Group.

LANGE, Rolf -- Doe87, Interlaboratory Task Group on Health and Environmental Aspects of the Soviet Nuclear Accident.

LEMAIRE, G. -- Unsc88, France Delegation.

LENTLE, B.C. -- Unsc88, Canada Delegation.

LeROY, George V. -- Ncrp80, Honorary member, full NCRP.

LETOURNEAU, E.G. -- Unsc82, Specialist Scientist, Canada Delegation. Unsc86, Unsc88, Canada Delegation.

LEVINTHAL, Cyrus -- Beir72, full Committee. Beir72, Ad Hoc Committee.

LEWIS, Edward B. -- Beir72, full Committee. Beir72, Subcommittee on Somatic Effects. Ncrp80, member, full NCRP.

LINCOLN, Thomas A. -- Ncrp80, member, full NCRP.

LINIECKI, J. -- Unsc77, Scientific Staff or Consultant to UNSCEAR. Icrp77, Member of the Main Commission of the ICRP. Icrp85-89, Member of the Main Commission of the ICRP. Unsc86, Unsc88, Poland Delegation.

LINDELL, Bo -- Unsc77, Specialist Scientist, Sweden Delegation. Icrp77, Member of the Main Commission of the ICRP. Unsc82, Specialist Scientist, Sweden Delegation. Icrp85-89, Member (Emeritus) of the Main Commission of the ICRP. Unsc86, Unsc88, Sweden Delegation.

LITTLEFIELD, Gayle -- Ncrp80, member, Scientific Committee 40.

LOHMAN, P. -- Unsc88, Belgium Delegation.

LOKAN, K.H. -- Unsc82, Australia Delegation. Unsc86,Unsc88, Australia Delegation.

LOWDER, W.M. -- Unsc77, Scientific Staff or Consultant to UNSCEAR.

LOWMAN, F. -- Unsc77, Specialist Scientist, United States Delegation.

LUNING, K.G. -- Unsc77, Specialist Scientist, Sweden Delegation. Unsc82, Specialist Scientist, Sweden Delegation. Unsc86, Unsc88, Sweden Delegation.

LUXIN, Wei. -- Unsc88, China Delegation.

LYSCOV, V. -- Unsc77, Scientific Staff or Consultant to UNSCEAR.

MACMAHON, Brian -- Beir72, consultant to the full Committee. Beir72, consultant to the Subcommittee on Somatic Effects.

MAGIDIN de NULMAN, Rebeca -- Unsc77, Specialist Scientist, Mexico Delegation.

MAISIN, J. -- Unsc82, Unsc86, Unsc88, Specialist Scientist, Belgium Delegation.

MARKO, A.M. -- Unsc82, Unsc86, Unsc88, Specialist Scientist, Canada Delegation.

MARTINEZ-BAEZ, M. -- Unsc77, Specialist
    Scientist, Mexico Delegation.

MASSE, R. -- Unsc86, Unsc88, France Delegation.

MATSUDAIRA, H. -- Unsc88, Japan Delegation.

MATSUOKA, Osamu -- Ircp85-89, Committee 2 -
    Secondary Limits.

MATTSSON, S. -- Unsc86, Unsc88, Sweden Delegation.

MAYS, Charles W. -- Beir80, full Committee.
    Beir80, Subcommittee on Somatic Effects.
    Ncrp80, member, Scientific Committee 40.
    Ncrp80, member, full NCRP.

McCLELLAN, Roger O. -- Ncrp80, member, full NCRP.

McCONNAUGHEY, David A. -- Beir80, Senior Staff
    Officer, BEIR Committee.

McLAUGHLIN, James -- Ncrp80, member, full NCRP.

McLEAN, A.S. -- Icrp77, Member of the Main
    Commission of the ICRP.

MEINHOLD, Charles B. -- Ncrp80, member, full
    NCRP. Icrp85-89, Member of the Main Commission
    of the ICRP. Icrp85-89, Chairman, Committee 2 -
    Secondary Limits.

MENDELSOHN, Mortimer M. -- Ncrp80, member, full
    NCRP.

MENOSSI, C.A. -- Unsc77, Specialist Scientist,
    Argentina Delegation.

MENZEL, Ronald G. -- Beir72, Subcommittee on
    Environmental Effects.

METTLER, F.A. -- Unsc82, Specialist Scientist,
    Unsc88, United States Delegation.

MILLER, Robert W. -- Beir72, full Committee.
    Beir72, Subcommittee on Somatic Effects.

MILLS, William A. -- Beir90, Sponsor's Project
    Officer.

MISONO, K. -- Unsc77, Specialist Scientist,
    Japan Delegation. Unsc82, Specialist Scientist,
    Japan Delegation.

MODAN, Baruch -- Icrp85-89, Member, Committee on
    Radiation Effects.

MOELLER, Dade W. -- Beir72, Subcommittee on
    Environmental Effects. Ncrp80, member, full
    NCRP. Beir80, full Committee. Beir80,
    Subcommittee on Somatic Effects. Beir80,
    Compromise Group. Nrc85, Co-Principal
    Investigator.

MOISEEV, A. -- Unsc77, Specialist Scientist,
    U.S.S.R. Delegation. Unsc82, Specialist
    Scientist, U.S.S.R. Delegation. Unsc86,
    Unsc88, U.S.S.R. Delegation.

MOORE, Carl V. -- Beir72, full Committee.
    Beir72, Subcommittee on Somatic Effects.

MORGAN, K.Z. -- Icrp77, Member (Emeritus) of the
    Main Commission of the ICRP. Ncrp80, Honorary
    member, full NCRP. Icrp85-89, Member (Emeritus)
    of the Main Commission of the ICRP.

MORGAN, RUSSELL H. -- Ncrp80, Honorary member,
    full NCRP.

MORLEY, F. -- Unsc77, Specialist Scientist,
    United Kingdom Delegation. Unsc82, Specialist
    Scientist, United Kingdom Delegation.

MORONEY, J.R. -- Unsc77, Specialist Scientist,
    Australia Delegation. Unsc82, Specialist
    Scientist, Australia Delegation.

MORONI, J.P. -- Icrp85-89, Member, Committee 2 -
    Secondary Limits.

MORREY, M. -- Unsc88, Consultant to UNSCEAR.

MORROW, Paul E. -- Ncrp80, member, full NCRP.

MOSELEY, R.D. Jr. -- Unsc77, Specialist
    Scientist, United States Delegation. Ncrp80,
    member, full NCRP. Unsc82, Specialist
    Scientist, United States Delegation. Unsc86,
    Unsc88, United States Delegation.

MOSKALEV, Yuri I.-- Icrp77, Member of the Main
    Commission of the ICRP. Icrp85-89, Member,
    Committee 2 - Secondary Limits. Unsc86,
    Unsc88, U.S.S.R. Delegation.

MULLER, E. -- Unsc82, Specialist Scientist,
    Canada Delegation.

MYERS, D.K. -- Unsc82, Unsc86, Unsc88,
    Specialist Scientist, Canada Delegation.

NAKATANI, Roy E. -- Beir72, Subcommittee on
    Environmental Effects.

NAKAI, S. -- Unsc77, Specialist Scientist, Japan
    Delegation. Unsc82, Specialist Scientist,
    Japan Delegation.

NEEL, James V. -- Ncrp80, member, full NCRP.

NELSON, Robert J. -- Ncrp80, member, full NCRP.

NEWCOMBE, H.B. -- Icrp77, Member of the Main
    Commission of the ICRP.

NOTANI, N.K. -- Unsc88, India Delegation.

NYGAARD, Oddvar F. -- Nih85, member, Ad Hoc
    Working Group.

O'BRIEN, B.J. -- Unsc77, Scientific Staff or
    Consultant to UNSCEAR.

OPPENHEIM, Bernard E. -- Beir80, Consultant to
    Subcommittee on Somatic Effects.

ORTIZ-MAGANA, J.R. -- Unsc77, Specialist
    Scientist, Mexico Delegation. Unsc82,
    Specialist Scientist, Mexico Delegation.
    Unsc86, Unsc88, Mexico Delegation.

PALACIOS, E. -- Unsc88, Argentina Delegation.

PARKER. Dean R. -- Beir80, full Committee.
    Ncrp80, Consultant to Scientific Committee 40.

==

PARKER, Frank -- Ncrp80, member, full NCRP.

PARKER, Herbert M. -- Ncrp80, Honorary member,
   full NCRP.

PARMENTIER, N. -- Icrp85-89, Member, Committee 2
   - Secondary Limits.

PAVLINOV, V. -- Unsc86, Unsc88, U.S.S.R. Delegation.

PAVLOVSKY, O. -- Unsc86, Unsc88, U.S.S.R. Delegation.

PELLERIN, P. -- Unsc77, Specialist Scientist,
   France Delegation. Unsc82, Specialist
   Scientist, France Delegation. Unsc86, Unsc88,
   France Delegation.

PENNA-FRANCA, E. -- Unsc77, Unsc82, Specialist
   Scientist, Brazil Delegation.
   Unsc86, Unsc88, Brazil Delegation.

PERSSON, R.B. -- Unsc82, Scientific Staff or
   Consultant.

PIATAK, O. -- Unsc88, U.S.S.R. Delegation.

PINILLOS ASHTON, L.V. -- Unsc86, Unsc88, Peru
   Delegation.

PLACER, Dr. A.E. -- Unsc77, Specialist
   Scientist, Argentina Delegation.

PLATT, Robert B. -- Beir72, Subcommittee on
   Environmental Effects.

POCHIN, Edward -- Unsc77, Specialist Scientist,
   United Kingdom Delegation. Icrp77, Member of
   the Main Commission of the ICRP. Unsc82,
   Specialist Scientist, United Kingdom
   Delegation. Icrp85-89, Member(Emeritus) of the
   Main Commission.

POZNANSKI, Andrew K. -- Ncrp80, member, full
   NCRP. Icrp85-89, Member of the Main Commission
   of the ICRP.

PRANTL, F. -- Unsc82, Specialist Scientist,
   Canada Delegation.

PRESTON, Dale -- Beir90, Scientific Advisor to
   the Committee.

QUIMBY, Edith H. -- Ncrp80, Honorary member,
   full NCRP.

RADFORD, Edward P. -- Beir72, full Committee.
   Beir72, Subcommittee on Somatic Effects. Beir72,
   Subcommittee on Environmental Effects. Beir80,
   Chairman, BEIR Committee. Beir80, Chairman,
   Subcommittee on Somatic Effects.

RALL, Joseph E. -- Beir72, full Committee.
   Beir72, Subcommittee on Somatic Effects. Beir72,
   Ad Hoc Committee. Nih85, Chairman, Ad Hoc
   Working Group.

RAMZAEV, P.V. -- Icrp85-89, Member of the Main
   Commission of the ICRP.

RAUSCH, L. -- Unsc77, Specialist Scientist, West
   Germany Delegation. Unsc82, Specialist
   Scientist, West Germany Delegation.

REDKIN. V.V. -- Unsc82, Specialist Scientist,
   U.S.S.R. Delegation. Unsc86, Unsc88,
   U.S.S.R. Delegation.

REINIG, William C. -- Ncrp80, member, full NCRP.

RICHMOND, Chester R. -- Ncrp80, member, full
   NCRP. Icrp85-89, Committee 2 - Secondary Limits.

RICKS, R.C. -- Unsc88, United States Delegation.

RIDWAN, M. -- Unsc86, Unsc88, Indonesia Delegation.

ROBERTSON, David -- Doe87, Interlaboratory Task
   Group on Health and Environmental Aspects of the
   Soviet Nuclear Accident.

ROSSI, Harald H. -- Unsc77, Specialist
   Scientist, United States Delegation. Beir80,
   full Committee. Beir80, Subcommittee on Somatic
   Effects. Ncrp80, member, full NCRP. Unsc86,
   Unsc88, United States Delegation.

ROTHSCHILD, H.C. -- Unsc77, Specialist
   Scientist, Canada Delegation. Unsc82,
   Specialist Scientist, Canada Delegation.

ROUSHDY, H. -- Unsc88, Egypt Delegation.

ROWLAND, Robert E. -- Ncrp80, member, full NCRP.

RUSSELL, Liane B. -- Beir80, full Committee.
   Beir80, Subcommittee on Somatic Effects.

RUSSELL, William L. -- Beir72, full Committee.
   Unsc77, Specialist Scientist, United States
   Delegation. Beir80, full Committee. Unsc82,
   Specialist Scientist, United States Delegation.
   Unsc86, Unsc88, United States Delegation.

RUST, John H. -- Ncrp80, Honorary member, full
   NCRP.

SAENGER, Eugene L. -- Beir72, full Committee.
   Beir72, Subcommittee on Somatic Effects.
   Ncrp80, member, full NCRP.

SANKARANARAYANAN, K. -- Unsc77, Scientiific
   Staff or Consultant to UNSCEAR. Icrp85-89,
   Member, Committee on Radiation Effects. Unsc86,
   Unsc88, Scientific Consultant to UNSCEAR.

SAUROV, M.M. -- Unsc77, Specialist Scientist,
   U.S.S.R. Delegation.

SCHLENKER, Robert -- Doe87, Interlaboratory Task
   Group on Health and Environmental Aspects of the
   Soviet Nuclear Accident.

SCHULL, William J. -- Icrp85-89, Member, Committee
   on Radiation Effects. Unsc88, United
   States Delegation.

SCHULTE, Harry F. -- Ncrp80, member, full NCRP.

SCHUTTMANN, W. -- Unsc77, Scientific Staff or
   Consultant to UNSCEAR.

SEAMAN, William B. -- Beir72, Subcommittee on
   Somatic Effects.

SEARLE, A.G. -- Unsc77, Specialist Scientist,
   United Kingdom Delegation. Unsc82, Specialist
   Scientist, United Kingdom. Unsc86, Unsc88,
   United Kingdom Delegation.

SELBY, Paul B. -- Beir80, full Committee.
Unsc86, Unsc88, United States Delegation.

SHAH, V.A. -- Unsc82, Specialist Scientist,
India Delegation.

SHEVCHENKO, V.A. -- Unsc82, Specialist
Scientist, U.S.S.R. Delegation. Unsc86,
Unsc88, U.S.S.R. Delegation.

SHIGEMATSU, Itsuzo -- Icrp85-89, Member,
Committee on Radiation Effects.

SHORE, Roy E. -- Beir80, Consultant to
Subcommittee on Somatic Effects.

SILINI, Giovanni -- Unsc77, Scientific Staff or
Consultant to UNSCEAR. Icrp85-89, Member of the
Main Commission of the ICRP. Unsc86, Unsc88,
Scientific Staff or Consultant to UNSCEAR.

SINCLAIR, Warren K. -- Unsc77, Specialist
Scientist, United States Delegation. Ncrp80,
President, NCRP. Unsc82, Specialist Scientist,
United States Delegation. Icrp85-89, Member of
the Main Commission of the ICRP. Icrp85-89,
Chairman, Committee on Radiation Effects.
Unsc86, Unsc88, United States Delegation.

SLOAN, Margaret H. -- Beir80, full Committee.
Beir80, Subcommittee on Somatic Effects.

SMITH, Harold -- Ncrp80, member, Scientific
Committee 40. Icrp85-89, Scientific Secretary
of the ICRP.

SNIHS, Jan O. -- Unsc77, Specialist Scientist,
Sweden Delegation. Icrp85-89, Member, Committee
2 - Secondary Limits. Unsc82, Specialist
Scientist, Sweden Delegation. Unsc86, Unsc88,
Sweden Delegation.

SOBELS, F.H. -- Unsc77, Specialist Scientist,
Belgium Delegation. Unsc82, Specialist
Scientist, Belgium Delegation. Unsc86,Unsc88,
Belgium Delegation.

SOKOLOWSKI, Evelyn -- Unsc77, Specialist
Scientist, Sweden Delegation.

SOMAN, S.D. -- Unsc82, Specialist Scientist,
India Delegation.

SOWBY, F.D. -- Icrp77, Scientific Secretary of
the International Commission on Radiological
Protection. Icrp77, Editor, Annals of the
ICRP. Unsc86, Unsc88, Scientific Staff or
Consultant to UNSCEAR.

STANNARD, J. Newell -- Ncrp80, Honorary member,
full NCRP.

STARR, Chauncey -- Ncrp80, member, full NCRP.

STEVENS, G.E. -- Unsc77, Specialist Scientist,
Australia Delegation.

STEWART, C.G. -- Icrp77, Member of the Main
Commission of the ICRP. Icrp77, Chairman,
International Commission on Radiological
Protection.

STIEVE, F.E. -- Unsc77, Specialist Scientist,
West Germany Delegation. Unsc82, Specialist
Scientist, West Germany Delegation. Unsc86,
Unsc88, West Germany Delegation.

STORER, John B. -- Beir72, Subcommittee on
Somatic Effects. Ncrp80, member, Scientific
Committee 40. Ncrp80, member, full NCRP.
Unsc82, Specialist Scientist, United States
Delegation.

STREFFER, C. -- Unsc82, Specialist Scientist,
West Germany Delegation. Unsc86, Unsc88, West
Germany Delegation.

SUGIARTO, C.J. -- Unsc88, Indonesia Delegation.

SUNDARAM, K. -- Unsc77, Specialist Scientist,
India Delegation. Unsc82, Unsc86, Unsc88,
Specialist Scientist, India Delegation.

SZOT, Z. -- Unsc88, Poland Delegation.

TADJUDIN, M.K. -- Unsc77, Specialist Scientist,
Indonesia Delegation.

TAJIMA, Eizo -- Icrp85-89, Member of the Main
Commission of the ICRP.

TAKAHASHI, S. -- Icrp77, Member of the Main
Commission of the ICRP.

TATES, A.D. -- Unsc86,Unsc88, Belgium Delegation.

TAYLOR, David M. -- Icrp85-89, Member, Committee
2 - Secondary Limits.

TAYLOR, F. -- Unsc82, Scientific Staff or
Consultant.

TAYLOR, L.S. Icrp77, Member (Emeritus) of the
Main Commission of the ICRP. Icrp85-89,
Member(Emeritus) of the Main Commission of the
ICRP.

TAZIMA, Y. -- Unsc77, Specialist Scientist,
Japan Delegation.

TELICH, J.R. -- Unsc82, Specialist Scientist,
Mexico Delegation.

TERASIMA, T. -- Unsc88, Japan Delegation.

THIESSEN, J.W. -- Unsc86, Unsc88, United States
Delegation.

THOMAS, Duncan C. -- Beir90, member, full
Committee.

THOMAS, Ralph H. -- Icrp85-89, Member, Committee
2 - Secondary Limits.

THOMPSON, Keith -- Ncrp80, Consultant to
Scientific Committee 40.

THOMPSON, Roy C. -- Ncrp80, member, full NCRP.

TRIMBLE, Benjamin K. -- Unsc77, Specialist
Scientist, Canada Delegation. Beir80, full
Committee. Beir80, Subcommittee on Somatic
Effects.

TUBIANA, M.R. -- Unsc88, France Delegation.

==

TUKEY, H.B., Jr. -- Beir72, Subcommittee on
Environmental Effects.

TURNER, James D. -- Ncrp80, member, full NCRP.

ULLRICH, Robert -- Ncrp80, member, Scientific
Committee 40.

UPTON, Arthur C. -- Beir72, full Committee.
Beir72, Chairman of the Subcommittee on Somatic
Effects. Beir72, Ad Hoc Committee. Beir80,
First Chairman, full Committee. Unsc77,
Specialist Scientist, United States Delegation.
Icrp77, Member of the Main Commission of the
ICRP. Nih85, member, Ad Hoc Working Group.
Icrp85-89, Member, Committee on Radiation
Effects. Beir90, Chairman of the Committee.

UZZAN, G. -- Unsc88, France Delegation.

VALENTIN, J. -- Unsc86,Unsc88, Sweden Delegation.

VENNART, J. -- Icrp77, Member of the Main
Commission of the ICRP.

VICHROV, A.I. -- Unsc82, Specialist Scientist,
U.S.S.R Delegation.

VILLFORTH, John C. -- Ncrp80, member, full NCRP.
Unsc82, Specialist Scientist, United Delegation.

VOELZ, George L. -- Ncrp80, member, full NCRP.

WALD, Neil -- Ncrp80, member, full NCRP.

WALINDER, G. -- Unsc77, Specialist Scientist,
Sweden Delegation. Unsc82, Specialist
Scientist, Sweden Delegation. Unsc86, Unsc88,
Sweden Delegation.

WALSH, R.J. -- Unsc77, Specialist Scientist,
Australia Delegation.

WARMAN, Edward -- Doe87, Interlaboratory Task
Group on Health and Environmental Aspects of the
Soviet Nuclear Accident.

WARREN, Shields -- Beir72, full Committee.
Beir72, Subcommittee on Somatic Effects.
Ncrp80, Honorary member, full NCRP.

WATSON-MUNRO, C.N. -- Unsc77, Specialist
Scientist, Australia Delegation.

WEBB, G.A.M. -- Unsc77, Unsc88, Scientific Staff
or Consultant to UNSCEAR.

WEBSTER, Edward W. -- Beir80, full Committee.
Beir80, Subcommittee on Somatic Effects. Beir80,
Compromise Group. Ncrp80, member, full NCRP.
Unsc88, United States Delegation.

WEISS, K. -- Unsc88, Consultant to UNSCEAR.

WELLMAN, Henry N. -- Beir80, full Committee.
Beir80, Subcommittee on Somatic Effects.

WILKENING, George M. -- Ncrp80, member, full
NCRP.

WINDEYER, B. -- Icrp77, Member of the Main
Commission of the ICRP.

WIRYOSIMIN, S.N. -- Unsc88, Indonesia Delegation.

WRENN, McDonald E. -- Ncrp80, member, full NCRP.

WYCKOFF, Harold O. -- Unsc77, Specialist
Scientist, United States Delegation. Ncrp80,
member, Scientfic Committee 40. Ncrp80,
Honorary member, full NCRP. Unsc82, Specialist
Scientist, United States Delegation. Unsc86,
Unsc88, United States Delegation.

XING-AN, Chen -- Icrp85-89, Member, Committee 2
- Secondary Limits.

YALOW, Rosalyn S. -- Nih85, member, Ad Hoc
Working Group.

YAMATO, A. -- Unsc86,Unsc88, Japan Delegation.

YOUSIF, A.A. -- Unsc86,Unsc88, Sudan Delegation.

ZAHARIA, M. -- Unsc82, Specialist Scientist,
Peru Delegation. Unsc86, Unsc88,
Peru Delegation.

ZEVE, Victor H. -- Nih85, Executive Secretary,
Ad Hoc Working Group.

37-empty, after 37-9.
===

References

Chapter 36 has its own Reference List.

Alex88a Alexander, Robert E., February 1988.
"Health Effects from Radiation," ENVIRONMENTAL
SCIENCE & TECHNOLOGY 22 No.2: 144-145.

Alex88b Alexander, Robert E., June 1988.
"A New Intellectual Atmosphere," guest editorial
by the 1988-89 president of the Health Physics
Society, HEALTH PHYSICS 54, No.6: 589-595.

Alex89 Alexander, Robert E., January 1989.
"More on Very Low Radiation Doses," letter in
HEALTH PHYSICS 56, No.1: 117.

And88 Anderson, R.E. + W.L. Williams + S. Tokuda,
1988.
"Effect of Low-Dose Irradiation upon T Cell Subsets
Involved in the Response of Primed A/J Mice to SaI
Cells," INTERNATIONAL JOURNAL OF RADIATION BIOLOGY
53, No.1: 103-118.

Ansp88 Anspaugh, Lynn R. + Robert J. Catlin + Marvin
Goldman, Dec. 16, 1988.
"The Global Impact of the Chernobyl Reactor
Accident," SCIENCE 242: 1513-1519.

As89 ASSOCIATED PRESS, series of reports filed from
Moscow.
July 30, 1989: "Larger Chernobyl-Area Evacuation
Urged."
August 9, 1989: "3,000 Told to Flee Chernobyl
Area."
August 15, 1989: "Radiation Study Based in
Chernobyl Area."

Bar85 Barendsen, G.W., 1985.
"Do Fast Neutrons at Low Dose Rate Enhance Cell
Transformation IN VITRO? A Basic Problem of
Microdosimetry and Interpretation," INTERNATIONAL
JOURNAL OF RADIATION BIOLOGY 47: 731-744.

Bara77 Baral, E. + L. Larsson + B. Mattson, 1977.
"Breast Cancer Following Irradiation of the
Breast." CANCER 40: 2905-2910.

Bau73 Baum, J.W., 1973.
"Population Heterogeneity Hypothesis on Radiation
Induced Cancer," HEALTH PHYSICS 25: 97-104.

Bav81 Baverstock, Kenneth F. + D. Papworth +
J. Vennart, Feb. 21, 1981.
"Risk of Radiation at Low Dose Rates," LANCET 1981,
1: 430-433.

Bav83 Baverstock, K.F. + J. Vennart, 1983.
"A Note on Radium Body Content and Breast Cancers
in U.K. Radium Luminisers," HEALTH PHYSICS 44,
SUPPL. No. 1: 575-577.

Bav85 Baverstock, K.F., September 1985.
"UK Luminizer Survey Misrepresented," letter in
JOURNAL OF OCCUPATIONAL MEDICINE 27, No.9: 613.

Bav87 Baverstock, K.F. + D.G. Papworth, 1987.
"The UK Radium Luminizer Survey," BRITISH JOURNAL
OF RADIOLOGY, Supplemental BIR Report 21, 71-76.
(BIR = British Institute of Radiology.)

Bav89 Baverstock, K.F. + R.B. Cundall, 1989.
"Are Solitons Responsible for Energy Transfer in
Oriented DNA?", letter in INTERNATIONAL JOURNAL OF
RADIATION BIOLOGY 55, No.1: 151-153.

Bee70 is also TR-11-70. Beebe, Gilbert W. + Hiroo
Kato + Charles E. Land, 1970.
JNIH-ABCC LIFE SPAN STUDY, HIROSHIMA-NAGASAKI,
REPORT 5. MORTALITY AND RADIATION DOSE, OCTOBER
1950-SEPTEMBER 1966. Technical Report TR-11-70.
(Current source today, Hiroshima: RERF.)

Bee71 is also TR-11-70, abbreviated. Beebe, Gilbert
W. + Hiroo Kato + Charles E. Land, 1971.
"Studies of the Mortality of A-Bomb Survivors 4.
Mortality and Radiation Dose, 1950-1966"
(TR-11-70). RADIATION RESEARCH 48: 613-649.

Bee77 is also TR-1-77. Beebe, Gilbert W.
+ Hiroo Kato + Charles E. Land, 1977.
LIFE SPAN STUDY REPORT 8. MORTALITY EXPERIENCE OF
ATOMIC BOMB SURVIVORS, 1950-1974. RERF Technical
Report TR-1-77. (Hiroshima: RERF.)

Bee78 is also TR-1-77, abbreviated. Beebe, Gilbert W.
+ Hiroo Kato + Charles E. Land, 1978.
"Studies of the Mortality of A-Bomb Survivors: 6.
Mortality and Radiation Dose, 1950-1974" (RERF
TR-1-77). RADIATION RESEARCH 75: 138-201.

Beir72 BEIR Committee, 1972.
THE EFFECTS ON POPULATIONS OF EXPOSURE TO LOW
LEVELS OF IONIZING RADIATION (also known as the
BEIR-1 Report). Report prepared by the Advisory
Committee on the Biological Effects of Ionizing
Radiation. Individual authors are acknowledged in
our Chapter 37. (Washington, DC 20418: National
Academy of Sciences, 2101 Constitution Avenue.)
No index.

Beir80 BEIR Committee, 1980.
THE EFFECTS ON POPULATIONS OF EXPOSURE TO LOW
LEVELS OF IONIZING RADIATION (also known as the
BEIR-3 Report). This report was issued by the
Committee on the Biological Effects of Ionizing
Radiations, Division of Medical Sciences, National
Research Council, National Academy of Sciences.
Individual authors are acknowledged in our Chapter
37. (Washington, DC 20418: National Academy
Press, 2101 Constitution Avenue, NW.) No index.
This report was issued in two formats, a large
book (typewriter edition) and later in the year, a
small book (typeset edition). Page numbers cited
in Go81 refer to pagination in the large format,
whereas pages cited in this book refer to the
small format.

Beir90 BEIR Committee, December 19, 1989.
HEALTH EFFECTS OF EXPOSURE TO LOW LEVELS OF
IONIZING RADIATION (also known as the BEIR-5
Report). This report was issued by the Committee
on the Biological Effects of Ionizing Radiations,
Board on Radiation Effects Research, Commission on
Life Sciences, National Research Council, National
Academy of Sciences. Individual authors are
acknowledged in our Chapter 37. (Washington, DC
20418: National Academy Press, 2101 Constitution
Avenue, NW.) Indexed.

Ben82 Bender, Michael A. + R.J. Preston, 1982.
"Role of Base Damage in Aberration Formation:
Interaction of Aphidicolin and X-Rays," in
PROGRESS IN MUTATION RESEARCH, VOLUME 4: pp.
37-46. Edited by A.T. Natarajan, G. Obe, and H.
Altmann. (Amsterdam, Netherlands: Elsevier
Biomedical Press.)

Ben84 Bender, Michael A., 1984.
"Significance of Chromosome Abnormalities,"
pp.281-289 in Boice84.

==

Ber85 Beral, Valerie + Hazel Inskip + Patricia
       Fraser + Margaret Booth + Derek Coleman + Geoffrey
       Rose, Aug. 17, 1985. "Mortality of Employees of
       the United Kingdom Atomic Energy Authority,
       1946-1979," BRITISH MEDICAL JOURNAL 291: 440-447.

Ber87 Beral, Valerie + Patricia Fraser + Margaret
       Booth + Lucy Carpenter, 1987. "Epidemiological
       Studies of Workers in the Nuclear Industry,"
       Chapter 8, pp.97-106 in Jones87.

Berry87 Berry, Roger J., 1987.
       "The International Commission on Radiological
       Protection -- A Historical Perspective," Chapter
       10, pp.117-123 in Jones87.

Boice77 Boice, J.D., Jr. + R.R. Monson, 1977.
       "Breast Cancer in Women after Repeated Fluoroscopic
       Examinations of the Chest," JOURNAL OF THE NATIONAL
       CANCER INSTITUTE 59: 823-832.

Boice78 Boice, John D. + Marvin Rosenstein + E. Dale
       Trout, 1978. "Estimation of Breast Doses and
       Breast Cancer Risk Associated with Repeated
       Fluoroscopic Chest Examinations of Women with
       Tuberculosis," RADIATION RESEARCH 73: 373-390.

Boice79 Boice, John D., Jr. + Charles E. Land + Roy
       E. Shore + J.E. Norman + Masayoshi Tokunaga, 1979.
       "Risk of Breast Cancer Following Low-Dose Radiation
       Exposure," RADIOLOGY 131: 589-597.

Boice81 Boice, John D., + Richard R. Monson + Marvin
       Rosenstein, 1981. "Cancer Mortality in Women after
       Repeated Fluoroscopic Examinations of the Chest,"
       JOURNAL OF THE NAT'L CANCER INSTITUTE 66: 863-867.

Boice84 Boice, John D. Jr. and Joseph F. Fraumeni
       (editors), 1984. RADIATION CARCINOGENESIS:
       EPIDEMIOLOGY AND BIOLOGICAL SIGNIFICANCE. (New
       York, NY: Raven Press.)

Boice85 Boice, J.D. + N.E. Day + A. Anderson + 33
       others, 1985.
       "Second Cancers Following Radiation Treatment for
       Cervical Cancer; An International Collaboration
       among Cancer Registries," JOURNAL OF THE NATIONAL
       CANCER INSTITUTE 74: 955-975.

Bon78 Bond, Victor P. + Charles B. Meinhold + Harald
       H. Rossi, May 1978.
       "Low-Dose RBE and Q for X-Ray Compared to Gamma
       Radiations," HEALTH PHYSICS 34: 433-438.

Bon84 Bond, Victor P., 1984.
       "Stochastic Basis for Dose-Response Curves, RBE,
       and Temporal Dependence," in Boice84, pp.387-402.

Bov14 Boveri, Theodore, 1914. English-language
       edition: 1929.
       THE ORIGIN OF MALIGNANT TUMORS. (Baltimore,
       Maryland, USA: Williams and Wilkins.)

Brack88 Brackenbush, L.W. and L.A. Braby, 1988.
       "Microdosimetric Basis for Exposure Limits,"
       HEALTH PHYSICS 55: 251-255.

Brod78 Brodsky, Allen B. (editor), 1978.
       CRC HANDBOOK OF RADIATION MEASUREMENTS AND
       PROTECTION. SECTION A, VOLUME I: PHYSICAL SCIENCE
       AND ENGINEERING DATA. (West Palm Beach, Florida:
       CRC Press.)

Burns81 Burns, Frederic J. + Edward V. Sargent, 1981.
       "The Induction and Repair of DNA Breaks in Rat
       Epidermis Irradiated with Electrons," RADIATION
       RESEARCH 87: 137-144.

Chris87 Christy, Robert F. + Eizo Tajima, 1987.
       "Executive Summary,", pp.14-25 in Roes87.

Co56 Cooperative Study of Lipoproteins and
       Atherosclerosis, Oct. 1956.
       "Evaluation of Serum Lipoprotein and Cholesterol
       Measurements as Predictors of Clinical
       Complications of Atherosclerosis," CIRCULATION
       1956, VOL XIV, No. 4, Part 2: 691-742. The four
       participating laboratories were from University of
       California (Berkeley), The Cleveland Clinic,
       Harvard University, and University of Pittsburgh.

Cohen87 Cohen, Jerry J., May 1987.
       "Conference on Radiation Hormesis: An Overview,"
       HEALTH PHYSICS 52, No.5: 519.

Cong87 Congdon, Charles C., May 1987.
       "A Review of Certain Low-Level Ionizing Radiation
       Studies in Mice and Guinea Pigs," HEALTH PHYSICS
       52, No.5: 593-597.

Dar87 Darby, S.C. + R. Doll + S.K. Gill + P.G.
       Smith, 1987.
       "Long Term Mortality after a Single Treatment
       Course with X-Rays in Patients Treated for
       Ankylosing Spondylitis," BRITISH JOURNAL OF CANCER
       55: 179-190.

Davis87 Davis, Faith G. + John D. Boice, Jr. +
       Jennifer L. Kelsey + Richard R. Monson, April 1987.
       "Cancer Mortality after Multiple Fluoroscopic
       Examinations of the Chest," JOURNAL OF THE
       NATIONAL CANCER INSTITUTE 78, No.4: 645-652.

Des89 DeSaia, Philip J. and William Creasman, 1989.
       CLINICAL GYNECOLOGIC ONCOLOGY, THIRD EDITION.
       (St. Louis, Missouri: C.V. Mosby Co.)

Doe87 U.S. Department of Energy, June 1987.
       HEALTH AND ENVIRONMENTAL CONSEQUENCES OF THE
       CHERNOBYL NUCLEAR POWER POWER PLANT ACCIDENT.
       DOE/ER-0332. Prepared by the Committee on the
       Assessment of Health Consequences in Exposed
       Populations: Marvin Goldman (Chairman) + Lynn
       Anspaugh + Robert J. Catlin + Jacob I. Fabrikant +
       Paul Gudiksen. (Washington, DC 20545: U.S. Dept. of
       Energy Office of Energy Research.) No index.

Doe88 (U.S.) Department of Energy, 1988. Doe88 is
       the same as Ansp88.

Dor51 Dorland, W.A. Newman, 1951.
       THE AMERICAN ILLUSTRATED MEDICAL DICTIONARY.
       (Philadelphia and London: W.B. Saunders Company.)

Elias78 Elias, H. + J.E. Pauly + E.R. Burns, 1978.
       HISTOLOGY AND HUMAN MICROANATOMY. (New York, NY:
       John Wiley & Sons.)

Elle87 Ellett, William H. (editor), 1987.
       AN ASSESSMENT OF THE NEW DOSIMETRY FOR A-BOMB
       SURVIVORS, by the Panel on Reassessment of A-bomb
       Dosimetry, Advisory Committee on the Radiation
       Effects Research Foundation, Commission on Life
       Sciences, National Research Council. (Washington,
       DC 20418: National Academy Press, 2101
       Constitution Avenue.)

Ev55 Evans, Robley D., 1955. "Stopping of Electrons
       by Thick Absorbers", Chapter 21, pp.611-631 in
       THE ATOMIC NUCLEUS. (New York: McGraw Hill.)

Eva79 Evans, H.J. + K.E. Buckton + G.E. Hamilton +
       A. Carothers, 1979.
       "Radiation-Induced Chromosome Aberrations in
       Nuclear-Dockyard Workers," NATURE 277: 531-534.

Eva87 Evans, H.J., 1987.
       "Cytogenetic Damage: Threshold Effects and
       Sensitivities," Chapter 14, pp.179-189, in Jones87.

Evans85 Evans, John S., 1985. See Nrc85.

Evans86 Evans, John S. + John E. Wennberg +
       Barbara J. McNeil, Sept. 25, 1986.
       "The Influence of Diagnostic Radiography on the
       Incidence of Breast Cancer and Leukemia," NEW
       ENGLAND JOURNAL OF MEDICINE 315: 810-815.

Fein87 Feinendegen, L.E. + H. Muhlensiepen + Victor
       P. Bond + C.A. Sondhaus, May 1987.
       "Intracellular Stimulation of Biochemical Control
       Mechanisms by Low-Dose, Low-Let Radiation," HEALTH
       PHYSICS 52, No.5: 663-669.

Fein88 Feinendegen, L.E. + Victor P. Bond + J. Booz
       + H. Muhlensiepen, 1988.
       "Biochemical and Cellular Mechanisms of Low-Dose
       Effects, " INTERNATIONAL JOURNAL OF RADIATION
       BIOLOGY 53, No.1: 23-37.

Free87a Freeman, Gordon R. (editor), 1987.
       KINETICS OF NONHOMOGENEOUS PROCESSES. (New York:
       John Wiley and Sons.)

Free87b Freeman, Gordon R., 1987.
       "Stochastic Model of Charge Scavenging in Liquids
       under Irradiation by Electrons or Photons," Chapter
       6, pp.277-304, in Free87a.

==

Frig76 Frigerio, N.A. + R.S. Stowe, 1976.
   "Carcinogenic and Genetic Hazard from Background
   Radiation," in BIOLOGICAL AND ENVIRONMENTAL
   EFFECTS OF LOW-LEVEL RADIATION, pp. 385-393.
   (Vienna, Austria: Internat'l Atomic Energy Agency.)

Fry81 Fry, R.J.M., 1981.
   "Experimental Radiation Carcinogenesis: What Have
   We Learned?", RADIATION RESEARCH 87: 224-239.

Fry87 Fry, R.J.M. + Warren K. Sinclair, 1987.
   "New Dosimetry of Atomic Bomb Radiations," LANCET,
   Oct. 10, 1987, 845-848.

Gar76 Gardner, D.L. + T.C. Dodds, 1976.
   HUMAN HISTOLOGY: AN INTRODUCTION TO THE STUDY OF
   HISTOPATHOLOGY. (Edinburgh: Churchill
   Livingstone.)

Gilb85 Gilbert, Ethel, July 1985.
   "Late Somatic Effects," Chapter 2 of Part 2 in
   HEALTH EFFECTS MODEL FOR NUCLEAR POWER PLANT
   ACCIDENT CONSEQUENCE ANALYSIS, NUREG/CR-4214.
   (See Nrc85).

Gilb89 Gilbert, Ethel, May 1989.
   "Late Somatic Effects," Chapter 3.0 in HEALTH
   EFFECTS MODELS FOR NUCLEAR POWER PLANT ACCIDENT
   CONSEQUENCE ANALYSIS, NUREG/CR-4214, Rev.1, Part
   2. (See Nrc89).

Gilm88 Gilman, E.A. + George W. Kneale + E.G. Knox +
   Alice M. Stewart, 1988.
   "Pregnancy X-Rays and Childhood Cancers: Effects of
   Exposure Age and Radiation Dose," JOURNAL RADIOL.
   PROTECTION 8: 3-8.

Go50a Gofman, John W. + Frank Lindgren + Harold
   Elliott + William Mantz + John Hewitt + Beverly
   Strisower + Virgil Herring, 1950.
   "The Role of Lipids and Lipoproteins in
   Atherosclerosis," SCIENCE 3: 166-171, 186.

Go50b Gofman, John W. + Hardin B. Jones + Frank T.
   Lindgren + Thomas P. Lyon + Harold A. Elliott +
   Beverly Strisower + the Ultracentrifugal Laboratory
   Group, 1950.
   "Blood Lipids and Human Atherosclerosis,"
   CIRCULATION 2, No.2: 161-177.

Go54 Gofman, John W. + J.W. Glazier + Arthur R.
   Tamplin + Beverly Strisower + Oliver DeLalla, July
   1954.
   "Lipoproteins, Coronary Heart Disease, and
   Atherosclerosis," PHYSIOLOGICAL REVIEWS 34 (3):
   589-607.

Go69 Gofman, John W. + Arthur R. Tamplin, Oct. 29,
   1969.
   "Low Dose Radiation and Cancer," paper presented
   at the IEEE Nuclear Science Symposium, San
   Francisco. In IEEE TRANSACTIONS ON NUCLEAR
   SCIENCE, Vol. NS-17 Number 1, Feb. 1970: 1-9.
   (New York, NY: Inst. of Electrical and Electronics
   Engineering.)

Go71 Gofman, John W. + Arthur R. Tamplin, July 20,
   1971.
   "Epidemiologic Studies of Carcinogenesis by
   Ionizing Radiation," in PROCEEDINGS OF THE SIXTH
   BERKELEY SYMPOSIUM ON MATHEMATICAL STATISTICS AND
   PROBABILITY: VOLUME 6: EFFECTS OF POLLUTION ON
   HEALTH: pp. 235-277. Edited by L.M. Lecam, J.
   Neyman, and E. Scott, 1972. (Berkeley, CA 94720:
   University of California Press.)

Go72 Gofman, John W. + John D. Gofman + Arthur R.
   Tamplin + Erma Kovich, 1972.
   "Radiation As an Environmental Hazard," in
   ENVIRONMENT AND CANCER (papers presented at the
   24th Annual Symposium on Fundamental Cancer
   Research, 1971, at the University of Texas, M.D.
   Anderson Hospital and Tumor Institute at Houston)
   pp. 157-186. (Baltimore, MD: Williams and Wilkins.)

Go79 Gofman, John W., November 1979.
   "The Question of Radiation Causation of Cancer
   in Hanford Workers," HEALTH PHYSICS 37: 617-639.

Go81 Gofman, John W., October 1981.
   RADIATION AND HUMAN HEALTH. (San Francisco, CA
   94109: Sierra Club Books, 730 Polk Street.)
   Available also from CNR Books, pob 11207, San
   Francisco, CA 94101, USA. Price is U.S. 30
   dollars. Orders must be prepaid in U.S. dollars.
   No extra fee for worldwide shipping by surface
   mail.

Go83 Gofman, John W. May 30, 1983.
   "The Cancer-Leukemia Risk from Ionizing Radiation:
   Let's Have a Closer Look," presentation as a
   panelist at the Symposium on Radiation Risk:
   Assessment and Applications (Charles B. Meinhold,
   presiding), Annual Meeting of the American
   Association for the Advancement of Science, held
   in Detroit, Michigan.

Go85 Gofman, John W. + Egan O'Connor, Sept. 1985.
   X-RAYS: HEALTH EFFECTS OF COMMON EXAMS. (San
   Francisco, CA 94109: Sierra Club Books.)
   Available also from CNR Books for U.S. 25
   dollars. See Go81 above.

Go86 Gofman, John W., Sept. 9, 1986.
   "Assessing Chernobyl's Cancer Consequences:
   Application of Four 'Laws' of Radiation
   Carcinogenesis," presentation as a panelist at the
   Symposium on Low-Level Radiation, 192nd National
   Meeting of the American Chemical Society, held in
   Anaheim, California.

Go87 Gofman, John W., May 1987.
   "Health Effects of Ionizing Radiation: Dr. Sagan's
   Paradigms," letter in HEALTH PHYSICS 52: 679-680.

Go88a Gofman, John W., February 1988.
   "Did You Write It, Len? Reply to Dr. Sagan,"
   letter in HEALTH PHYSICS 54, No.2: 226.

Go88b Gofman, John W., September 1988.
   "A Proposal Concerning 'the New Dosimetry'",
   letter in HEALTH PHYSICS 55, No.3: 580-581.

Go88c Gofman, John W., June 1988.
   "Cancer-Risk among A-Bomb Survivors in Both the
   'Old' and 'New' Dosimetries" ("Das Krebsrisiko
   unter den Ueberlebenden der Atombombenabwuerfe auf
   Grund der 'Alten' und 'Neuen'
   Dosimetrieberechnungen," pp.57-73 in DIE WIRKUNG
   NIEDRIGER STRAHLENDOSEN: BIOLOGISCHE UND
   MEDIZINISCHE ASPEKTE. Edited proceedings of a
   symposium, "Effects of Low-Level Radiation on
   Humans," sponsored by the Institute for
   Radiobiology of the Westfaelischen
   Wilhelms-Universitaet and the Institute for
   Nuclear Medicine of the Staedtischen Kliniken
   Kassel, and held 26-27 February 1988. Papers
   edited by Wolfgang Koehnlein, Horst Traut, and
   Manfred Fischer, printed 1989. (Berlin, New York:
   Springer-Verlag.)

Go89a Gofman, John W., January 1989.
   "Warning from the A-Bomb Study about Low and Slow
   Radiation Exposures," letter in HEALTH PHYSICS 56,
   No.1: 117-118.

Go89b Gofman, John W., December, 1989.
   "Supra-Linear Dose-Response in the A-Bomb Study,"
   letter in HEALTH PHYSICS 57, No.6: 1037-1038.

Gold87 Goldman, Marvin + Lynn Anspaugh + Robert J.
   Catlin + Jacob I. Fabrikant + Paul Gudiksen, June
   1987.
   HEALTH AND ENVIRONMENTAL CONSEQUENCES OF THE
   CHERNOBYL NUCLEAR POWER PLANT ACCIDENT,
   DOE/ER-0332. See Doe87.

Goldsc85 Goldschmidt, Herbert + William K.
   Sherwin, 1985. "Dermatologic Radiation Therapy," in
   Chapter 38 of DERMATOLOGY, Volume 2, edited by Samuel
   L. Moschella and Harry J. Hurley. (Philadelphia:
   W.B. Saunders Company.)

Good88 Goodhead, D.T., 1988.
   "Spatial and Temporal Distribution of Energy,"
   HEALTH PHYSICS 55: 231-240.

Gui56 Guilford, J.P. 1956. "Multiple Prediction,"
    p.423 in FUNDAMENTAL STATISTICS IN PSYCHOLOGY
    AND EDUCATION. (New York, N.Y.: McGraw-Hill.)
Ha81 Hall, Eric J. + Richard C. Miller, 1981.
    "The How and Why of In Vitro Oncogenic
    Transformation," RADIATION RESEARCH 87: 208-223.
Ham85 Hammersen, F., 1985.
    SOBOTTA/HAMMERSEN HISTOLOGY; COLOR ATLAS OF
    MICROSCOPIC ANATOMY. (Baltimore, MD: Urban &
    Schwarzenberg.)
Har83 Harvey, E. + J. Boice + M. Honeyman +
    J. Flannery, 1983.
    "Prenatal X-Ray and Childhood Cancer in Twins,"
    AMERICAN JOURNAL OF EPIDEMIOLOGY 118: 424-425.
Har85 Harvey, Elizabeth B. + John D. Boice Jr. +
    Merton Honeyman + John T. Flannery, Feb. 28, 1985.
    "Prenatal X-Ray Exposure and Childhood Cancer in
    Twins," New England Journal of Med. 312 (No.9):
    541-545.
Harpe57 Harper, Floyd Arthur, 1957.
    "To Shoot a Myth," (essay, Nov. 1957), pp.537-542
    in THE WRITINGS OF F.A. HARPER, VOLUME 2: SHORTER
    ESSAYS, 1979. (Institute for Humane Studies,
    George Mason University: Fairfax, Virginia, USA.)
Hay87 Hayek, L. + A. Cheetham, May 1987.
    "Curvilinear Regression, in Release 2," LOTUS:
    COMPUTING FOR MANAGERS AND PROFESSIONALS: (May) 78.
Hi84 Hill, C.K. + A. Han + M.M. Elkind, 1984.
    "Fission-Spectrum Neutrons at Low Dose Rate
    Enhance Neoplastic Transformation in the Linear,
    Low Dose Region (0-10 Gy)," INTERNATIONAL JOURNAL
    OF RADIATION BIOLOGY 46: 11-15.
Hic81 Hickey, Richard J. + E.J. Bowers + D.E. Spence
    + B.S. Zemel + A.B. Clelland + R.C. Clelland, 1981.
    "Low Level Ionizing Radiation and Human Mortality:
    Multi-Regional Epidemiological Studies. A
    Preliminary Report," HEALTH PHYSICS 40: 625-641.
Hic85 Hickey, Richard J., November, 1985.
    "Risks Associated with Exposure to Radiation:
    Science, Pseudoscience, and Opinion," HEALTH
    PHYSICS 49, No.5: 949-952.
Hic88 Hickey, Richard J., May 23, 1988.
    "Health and Nuclear Power Plants," letter in
    CHEMICAL AND ENGINEERING NEWS, May 23, 1988,
    p.2,47.
High80 High Background Radiation Research Group
    (China), 1980.
    "Health Survey in High Background Radiation Areas
    in China," SCIENCE 209: 877-880.
Hild83 Hildreth, Nancy G. + Roy E. Shore + Louis H.
    Hempelmann, July 30, 1983.
    "Risk of Breast Cancer among Women Receiving
    Radiation Treatment in Infancy for Thymic
    Enlargement," LANCET, July 30, 1983, 273.
Hild85 Hildreth, N.G. + R.E. Shore + L. Hempelmann +
    M. Rosenstein, 1985.
    "Risk of Extrathyroid Tumors Following Radiation
    Treatment in Infancy for Thymic Enlargement,"
    RADIATION RESEARCH 102: 378-391.
Hild89 Hildreth, Nancy G. + Roy E. Shore + Philip M.
    Dvoretsky, November 9, 1989.
    "The Risk of Breast Cancer after Irradiation of
    the Thymus in Infancy," NEW ENGLAND JOURNAL OF
    MEDICINE 321, No.19: 1281-1284.
Hoff85 Hoffman, Daniel A. and Edward P. Radford,
    April 1985.
    A REVIEW OF THE CARCINOGENIC EFFECTS OF LOW DOSES
    OF IONIZING RADIATION. (Philadelphia, PA 19103:
    Three Mile Island Public Health Fund, 1622 Locust
    Street.)
Hogue89 Hogue, Mark G., September 26, 1989.
    "Radiation Exposure: A Little Might Be Good,"
    letter to the editor in the WALL STREET JOURNAL,
    September 26, 1989.
Hol75 Holford, R.M., 1975.
    "The Relationship between Juvenile Cancer and
    Obstetric Radiography," HEALTH PHYSICS 28: 153-156.

Holm80a Holm, Lars-Erik + Goran Lundell + Gunnar
    Walinder, May 1980.
    "Incidence of Malignant Thyroid Tumors in Humans
    after Exposure to Diagnostic Doses of Iodine-131.
    (1) Retrospective Cohort Study," JOURNAL OF THE
    NATIONAL CANCER INSTITUTE 64, No.5: 1055-1059.
Holm80b Holm, Lars-Erik + Gunnar Eklund + Goran
    Lundell, December 1980.
    "Incidence of Malignant Thyroid Tumors in Humans
    after Exposure to Diagnostic Doses of Iodine-131.
    (2) Estimation of Thyroid Gland Size, Thyroid
    Radiation Dose, and Predicted versus Observed
    Number of Malignant Thyroid Tumors," JOURNAL OF
    THE NATIONAL CANCER INSTITUTE 65, No.6: 1221-1224.
Holm88 Holm, L.E. and eleven co-workers, 1988.
    "Thyroid Cancer after Diagnostic Doses of
    Iodine-131: A Retrospective Cohort Study," JOURNAL
    OF THE NATIONAL CANCER INSTITUTE 80: 1132-1138.
Howe84 Howe, Geoffrey R., 1984.
    "Epidemiology of Radiogenic Breast Cancer,"
    pp.119-129 in Boice84.
Hru89 Hrubec, Zdenek + J. D. BOice, Jr. + R. R. Monson
    + M. Rosenstein, 1989. "Breast Cancer after Multiple
    Chest Fluoroscopies," CANCER RESEARCH 49: 229-234.
Icrp77 International Commission on Radiological
    Protection, 1977.
    "Recommendations of the International Commission on
    Radiological Protection," adopted January 17, 1977,
    ICRP Publication 26. Individual members of the
    Main Commission are acknowledged in our Chapter 37.
    In ANNALS OF THE ICRP, Vol.1, No.3, 1977. (Oxford,
    England: Pergamon Press Ltd.)
Ilyin87 Ilyin, L.A. + O.A. Pavlovski, Sept. 1987.
    Ilyin87 is the same as Ussr87b.
    "Radiological Consequences of the Chernobyl
    Accident in the Soviet Union and Measures Taken to
    Mitigate Their Impact," pp. 149-166 in PROCEEDINGS
    OF THE INTERNATIONAL CONFERENCE ON NUCLEAR POWER
    PERFORMANCE AND SAFETY, VOLUME 3, Sept.28-October
    2, 1987, Vienna. IAEA-CN-48/33. (Vienna:
    International Atomic Energy Agency.)
Ilyin88 Ilyin, L.A., May 13, 1988.
    "The Chernobyl Experience and the Contemporary
    Problems of Radiation Protection," in PROCEEDINGS
    OF THE SCIENTIFIC CONFERENCE ON THE MEDICAL
    ASPECTS OF THE CHERNOBYL ACCIDENT, May 11-13, 1988
    in Kiev. (Moscow: USSR Ministry of Public Health.)
Ins87 Inskip, Hazel + Valerie Beral + Patricia
    Fraser + Margaret Booth + D. Coleman + Ann Brown,
    1987. "Further Assessment of the Effects of
    Occupational Radiation Exposure in the United Kingdom
    Atomic Energy Authority Mortality Study," BRITISH J.
    OF INDUSTRIAL MEDICINE 44: 149-160.
Jab63 is also TR-15-63. Jablon, Seymour + M. Ishida
    + M. Yamasaki, 1963.
    JNIH-ABCC LIFE-SPAN STUDY, HIROSHIMA-NAGASAKI.
    REPORT 3, MORTALITY OCTOBER 1950-SEPTEMBER 1960.
    Technical Report TR-15-63. (Current source
    today, Hiroshima: RERF.)
Jab65 is also TR-15-63. Jablon, Seymour + M. Ishida
    + M. Yamasaki, 1965. Same as Jab63, but published in
    RADIATION RESEARCH 25: 25-52.
Jab71 is also TR-10-71. Jablon, Seymour + Hiroo
    Kato, 1971.
    JNIH-ABCC LIFE SPAN STUDY, REPORT 6: MORTALITY
    AMONG ATOMIC BOMB SURVIVORS, HIROSHIMA-NAGASAKI
    1950-1970. Technical Report TR-10-71.
    (Current source today, Hiroshima: RERF.)
Jab72 is also TR-10-71. Jablon, Seymour + Hiroo
    Kato, 1972.
    "Studies of the Mortality of A-Bomb Survivors 5.
    Radiation Dose and Mortality, 1950-1970"
    (TR-10-71). RADIATION RESEARCH 50: 649-698.
Jab80 Jablon, Seymour + John C. Bailar III, 1980.
    "The Contribution of Ionizing Radiation to Cancer
    Mortality in the United States," PREVENTIVE MED 9:
    219-226.

==

James88 James, S.I. + T. Makinodan, 1988.
"T Cell Potentiation in Normal and
Autoimmune-Prone Mice after Extended Exposure to
Low Doses of Ionizing Radiation and/or Caloric
Restriction," INTERNATIONAL JOURNAL OF RADIATION
BIOLOGY 53, No.1: 137-152.

Jo85 Johannessen, J.V. (editor), 1985.
ELECTRON MICROSCOPY IN HUMAN MEDICINE. In twelve
volumes through 1985. (New York, NY: McGraw-Hill
International Book Co.)

Jones87 Jones, Robin Russell and Richard Southwood
(editors), 1987.
RADIATION AND HEALTH: THE BIOLOGICAL EFFECTS OF
LOW-LEVEL EXPOSURE TO IONIZING RADIATION. Edited
proceedings of a symposium, "The Biological
Effects of Radiation," sponsored by Friends of the
Earth U.K. and Greenpeace International, and held
24-25 November 1986 at the Hammersmith Hospital,
London; Sir Richard Southwood, Chairman. (London:
John Wiley & Sons.)

Kato80 is also TR-12-80. Kato, Hiroo + William J.
Schull, 1980.
LIFE SPAN STUDY REPORT 9, PART 1. CANCER MORTALITY
AMONG ATOMIC BOMB SURVIVORS, 1950-1978. RERF
Technical Report TR-12-80. (Hiroshima: RERF.)

Kato82 is also TR-12-80. Kato, Hiroo + William J.
Schull, 1982.
"Studies of the Mortality of A-Bomb Survivors, 7.
Mortality, 1950-1978: Part I, Cancer Mortality"
(RERF TR-12-80). RADIATION RESEARCH 90: 395-432.

Kato82b Kato, H. + C.C. Brown + D.G. Hoel. 1982.
"Life Span Study Report 9, Part2: Mortality from
Causes Other Than Cancer among A-Bomb Survivors,
1950-1978. RADIATION RESEARCH 91: 243-264.

Kato87 Kato, Hiroo + William J. Schull + Akio Awa +
Mitoshi Akiyama + Masanori Otake, May 1987.
"Dose-Response Analyses among Atomic Bomb Survivors
Exposed to Low-Level Radiation," HEALTH PHYSICS 52,
No.5: 645-652.

Kau87 Kaul, Dean C. + Stephen D. Egbert + Mark D.
Otis + Thomas Kuhn + George D. Kerr + Keith F.
Eckerman + Mark Cristy + Takashi Maruyama + Jeffrey
C. Ryman + Jabo S. Tang, 1987.
"Organ Dosimetry" Chapter 8, pp.306-404 in Roes87.

Kelle87 Kellerer, Albrecht M., 1987.
"Models of Cellular Radiation Action," Chapter 7,
pp.305-375, in Free87a.

Kelle88 Kellerer, Albrecht M., 1988.
"Die neue Bewertung der Strahlenrisiken:
Folgerungen aus der Revision der Dosimetrie in
Hiroshima und Nagasaki," pp.37-56 in DIE WIRKUNG
NIEDRIGER STRAHLENDOSEN: BIOLOGISCHE UND
MEDIZINISCHE ASPEKTE. Edited proceedings of a
symposium, "Effects of Low-Level Radiation on
Humans," sponsored by the Institute for
Radiobiology of the Westfaelischen
Wilhelms-Universitaet and the Institute for
Nuclear Medicine of the Staedtischen Kliniken
Kassel, and held 26-27 February 1988. Papers
edited by Wolfgang Koehnlein, Horst Traut, and
Manfred Fischer, printed 1989. (Berlin, New York:
Springer-Verlag.)

Kenn78 Kennedy, A.R. + G. Murphy + S. Mondal + C.
Heidelberger + J.B. Little, 1978.
"Enhancement of X-Ray Transformation by
12-O-tetradecanoyl-phorbol-13-acetate in a Cloned
Line of C3H Mouse Embryo Cells," CANCER RESEARCH
38: 439-443.

Kerr79 Kerr, George D., 1979.
"Organ Dose Estimates for the Japanese Atomic Bomb
Survivors," HEALTH PHYSICS 37: 487-508.

Kerr87a Kerr, George D. + Tadashi Hashizume + Charles
W. Edington, 1987.
"Historical Review," pp.1-13 in Roes87.

Kerr87b Kerr, George D. + eleven others, 1987.
"Transport of Initial Radiations in Air over
Ground," Chapter 3, pp.66-142 in Roes87.

Kerr88 Kerr, George D., August 1988.
"Quality Factors," HEALTH PHYSICS 55, No.2:
pp.241-249.

Knea86 Kneale, George W. + Alice M. Stewart, 1986.
"Prenatal X-Rays and Cancers: Further Tests of
Data from the Oxford Survey of Childhood Cancers,"
HEALTH PHYSICS 51: 369-376.

Knea87 Kneale, George W. + Alice M. Stewart, 1987.
"Childhood Cancers in the UK and Their Relation to
Background Radiation," Chapter 16, pp.203-219, in
Jones87.

Knox87 Knox, E.G. + Alice M. Stewart + George W.
Kneale + E.A. Gilman, 1987.
"Prenatal Radiation and Childhood Cancer," J. SOC.
RADIOL. PROT. 8: 3-8.

Kondo75 Kondo, Sohei, 1975.
"DNA Repair and Evolutionary Considerations,"
pp.91-162 in ADVANCES IN BIOPHYSICS, VOLUME 7.
Edited by M. Kotani. (Tokyo/Baltimore: University
of Tokyo Press/University Park Press.)

Kondo84 Kondo, Sohei + H. Ryo + K. Fujikawa + A.
Fukunaga, 1984.
"The Threshold Effect in Mutagenesis by Radiation
and Chemicals in Relation to DNA Repair and Cell
Replacement," pp.121-131 in PROBLEMS OF THRESHOLD
IN CHEMICAL MUTAGENESIS. Edited by Y. Tazima + S.
Kondo + Y.Kuroda. (Mishima: Environmental Mutagen
Society of Japan.)

Kondo88 Kondo, Sohei, 1988.
"Altruistic Cell Suicide in Relation to Radiation
Hormesis," INTERNATIONAL JOURNAL OF RADIATION
BIOLOGY 53, No.1: 95-102.

Ku88 Kusunoki, Yoichiro + Mitoshi Akiyama + Seishi
Kyoizumi + Eda T. Bloom + Takashi Makinodan, 1988.
"Age-Related Alteration in the Composition of
Immunocompetent Blood Cells in Atomic Bomb
Survivors," INTERNATIONAL JOURNAL OF RADIATION
BIOLOGY 53, No.1: 189-198.

Lanc89 LANCET, anonymous. August 26, 1989.
"Who's for Hormesis," in the "Notes and News"
Section of the LANCET, August 26, 1989, p.518.

Land79 Land, Charles E. + Douglas H. McGregor,
1979.
"Breast Cancer Incidence among Atomic Bomb
Survivors: Implications for Radiobiologic Risk at
Low Doses," JOURNAL OF THE NATIONAL CANCER
INSTITUTE 62: pp.17-21.

Land80 Land, Charles E. + John D. Boice, Jr. + Roy
E. Shore + J.E. Norman + Masayoshi Tokunaga, 1980.
"Breast Cancer Risk from Low-Dose Exposures to
Ionizing Radiation: Results of Parallel Analysis
of 3 Exposed Populations of Women," JOURNAL OF THE
NATIONAL CANCER INSTITUTE 65: 353-376.

Land80b Land, Charles E., 1980.
"Estimating Cancer Risk from Low Doses of Ionizing
Radiation," SCIENCE 209: 1197-1202.

Land84 Land, Charles E. + Masayoshi Tokunaga, 1984.
"Induction Period,", pp.421-436 (esp. Figs. 3, 5,
6) in Boice84.

Land88 Land, Charles E., 1988.
"New Understanding from Epidemiology -- The Next 25
Years," HEALTH PHYSICS 55: 269-278.

Lang71 Langley, Russell, 1971.
"Significance Tests", Chapter 6, in "Practical
Statistics, Simply Explained" (New York, N.Y.:
Dover Publications.)

Le65 Lesher, S. + George A. Sacher + Douglas Grahn +
K. Hamilton + A. Gallese, 1965.
"Survival of Mice under Duration-of-Life Exposure
to Gamma Rays," RADIATION RESEARCH 24: 239-277.

Lee82 Lee, W. + R.P. Chiaccierini + B. Shleien et
al, 1982.
"Thyroid Tumours Following Iodine-131 or Localized
X-Irradiation to the Thyroid and Pituitary Glands
in Rats," RADIATION RESEARCH 92: 307-319.

Li81 Little, John B., 1981.
  "Influence of Noncarcinogenic Secondary Factors on
  Radiation Carcinogenesis," RADIATION RESEARCH 87:
  240-250.

Lie60 Liebhafsky, H.A. + H.G. Pfeiffer + E.H.
  Winslow + P.D. Zemany, 1960.
  "Reliability of X-Ray Emission Spectrography,"
  Chapter 10 in X-RAY ABSORPTION AND EMISSION IN
  ANALYTICAL CHEMISTRY. (New York, NY: John Wiley and
  Sons.)

Lin80 Linos, Athena + Joel E. Gray + A.L. Orvis +
  R.A. Kyle + W.M. O'Fallon + L.T. Kurland, 1980.
  "Low Dose Radiation and Leukemia," NEW ENGLAND J.
  OF MED. 302: 1101-05.

Linde89 Lindell, Bo, July 1989.
  "Comments on Various Views on the Concept of 'de
  Minimis'," letter in HEALTH PHYSICS 57, No.1:
  211-212.

Liu87 Liu, Shu Zheng + W.H. Liu + J.B. Sun, May 1987.
  "Radiation Hormesis: Its Expression in the Immune
  System," HEALTH PHYSICS 52, No.5: 579-583.

Lloyd80 Lloyd, D.C. + R.J. Purrott + E.J. Reeder,
  1980.
  "The Incidence of Unstable Chromosome Aberrations
  in Peripheral Blood Lymphocytes from Unirradiated
  and Occupationally Exposed People," MUTATION
  RESEARCH 72: 523-532.

Lloyd88 Lloyd, D.C. + A.A. Edwards + A. Leonard +
  Gh. Deknudt + A. Natarajan + G. Obe + F. Palitti +
  C. Tanzarella + E.J. Tawn, 1988.
  "Frequencies of Chromosomal Aberrations Induced in
  Human Blood Lymphocytes by Low Doses of X-Rays,"
  INTERNATIONAL JOURNAL OF RADIATION BIOLOGY 53,
  No.1: 49-55.

Lo80 Loewe, William E. + Edgar Mendelsohn, 1980.
  "Revised Estimates of Dose at Hiroshima and
  Nagasaki, and Possible Consequences for Radiation
  Induced Leukemia (Preliminary)", Report D-80-14.
  (Livermore, CA: Lawrence Livermore National
  Laboratory.)

Lo81 Loewe, William E. + Edgar Mendelsohn,
  October 1981.
  "Revised Dose Estimates at Hiroshima and Nagasaki,"
  HEALTH PHYSICS 41, No.4: 663-666.

Lo82 Loewe, William E. + Edgar Mendelsohn, 1982.
  "Neutron and Gamma-Ray Doses at Hiroshima and
  Nagasaki," NUCLEAR SCIENCE AND ENGINEERING 81:
  325-350.

Loken87 Loken, Merle K., August 7, 1987.
  "Physicians' Obligations in Radiation Issues," a
  Commentary article in JOURNAL OF THE AMER. MEDICAL
  ASSN. 258 (5): 673-676.

Lor55 Lorenz, Egon + J.W. Hollcroft + E. Miller +
  Charles C. Congdon + R. Schweisthal, 1955.
  "Long-Term Effects of Acute and Chronic Irradiation
  in Mice. I. Survival and Tumor Incidence Following
  Chronic Irradiation of 0.11 R per Day," JOURNAL OF
  THE NATIONAL CANCER INSTITUTE 15: 1049-1058.

Luc80 Luckey, Thomas D., 1980.
  HORMESIS WITH IONIZING RADIATION. (Boca Raton, FL:
  CRC Press.)

Luc82 Luckey, Thomas D., 1982.
  "Physiological Benefits from Low Levels of Ionizing
  Radiation," HEALTH PHYSICS 43: 771-789.

Mac62 MacMahon, Brian, 1962.
  "Prenatal X-Ray Exposure and Childhood Cancer,"
  JOURNAL OF THE NATIONAL CANCER INSTITUTE 28:
  1173-1191.

Magee87 Magee, John L. + Aloke Chatterjee, 1987.
  "Track Reactions of Radiation Chemistry," Chapter
  4, pp.171-214, in Free87a.

Maki68 is also TR-24-68. Maki, H. + T. Ishimaru +
  Hiroo Kato + T. Wakabayashi, 1968.
  CARCINOGENESIS IN ATOMIC BOMB SURVIVORS. Technical
  Report TR-24-68. (Hiroshima: RERF, today.)

Mart70 Martin, H. + E. Strong + R.H. Spiro, January
  1970.
  "Radiation-Induced Skin Cancer of the Head and
  Neck," CANCER, January 1970, 61-71.

Marte89 Martell, Edward A., 1989.
  Production of 'Spontaneous' Chromosomal Aberrations
  by Primordial and Cosmogenic Radionuclides."
  Submitted for publication.

McGr77 McGregor, Douglas H. + Charles E. Land + K.
  Choy + S. Tokuoka + P.I. Liu + T. Wakabayashi +
  Gilbert W. Beebe, 1977.
  "Breast Cancer Incidence among Atomic Bomb
  Survivors, Hiroshima and Nagasaki, 1950-1969,"
  JOURNAL OF THE NATIONAL CANCER INSTITUTE 59:
  799-811.

McTier84 McTiernan, Anne M. + Noel S. Weiss + Janet
  R. Daling, Sept. 1984.
  "Incidence of Thyroid Cancer in Women in Relation
  to Previous Exposure to Radiation Therapy and
  History of Thyroid Disease," JOURNAL OF THE
  NATIONAL CANCER INSTITUTE 73, No.3: 575-581.

Mi89 Miller, Anthony B. + Geoffrey R. Howe + Gregory
  J. Sherman + Joan P. Lindsay + Martin J. Yaffe +
  Paul J. Dinner + Harvey A. Risch + Dale L.
  Preston, Nov. 9, 1989.
  "Mortality from Breast Cancer after Irradiation
  during Fluoroscopic Examinations in Patients Being
  Treated for Tuberculosis," NEW ENGLAND JOURNAL OF
  MEDICINE 321, No.19: 1285-1289.

Modan77 Modan, Baruch + E. Ron + A. Werner, 1977.
  "Thyroid Cancer Following Scalp Irradiation,"
  RADIOLOGY 123: 741-744.

Modan89 Modan, Baruch + Angela Chetrit + Esther
  Alfandary + Leah Katz, March 25, 1989.
  "Increased Risk of Breast Cancer after Low-Dose
  Irradiation," LANCET 1, 1989: 629-631.

Mog89 Moghissi, A. Alan + Dixy Lee Ray, Nov. 1989.
  "Reply to Radiation Cancer Risk Series," letter in
  HEALTH PHYSICS 57, No.5: 841-842.

Mole74 Mole, Robin H., 1974.
  "Antenatal Irradiation and Childhood Cancer;
  Causation or Coincidence?" BRITISH JOURNAL OF
  CANCER 30: 199-208.

Mole78 Mole, Robin H., June 1978.
  "Review Article. The Sensitivity of the Human
  Breast to Cancer Induction by Ionizing Radiation,"
  BRITISH JOURNAL OF RADIOLOGY 51 No.606: 401-405.

Mole79 Mole, Robin H., 1979.
  "Radiation Effects on Pre-Natal Development and
  Their Radiological Significance," BRITISH JOURNAL
  OF RADIOLOGY 52: 89-101.

Mole87 Mole, Robin H., December 12, 1987.
  "Radiation, Cancer Risk, and the New Dosimetry,"
  letter in LANCET, Dec. 12, 1987, 1403-4.

Mole88 Mole, Robin H., March 5, 1988.
  "Assessing Radiation Risks," letter in LANCET 1,
  1988: p.531.

Mon84 Monson, R.R. + Brian MacMahon, 1984.
  "Prenatal X-Ray Exposures and Cancer in Children,"
  pp.97-106 in Boice84.

Mu89 Muirhead, Colin R. + Barbara K. Butland,
  December, 1989.
  "Dose-Response Analyses for the Japanese A-Bomb
  Survivors," letter in HEALTH PHYSICS 57, No.6:
  1035-1036.

My69 Myrden, J.A. + Hiltz, J.E., 1969.
  "Breast Cancer Following Multiple Fluoroscopies
  during Artificial Pneumothorax Treatment of
  Pulmonary Tuberculosis," CANADIAN MEDICAL
  ASSOCIATION JOURNAL 100: 1032-1034.

Naor87 Naor, D., 1987.
  "Suppressor Cells and Human Malignancy," CLINICAL
  IMMUNITY NEWSLETTER 8, No.5: 65-69.

Nas80 See Beir80.

===

Ncrp80 National Council on Radiation Protection and
    Measurements, 1980.
    INFLUENCE OF DOSE AND ITS DISTRIBUTION IN TIME ON
    DOSE-RESPONSE RELATIONSHIPS FOR LOW-LET
    RADIATIONS. NCRP Report 64. Prepared by NCRP's
    Scientific Committee 40. Individual authors are
    acknowledged in our Chapter 37. (Bethesda,
    Maryland, USA: NCRP.) Indexed.
Ncrp85 National Council on Radiation Protection and
    Measurements, 1985.
    INDUCTION OF THYROID CANCER BY IONIZING RADIATION.
    NCRP Report 80. (Bethesda, Maryland, USA: NCRP.)
New71 Newcombe, H.B. + McGregor, J.F., 1971.
    "Childhood Cancer Following Obstetric Radiography,"
    LANCET 1971, 2: 1151-1152.
Nih85 National Institutes of Health, January 4, 1985.
    REPORT OF THE NATIONAL INSTITUTES OF HEALTH AD HOC
    WORKING GROUP TO DEVELOP RADIOEPIDEMIOLOGICAL
    TABLES. Individual authors are acknowledged in our
    Chapter 37. NIH Publication No. 85-2748.
    (Washington, DC 20402: U.S. Government Printing
    Office.) No Index.
NOVA, October 25, 1988.
    "Do Scientists Cheat?", a one-hour broadcast of
    the PBS science series NOVA. Transcript # 1517.
    (Boston, MA 02134, USA: WGBH Educational
    Foundation, 125 Western Ave.)
Nrc85 U.S. Nuclear Regulatory Commission, July 1985.
    HEALTH EFFECTS MODEL FOR NUCLEAR POWER PLANT
    ACCIDENT CONSEQUENCE ANALYSIS. NUREG/CR-4214. The
    report was prepared by the Harvard School of
    Public Health under sub-contract to the Sandia
    National Laboratories. Principal investigators:
    John S. Evans + Dade W. Moeller + Douglas W.
    Cooper. (Washington, DC 20555: U.S. Nuclear
    Regulatory Commission, Division of Risk Analysis
    and Operations.) No index.
Nrc87 U.S. Nuclear Regulatory Commission, January
    1987.
    REPORT ON THE ACCIDENT AT THE CHERNOBYL NUCLEAR
    POWER STATION. NUREG-1250. The report was
    prepared by: Department of Energy.
    Electric Power Research Institute (industry group).
    Environmental Protection Agency.
    Federal Emergency Management Agency.
    Institute of Nuclear Power Operations (industry
    group).
    Nuclear Regulatory Commission.
    The section on Health and Environmental
    Consequences was prepared by J. Pushkin + C.
    Nelson + D. Janes + S. Myers of the Environmental
    Protection Agency.
    No index.
Nrc89 U.S. Nuclear Regulatory Commission, May 1989.
    HEALTH EFFECTS MODELS FOR NUCLEAR POWER PLANT
    ACCIDENT CONSEQUENCE ANALYSIS. NUREG/CR-4214,
    Rev.1, Part 2, "Scientific Bases for Health
    Effects Models." This revision was prepared under
    contract with the Sandia National Laboratories,
    Albuquerque, New Mexico. (Washington, DC 20555:
    U.S. Nuclear Regulatory Commission.)
NUREG-1250 is the same as Nrc87.
NUREG/CR-4214 is the same as Nrc85.
Nyt82 NEW YORK TIMES, September 26, 1982.
    "Peking Is Ready to Negotiate but Hong Kong Is
    Still Jittery," by Steve Lohr. Filed from Hong
    Kong. Page E-3.
Nyt88 NEW YORK TIMES, July 14, 1988.
    Wald, Matthew L., "Cleanup Estimate for A-Bomb
    Plants Is Called Low," p.A16.
Nyt89a NEW YORK TIMES, February 25, 1989.
    Associated Press, "Rise in Cleanup Cost Seen."
Nyt89b NEW YORK TIMES, April 27, 1989.
    "Soviets Curb News about Disasters: Reporting
    Nuclear Accidents To Be Restricted by Ruling Given
    by Energy Chief," by Esther B. Fein, filed from
    Moscow.

Nyt89c NEW YORK TIMES, June 6, 1989.
    "Errors Prompt Proposals to Improve 'Peer Review'
    at Science Journals," by Lawrence K. Altman, M.D.
    Page C-3.
Ober89 Oberfield, Richard A. + Glenn Steele, Jr. +
    John L. Gollan + David Sherman, July/Aug. 1989.
    "Liver Cancer," CA - A CANCER JOURNAL FOR
    CLINICIANS 39 (No.4): 206-218.
Oka87 Okajima, Shunzo + Shoichiro Fujita (+ John H.
    Harley, consultant), 1987.
    "Radiation Doses from Residual Radioactivity,"
    Chapter 6, pp.205-226 in Roes87.
Oli84 Olivieri, Gregorio + Judy Bodycote + Sheldon
    Wolff, February 10, 1984.
    "Adaptive Response of Human Lymphocytes to Low
    Concentrations of Radioactive Thymidine," SCIENCE
    223: 594-597.
Par87 Paretzke, Herwig G., 1987.
    "Radiation Track Structure Theory," Chapter 3,
    pp.89-169, in Free87a.
Phs80 Public Health Service, 1980.
    "X-Rays: Get the Picture on Protection." Folder
    published by the U.S. Dept. of Health & Human
    Services, Public Health Service, in cooperation
    with the American College of Radiology and the
    American Society of Radiologic Technologists. HHS
    Publication (FDA) 80-8088.
Pier87 Pierce, Donald A., October 1987.
    "A Summary of Some Results of the Dosimetry
    Revisions for the Atomic Bomb Survivors," paper
    presented at the OECD Workshop on Epidemiology and
    Radiation Protection, Paris.
Pier88 Pierce, Donald A. August 11, 1988.
    Letter from Donald A. Pierce, Chief of the
    Department of Statistics at RERF, to John W.
    Gofman, in reply to a request for additional data.
Poh83 Pohl-Ruling, J. and 17 co-authors, 1983.
    "Effect of Low-Dose Acute X-Irradiation on the
    Frequencies of Chromosomal Aberrations in Human
    Peripheral Lymphocytes IN VITRO," MUTATION
    RESEARCH 110: 71-82.
Pr85 Preston, Dale L., March 1985.
    Report presented at the Third U.S.-Japan Joint
    Workshop for Reassessment of Atomic Bomb Radiation
    Dosimetry in Hiroshima and Nagasaki, March 12-14,
    1985, Pasadena, California.
Pr86 is also TR-1-86. Preston, Dale L. + Hiroo Kato
    + Kenneth J. Kopecky + Shoichiro Fujita, 1986.
    LIFE SPAN STUDY REPORT 10, PART 1, CANCER
    MORTALITY AMONG A-BOMB SURVIVORS IN HIROSHIMA AND
    NAGASAKI, 1950-1982. RERF Technical Report
    TR-1-86. (Hiroshima: RERF.)
Pr87a is TR-1-86 abbreviated. Preston, Dale L. +
    Hiroo Kato + Kenneth J. Kopecky + Shoichiro Fujita,
    1987.
    "Studies of the Mortality of A-Bomb Survivors,
    Report 8; Cancer Mortality 1950-1982" (RERF
    TR-1-86). RADIATION RESEARCH 111: pp.151-178.
Pr87b is also TR-9-87. Preston, Dale L. + Donald A.
    Pierce, 1987.
    THE EFFECT OF CHANGES IN DOSIMETRY ON CANCER
    MORTALITY RISK ESTIMATES IN THE ATOMIC BOMB
    SURVIVORS. RERF Technical Report TR-9-87.
    (Hiroshima: RERF.)
Pr88 is TR-9-87 abbreviated. Preston, Dale L. +
    Donald A. Pierce, 1988.
    "The Effect of Changes in Dosimetry on Cancer
    Mortality Risk Estimates in the Atomic Bomb
    Survivors" (RERF TR-9-87). RADIATION RESEARCH 114:
    437-466.
Pre87 Preston-Martin, S. + L. Bernstein + M.C. Pike
    + A.A. Maldonado + B.E. Henderson, February 1987.
    "Thyroid Cancer among Young Women Related to Prior
    Thyroid Disease and Pregnancy History," BRITISH
    JOURNAL OF CANCER 55, No.2: 191-195.

Pres73 Preston, R.J. + J.G. Brewen, 1973.
"X-Ray Induced Translocation in Spermatogonia. I.
Dose and Fractionation Responses in Mice," MUTATION
RESEARCH 19: 215-223.

Pres80 Preston, R.J., 1980.
"The Effect of Cytosine Arabinoside on the
Frequency of X-Ray-Induced Chromosome Aberrations
in Normal Human Leukocytes," MUTATION RESEARCH 69:
71-79.

Rad82 Radford, Edward P., Sept. 26, 1982.
In "A Roundtable: With Radiation, How Little Is
Too Much?" NEW YORK TIMES, WEEK IN REVIEW, SECTION
4: p. EY 19.

Ras74 Rasmussen, Norman C., August 1974.
Rasmussen was director of the Atomic Energy
Commission's study, in 14 volumes:
AN ASSESSMENT OF ACCIDENT RISKS IN U.S. COMMERCIAL
NUCLEAR POWER PLANTS, WASH-1400, widely called "The
Rasmussen Report."

Ras89 Rasmussen, Norman C., April 1989.
Quoted at p.411 in "Living with Radiation," by
Charles E. Cobb, Jr., in NATIONAL GEOGRAPHIC 175,
No.4: pp.403-437.

Ray86 Ray, Dixy Lee, October 27, 1986.
Book review by Ray of UNDER THE NUCLEAR CLOUD: THE
DECADES OF NUCLEAR TESTING (by Richard L. Miller).
In the newspaper THE WASHINGTON TIMES (Washington,
D.C.), Section M, p.1, 4.

Ray87 Ray, Dixy Lee, April 30, 1987.
Quoted by Joel Connelly in "Dixy: Chernobyl
Accident 'Was Not a Catastrophe'," in the
newspaper SEATTLE POST-INTELLIGENCER, April 30,
1987, p.A9.

Renn86 Rennie, Drummond, November 7, 1986.
"Guarding the Guardians: A Conference on Editorial
Peer Review," JOURNAL OF THE AMERICAN MEDICAL
ASSOCIATION 256, No.17: 2391-2392.

Renn88 Rennie, Drummond + Elizabeth Knoll, August
1, 1988. "Investigating Peer Review," ANNALS OF
INTERNAL MEDICINE 109, No.3: 181.
See also "Guarding the Guardians" Proceedings
in JOURNAL OF THE AMERICAN MEDICAL
ASSOCIATION, ENTIRE ISSUE, March 9,1990.

Roes68 Roesch, William C., 1968.
"Mathematical Theory of Radiation Fields," Chapter
5, pp.229-274 in RADIATION DOSIMETRY, Vol. 1.
(New York: Academic Press.)

Roes87 Roesch, William C. (editor), 1987.
U.S.-JAPAN JOINT REASSESSMENT OF ATOMIC BOMB
RADIATION DOSIMETRY IN HIROSHIMA AND NAGASAKI:
FINAL REPORT, VOL. 1., DS86 DOSIMETRY SYSTEM
1986. (Hiroshima: RERF.) No index.

Ron87 Ron, Elaine + Ruth A. Kleinerman + John D.
Boice, Jr. + Virginia A. LiVolsi + John T.
Flannery + Joseph F. Fraumeni, Jr., July 1987.
"A Population-Based Case-Control Study of Thyroid
Cancer," JOURNAL OF THE NATIONAL CANCER INSTITUTE
79, No.1: 1-12.

Ron88 Ron, E. + Baruch Modan + J.D. Boice, Jr., 1988.
"Mortality after Radiotherapy for Ringworm of the
Scalp," AMERICAN JOURNAL OF EPIDEMIOLOGY 127:
713-725.

Rossi84 Rossi, Harald H. + E.J. Hall, 1984.
"The Multicellular Nature of Radiation Carcinogenesis," pp.359-367 in Boice84.

Ru66 Rust, J.H. + R.J. Robertson + E.F. Staffeldt +
George A. Sacher + Douglas Grahn + R.J.M. Fry,1966.
"Effects of Lifetime Periodic Gamma-Ray Exposure on
the Survival and Pathology of Guinea Pigs," in
RADIATION AND AGING, edited by P.J. Lindop and
George A. Sacher. (London: Taylor and Francis.)

Run85 Runyon, R., 1985.
FUNDAMENTALS OF STATISTICS IN THE BIOLOGICAL,
MEDICAL, AND HEALTH SCIENCES. (Boston, MA:
Duxbury Press.)

Sa64 Sacher, George A. + Douglas Grahn, 1964.
"Survival of Mice under Duration-of-Life Exposure
to Gamma Rays," JOURNAL OF THE NATIONAL CANCER
INSTITUTE 32: 277-321.

Sag87 Sagan, Leonard A., May 1987.
"Reply to Dr. Gofman's Comments on the Health
Effects of Ionizing Radiation," letter in HEALTH
PHYSICS 52, No.5: 680.

Sag89 Sagan, Leonard, August 11, 1989.
"On Radiation, Paradigms, and Hormesis," in
the Policy Forum Section, SCIENCE 245: 574,
621.

Sas68 Sasaki, M.S. + H. Miyata, 1968.
"Biological Dosimetry in Atomic Bomb Survivors,"
NATURE 220: 1189.

Shad87a Shadley, Jeffery D. + Sheldon Wolff, 1987.
"Very Low Doses of X-Rays Can Cause Human
Lymphocytes to Become Less Susceptible to Ionizing
Radiation," MUTAGENESIS 2, No.2: 95-96.

Shad87b Shadley, Jeffery D. + Veena Afzal + Sheldon
Wolff, 1987.
"Characterization of the Adaptive Response to
Ionizing Radiation Induced by Low Doses of X Rays
to Human Lymphocytes," RADIATION RESEARCH 111:
511-517.

Shi87 is also TR-12-87. Shimizu, Yukiko + Hiroo Kato
+ William J. Schull + Dale L. Preston + Shoichiro
Fujita + Donald A. Pierce, 1987.
LIFE SPAN STUDY REPORT 11, PART 1. COMPARISON OF
RISK COEFFICIENTS FOR SITE-SPECIFIC CANCER
MORTALITY BASED ON THE DS86 AND T65DR SHIELDED
KERMA AND ORGAN DOSES. RERF Technical Report
TR-12-87. (Hiroshima: RERF.)

Shi88 is also TR-5-88. Shimizu, Yukiko + Hiroo Kato
+ William J. Schull, 1988.
LIFE SPAN STUDY REPORT 11, PART 2. CANCER
MORTALITY IN THE YEARS 1950-1985 BASED ON THE
RECENTLY REVISED DOSES (DS86). RERF Technical
Report TR-5-88. (Hiroshima: RERF.)

Sho77 Shore, R.E. + L.H. Hempelmann + E. Kowaluk +
P.S. Mansur + B.S. Pasternack + R.E. Albert + G.E.
Haughie, 1977.
"Breast Neoplasms in Women Treated with X-Rays for
Acute Postpartum Mastitis," JOURNAL OF THE NATL.
CANCER INST. 59: 813-822.

Sho80 Shore, R.E. + E.D. Woodard + L.H. Hempelmann +
B.S. Pasternack, 1980.
"Synergism between Radiation and Other Risk Factors
for Breast Cancer," PREV. MED. 9: 815-822.

Sho84 Shore, R.E. + R.E. Albert + M. Reed + N.
Harley + B.S. Pasternack, 1984.
"Skin Cancer Incidence among Children Irradiated
for Ringworm of the Scalp," RADIATION RESEARCH
100: 192-204.

Sho85 Shore, R.E. + E. Woodard + N. Hildreth + P.
Dvoretsky + L. Hempelmann + B. Pasternak, 1985.
"Thyroid Tumors Following Thymus Irradiation, "
JOURNAL OF THE NATIONAL CANCER INSTITUTE 74:
1177-1184.

Sho86 Shore, R.E. + N. Hildreth + E. Woodard + P.
Dvoretsky + L. Hempelmann + B. Pasternak, 1986.
"Breast Cancer among Women Given X-Ray Therapy for
Acute Postpartum Mastitis," JOURNAL OF THE
NATIONAL CANCER INSTITUTE 77: 689-696.

Sies85 Sies, Helmut (editor), 1985.
OXIDATIVE STRESS. (New York: Academic Press.)

Silver90 Silverberg, Edwin + Catherine C. Boring +
Teresa S. Squires, Jan-Feb. 1990.
"Cancer Statistics 1990," CA - A CANCER JOURNAL FOR
CLINICIANS 40, No.1: 9-26.

Sin85 Sinclair, Warren K., 1985.
"Experimental RBE Values of High LET Radiations at
Low Doses and the Implications for Quality Factor
Assignment," RADIATION PROTECTION AND DOSIMETRY 13:
319-326.

Sin88 Sinclair, Warren K., August 1988.
"Trends in Radiation Protection - A View from the
National Council on Radiation Protection and
Measurements (NCRP)", HEALTH PHYSICS 55, No.2:
149-157.

Smith79 Smith, P.G. and R. Doll, 1979.
"Age- and Time-Dependent Changes in the Rates of
Radiation-Induced Cancers in Patients with
Ankylosing Spondylitis Following a Single Course
of X-ray Treatment," in LATE BIOLOGICAL EFFECTS
OF IONIZING RADIATION, VOLUME 1. (Vienna, Austria:
International Atomic Energy Agency.)

Smith84 Smith, P.G., 1984.
"Late Effects of X-ray Treatment of Ankylosing
Spondylitis," pp. 107-118 in Boice 84.

So81 Society for Promotion of Cancer Research, 1981.
FIGURES ON CANCER IN JAPAN. Data from Japan Vital
Statistics, Ministry of Health and Welfare.
(Tokyo, Japan: Society for Promotion of Cancer
Research.)

South87 Southwood, Richard, 1987.
"Opening Remarks," [for the conference], pp.3-6 in
Jones 87.

Spen83 Spengler, R.F. + D.H. Cook + E.A. Clarke +
P.M. Olley + A.M. Newman, 1983.
"Cancer Mortality Following Cardiac
Catheterization: A Preliminary Follow-Up Study on
4,891 Irradiated Children," PEDIATRICS 71: 235-239.

Steer73 is also TR-16-73. Steer A. + I.M. Moriyama +
K. Shimizu, 1973.
ABCC-JNIH PATHOLOGY STUDIES, HIROSHIMA AND
NAGASAKI. REPORT 3. THE AUTOPSY PROGRAM AND THE
LSS STUDY: JANUARY 1951-DECEMBER 1970. Atomic
Bomb Casualty Commission Technical Report
TR-16-73. (Hiroshima: RERF.)

Stew56 Stewart, Alice M + J.W. Webb + B.D. Giles +
D. Hewitt, 1956.
"Preliminary Communication: Malignant Disease in
Childhood and Diagnostic Irradiation In-Utero,"
LANCET 1956, 2: 447.

Stew58 Stewart, Alice M. + J.W. Webb +
D. Hewitt, 1958.
"A Survey of Childhood Malignancies," BRITISH
MEDICAL JOURNAL 1958, 2: 1495-1508.

Stew70 Stewart, Alice M. + George W. Kneale, 1970.
"Radiation Dose Effects in Relation to Obstetric
X-Rays and Childhood Cancers," LANCET 1970, 1:
1185-1188.

Strom58 Strominger, D. + J.M. Hollander + Glenn T.
Seaborg, April 1958.
"Table of Isotopes," REVIEWS OF MODERN PHYSICS 30,
No.2, Part 2: 585-904.

Sz78 Sztanyik, L.B., 1978.
"Late Radiobiological Effects of A-Bombing in
Japan," in LATE BIOLOGICAL EFFECTS OF IONIZING
RADIATION, VOL I. (Vienna, Austria: Internatl.
Atomic Energy Agency.)

Tay80 Taylor, Lauriston S., 1980.
"Some Nonscientific Influences on Radiation
Protection Standards and Practice. The 1980
Sievert Lecture," HEALTH PHYSICS 39: 851-874.

Terz76 Terzaghi, M. + J.B. Little, 1976.
"X-Radiation-Induced Transformation in a C3H Mouse
Embryo-Derived Cell Line," CANCER RESEARCH 36:
1367-1374.

Time89 TIME MAGAZINE, November 13, 1989, p.73.
"The Chernobyl Cover-Up: Are Soviet Officials
Still Concealing the Truth about the Disaster?"
Written by Michael Lemonick. Reported by Glenn
Garelik (Washington DC) and Paul Hofheinz (Moscow).

Toku84 Tokunaga, Masayoshi + Charles E. Land +
Tsutomu Yamamoto + Mashahide Asano + Shoji Tokuoka
+ Haruo Ezaki + Issei Nishimora + T. Fujikura,1984.
"Breast Cancer among Atomic Bomb Survivors,"
pp.45-56 (esp. Fig.2 p.49), in Boice84.

Toku85 Tokunaga, Masayoshi + C.E. Land + T. Yamamoto
+ M. Asano + S. Tokuoka + H. Ezaki + I. Nishimori,
October 1985.
INCIDENCE OF FEMALE BREAST CANCER AMONG A-BOMB
SURVIVORS, HIROSHIMA AND NAGASAKI, 1950-1980. RERF
Technical Report TR-15-84. (Hiroshima: RERF.)

TR-15-63. See Jab63.
TR-24-68. See Maki68.
TR-11-70. See Bee70 and Bee71.
TR-10-71. See Jab71 and Jab72.
TR-16-73. See Steer73.
TR-1-77.   See Bee77 and Bee78.
TR-12-80. See Kato80 and Kato82.
TR-15-84. See Toku85.
TR-1-86.   See Pr86 and Pr87a.
TR-9-87.   See Pr87b and Pr88.
TR-12-87. See Shi87.
TR-5-88.   See Shi88.

Tusc80 Tuschl, Helga + Hans Altmann + Rozi Kovac +
Alexander Topaloglou + Dietmar Egg + Robert
Gunther, 1980.
"Effects of Low-Dose Radiation on Repair Processes
in Human Lymphocytes," RADIATION RESEARCH 81: 1-9.

Un77 UNSCEAR or United Nations Scientific Committee
on the Effects of Atomic Radiation, 1977.
SOURCES AND EFFECTS OF IONIZING RADIATION.
Individual authors are acknowledged in our Chapter
37. (New York, NY: United Nations.) No index.

Un82 UNSCEAR or United Nations Scientific Committee
on the Effects of Atomic Radiation, 1982.
IONIZING RADIATION: SOURCES AND BIOLOGICAL
EFFECTS. Individual authors are acknowledged in
our Chapter 37. (New York, NY 10017: United
Nations.) No index.

Un86 UNSCEAR or United Nations Scientific Committee
on the Effects of Atomic Radiation, 1986.
GENETIC AND SOMATIC EFFECTS OF IONIZING RADIATION.
Individual authors are acknowledged in our Chapter
37. (New York, NY 10017: United Nations.) No
index. Sales Number E.86.IX.9. ISBN
92-1-142123-3. 004800P.

Un88 UNSCEAR or United Nations Scientific Committee
on the Effects of Atomic Radiation, 1988.
SOURCES, EFFECTS AND RISKS OF IONIZING RADIATION.
Individual authors are acknowledged in our Chapter
37. (New York, NY 10017: United Nations.) No
index. Sales Number E.88.IX.7. ISBN
92-1-142143-8. 09000P.

Undemo86 United Nations Statistical Office of the
Dept. of International & Social Affairs, 1986.
DEMOGRAPHIC YEARBOOK 1984. (New York, NY 10017:
United Nations.)

Uni89 University of California Academic Senate,
November 1989.
"Science Wrestling with Question of Fraudulent
Research," NOTICE: NEWS FOR THE UC FACULTY, Volume
14, No.2: 1-4.

Up87 Upton, Arthur C., 1987.
"Prevention of Work-Related Injuries and Diseases:
Lessons from Experience with Ionizing Radiation,"
AMER. JOURNAL OF INDUSTRIAL MED. 12: 291-309.

Up88 Upton, Arthur C., 1988.
"Evolving Perspectives on the Concept of Dose in
Radiobiology and Radiation Protection," HEALTH
PHYSICS 55: 605-614.

Up89 Upton, Arthur C., April 1989.
As quoted in "Living with Radiation" (at pages 418,
420), by Charles E. Cobb, Jr. in NATIONAL GEOGRAPHIC
175, No.4: 403-437.

===

Ussr86 U.S.S.R. State Committee for Using the Atomic
  Energy.
  THE ACCIDENT AT THE CHERNOBYL ATOMIC ENERGY
  STATION AND ITS CONSEQUENCES; DATA PREPARED FOR
  THE INTERNATIONAL ATOMIC ENERGY AGENCY EXPERT
  CONFERENCE 25-29 AUGUST 1986 IN VIENNA.
  (Translated by U.S. Dept. of Energy.)
Ussr87a U.S.S.R. Ministry of Health, May 1987.
  ANALYSIS OF THE RADIOLOGICAL CONSEQUENCES OF THE
  ACCIDENT AT THE CHERNOBYL NUCLEAR POWER PLANT FOR
  THE POPULATION OF THE EUROPEAN REGIONS OF THE USSR.
  (Moscow: Ministry of Health. Also [U.N] World
  Health Organization Information Document
  A40/INF.DOC./9, May 1987.)
Ussr87b See Ilyin87.
Ussr88 See Ilyin88.
Vir82 Virsik, R.P. + R. Blohm + K.P.Herman + H.
  Modler + D. Harder, 1982.
  PROCEEDINGS OF THE EIGHTH SYMPOSIUM ON
  MICRODOSIMETRY, edited by J. Booz and H.G. Ebert,
  pp.409-422. (Luxembourg 8395: Euratom.)
Wag89 Wagner, Henry N., Jr., and Linda E. Ketchum,
  1989.
  LIVING WITH RADIATION: THE RISK, THE PROMISE.
  (Baltimore and London: The Johns Hopkins University
  Press.)
Waka83 Wakabayashi, T. + Hiroo Kato + T. Ikeda +
  William J. Schull, 1983.
  "Studies of the Mortality of A-Bomb Survivors,
  Report 7, Part 3. Incidence of Cancer in 1959-1978,
  Based on the Tumor Registry, Nagasaki," RADIATION
  RESEARCH 93: 112-146.
Wat89a Watkins, James, June 28, 1989.
  Quoted in "Energy Chief Raps Nuclear Waste Setup,"
  WASHINGTON POST NEWS SERVICE, as published in the
  SAN FRANCISCO CHRONICLE, June 28, 1989, page A-14.
Wat89b Watkins, James, December 13, 1989.
  Quoted in "Problems Plague U.S. Bomb Plants," by
  Matthew L. Wald, NEW YORK TIMES NEWS SERVICE, as
  published in the SAN FRANCISCO CHRONICLE, Briefing
  Section, page 8, December 13, 1989.
Webs81 Webster, Edward W., 1981.
  "On the Question of Cancer Induction by Small X-Ray
  Doses," AMERICAN JOURNAL OF ROENTGENOLOGY 37:
  647-666.
Webs82 Webster, Edward W., September 26, 1982.
  Quoted in 3-way colloquium (John Gofman, Edward
  Radford, Edward Webster) entitled "A Roundtable:
  With Radiation, How Little Is Too Much?", NEW YORK
  TIMES Week in Review Section (4), September 26,
  1982, p.EY-19.
Webs87 Webster, Edward W., April 1987.
  "Chernobyl Predictions and the Chinese
  Contribution," in the Newsline Section,
  "Commentary" feature, JOURNAL OF NUCLEAR MEDICINE
  28, No.4: 423-425. Based on an invited paper
  delivered at the 4th World Congress of Nuclear
  Medicine and Biology, Nov. 6, 1986, in Buenos
  Aires, Argentina.
Wien86 Wiencke, John K. + Veena Afzal + Gregorio
  Olivieri + Sheldon Wolff, 1986.
  "Evidence that the [3H]thymidine-induced Adaptive
  Response of Human Lymphocytes to Subsequent Doses
  of X-rays Involves the Induction of a Chromosomal
  Repair Mechanism," MUTAGENESIS 1, No.5: 375-380.
Wolfe86 Wolfe, Bertram, Sept. 27, 1986.
  "Public Has Exaggerated Fears of Exposure to
  Radiation," article in THE DENVER POST, Sept. 27,
  1986, p.4-B.

Wolff84 Wolff, Sheldon, June 1984.
  As quoted in "Low Doses of Radiation May Protect
  against Later Damage," by Robert Sanders, in UCSF
  MAGAZINE 7, No.2: 52. (San Francisco: University
  of California at San Francisco, Medical Center.)
Wolff88 Wolff, Sheldon + Veena Afzal + J.K. Wiencke
  + Gregorio Olivieri + A. Michaeli, 1988.
  "Human Lymphocytes Exposed to Low Doses of
  Ionizing Radiations Become Refractory to High
  Doses of Radiation As Well As to Chemical Mutagens
  That Induce Double-Strand Breaks in DNA,"
  INTERNATIONAL JOURNAL OF RADIATION BIOLOGY 53,
  No.1: 39-48.
Wolff89 Wolff, Sheldon, August 11, 1989.
  "Are Radiation-Induced Effects Hormetic?" in the
  Policy Forum section, SCIENCE 245: 575, 621.
Woo87 Woolson, William A. + Stephen D. Egbert +
  Michael L. Gritzner, 1987.
  "Dosimetry System 1986," Chapter 9, pp.405-431 in
  Roes87.
Wsj87 WALL STREET JOURNAL, April 13, 1987.
  "Few in Hong Kong Still Trust Promises of Britain
  and China," by June Kronholz, filed from Hong
  Kong. Pages A-1 and A-15.
Wsj89 WALL STREET JOURNAL, March 6, 1989.
  "Villagers Suffering Chernobyl's Fallout Face
  Soviet Silence," by Peter Gumbel, filed from
  Kiev. Pages A-1 and A-8.
Ya80 Yalow, Rosalyn S., March 9, 1980.
  "Science: Our Hope, Not Our Foe," in the Long
  Island newspaper NEWSDAY, "Idea" Section, p.1,
  March 9, 1980.
Ya81 Yalow, Rosalyn S., February 24, 1981.
  Quoted in story by Linda Sillitoe, "A-tests and
  Cancer: Nobelist Objects to Link," DESERET NEWS
  (Salt Lake City), p.2-B.
Ya82 Yalow, Rosalyn S., December 1982.
  "Psychology Tomorrow," in PSYCHOLOGY TODAY,
  December 1982, p.26.
Ya83 Yalow, Rosalyn S., 1983.
  "Reply to K.Z. Morgan's Comments," COMMENTS MOL.
  CELL BIOPHYSICS 2: 49-55.
Ya84 Yalow, Rosalyn S., April 1984.
  "Nuclear Nonsense," in SAVVY magazine, April 1984,
  p.21.
Ya88 Yalow, Rosalyn S., June 13, 1988.
  "Unwarranted Fear about the Effects of Radiation
  Leads to Bad Science Policy," in THE SCIENTIST
  ("The Newspaper for the Science Professional,"
  Philadelphia) June 13, 1988, pp.11-12.
Ya89 Yalow, Rosalyn S., March/April 1989.
  "The Contributions of Medical Physicists to
  Radiation Phobia," a guest editorial invited by
  John S. Laughlin, in MEDICAL PHYSICS 16, No.2:
  159-161.
Yoshi88 Yoshimoto, Yasuhiko + Hiroo Kato + William
  J. Schull, Sept. 17, 1988.
  "Risk of Cancer among Children Exposed In-Utero to
  A-Bomb Radiations, 1950-84," LANCET, Sept. 17,
  1988, pp.665-669.
Zu86 Zufan, Tao + Wei Luxin, 1986.
  "An Epidemiological Investigation of Mutational
  Diseases in the High Background Radiation Area of
  Yangjiang, China," in JOURNAL OF RADIATION RESEARCH
  (JAPAN) 27: 141-150. Presented by Tao Zufan at the
  28th Annual Meeting of the Japan Radiation Research
  Society, Oct. 16, 1985, Nara City.

Index and Glossary

● -- Format of Exponents and Subscripts in This Book :
==

In this book, "raised to a power" is most often expressed by the symbol ^. Thus, Dose^2 means Dose Squared. Dose^1.4 means Dose raised to the power 1.4 . Dose^0.5, which is Dose raised to the power (1/2), is of course the same as the square root of Dose. 10^6 means million, and 10^-6 means "per million." Rad^-1 means "per rad,", and cm^-3 means "per cubic centimeter."

Less frequently, we use the common computer notation in which E+ or E- signifies the base "10" and the next number signifies the power. Thus 2.3E+13 means 2.3 x 10^13, and 2.3E-13 means 2.3 x 10^-13. Our table 20-C illustrates the conversion from one format to another.

For the "prime" and "double-prime" superscripts, we use the single and double quote-marks.
Subscripts in this book are indicated by their position, not by their size. In Chapter 15, for instance D2 means D-sub-two. By contrast, 2D means (2 times D).

● -- Significant Figures, Trailing Digits, Rounding-Off :
==

Sometimes entries in our tables appear to be "wrong" in the last digit. This is a common nuisance in the computer age, where analysts are routinely working with many more "trailing digits" than the readers can see. The "trailing digit" phenomenon is illustrated in our Table 11-A, Step 1.

In efforts to reduce the ostensible discrepancies, analysts are discarding the past rules about rounding-off and about showing only "significant figures." For instance, the BEIR-3 Report shows lots of non-significant digits, and comments (Beir80, p.145) that "... the intention is to facilitate the reconstruction of the final results by readers who may wish to reconstruct them, rather than to suggest an unwarranted accuracy of the estimates." The BEIR-5 Report makes exactly the same comment (Beir90, p.192).

We think that this BEIR decision is a piece of good common sense, and we also show many digits in this book which are not formally "significant." Some small discrepancies develop no matter what one does, however, since input sometimes comes from a "rounded-off" hard-copy, and sometimes from the digit-rich computer memory. Readers should just not worry over small discrepancies, but of course we encourage readers to tell us if any big ones turn up.

● -- Format of the Index :
==

THE STAR FLAG. For readers whose first language is not English, or who are new to this particular field, the entries flagged by a star locate the meaning of a term or phrase in context. Some definitions, if brief, are provided right in the Index. For easy reference, the Index decodes abbreviations too.

SEQUENCE. Our alphabetical sequence of entries ignores space and punctuation. Thus an entry like "K-values, by age" would be alphabetized as if it were a single word: Kvaluesbyage.
The "star flag" comes ahead of any comparable entries.

INDEX ABBREVIATIONS. Ta means Table. Pt means Part. T means through.
Thus 23-12 T 15 means "Chapter 23, pages 12 through 15."

IMAGES OR PHRASES: For readers who recall an image but not the context, some specific words and phrases receive their own entries (for instance: Canary; Peoria; Lizzie Borden; "Radiobiological grounds"; "Tortured mathematics"; "Violent disassembly").

===

===
● -- "To believe with certainty, we must begin with
doubting." -- Stanilaus, King of Poland
===

==
● -- "If at first you don't succeed, you are
running about average." -- M.H. Alderson
==

==
● -- "If you have an important point to make, don't
try to be subtle or clever. Use a pile-driver.
Hit the point once. Then come back and hit it
again. Then hit it a third time -- a tremendous
whack!" -- Winston Churchill
==

==

==
● -- "If you have anything to tell me of
importance, for God's sake begin at the end."
-- Sara Jeanette Duncan
==

==
● -- "If you keep your mind sufficiently open,
people will throw a lot of rubbish into it."
-- William A. Orton
==

●   ==

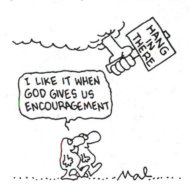

===
● -- "When your work speaks for itself, don't
interrupt." -- Henry J. Kaiser
===

===
● -- "What is research, but a blind date with
knowledge." -- Will Henry
===

● ===

===
● -- "The larger the island of knowledge, the
longer the shore of wonder." -- Ralph Sockman
===

===

===
● -- "It makes all the difference in the world
whether we put truth in the first place, or in the
second place." -- John Morley
===

==

==

==
● -- "To get maximum attention, it's hard to beat a
good, big mistake!" -- Unknown
==

● ==

===
● -- "In nature, there are neither rewards nor
punishments -- there are consequences." -- Robert
G. Ingersoll
===

==

==
● -- "We cannot command nature except by obeying
her." -- Francis Bacon
==

==
● -- "For peace of mind, resign as general manager
of the universe." -- Larry Eisenberg
==

● ==

===
● -- "If the shepherds do not believe that wolves
exist, then some of the sheep are going to have a
bad time." -- David F. Horrobin
===

● ===

The occurrence of major radioactivity releases from the Chernobyl accident has made the use of the (S.I.) Becquerel unit somewhat awkward. The release of 2 million Curies (2 megacuries) of 137-Cs is the same release as 2 x 3.7 x 10^10 x, 10^6; or 7.4 x 10^16 Becquerels. The reader will encounter units such as the peta-Becquerel, which is 10^15 Becquerels. Therefore there are 74 peta-Becquerels per 2 megacuries of 137-Cs. Some of the additional units used with Becquerels are as follows:

1 exa-Becquerel = 10^18 Becquerels;	1 peta-Becquerel = 10^15 Becquerels;
1 tera-Becquerel = 10^12 Becquerels;	1 giga-Becquerel = 10^9 Becquerels;
1 mega-Becquerel = 10^6 Becquerels ;	1 kilo-Becquerel = 10^3 Becquerels.

For many years and with limited success, journals have been trying to replace rads and rems by the International System of Units (SI Units) -- which are Grays and Sieverts.

There is 1 centi-gray (cGy) per 1 rad. There is 1 centi-sievert (cSv) per 1 rem.

WE USE THIS ONE-FOR-ONE EQUIVALENCE, and intentionally avoid Grays (Gy), milligrays (mGy), Sieverts (Sv) and millisieverts (mSv) in our own writing.

1	Gy .... per 100 rads		1	Sv .... per 100 rems	
1	cGy ********** per 1 rad		1	cSv ********** per 1 rem	
0.01	Gy .... per 1 rad		0.01	Sv .... per 1 rem	
10	mGy .... per 1 rad		10	mSv .... per 1 rem	
1	mGy .... per 100 millirads		1	mSv .... per 100 millirems	

Relative Biological Effectiveness (RBE) is a factor expressing the relative biological potency of one radiation compared with some standard low-LET radiation (usually orthovoltage X-rays). If a dose of neutrons, for instance, produces radiogenic cancer equal to the impact from a ten-fold higher dose of X-rays, neutrons are more potent by a factor of 10, and their RBE for carcinogenesis is 10. In radiation protection, RBE is usually called Quality factor, or Q. Thus dose in centi-grays times Q = dose-equivalent in centi-sieverts. Thus dose in rads times Q = dose-equivalent in rems.

When doses are expressed in centi-sieverts instead of centi-grays, or in rems instead of rads, it is a signal that the adjustment for different RBE has already been incorporated. Thus a dose already in rems (or cSv) is directly comparable with a dose in rads (or cGy). Readers will see a conversion from centi-grays to centi-sieverts performed in our Tables 9-C and 10-E.